David Morgan

November 1989

PHYSIOLOGICAL BASIS OF GERIATRICS

PHYSIOLOGICAL BASIS OF GERIATRICS

Paola S. Timiras, M.D., Ph.D.

Professor of Physiology
Department of Physiology-Anatomy
University of California, Berkeley
Berkeley, California

MACMILLAN PUBLISHING COMPANY
New York
COLLIER MACMILLAN CANADA, INC.
Toronto
COLLIER MACMILLAN PUBLISHERS
London

Printed in the United States of America

Macmillan Publishing Company
866 Third Avenue, New York, New York 10022

Collier Macmillan Canada, Inc.
Collier Macmillan Publishers · London

Library of Congress Cataloging-in-Publication Data

Physiological basis of geriatrics.

Includes bibliographies and index.
1. Aging—Physiological aspects. 2. Geriatrics.
I. Timiras, Paola S. [DNLM: 1. Aging—physiology.
2. Geriatrics. WT 104 P578]
QP86.P557 1988 612′.67 87-34884
ISBN 0-02-420810-8

Printing: 1 2 3 4 5 6 7 8 Year: 8 9 0 1 2 3 4 5

PREFACE

AGING is an inevitable aspect of living. How does it affect body and organ functions? This book addresses this question from several perspectives. Using the traditional physiologic approach, it presents aging of the various systems, focusing on the human, but drawing, when necessary, on animal research. A more comprehensive understanding of the basic aspects of aging is educed by exploring the molecular and cellular mechanisms underlying systemic and organismic aging. Inasmuch as one of the characteristics of aging is the increasing incidence of disease, clinical correlations are included both as a practical reference for the geriatrician and as a comparison with pathologic aging for the gerontologist. Discussion of various theories of aging as well as demographic, comparative, and differential aging is intended to provide further knowledge of the aging processes. As more is learned of these processes, the possibility of intervening is within reach, not only to treat medically the diseases associated with old age, but, more importantly, to strengthen the physiologic competence of the elderly. Therefore, current measures of intervention are presented with the expectation of further progress of life extension technology to improve the quality of life as well as prolong its duration.

In 1972, I published an earlier text entitled *Developmental Physiology and Aging* purposely designed to call attention to the continuum of physiologic events throughout the lifespan, including early developmental and late senescent stages. Since then, the concept of aging as a "normal" physiologic sequence of events has been generally accepted. In addition, the wealth of information on aging that has been accumulating since 1972 warrants extracting and updating the section on aging from the earlier text. This book is the result of such an attempt.

My goal has been to provide a book that will be useful to a broad spectrum of individuals with varying biologic backgrounds. This intent to attract a broad readership may seem too ambitious. The fields of gerontology and geriatrics are rapidly expanding and they attract people from many disciplines who require a common understanding of the biology of aging. The present work, using physiology as the unifying concept, attempts to assimilate and distill information from multiple sources in an understandable, comprehensive text. Psychologic and social aspects of aging are important, particularly for the geriatrician who deals with the whole individual. While these aspects are the subject of many other texts, this volume is limited to biologic concerns.

I have been aided in my task by a number of outstanding collaborators who are also good friends, some of them former students. To each of them I offer my most heartfelt thanks not only for contributing one or several chapters or sections of chapters but also for their encouragment throughout the preparation of the book. Special thanks go to: Dr. D.B. Hudson, who has evaluated each chapter for content and style and helped to improve them. I want to express to her my appreciation and enduring friendship; to Dr. M.L. Timiras, for providing pertinent clinical correlations throughout; to Dr. S. Oklund, for her many drawings, which have presented an effective visual interpretation of complex material; and to Darla Wigginton, who has competently prepared the manuscripts, and dealt with the bibliography and editing. My thanks also to my students—undergraduate, graduate, and postdoctoral—who, while enduring my preoccupation with this book, provided their enthusiasm and criticism and have spurred me on to complete this work.

CONTRIBUTORS

Anne M. Holehan
The Wolfson Institute
The University of Hull
North Humberside, HU6 7RX, England

Brian J. Merry
The Wolfson Institute
The University of Hull
North Humberside, HU6 7RX, England

Jerome S. Tobis
Department of Physical Medicine
and Rehabilitation
Irvine Medical Center
University of California
Orange, CA 92668

Rolf J. Mehlhorn
Department of Physiology-Anatomy
University of California
Berkeley, CA 94720

Trudy M. Forte
Donner Laboratory
University of California
Berkeley, CA 94720

Chang-Zern Hong
Department of Physical Medicine
and Rehabilitation
Irvine Medical Center
University of California
Orange, CA 92668

Robert W. Atherton
Department of Zoology and Physiology
University of Wyoming
Laramie, WY 82070

Ramesh Sharma
Fels Research Institute
School of Medicine
Temple University
Philadelphia, PA 19140

Esmail Meisami
Department of Physiology and Biophysics
University of Illinois
Urbana, IL 61801

Hal Sternberg
Department of Physiology-Anatomy
University of California
Berkeley, CA 94720

Mary L. Timiras
Older Adults Clinic
3052 Willow Pass Road
Concord, CA 94519

Doherty B. Hudson
Department of Physiology-Anatomy
University of California
Berkeley, CA 94720

Paul E. Segall
Department of Physiology-Anatomy
University of California
Berkeley, CA 94720

CONTENTS

PART
IV
Prevention and Rehabilitation

PHYSIOLOGICAL BASIS OF GERIATRICS

PART I
General Perspectives

CHAPTER 1 INTRODUCTION: AGING AS A STAGE IN THE LIFE CYCLE

Underlying the increased concern of the biomedical community for the problems of the aged and the understanding of the aging process is the fact that the elderly now comprise a significant proportion of the population in many leading nations of the world: in the United States, 20 million out of a population of 200 million are over 65 years of age—a ratio that is even higher in France and Sweden. Although the pathology of aging has been studied extensively in terms of combating specific diseases associated with this "high-risk" group, the physiology of aging has not been of primary interest, partly because of the difficulty of isolating "normal" from "abnormal" aging processes. Old age in humans is conventionally accepted as the stage of the life cycle that starts around 65 years of age and terminates with death, but it is extremely difficult to circumscribe its temporal boundaries in physiologic terms. Thus, aging is commonly described as having its onset at some indeterminate point following maturity, in contrast to other periods of the life cycle in which the onset is clearly marked by specific physiologic events—such as menarche at puberty. Aging has, so far, defied all attempts to establish objective landmarks that would precisely characterize its earlier stages.

Bases and Organization of Subject Material

The breadth of the included material reflects the wealth of information on aging since publication of the earlier text by the same author (Timiras, 1972). Historically, physiology focuses on the structure and function of bodily biological systems. A prominent part of the book is therefore concerned with systemic and organismic aging. Herein, we attempt to present the aging of the various systems in the traditional manner, focusing on the human but drawing, where necessary, on animal research. To provide a more comprehensive understanding of these basic aspects, clinical correlations are included. This book is not considered to be a textbook of medicine but will, however, include therapies that employ physiological concepts.

Clearly, any consideration of aging should not ignore the psychological and social components. As briefly discussed in Chapter 27, we recognize the importance of these fields, particularly to the geriatrician who deals with the individual as a whole. We do not have expertise in these areas, however, and have, therefore, not included such subject material.

Understanding systemic and organismic aging can only be achieved based on current knowledge of molecular and cellular aging. The various theories of aging are also necessary background for comprehending aging processes. All of these, together with demographics and comparative and differential aspects of aging, are considered in the first eight chapters.

Our anticipated goal is to provide a book that will be useful to a broad spectrum of individuals with different degrees of biologic background. Therefore each chapter is organized to begin with *structure,* then move to *function,* considered first in the adult (a brief synopsis) and then in the aged. Essential material is presented in normal text size; smaller type furnishes additional information, in-depth discussion, or less well-accepted or controversial matters.

The intent to attract a broad readership may seem too ambitious. The studies of aging and geriatrics are fast expanding and attracting people from many disciplines who require a common understanding of the biology of aging. Current texts are directed to very specific aspects of aging or are designed for a particular group of readers. The present work, using physiology as the unifying concept, assimilates and distills information from multiple sources to produce an understandable, comprehensive text.

Table 1–1. STAGES OF THE LIFESPAN

STAGE	DURATION
Prenatal life	
Ovum	Fertilization through week 1
Embryo	Weeks 2–8
Fetus	Lunar months 3–10
Birth	
Postnatal life	
Neonatal period	Newborn; birth through week 2
Infancy	3 weeks until end of first year
Childhood	
Early	Years 2–6
Middle	Years 7–10
Later	Prepubertal; females 9–15; males 12–16
Adolescence	The 6 years following puberty
Adulthood	Between 20 and 65 years
Senescence	From 65 years on
Death	

PRE- AND POSTNATAL STAGES

In the broadest sense, the lifespan of the individual is divided into two main periods: prenatal life and postnatal life. For a long time, attention was focused on the period before birth, when the most striking physiologic events occur. That important changes continue to occur even in the adult state is recognized, and, indeed, systematic studies have now been extended to embrace old age. The necessity for caution and prudence in establishing "chronologic boundaries" for life stages is abundantly clear: not only are there numerous examples of individual variation in any species, but the limits of life periods also shift forward and backward.

Although many animal species are capable of an independent existence at relatively immature stages, others, including mammals, are not. The human newborn, fully formed anatomically, is still utterly dependent on adults for food and care. Throughout infancy, childhood, and adolescence, a gradual remolding of body shape continues, together with the acquisition of new functions and the perfecting of already established functions. At about 25 years, the last of these changes is completed and the body is stabilized in the adult condition. The mature adult period lasts for approximately another 40 years and encompasses the period of maximal physiologic competence. The progressive decline of physiologic potentialities with age leads to senescence and death.

Both prenatal and postnatal stages can be subdivided into several periods, each of which may be distinguished by identifiable morphologic, physiologic, biochemical, and psychologic features. The main divisions and the approximate time periods of the life-span in humans are listed in Table 1–1. The prenatal period includes three main stages: the stage of the ovum, the embryonic stage, and the fetal stage. The postnatal period commences with birth and continues into stages of neonatal life, infancy, childhood, adolescence, adulthood, and old age. The practical necessity of research to fragment the biologic study of living organisms, however, has a tendency to obscure the dynamic relationships that obtain at many levels of organization. This is true whether we speak of the morphology and function of a single system or of the effects of environmental stress from one age period to another. The physiologic profile of a given individual must be assessed with regard to his particular life history in all its biosocial complexity. Succeeding stages of the lifespan cannot help but reflect on the events that have occurred in the preceding stages. The concept that attained growth tells of past growth processes and foretells growth yet to be achieved can even more appropriately be applied to the later stages of the lifespan when function most certainly depends on past physical history. Indeed, as the saying goes—growing old gracefully is the work of a lifetime.

HEREDITY AND ENVIRONMENT

Developmental processes and the significant influences of environment and heredity on adaptations made by the organism have engaged biologists for many decades. At all stages of life, the directing force of heredity and the molding influences of the internal and external environment play important roles in regulating development and in determining the length of the lifespan. All physiologic changes occurring with time involve interactions between genetic and environmental factors, and to weigh the value of one against the other is to disturb the integrity of the whole. Heredity operates through internal factors, present in the fertilized egg itself. Chief among these are the genes, or hereditary determiners, located in the chromosomes, which contain the genetic contribution of each parent. Environment supplies the external factors that make development possible and allow inherited potentials to find expression. Environmental factors include temperature, humidity, atmospheric gases, nutrition, drugs, infections, radiation, and so forth. Without doubt, environmental factors can condition the appearance and modify the type of genetic characters, influence their expression, and alter their composition to make possible the creation of new inheritable characters (mutation). Such external factors are operative throughout the lifespan. Indeed, one of the basic characteristics of humans and animals is their capacity to adapt to an ever-changing environment. Adaptation is attained through a series of physiologic adjustments that serve to restore the normal state once it has been disturbed. These adjustments are grouped under the term *homeostasis,* and a large part of physiology is concerned with regulatory mechanisms (such as negative and positive feedback) that act to maintain constant the internal environment. By the time of maturity, numerous such adjustments already have been accomplished. Homeostatic regulation, together with inherited traits, defines the competence with which the individual will continue to respond to environmental challenges; it is in this sense that aging has been viewed as a general decline in the capacity to adapt to continuing stress and that external factors have been related to the length of the lifespan. After consideration of all these influences, the best assurance for a long lifespan remains the thoughtful selection of long-lived parents.

STEPS OF DEVELOPMENT

As already indicated, the global view of the lifespan should encompass all stages of the life cycle; therefore, any text on aging must take into consideration developmental events. From a practical point of view, however, the focus here is on aging, but we will not hesitate to broaden our horizons to consider the contribution of development to the total lifespan. Indeed, the changes that come with aging might depend on occurrences during development as well as in maturity.

It is in the years before maturity that the gradual acquisition of physiologic competence is clearly recognized in discrete but critical phenomena appearing at specific ages. The whole process of growth and development starts with fertilization, when the genetic "code" of the individual is laid down. From this period on, the general course of growth proceeds in a continuous and orderly sequence throughout the prenatal and postnatal periods. Whether physical or mental, growth and development represent an orderly, although not uniform, process; rather, both are characterized by accelerated and slow cycles.

STAGES OF MATURITY AND AGING

The mature years, those that follow the acquisition of sexual and reproductive capacity, are considered a major life stage. However, with the exception of menopause in women, this period is not marked by any sequence of precisely timed physiologic events, as is the developmental period. On the contrary, adulthood is characterized by great functional stability; it connotes the attainment of optimal, integrated function of all body systems and is a standard against which to measure any degree of physiologic or pathologic deviation. Most textbooks in human physiology take the mature 25-year-old, 70-kg, 170-cm man as their model. In the present text, this period and this average man will serve mainly as a reference point for the discussion of aging and the aged.

Yet, it must be recognized that functional competence is multifaceted and that optimal performance may differ from age to age and from one parameter to another. In other words, it would be unsound, if not physiologically incorrect, to assume that a function is maximally efficient only during adulthood and that differences in the earlier or later years necessarily represent functional immaturity or deterioration, respectively. Rather, one must view physiologic competence as having several levels of integration, depending on the requirements of the organism at any specific age and the type and severity of the challenges to which the organism is exposed. Evidence for conceptualizing physiological competence along a continuum throughout the lifespan emerges from the study of developmental physiology and aging. Although the age of 65 has been accepted as the demarcation line between maturity and old age, a person of 65 may be quite healthy and a long way from "retiring" from life—a situation about which social scientists frequently express concern.

If the adult years are difficult to subdivide into physiologic stages, aging or senescence is even more of a challenge. Inasmuch as the "winter years" are increasingly besieged by pathologic events, the study of aging is diversely approached, i.e., in terms of the extent to which physiologic competence is retained. In this respect, however, it must be kept in mind that despite the absence of sequential stages of decline from maturity to death, in aging as in development, the changes that do take place do not occur simultaneously at all levels of functional organization, nor do they involve all functions to the same degree. It appears more likely that each change, whether at the molecular, cellular, tissular, or organismic level, follows its own timetable and that the latter is differentially susceptible to specific intrinsic and extrinsic factors. Indeed, gerontology is not restricted to the identification of pathologic factors. Old age cannot be regarded simplistically as a "disease," but involves a complexity of physiologic and pathologic phenomena, all of which are subject to numerous environmental influences. Thus, as a life stage, aging is presented here not only as it affects the whole organism, but also on the basis of alterations occurring at the level of cellular and subcellular elements, tissues, organs, and systems.

Table 1–2. BRIEF GLOSSARY OF AGING-RELATED TERMS

TERM	DEFINITION
Aging	Latin "aetas," age or lifetime The condition of becoming old
Geriatrics	Greek "geron," old man, and "iatros," healer A medical specialty dealing with the problems and diseases of old age and aging people
Gerontology	Greek "geron," old man, and "logos," knowledge A branch of biology dealing with aging and the problems of old age
Senescence	Latin "senex," old man The condition of being old, used interchangeably with aging

The interpretation of aging as a physiologic process upon which pathology and disease have been superimposed has been formalized under the separate disciplines of *gerontology*—the study of aging processes—and *geriatrics*—the treatment of the debilitating symptoms and diseases associated with old age (Table 1–2). Both disciplines are relatively new, are growing rapidly, and are affected by the growing pains that afflict all neophyte fields. The terms aging and senescence are often used interchangeably (Table 1–2) despite some minor interpretative differences: *aging* refers more appropriately to the process of growing old regardless of chronologic age, whereas *senescence* is restricted to the state of old age characteristic of the late years of the lifespan.

DEATH VERSUS IMMORTALITY

While aging is approached gradually without any specific physiologic markers of its onset, death is the terminal event of this stage in the lifespan. Various types of death terminate the aging process. In broad terms, these include trauma, accidents, and disease. Trauma and accidents (e.g., high-speed vehicle crashes, dangerous occupations, drug abuse, smoking) are the major causes of death in young adulthood. Disease processes that overwhelm the defense or repair systems of the body affect all ages but are particularly life-endangering in the very young and in the old. Many diseases that lead to death in the perinatal period—a period of high risk—have been conquered in developed countries, including the United States. Today the majority of deaths from disease occur in the elderly, in whom diminished function makes the accumulation of pathology less tolerable than in the young. Indeed, some diseases occur almost exclusively in the old, and this linkage of pathology with old age justifies the argument of some investigators that aging itself is a disease. It should be noted, however, that senescence is not an accepted cause of death and is not so noted on the death certificate. Whether death is a natural event has never been validated scientifically. The attitude of tacit acceptance of a debilitating old age, prevalent even among biologists, is now being replaced by one that regards senescence as the "subversion of function," the inevitability of which is open to question.

Nostalgically we consider immortality in the light of extending our life through our offspring; however, this sense of immortality is no longer adequate. It is frustrating that in a time when humans have gone into and returned from outer space and can manipulate DNA, they have not conquered death. Death, indeed, remains the last "sacred" enemy.

PHYSIOLOGIC, CLINICAL, AND INTERVENTIVE CONSIDERATIONS

Biologists working in the area of aging have defined two major goals to guide their research programs: one entails the effort to prolong human life, and the other the effort to significantly enhance viability, the so-called quality of life, throughout the lifespan. Organ transplantation, perhaps, encompasses both objectives, but it represents a "crude and clumsy" approach in either case. Pharmacologic and genetic research, on the other hand, has startling potential for the amelioration and prolongation of life and is currently attracting increasing support. Nevertheless, the fact that the answers remain obscured need not deter our search, for only by continually posing bold new questions can we hope to accomplish the spirited goals of the gerontologists, whose motto—"to add years to life and life to years"—emphasizes for all of us the importance of the quality of life.

Whether specific age-related changes are the cause or consequence of the aging process remains to be established. The concept of a single causative factor pervades many areas of biologic study, and gerontology is no exception. It is unlikely that a single "triggering" event is responsible for the aging of the organism but, rather, aging probably entails numerous and complex interactions at different levels.

Viewing aging, therefore, as the consequences of many diverse factors, we shall consider, first, the aging of human and animal populations. This comparative and demographic section will be followed by consideration of the molecular and cellular aspects of aging. Inasmuch as our major concern is with the human, the aging of systems and organs will be discussed along with selected relevant clinical aspects. And finally, in the desire to actively improve the quality of life of the elderly, we shall emphasize prevention and rehabilitation.

References

Bergener, M.; Ermini, M.; and Stahelin, H. B. (eds.): *Thresholds in Aging*, Academic Press, New York, **1985.**

Calow, P.: *Life Cycles: An Evolutionary Approach to the Physiology of Reproduction, Development and Aging*, Chapman and Hall, London, **1978.**

Carter, N. (ed.): *Development, Growth and Aging*, Croom Helm, London, **1980.**

Comfort, A.: *The Biology of Senescence*, 3rd ed., Elsevier, New York, **1979.**

Coni, N.; Davison, W.; and Webster, S.: *Ageing: The Facts*, Oxford University Press, Oxford, New York, Toronto, **1984.**

Danon, D.; Shock, N. W.; and Marois, M.: *Aging: A Challenge of Science and Society*, Vol. 1, Biology. Oxford University Press, Oxford, **1981.**

Davis, B. B., and Wood, W. G. (eds.): *Homeostatic Function and Aging,* Vol. 30, Raven Press, New York, **1985.**

Frolkis, V. V.: *Aging and Life-Prolonging Processes,* Springer-Verlag, New York, **1982.**

Johnson, H. A. (ed.): *Relations Between Normal Aging and Disease,* Aging, Vol. 28, Raven Press, New York, **1985.**

Kenney, R. A.: *Physiology of Aging: A Synopsis,* Year Book Medical Publishers, Chicago, IL, **1982.**

Kimmel, D. C.: *Adulthood and Aging: An Interdisciplinary Developmental View,* 2nd ed., John Wiley & Sons, New York, **1980.**

Masoro, E. J.; Adelman, R. C.; and Roth, G. S.: *CRC Handbook of Physiology of Aging,* CRC Press, Boca Raton, FL, **1981.**

Perlmutter, M., and Hall, E.: *Adult Development and Aging,* John Wiley & Sons, New York, **1985.**

Rockstein, M., and Sussman, M.: *Biology of Aging,* Wadsworth Publishing Co., Belmont, CA, **1979.**

Smith, D. W.; Bierman, E. L.; and Robinson, N. M. (eds.): *The Biologic Ages of Man: From Conception Through Old Age,* 2nd ed., Saunders, Philadelphia, **1978.**

Timiras, P. S.: *Developmental Physiology and Aging,* Macmillan, New York, **1972.**

Vernadakis, A., and Timiras, P. S.: *Hormones in Development and Aging,* SP Medical & Scientific Books (Spectrum Publications), Jamaica, NY, **1982.**

Young, J. Z.: *An Introduction to the Study of Man,* Oxford University Press, London, **1971.**

CHAPTER

2 DEFINITIONS: DEMOGRAPHIC, COMPARATIVE AND DIFFERENTIAL AGING

DEFINITIONS

At our present state of knowledge, we cannot present an all-encompassing definition of aging—indeed there are as many definitions as there are theories of aging. Those presented here are arbitrarily selected on the basis of their relevance to the physiologic aspects of aging and focus on decrements in physiologic competence following maturity (Table 2–1). During the years following maturity, physiologic change is far less rapid than during development. Indeed, in the absence of pathology, aging may be superimposed on maturity as an integral aspect of the continuous development of the organism. Accordingly, a first definition of aging is *the sum of all changes that occur in an organism with the passage of time.* This definition visualizes the lifespan as an orderly unfolding of precisely timed events from fertilization to death, with aging as a stage of the lifespan (see Chapter 1).

Aging as a Consequence of Growth Cessation

Based on the "global appreciation" of aging as an integral part of development but differentiated from it in time, several theories have postulated that aging may best be understood by studying development. Thus, cessation of normal growth and/or initiation of abnormal (tumor) growth have been suggested as causative factors in the aging of the organism. This view, still speculative rather than substantive, has led to a number of theories some of which have fallen into disrepute while others are still being actively supported.

From comparative studies, discussed later, the duration of life can be equated to some extent with the growth period: an animal that acquires all its growth in a short time would perish much sooner than another that takes longer in growing. Among the less complex organisms, the rotifer (*Philodina citrina*) has been utilized as a model for studying the relationship between aging, parental age, and growth cessation (Lansing, 1954; Lints, 1985). In culture, this species demonstrates remarkable constancy in egg production and longevity. The life cycle of the rotifers is: hatching, day 1; onset of egg laying, day 5; adult size attained, day 6; onset of senescence, day 15; death, day 25. Eggs laid on day 5 produce orthoclones (generations) that have long survival and appear capable of reproducing indefinitely. The later in the life cycle that the eggs are laid, that is, the older the parental age, the shorter the lifespan of the offspring, which, in fact, die out after a number of generations. These data have been interpreted to mean that, in these organisms, aging commences after day 5 and is signaled by the cessation of growth.

In mammals, the slowing of growth during the prenatal period as the embryo matures has been interpreted as the onset of aging, and the decline in the rate of growth has been extrapolated to indicate that aging is most rapid early in embryonal life. Another extrapolation, by the physiologist Minot (1908), considers aging and death as the price paid for differentiation.

Because of the inverse relationship between mitotic activity (as an index of growth) and cell differentiation (as an index of functional specialization), the hypothesis relating growth cessation to aging has been further elaborated to imply that cell differentiation, associated with a reduced capacity for growth, represents a step toward cellular aging.

Further arguments in support of a causal relationship between growth cessation and aging are based on the continual renewal and increase of cell constituents characteristic of the growing cell (Kohn, 1965). Substances that are continually turning over and being replaced would not be expected to contribute to aging. For a system to change with time, either new compounds must be added or subtracted at different times, or changes must take place in the components that remain. It follows that the aging rate of cells and cellular components, as with discrete tissues or the intact organism, depends on the ratio between biologically important nonrenewable and renewable materials and the changes occurring in this ratio with time. In humans, neurons are capable of living as long as the individual, whereas certain blood cells have a lifespan of days or even hours; on the organismic level, the thymus undergoes marked involution at adolescence and the ovary ceases to function long before the age of 65, when aging "officially" begins. On the other hand, it is well known that the reserve of cells in various organs is enormous and that a human being can survive with less than 40 percent of his liver, part of one kidney, one lung, fractions of stomach and intestine, and so forth. Consequently, if aging of the intact animal results from aging of its cells, we should expect to find death or loss of function in

Table 2–1. DEFINITIONS OF AGING

Aging as a stage of the lifespan	• the sum of all changes occurring in an organism with the passage of time
Aging as a deteriorative process	• the sum of all changes occurring with time and leading to functional impairment and death
Aging as cellular and molecular damage	• changes in membranes, cytoplasm, and/or nucleus

a large percentage (50 percent or more) of cells in organs throughout the aging body. Yet, this is not the case: many cells are continually being renewed (e.g., epithelial cells of the skin and gastrointestinal mucosa), and even in neurons, cellular death is not a common finding; in fact, the rate of metabolic turnover in these elements indicates a continuing renewal of cellular components.

Retardation of Growth and Maturation as Interventions to Delay Aging

It should be noted that the relationship between developmental phenomena and chronologic aging in general has not been experimentally validated and, for many biologists, represents an untenable working hypothesis (Strehler, 1977). On the other hand, from this conceptual framework have derived some peripheral speculations that suggest that this approach may yet be profitable to our knowledge of aging processes. For example, this approach raises the question of which regulatory mechanisms trigger the progression from one stage of the life cycle to the next; it focuses attention on the significance of the cessation of a given function (e.g., cessation of growth) or the role of initiation or transformation of another function (e.g., higher incidence of autoimmunity) to aging processes; it postulates the existence of a precise genetic programming of the lifespan; it invites research on the role that environmental factors may play in regulating the course of development and aging, and finally, it suggests the possibility of prevention or control of aging by delaying or accelerating specific developmental events at critical periods.

The concepts discussed remain to be substantiated by solid experimental or clinical evidence and would have been abandoned were it not for a resurgence of interest in the relationship between growth, development, and aging as illustrated by the delay in development and aging induced by food restriction in rodents. Starting with the work of McCay (1952) and extending to the present numerous investigations, reports show that food restriction inhibits growth and maturation and delays aging. This type of life-extension intervention will be discussed in Chapter 25.

As a consequence of the concept that aging has its genesis during development, it may be postulated that any measure taken to ameliorate or prolong life—whether hygienic, pharmacologic, nutritional, or environmental—is most likely to be effective when applied before the signs of aging become manifest. Paradoxic as it may seem, then, the goal of gerontologists—to "add life to years and years to life"—in practical terms may have to be accomplished far earlier in the lifespan than has been customarily thought. Indeed, it is true that many measures utilized during early life to protect or enhance the functional competence of the infant have long-term implications for health in old age, and it may be that amelioration of the quality of life and its prolongation should properly be sought through ontogenetic conditioning.

Despite the many differences that are the consequence of heredity, sex, past history, and life experience, it is undeniable that older persons share certain traits with respect to the onset, rate, and characteristics of the aging process. Indeed, we cannot ignore the fact that aging is a deteriorative process characterized by increased vulnerability and decreased viability. The first definition, therefore, must be amended to indicate that, with advancing age, functional impairment increases as does the probability of death. Thus, in humans, aging takes the form of morphologic and functional involution, always progressive and often silent, which affects most organs, tissues, and cells and results in a gradual decline in performance, leading to *"functional impairment and death."*

Adaptation to environmental stress is one of the major functions of the organism, and as the capacity for adaptation progressively fails with age, so aging may be further defined as *a decreasing ability to survive stress*. At the organismic and systemic levels, then, aging is recognized as the progressive deterioration of the physiologic processes necessary for the maintenance of a constant "milieu intérieur" and death as the ultimate failure of the organism to maintain this constancy, that is, to sustain homeostasis. Other definitions of aging focus on cellular and molecular changes, and aging and death would result from alterations therein. Proponents of this view ascribe aging to progressive cellular changes in the plasma and intracellular membranes (fluidity, permeability, transport), cytoplasm (formation of free radicals, cross-linking, lipofuscin), and nucleus (DNA damage and DNA repair failure, mRNA error catastrophe, alterations in replication and histocompatibility complex).

DEMOGRAPHIC AGING

LIFE TABLES

One way of expressing and studying aging is to construct life tables from census and vital statistics. A life table represents the action of mortality on a conventional cohort of newborn individuals as they proceed through successive ages. A life table represents, therefore, the number of survivors at each birthday out of an initial cohort of size 10^n (commonly 10,000 or 100,000) at age 0, until the last survivor is eliminated by death (Table 2–2). A life table consists, also, of a series of probabilities of death, or the risk that a group of individuals, upon reaching their xth birthday, have to die before the next xth + 1 birthday. Other functions of the life table (such as the number of deaths in each interval or the life expectancy at each birthday) can be easily derived. Thus, the life table is a precise tool for measuring the level of mortality—and therefore the length of life—of any population.

A life table, however, does not offer any indication as to the process of aging of a real population, since this depends on the past history (i.e., during the preceding 100 years), fertility, mortality, and migration of that population. Indeed, if we rule out migration and consider a population that gains or loses elements only because of birth and death, the age structure of a population (or, in other words, the percentage of the total population in the various age groups) is determined more by the changing level of the birth rate than by the trend of mortality.

A decline in the number of births, for instance, determines the reduction of the size of each newborn cohort and, if sustained for one or more decades, induces a reduction of the proportional importance of infants and of children and the young, and, conversely, an increased proportional importance of the aged. Thus, aging of a population would occur when its age structure is altered in such a way as to favor an increased proportion of the older versus the younger individuals. A decline in mortality, on the other hand, such as the continuous one witnessed by the developed countries during the last 100 years, proportionally enhances the chances of survival from birth to all ages; it does not greatly change the age structure of the population concerned if, in the meantime, fertility has remained constant. It is therefore important to distinguish the process of increasing longevity, produced by a decline of the risks of mortality at the various ages, from the process of aging of a population.

A number of survival curves are portrayed graphically in Figure 2–1, where the abscissa measures chronologic age and the ordinate indicates that portion of the original population surviving (percentage of survivors). The straight portion of Curve 2 indicates a very low rate of death—approximately 100% survival—at early ages, but with increasing age, the number of survivors decreases, as shown by the shoulder of the curve, and the 50% survival is the median age at death; the tail of the curve indicates the maximum lifespan or maximum longevity in the population.

Cumulative genetic or environmental hazards may lead to a more rapid decrease in the number of survivors. In this case the curve will shift to the left, as shown in Curve 1. Although the average lifespan is shortened, the maximum lifespan does not necessarily change. If conditions are improved, more people will survive longer, the curve becomes more rectangular, and the average lifespan is shifted to the right, as shown in Curve 3. The maximum lifespan, however, is little affected. To increase the maximum lifespan—the length of life of the oldest members of a population (Curve 4)—is one of the goals of gerontologists, but to date is the most difficult to achieve.

Survival data provide a concrete measure against which any theory of aging eventually must be measured. Thus, removal of a particular cause or a number of factors causing aging may cause a shift in the average longevity of a population, producing a more rectangular curve. In contrast, add-

Table 2–2. SELECTED DATA TAKEN FROM LIFE TABLES*

AGE(X)	PROBABILITY OF DYING BETWEEN TWO BIRTHDAYS 1000 Q(X)	NUMBER OF DEATHS BETWEEN TWO BIRTHDAYS D(X)	SURVIVORS AT EACH BIRTHDAY L(X)	EXPECTATIONS OF LIFE AT EACH BIRTHDAY E(X)
		Females		
0	4.45	445	100000	80.000
1	0.32	32	99555	79.358
5	0.24	24	99522	75.383
10	0.21	21	99499	70.400
15	0.38	38	99478	65.414
20	0.57	57	99440	60.438
25	0.78	77	99384	55.471
30	1.09	109	99306	50.512
35	1.78	176	99198	45.565
40	3.28	325	99022	40.641
45	6.70	661	98697	35.766
50	11.55	1132	98036	30.990
55	20.18	1956	96904	26.322
60	34.63	3288	94948	21.810
65	67.43	6181	91660	17.499
70	126.45	10809	85479	13.577
75	229.32	17123	74670	10.166
80	362.56	20865	57547	7.447
85	538.55	19756	36683	5.238
90	735.07	12443	16927	3.544
95	897.85	4026	4484	2.311
100	1000.00	458	458	1.461
		Males		
0	7.11	711	100000	76.647
1	0.58	58	99289	76.195
5	0.61	60	99231	72.239
10	0.57	57	99171	67.281
15	1.30	129	99114	62.318
20	1.77	175	98985	57.396
25	1.63	161	98810	52.493
30	1.83	180	98648	47.575
35	2.55	251	98468	42.657
40	4.51	443	98217	37.759
45	9.39	918	97775	32.919
50	18.08	1751	96857	28.206
55	35.40	3367	95106	23.677
60	60.86	5583	91738	19.451
65	104.82	9031	86155	15.543
70	175.83	13561	77124	12.059
75	282.05	17928	63564	9.077
80	422.30	19272	45636	6.660
85	596.40	15723	26364	4.714
90	776.95	8267	10640	3.228
95	916.34	2175	2373	2.145
100	1000.00	199	199	1.390

*Source: Coale, A.Y., and Demeny, P.: *Regional Model Life Tables and Stable Populations*. Academic Press, New York, 1983.

ing risk factors results in decreased survivorship at early ages, and the curve becomes less rectangular. Of course, one must also consider side effects—if the removal of a damaging factor doubled the lifespan but rendered people impotent, not many people would choose longer life. Accordingly, in weighing the value of a given intervention to delay aging and improve the quality of life of the elderly, we must also consider the practical consequences involved in any suggested remedies or preventives adopted on a wide scale.

The beneficial influence of improved environment and health on life expectancy at birth is reflected in the progressive increase

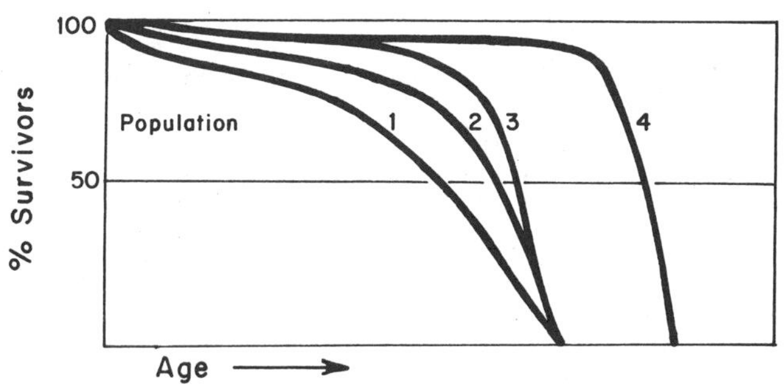

Figure 2–1. *Population survival curves.*

Flat portion of curve indicates very low death rate; 50% survival is median age at death; tail of curve indicates maximum lifespan (longevity). Curve 2—representative survival curve. Curve 1—increased genetic or environmental hazards. Curve 3—improved health or living conditions. Curve 4—goal of gerontologists. Increased or decreased risk factors shift average lifespan but do not extend maximum lifespan, the goal of gerontologists.

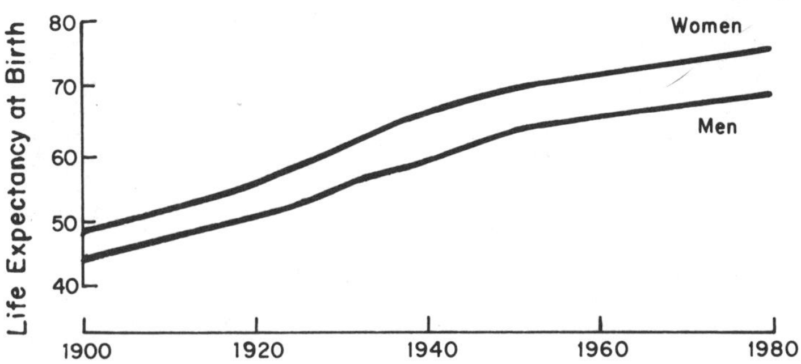

Figure 2–2. *Life expectancy at birth (1900–1980).*

Note progressive increase in life expectancy since 1900 and the greater life expectancy of women.

of this measurement in the United States population from 1900 to 1982 (Figure 2–2). Indeed, the life expectancy at birth, that is, the number of years an individual in a given population is expected to live, can be a useful indication of the health status of a population. In 1900, the average life expectancy was less than 50 years, whereas a child born in 1982 can expect to live almost to 80 years, with women living 5 or more years longer than men. This dramatic lengthening of the lifespan has been ascribed to progress in the standard of living, particularly in sanitation, nutrition, and medicine.

A direct consequence of the increase in the number of individuals reaching old age is reflected in the increased proportion of the elderly in the U.S. population. In 1910, 4% of the population was over 65 years of age; in 1980, 11%, and in 2030, it is predicted that 18% of the population will be over 65. Even more rapid is the increase in the population over 75 years of age, increasing from 1% in 1910 to an expected 8% in 2030 (Figure 2–3). The 85-year-old and older group represents, in fact, the fastest growing segment of the population. Between 1960 and 1980, their numbers increased 164% (Rabbin, 1985), more than six times the rate of growth of the U.S. population as a whole. It is predicted that, by the year 2000, almost half of the deaths in the United States will occur after age 80 (Brody *et al.*, 1987). It is probably safe to state that every one of these elderly individuals is sick in some way or in need of some type of assistance (Chapter 3). The social, economic, and psychologic as well as the medical problems of the elderly segment of the population are indeed overwhelming; these problems demand attention and should be dealt with expeditiously.

AGING IN PRIMITIVE AND ANCIENT POPULATIONS

The importance of intrinsic (genetic) and extrinsic (environmental) factors in determining the length of the lifespan can be ex-

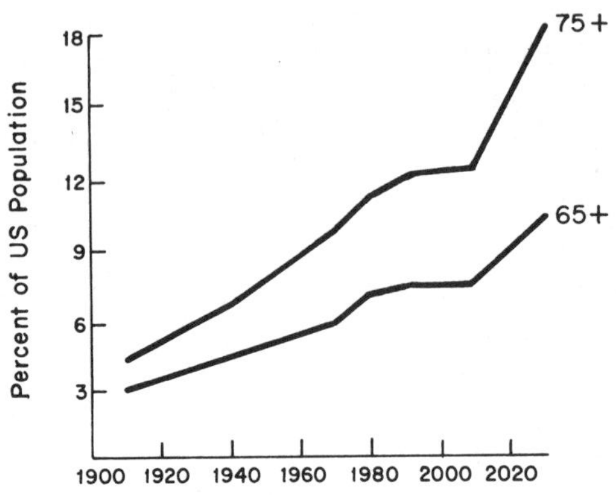

Percent of US Population

	1910	1940	1970	1980	1990	2010	2030
65+ Yrs.	4.3	6.8	9.9	11.3	12.3	12.6	18.3
75+ Yrs.	1.3	2.0	3.8	4.4	5.0	5.5	7.7

Figure 2–3. *Percentage of elderly in U.S. population (1900–2020).*

Note approximately sixfold increase in percentage of population over 75 years.

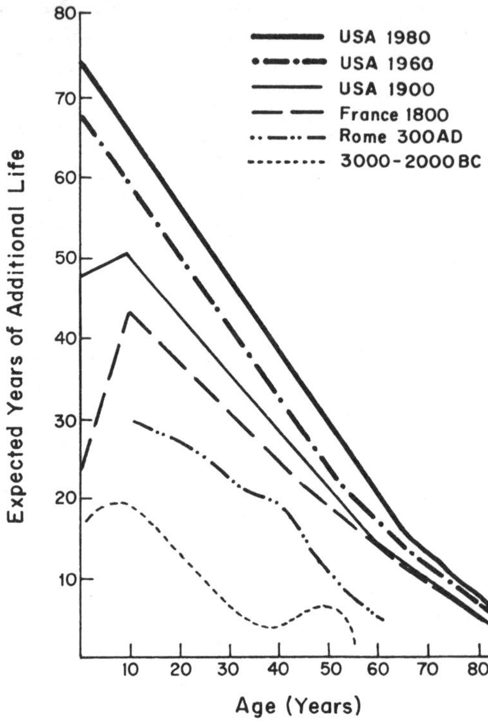

Figure 2–4. *Lifespan through the ages in various populations.*

Life expectancy at birth has increased dramatically since neolithic times. The conquest of infectious diseases has also raised the lifespan expectancy during childhood years, but nothing has effectively prolonged lifespan beyond age 65, although more people now reach this age.

amined by comparing the aging status of ancient and primitive populations. Extremely ancient human populations take us back to the neolithic and paleolithic eras of the old world, millennia before the beginning of history. The information we have concerning survivorship in the prehistoric old world prior to 10,000 years ago is derived entirely from skeletal material and can be expressed only in terms of age of death. According to the limited number (less than 100 specimens) of studies, it is evident that few persons survived past the age of 40. As shown in Figure 2–4, in the neolithic period, a 5-year-old had a life expectancy of 20 more years; at 20 years of age, perhaps 14 more years; and at 60 there were no survivors.

Despite the sketchy data, the findings of several investigators show that in the Stone Age, before the rise of the Mesopotamian and Egyptian civilizations, aging, as we know it today, simply did not exist. Not all investigators agree with this point of view. In their opinion, the evidence for the paleolithic and neolithic eras would be little more than a guess. Many, perhaps with reason, say that the incidence of infectious diseases has grown with the increased density of population made possible by the development of agriculture. Thus, early humans may have had a longer average lifespan than revealed by the few fossils available. Indeed, there is little evidence of progress in lowering mortality until perhaps the 18th century. Nevertheless, some reports suggest that, with continually improving conditions of life, life expectancy progressively increased. A Roman at 10 years of age had 30 more years of life to look forward to and at 60, perhaps 5 more years of life to enjoy (Figure 2–4).

It is a major achievement of civilization that life expectancy of humans has increased throughout history and particularly

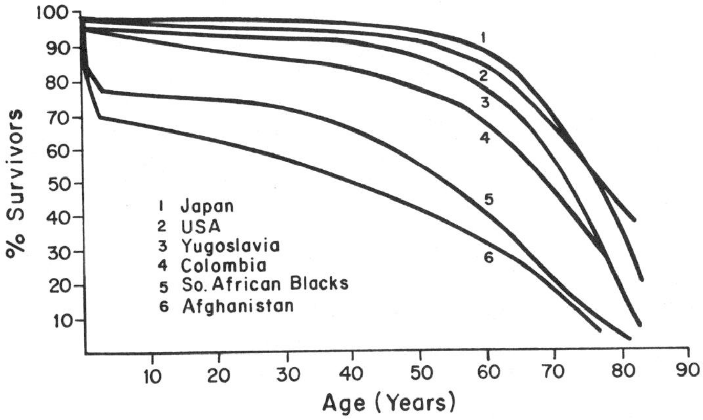

Figure 2–5. *Percentage survival in countries with different levels of socioeconomic status and industrialization.*

High levels of industrialization and socioeconomic status, 1 and 2; medium levels; 3 and 4; low levels, 5 and 6.

since the turn of this century. Taking only a few selected examples throughout the centuries, we see that in the France of 1800 and up to 1900 in the United States, life expectancy was relatively short until 10 years of age, a sign of high mortality due to childhood diseases. As shown for 1960 and 1980, life expectancy is considerably improved. The maximum lifespan, however, has remained essentially unchanged in the last few centuries.

CURRENT COMPARATIVE LIFESPAN IN VARIOUS COUNTRIES

Prolongation of life expectancy from prehistoric through historic times and its marked increase in the last 80 years are not equally shared by all world populations today. In Figure 2–5, survivorship at progressive age is compared in a few, representative countries with varying economic levels.

Japan and the United States, industrialized countries with relatively prosperous economies, show a slow decline of the survivors until 65 years, when a rapid decline begins. In Colombia and Yugoslavia, less prosperous countries, the survivorship is slightly lower and the rapid decline begins at about 50 years. The black South Africans and the Afghans, still part of the underdeveloped Third World, have an abrupt drop in rate of survival during early childhood, owing to high mortality before the age of 4 to 5 years, and then continuing declining survivorship. As indicated earlier, the standard of living, particularly in terms of sanitation and nutrition, is very important in the survivorship of human populations. Indeed, the socioeconomic and public health conditions of a population can be inferred from data regarding early childhood mortality and the average length of lifespan: the lower the former, the higher the childhood mortality and the shorter the lifespan.

If we consider, however, the extreme right of the curves, we see that they converge around 80 years of age. Thus, essential differences among countries are manifested in early age rather than later in the lifespan. Even in populations with a shorter average lifespan, a few individuals are capable of living as long a life as those from populations with a longer average lifespan. Indeed, individuals with unusually long lifespan have been found in populations living in a rather hostile environment and under marginal economic conditions.

It is to be noted that in some of the Third World countries, life expectancy, although still remaining well below that of economically advanced countries, has shown extraordinary progress since the 1950s. In India, for example, life expectancy, which at the end of World War II ranged from 27 to 30 years, has now increased to 55 to 58 years. The difficulties of collecting reliable census data in such a large country with such varied populations are obviously enormous, and any demographic study should be carefully evaluated. Nevertheless, some of the available figures are striking. According to some estimates of the sample registration system from the 1981 census (*Directory and Yearbook,* 1981; Hande,

1985), life expectancy at birth for 1970 to 1975 was 50.5 years for males and 49 years for females, and this has increased in 1981 to 58 years for males and 55 for females. Keeping in mind that India's total population is about 700 million, and that this population will soon witness a marked increase in the number of individuals 50 years old and older, one can appreciate the enormous impact that such an increase will have on that country's resources. Although we can view with some satisfaction the considerable progress in sanitation and medical care that this increased life expectancy represents, we can only be overwhelmed by the economic and social implications that such a lengthening of the lifespan implies for such a large population. Clearly, it is none too soon for planning a vigorous and effective program for the support of this so far minor, but rapidly expanding, segment of the population. While the major concern remains survival of the young during their early years (together with reduction in the number of births) and improvement of the health of the general population, the realization of an increased number of individuals over 50 who will compete for medical and welfare benefits must be addressed immediately.

MAXIMUM LIFESPAN IN HUMANS

Among mammals, humans represent the longest-living species. Accurate records of human longevity (longevity meaning length of life or long life) are difficult to collect; not only are they subject to unavoidable recording errors, especially in countries where demographic records are not kept consistently, but it is well known that, beyond a certain age, elderly individuals show a tendency to exaggerate their age (Mazess and Forman, 1979).

Claims of extreme longevity abound in particular regions (Leaf, 1982). For example, Russian investigators have frequently reported the celebrated longevity of some inhabitants of the Caucasus and of Siberia who claim to be 130 years old. Other, unusually long-lived populations have been studied in the high valley of Ecuador and in the Karakoram Mountains, west of Tibet. Although there is no question that many of the subjects interviewed were very old individuals, even centenarians, their exact age and their proportion in the total population have been questioned (Medvedev, 1974). In these populations, conditions are generally extremely arduous and caloric intake is low; genetic isolation and separation from urban viruses and pollution may be some of the key factors in the longevity of these populations. Again, a note of caution is needed. It has been clearly demonstrated that age in these populations has been grossly overstated, and therefore, it is dangerous to attempt to find any cause-to-effect relationship (Bennett and Garson, 1986).

Documented records have fixed the longest human lifetime at 114 years. Apart from examination of the observed records, attempts have been made to predict the maximum lifespan from statistical analysis of the life tables. In these terms, the actuarial probability of an individual exceeding the age of 150 years is probably zero. Indeed, the number of persons reaching even 100 years is too limited to permit statistically significant estimates to be made of the duration of the lifespan beyond 90 years of age.

COMPARATIVE PHYSIOLOGY OF AGING

Senescence may be viewed as a manifestation of the process of adaptation. In this sense the survival of the species demands the aging and death of its members. Survival beyond the period of reproductive activity represents a luxury that few species can afford. Contrasting the immortality of the germ line with the mortality of somatic cells suggests that, at least in some species, limiting the individual lifespan may be a positively beneficial adaptation. However, in many species, and certainly in humans, longevity can theoretically be subject to positive selection based on criteria of fitness other than reproductive capacity. Although much has been written about such reasoning, the question still remains—why is the lifespan of most species finite? One approach to this question is to compare life duration among several phyla and from this

Table 2–3. PHYSIOLOGIC CORRELATES WITH LONGEVITY

INDEX STUDIED	CORRELATION
Body weight	Direct
Brain/body weight	Direct
Basal metabolic rate	Inverse
Stress	Inverse
Reproductive function	Inverse
Fecundity	Inverse
Length of growth period	Direct
Evolution	Uncertain

comparison to extract principles applicable to the aging process in general (Table 2–3). Although the interest of gerontologists in obtaining accurate information on the lifespan of animals has increased considerably in the last few decades, much of the literature and knowledge of the nature of aging in animal and plant species is still incomplete. The available information has been reviewed by Comfort (1979) and Finch and Schneider (1985).

Among common factors governing aging in animals is brain weight and its relation to body weight. Data from several orders of placental mammals show a highly significant relationship between lifespan and body weight: the bigger the animal, the longer the lifespan. For example, the elephant may reach or exceed 70 years in captivity, whereas the rat seldom lives more than 3 years. There are, however, many exceptions to this generalization: humans may reach 114 years of age, whereas other, larger mammals show a shorter potential longevity (horse: approximately 60 years; hippopotamus and rhinoceros: approximately 50 years; bear: 30 years; camel: 25 years). Among domestic carnivores, cats, although generally smaller in size than dogs, live longer. The same data show an even more significant relationship between lifespan and brain weight. For example, insectivores with a smaller, simpler brain have a shorter lifespan than ungulates, and these have a simpler brain and shorter lifespan than humans. Humans with the longest lifespan have the heaviest brain in relation to body weight and also the most complicated structurally (Sacher, 1959). Important physiologic implications can be extrapolated from these data, such as the relation between brain size and longevity. The higher the brain weight is relative to the body weight (the higher the brain/body weight ratio) and, particularly, the greater the degree of cerebral cortical expansion, that is, the increase in size of the cerebral cortex, the more precise are the physiologic regulations and thus the greater chance for longer survival (Salk, 1973). Such an interpretation seems well justified by the essential role the nervous system plays in regulating vital physiologic adjustments, especially responses to environmental demands. Maintenance of the physiologic optimum and reduction of the magnitude of the fluctuations occurring over time diminish the probability of irreversible changes per unit time and, thus, the rate of aging and the incidence of death.

Another criterion of the relationship between a physiologic parameter and the length of the lifespan is basal metabolic rate: the higher the metabolic rate, the shorter the lifespan (Sacher, 1977). Metabolic rate represents the amount of energy liberated per unit time by the catabolism of food and physiologic processes in the body. The energy thus liberated appears as external work, heat, and energy storage. When metabolic rate is measured at rest, in a comfortable ambient temperature and at least 12 hours from the last meal, it is called basal metabolic rate; as such it is expressed in kilocalories per unit of body surface area and can be compared among different individuals and species. For example, comparison of shrews and bats shows that shrews, with the highest metabolic rate of all mammals, have a lifespan of 1 year compared with bats with a much lower metabolism and a lifespan of over 15 years (Kirkwood, 1985; Hart and Setlow, 1974). The higher metabolic rate would accelerate the accumulation of nuclear errors (DNA damage) or of cellular damage (accumulation of damage by free radicals) and thereby shorten the lifespan. The Pacific salmon and the Atlantic eel are prime examples of the inverse relationship between accumulation of damage, stress, and length of lifespan. Both fish age rapidly at the time of spawning and die shortly thereafter. However, if spawning and the associated stress are prevented, they will continue to live for several years (Robertson and Wexler, 1961). Lower temperature would increase longevity by decreasing immune responsivity and thereby preventing autoimmune disorders (Liu and Walford, 1970).

Fecundity, measured by the number of young born per year of mature life, appears also to be inversely related to longevity. Thus, shrews, with a short lifespan, have a large litter size and produce two litters per year, whereas the longer-lived bats have only one young per year.

Duration of growth also has been related to the lifespan. For example, comparison of the chimpanzee to humans shows that growth periods last approximately 10 years in the chimpanzee and 20 years in humans, and their respective lifespans are approximately 40 and 100 years. Duration of the growth period can be prolonged in experimental animals, primarily rodents, and the onset of maturation can be delayed by restricting food intake in terms of total calories or of some specific dietary components. With these dietary manipulations, not only is the lifespan prolonged, but some specific functions, such as reproduction and thermoregulation, are maintained until advanced age; also, the onset of aging-related pathology is delayed and its severity reduced (Segall and Timiras, 1976; Segall *et al.*, 1983).

Several factors, including body and brain size, metabolic rate, fecundity, duration of growth as well as stress and conditions of life, superimposed on the genetic makeup, undoubtedly contribute to the difference in longevity among species. As discussed above, natural selection suggests that the individual member of a group must survive through the reproductive period to ensure continuation of the species; thereafter, survival of the postreproductive individual becomes indifferent or detrimental (e.g., food competition) to the group. In this sense, a gene that acted to ensure a maximum number of offspring in youth but produced disease at later ages might be positively selected. In modern times, not only is life expectancy increased, but humans live well beyond the reproductive years, women some 40 years beyond the childbearing period. Longevity of a species beyond the reproductive years must be incidental to some earlier events, or the infertile individual must confer some advantage to the fertile. In our society, this must be the case, for older members do contribute to the maintenance of the entire population structure and to the development and progress of our society (de Beauvoir, 1972).

Selective Immortality

Senescence is assumed to occur in all vertebrates and leads to death, hence its qualification as being *universal, progressive, deleterious, and irreversible* (Strehler, 1977). As already indicated, it is that period of the lifespan characterized by an exponential increase in mortality and is terminated by death. However, there are certain life forms—particularly plants and invertebrates—in which aging may not occur at all. Among the unicellular organisms, protozoa have received considerable attention, but no one has definitively demonstrated or negated their immortality. For example, certain strains of *Paramecium* maintained in culture may be capable of surviving indefinitely without conjugation and cross-fertilization, whereas other strains do not survive unless periodically cross-fertilized. Other unicellular organisms, such as some *ciliates,* undergo age-related changes that involve not only cell size and a change in cell shape, but also alterations in cell skeleton and cell behavior. Bacteria, yeast, and clones of many kinds of plants may not exhibit senescence. Similarly, metazoa, such as sea anemones, appear to be ageless; in these jellyfish, the individual "jellies" have a fixed lifespan, but the larval "stub" produces a constant supply of new blanks as old ones are removed and the specimens remain vigorous indefinitely. Even in some vertebrates, such as large fish and tortoises, the process of aging is so slow as to be almost undetectable. From these and similar studies, it may be concluded that there is no inherent factor common to all forms of life that automatically produces senescence, but rather that some organisms could live indefinitely.

It must be recognized, however, that the absence of signs of aging cannot be equated with immortality; the advantage of an ageless organism consists simply in the fact that its lifespan is not affected by the passage of time. That is, it still may die but from a cause that can kill it at any age. In contrast, among the animals that undergo the characteristic age-dependent loss of vigor with advancing age, the mortality rate steadily increases at a rate typical for each species, thus producing a finite lifespan.

DIFFERENTIAL AGING IN HUMANS

Chronologic age, or age in number of years, and physiologic age, or age in terms of functional capacity, do not always coincide, and physical appearance and health status often belie chronologic age. Although no specialized knowledge is required to estimate an individual's age, in many cases a person may look younger or older than his/her chronologic age. From a physiologic standpoint, such disparities in the timetable of aging may occur among individuals or among selected populations; they result from complex interactions between genetic and environmental factors that operate on the individual as the child of her/his parents and also as a member of a societal group.

Studies on aging have often ignored or attributed differences among individuals of the same age to specific genetic endowment. Yet, one of the characteristics of the aging human population is its substantive heterogeneity. That is, some individuals "age" at a much slower or faster rate than others. Accordingly, aging processes have been divided into "usual" aging, referring to the average physiologic changes, and "successful" aging, referring to those individuals who show minimal functional decrements with aging (Rowe and Khan, 1987). The distinction between usual, that is, average aging and successful, that is, better than average aging supports the hypothesis that extrinsic factors play an important role in age-associated functional decline. As we consider the many cross-cultural differences that greatly influence aging, it is difficult to ascribe change to age alone. Attributing change to age, per se, may often be exaggerated, and factors such as diet, exercise, drugs, and psychosocial environment should not be underestimated or ignored as potential moderators of the aging process. Taking these elements into account, the prospects for avoidance, or eventual reversal, of functional loss with age are vastly improved and the risks of adverse consequences are reduced (Rowe and Khan, 1987).

Changes with aging lack uniformity not only among individuals of the same species, but also within the same individual, where onset, rate, and magnitude of the changes vary depending on the cell, tissue, organ, or system considered (Shock, 1960). In certain functions, regulation remains quite efficient until advanced age; in others, functional decrements appear at an early age. Examples of this type of differential aging include fasting blood glucose levels and acid-base balance, which remain stable as late as 70 to 90 years. In contrast, the basal metabolic rate declines continuously throughout the lifespan. Certain sensory modalities, such as vision and hearing, show functional decrements beginning in early adulthood. One classic example of a unique timetable involving an organ that develops and ages during a specific period of the lifespan is the ovary, which begins to function at adolescence (in humans, approximately, 10 to 12 years) and ceases to function at menopause (in humans, as long as 40 years before death) (Chapter 13). Other classic examples include embryonal structures, such as the placenta, which develop and age within a relatively short period of time as compared to the total length of the lifespan. Whatever the organ or tissue considered, timetables of aging represent an approximation, as already indicated above, for the onset of aging is not a precise event that can be pinpointed by a specific physiologic sign.

AGING OF THE PLACENTA: A MODEL FOR ORGAN AGING

In considering differential timetables of aging in different organs and tissues, the placenta offers the unique example of a structure fulfilling its function, aging, and disappearing within a short period of time from a few days to several months, depending on the animal species. The aging of the placenta has been studied in humans and other animals, both morphologically and functionally, although most of the research conducted has been primarily related to the possible implications of age-related changes for the health of the fetus. Morphologically, the aging placenta is characterized by the accumulation of metabolically less active material, such as deposition of fibrinoid substance, hyaline degeneration, calcification, formation of cysts, as well as by a decrease in protein synthesis and decline in enzymatic activity. Functionally, its degeneration is reflected in a decline in secretory activity, particularly of hormones, and in impairment of the transfer mechanisms operating between mother and fetus. In humans, several pathologic conditions can either delay or accelerate aging of the placenta. For example, in erythroblastosis fetalis (a disease of red blood cell maturation in the fetus) fetal erythropoiesis (red blood cell production) is greatly stimulated as a result of increased red cell destruction; this induces the placenta to continue to produce red blood cells throughout gestation—a function it normally loses in the first trimester. Conversely, such conditions as toxemia of pregnancy (a toxic disturbance of late pregnancy with hypertension) result in hormonal insufficiency due to early degenerative changes in the endocrine cells of the placenta. It seems worthwhile to determine whether less severe abnormalities than those mentioned above are capable of disturbing the aging processes of the placenta and to investigate their mechanisms and the consequences for the fetus. Studies of this type have already implicated endocrine or nutritional deficiencies, moderate hypoxia, and a variety of toxic substances and drugs (e.g., nicotine, carbon dioxide, alcohol) in the acceleration of placental aging and the development of fetal abnormalities. In addition to the placenta, other organs (e.g., yolk sac, allantois) and tissues (hemopoietic cells of liver and spleen) complete a life cycle during pregnancy—appearing, fulfilling their respective functions, and disappearing—within variable periods of time. Although these represent illustrations of organ aging unique to pregnancy, other structures of the body undergo similar age-related changes at different periods of life. Two prominent examples to be discussed fully in their respective chapters are the thymus, which ages at adolescence (Chapter 8), and the ovary which ceases to function at menopause (Chapter 13).

Because aging is a slow and continuous process, some of its effects can be observed only when they have progressed sufficiently to induce alterations that can be identified and validated by available testing methods. An illustrative example is atherosclerosis, the consequences of which become manifest in middle and old age even though the atherosclerotic lesion may start early in infancy (Chapter 17).

Comparison of several functions from young to old age shows a gradation of decrements with old age (Figure 2–6). Fasting blood glucose and acid-base balance (the latter not shown) remain relatively stable under basal conditions; these two functions are regulated by a number of mechanisms involving several organs and systems and providing alternate controls. If, however, these functions are tested after increased physiologic demand (e.g., sugar load, sustained physical exercise, environmental changes), the efficiency with which the organism is capable of maintaining levels within normal limits or the rapidity with which these levels return to normal demonstrates marked differences between adult and old. Thus, placing a system under stress brings to light age differences not otherwise detectable. It also clearly demonstrates the declining ability of the aging organism to withstand or respond adequately to stress (Chapter 12).

This inability of the aged organism to withstand stress may be the consequence of the overall functional decline in the major functions of the organism, as illustrated in a number of examples in Figure 2–6. While conduction velocity in nerves decreases moderately with aging, the cardiac index, that is, cardiac output/minute/squaremeter of body surface, decreases by 30% between ages 30 and 80. Similarly, tests of renal function—filtration rate, blood flow—and respiratory function—vital capacity and maximum breathing capacity—undergo 35 to 65 percent decline with aging. A detailed description of the aging-related changes in these functions is presented in the respective chapters (Chapters 19, 20, and 22).

Other functions of the body begin to age relatively early in adult life and fall to a minimum before the age of 65, officially heralding the stage of senescence. For example, in the eye, accommodation begins to decline in the teens and regresses to a minimum in the midfifties. Similarly, the auditory function begins to deteriorate at adolescence and deterioration continues steadily thereafter, culminating around 50 years of age. This auditory deterioration may also be hastened by the environmental noise to which, in our civilization, individuals are continuously exposed from young age. Some comparative studies in isolated populations living in a quiet environment (e.g., forest-dwelling African tribes) and maintaining a good auditory function into old age seem to support the view that continuous exposure to noise may be harmful to the auditory function. However, many other factors in the life style (e.g., rural versus urban living; modern versus primitive populations) may also be operative, and a definitive association between excess noise and loss of hearing with aging cannot be drawn at the present time. In the locomotor system, different muscle groups show different aging patterns. Irrespective of the muscle considered, the peak of muscle strength occurs between 20 and 30 years of age; the decline is continuous thereafter, but the rate of aging varies depending on

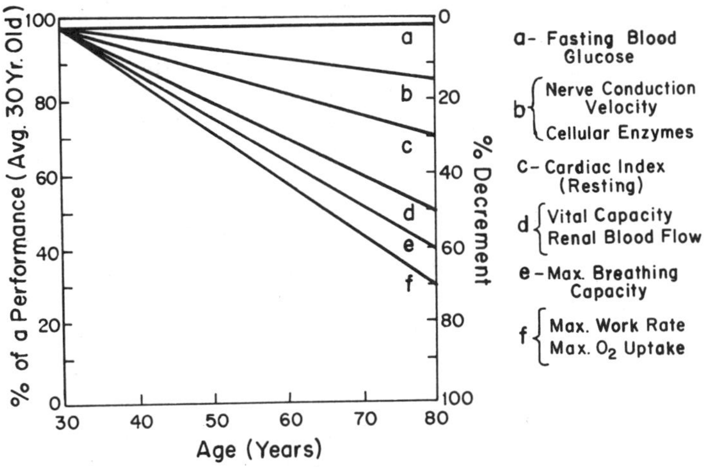

Figure 2–6. *Age decrements in physiological performance.*

Decline in various human functional capacities and physiologic measurements with age. (Courtesy of Dr. N.W. Shock.)

the muscular group considered (for example, the muscles of the leg are generally compromised earlier than those of the arm) as well as the test used for measuring muscle function (for example, short exercise is less affected than sustained work). To what extent the decline in muscle function can be prevented or reduced by physical exercise is a question of considerable interest; the possibility of maintaining muscular activity in the elderly is relevant not only to the function of the skeletal muscle but, more particularly, to that of the heart (Chapter 22).

CHANGES IN BODY AND ORGAN WEIGHTS

Morphologic impairments associated with functional decline also show great variability with respect to age of onset, structure examined, and the individual's sex and history. Some prominent changes that occur in body morphology with aging include: stature (or standing height), sitting height, breadth of shoulder, and depth of chest—all of which show a progressive reduction with aging in contrast to cephalic diameters, which remain practically unchanged. The considerable and progressive dimunition in stature that appears to occur in all human populations may be ascribed, at least in part, to alterations (osteoporosis) in bone structure to be discussed in Chapter 13.

Other age-related changes in external morphology are represented by an increase in fat deposition, particularly evident in the subcutaneous layer, where it is easily quantifiable by measuring the thickness of the skinfold at a number of points in the body. These measurements have shown that fat deposition increases with aging in parallel with body weight, reaching a peak at approximately 50 years, when it begins progressively to decline. Thus, although body weight characteristically increases during the initial stages of senescence, it decreases in advanced age.

In association with the decrease in body weight, the weight of organs also declines with aging. Although a comprehensive tabulation of changes in organ weight with age exists only for humans (Figure 2–6), it is probable that some features, such as skeletal muscle atrophy, are typical of mammalian aging. In humans, as in other mammals, this skeletal atrophy may be due not only to degenerative changes in the muscle itself, but also to the decreased use (disuse) of the muscles due to impairment of other functions (e.g., sensory, peripheral, and central nervous motor) as well as the changing life style of the older individual (Chapter 22).

Weight loss begins in humans between the fifth and seventh decades, a period of increased mortality, and involves primarily the skeletal muscles, liver, kidney, and adrenal. Brain weight declines significantly, but less than that of the above organs except in pathologic conditions in which brain atrophy may be quite severe, as in most cases of senile dementia of the Alzheimer type (Chapter 9). In contrast, heart weight does not change and, in fact, may even increase, especially when measured relative to whole-body weight. This is an indication of the attempt by cardiac muscle to compensate for its declining functional activity and the increased peripheral resistance (as a consequence of atherosclerosis). Compensation is achieved through hypertrophy of contractile cells (myocytes) and/or of interstitial cells (connective, conductive, and endothelial cells). The weight of some bones, such as the ribs, decreases with aging, whereas that of others, such as the sternum, increases with age.

In view of the high incidence of pathology with aging, sudden or progressive changes in body weight, abnormal in severity and timing, may also be indicative of onset and course of disease. In this manner, body weight represents a relatively simple measure of the physiologic and, eventually, pathologic assessment of the health status of the elderly (as it is also an indicator of the growth progress during development).

ASSESSMENT OF PHYSIOLOGIC AGE IN HUMANS

Evaluation of physiologic aging in humans requires quantitative measurements of numerous parameters selected as indices of physical (e.g., tests of physiologic performance) and mental (e.g., psychologic and psychiatric tests) competence at progressive ages (Bourlière, 1970; Kane and Kane, 1981). In order to establish an accurate profile that will reflect the different aging timetables for the body systems discussed above and will also combine them to represent the health status of the individual, a number of criteria must be satisfied. Such criteria must take into account the many variables among individuals and within the same individual. It is generally accepted that assessment of physiologic competence in humans, at any age, is a multifactorial process. The validity of any assessment lies in the choice of the right test or battery of tests best qualified to provide an overall picture of current health and to eventually serve as a basis for prediction of future health and length of the lifespan. Indeed a global measure of physiologic status may be derived from many different combinations of tests; the combination selected will depend on the purpose of the assessment and who will use these data. With respect to purpose, measurements may be expected:

- to describe the physiologic status of an individual at progressive chronologic ages,
- to screen a selected population for assessment of overall physiologic competence or competence of specific functions using either cross-sectional or longitudinal sampling methods (see below).
- to monitor the efficacy of specific treatments, drugs, exercise, special dietary regimens,
- to predict persistence or loss of physiologic competence, to determine incidence of disease, and to evaluate life expectancy.

With respect to the user of this derived information, the choice of tests will depend on whether he/she is a health provider, specialist, researcher, or case manager.

However, even with a precise identification of the nature of the assessment needed and of the user who needs it, it still remains difficult to choose the most significant and feasible tests, and no consensus is available on the usefulness of any of the current geriatric assessment and screening programs. This choice is further complicated by the need to take into account also the financial feasibility and the facilities available for the testing. Thus, failure to agree on the best checklist for assessing physiologic competence and health status in the elderly is reflected by the relative large number of such lists. Some of the most current used in this country are listed in Table 2–4.

Geriatric assessment can be defined as a multidimensional diagnostic process designed to qualify an elderly individual's medical, psychosocial, and functional capabilities and disabilities—usually using an interdisciplinary team—with the intention of arriving at a comprehensive plan for therapy and long-term follow-up. Thus, the major purposes of such an assessment are to improve diagnosis (medical and psychosocial), plan appropriate rehabilitation and other therapy, determine optimal living location, arrange for high-quality follow-up care and case management, and establish baseline information useful for future comparison.

In general, most of these assessment programs include several tests, which have been grouped into three categories:

- tests that examine general physical health as represented by physiologic competence and the absence of disease,
- tests that measure the ability to perform basic self-care activities, and
- tests that also measure, in addition to basic activities, the ability to perform more complex (instrumental) activities of daily living (Table 2–5).

Selection of the physiologic variables to be tested must be based on several prerequisites, including:

Table 2–4. SELECTED MEASURES OF PHYSICAL HEALTH

MEASURE/SOURCE	ITEMS COVERED	TYPE OF TEST
Cornell Medical Index	Multiple categories of physical and mental health	Self-completion tests of yes-no answers
Cumulative Illness Rating Score	Covers all organ systems including endocrine-metabolic and psychiatric	Physician ratings
Health Index	Common ailments and consequences (bed, hospital, etc.) and duration	Interview
PACE II: Medical Data	Checklist of diagnostic categories and medical status measures	Review of history, physical examination, and tests
Patient Classification for Long-Term Care (LTC): Impairments and Medical Status	Physical impairments, health risk factors	Physician and nursing staff rating
OARS: Physical Health (Old Age Retirement System)	In- and outpatient care, medications, illnesses and disabilities, self-ratings of health	Interview

Table 2–5. CATEGORIES OF PHYSICAL HEALTH INDEX MEASURING PHYSICAL COMPETENCE*

PHYSICAL HEALTH	ACTIVITIES OF DAILY LIVING	INSTRUMENTAL ACTIVITIES OF DAILY LIVING
Bed days	Feeding	Cooking
Restricted-activity days	Bathing	Cleaning
Hospitalizations	Toileting	Using telephone
Physician visits	Dressing	Writing
Pain and discomfort	Ambulation	Reading
Symptoms	Transfer from bed	Shopping
Signs on physical exam	Transfer from toilet	Laundry
Physiologic indicators (e.g., lab tests, x-rays, pulmonary and cardiac functions)	Bowel and bladder control	Managing medications
Permanent impairments (e.g., vision, hearing, speech, paralysis, amputations, dental)	Grooming	Using public transportation
Diseases/diagnoses	Communication	Walking outdoors
Self-rating of health	Visual acuity	Climbing stairs
Physician ratings of health	Upper extremities (e.g., grasping and picking up objects)	Outside work (e.g., gardening, snow shoveling)
	Range of motion of limbs	Ability to perform in paid employment
		Managing money
		Traveling out of town

*Many of the items presented are components of the Selected Measures of Physical Health shown in Table 2–4.

- the variables must be indicative of a function important to the competence or general health of the individual and capable of influencing the rate of aging;
- they must correlate with chronologic age.
- they must change sufficiently and with discernible regularity over time to reveal significant differences over a 3-to-5 year interval between tests, and
- they must be practically measurable in an individual or cohort of individuals without hazard, discomfort, or expense to the participant or excessive labor or expense for the investigator.

In most testing, the degree of wellness, that is, the absence of disease, is also recorded and, reciprocally, the presence of diseases and their severity are recorded as well. The incidence of disease and pathology in the elderly is discussed in Chapter 3. Examples of tests grouped under the previously mentioned categories are presented in Table 2–5, and an example of a geriatric

Table 2–6. GERIATRIC SCREENING AND ASSESSMENT PROGRAMS*

GERIATRIC SCREENING	GERIATRIC ASSESSMENT
History and physical examination Laboratory tests Speech and hearing tests Social worker interview Dental evaluation	History and physical examination Laboratory tests Speech and hearing tests Social worker interview Psychiatric evaluation Instrumental activities of daily living Interdisciplinary conference for disposition
Free service Individuals 60+ not seen by physician in previous year Generally ambulatory, relative good health, minor complaints 4 patients/week involves 4–5 health professionals	*Paid service* Individuals 60+ years, physician or family referral for specific problem and disposition Frequently demented 2 patients/week involves 6 health professionals

*Source: Geriatric Services, Dr. H. Brownstein, Director, Mount Zion Hospital and Medical Center, San Francisco, California 94120.

screening and assessment program is summarized in Table 2–6.

Evaluation of Geriatric Screening and Assessment Programs

Geriatric assessment traces its origins to the pioneering work of British geriatricians in the 1930s and 1940s. They demonstrated that end-stage, bed-bound, geriatric patients could be dramatically mobilized and many discharged to community settings following careful assessment and rehabilitation. Today, there are in this country several assessment programs within a variety of health care structures, ranging from hospital, to outpatient clinic, to nursing home.

Cross-Sectional and Longitudinal Studies of Physiologic Aging

The two basic approaches to the study of human aging, using the tests discussed above, are the *cross-sectional study* and the *longitudinal study*. With cross-sectional methods, physiologic characteristics are compared among different age groups at one time. Studies of this type can be conducted with relative rapidity and accuracy in a large group of people: for example, a population with a broad span of ages, perhaps birth to 90 years, is sectioned into narrow, age-defined subsets and measurements are made in identical fashion in each group. This type of study has been used in gerontologic research for such programs as short-term testing of new drugs or regimens capable of influencing some aspects of the aging process. This method has also been used profitably in animal studies conducted in such species as rats and mice, which can be raised and maintained under special, but standardized conditions (e.g., diet, drugs, exercise).

Human populations, however, live under widely different environmental conditions, and the same measurements obtained in cohorts of individuals of the same age are subject to multifactorial influences only one of which is aging per se. Thus, the cross-sectional study, although less time consuming, is subject to a number of errors. For example, because of the secular trend in stature (that is, changes that occur in a population as a whole over time) the 20-year-old in 1980 is taller than was the 20-year-old in 1910, suggesting an aging-related decrease in height, the oldest people in the comparison being born when body height was lower. Similarly, differential survivorship depends on the selected survival only of those individuals with a particular characteristic. To continue with the example of stature, it is possible that tall, lean individuals tend to live longer than short and obese; if true, this would bias the outcome of the study.

The longitudinal study avoids some of these errors and therefore is the preferred method of many gerontologists. In the longitudinal study, the same individuals are examined at regular intervals throughout the lifespan so that the process of aging can be compared in a dynamic fashion, each individual being his/her own control between two or several ages. Longitudinal studies have been used with great success in the study of growth processes. In aging, however, this method has many obvious disadvantages, especially in the study of human populations: not only is the human lifespan relatively long, but in industrialized countries, human populations are extremely mobile and many of the components of the cohort are lost during the study.

A compromise approach combining cross-sectional and longitudinal studies is often used; in this type of study, initial data from cross-sectional studies are supplemented and corrected by data from longitudinal follows-up. Another practical approach is to restrict the longitudinal survey to "critical" life periods (for example, 5 years before and 5 years after menopause or retirement).

With the continuing progress being made in the techniques and statistical analyses employed for measuring physiologic parameters, it is expected that more sensitive, accurate, and practicable tests will soon be implemented in clinical screening as well as in research programs. A further consideration concerns the validity of the standards accepted for assessing general health and functional competence, which are based on values obtained in the young. An example is the abnormal glucose tolerance test reported in 50% of the individuals aged 65 years or older; such abnormal response may be viewed as a pathologic condition or may appear normal when measured with age-related constructed nomograms. Indeed, formulation of reliable charts of physiologic aging comparable to those used to assess growth and development in children is one of the fundamental prerequisites to establish a rational and workable health care program for the elderly.

IN VITRO MEASUREMENTS OF BIOLOGIC AGE

The complexities and difficulties of formulating indices of biologic age in humans and, eventually, other animals involve, as discussed above, the differential aging of organ systems, cells, and molecules and their changing responses to internal (e.g., hormonal) and external (e.g., environmental) demands. An alternative approach utilizes single cell types removed from the body and cultured under *in vitro* conditions. Such studies compare cells derived from individuals of different chronologic ages, establish standardized conditions of culture of these cells, and measure specific parameters of cell function (e.g., replicative capability, metabolism).

One example is the systematic study of human skin fibroblast cell cultures established from skin biopsies from members of a human longitudinal study (the Baltimore Longitudinal Study) (Schneider, 1981). Cell doubling capacity was taken as one index (from several) of cell reproductive capability: the initial culture flask when the cells had reached confluency (i.e., formed a monolayer of tightly packed cells covering the entire flask bottom) was designated as cell population doubling 1 and the subsequent flasks with the correspondingly subsequent doublings were given progressive numbers. It is known that in cultured fibroblasts the number of doublings is about 50 and that this number may be influenced by genetic and environmental factors (Hayflick, 1965; Cristofalo and Balin, 1981; Martin *et al.*, 1981). Cell replication was slower and the number of doublings was reduced in cultures derived from old as compared to young donors. Similarly, other parameters of replicative capability showed a significant decline in the cultures from old donors.

These studies suggest that tissue culture can be utilized to examine human cellular aging. They provide useful correlations with *in vivo* physiologic measurements and may serve as models for the longitudinal analysis of cellular aging. Tissue culture models may also prove useful in mimicking aging pathologies characteristic of specific types of cellular aging (Chapter 3).

THE ELDERLY AS AN ASSET

This segment of society constitutes a group of skilled, literate, often well-informed individuals who are the products of a full, active, and, hopefully, useful life. This has involved many years of coping with life and surviving its many problems. Surely, such individuals can only be considered an asset.

One can find impressive examples of elderly people who are successful in public and political life, not only in early history (e.g., Roman senators) and many civilizations (e.g., Chinese elders), but also in current times (e.g., Ronald Reagan, born in 1911 and U.S. President for two terms, 1980–1988; whether success in politics is a creditable achievement depends on a personal point of view). Other examples of long and productive lives exist in the arts, humanities, and sciences (to quote only a few recent examples, Pablo Picasso, Arthur Rubenstein, Bertrand Russell). As old age is the final phase of growth and development, the longer the individual's life, the greater are the opportunities for the greatest progress. As written almost 2000 years ago, "Nor is age any bar to pursuits of every other kind . . . to the verge of extreme old age" (Cicero, c. 44 B.C.). To live into old age, therefore, gives the greatest chance of fulfillment of potential not only for those individuals with extraordinary talents, but also for ordinary people whose contributions to society, minor as they may be, will be of benefit in the planning of the future of mankind (Comfort, 1976). As written by an active centenarian, "At my age, I stand, as it were, on a peak alone. . . . But that very isolation gives me a less biased view of the vast panorama of human life which is spread before the eyes of a centenarian . . . and can see clearly the advance of mankind" (Murray, 1963).

Yet there is a tendency among the general public to concentrate on the negative aspects of age. We bemoan the stresses and strains placed on our social services as well as on the family finances and good-will by the elderly, the victims of increased pathology.

Despite the remarkable lengthening of the lifespan over the last 80 years, we dwell on the transitory nature of life and the rapid passage of time; from among many similar ones, one quotation of Edward Young (*Night Thoughts,* 1742–1746, quoted in Sampson and Sampson, 1985)—"Our birth is nothing but our death begun"—seems to embody and encourage this pessimistic obsession with aging. In our dislike and dread of aging, we overlook the positive contributions that can be made by the "third age" of life.

In a scholarly and compassionate treatise on old age, Simone de Beauvoir (1972) rests the analogy between "the infant scarcely come to life and the old man scarcely alive" on the dependency shared by both on the young and powerful members of society who possess the vigor and fertility necessary for the survival and perpetuation of social organization. Thus, whether the elderly members of society are neglected as a group or are integrated into the social structure varies with respect to the values of the society as established by its adult members. We find wide variation in living conditions and active social participation of the elderly in rural versus urban environment, primitive versus technologically advanced societies, nomadic versus sedentary life styles—all of which, in turn, show significant differences depending on the historic era and specific culture considered. In the strongly organized society of Western civilization, it is expected that the contributions of the elderly, mainly experience and various degrees of technical skills, represent a useful commodity; yet, in the view of many, these qualities are often devalued. Practical skills can easily become redundant with technologic advances. What remains of value are the organizational, advisory, educational activities in which the elderly excel. Knowledge of the past is a great asset in these activities, for it may be used to understand the present and foretell the future.

The "third age" should be viewed as a time of opportunity, a phase of life for reviewing one's goals and for making changes. "My remaining days, I may now consider a free gift," wrote Goethe at 81, and a year later, "Even at my great age, ideas come to me the pursuit and development of which would require another lifetime" (quoted in Sampson and Sampson, 1985). The special skills and talents of the elderly are valuable assets that can be used to the advantage of the remainder of society. It should be the duty and interest of the young and adult to assure that these talents and skills are fully utilized. There is a need to incorporate older people into meaningful societal roles and establish a clear progression of occupational steps that one ascends with age. Modern societies, despite the concern of many social scientists working in gerontology/geriatrics, have not been successful, so far, in making the necessary innovations that would provide adequately for the elderly. The "leisure town" communities constructed in the United States and other Western societies for retired persons of adequate income represent an entrepreneurial venture, more lucrative to business speculators than beneficial to the persons they purportedly serve. Another entrepreneurial venture is the nursing home, which is neither a hospital nor a "home," but has combined the negative aspects of both in confining and restricting the elderly.

In the view of Maddox (1969), the aged should not be isolated as a recipient group for purposes either of living or of policy making. Rather they present problems that are "likely to be the general problems of society, only more intensified." Not all elderly persons are handicapped by illness (as not all young and adult persons are in excellent health!), institutionalized, or dependent on public support. For this large segment of the aged population, the problems of adjusting to a "roleless role" may in large measure be solved by the aged themselves, particularly in a country like the United States in which private resources offer a viable adjunct to governmental social services agencies. The chief obstacle to such a self-help group among the aged is the fact that, given such qualifications as physical and mental health and economic independence, one refuses to view oneself as a member of the "subculture" of the elderly. Quite to the contrary, the elderly have much to offer and we should not hesitate to use them. We should be proud to learn from their previous experience, including mistakes. In many cases, the older the person, the more precious his/her knowledge and the greater the need to use it for the advantage of the entire society.

Unfortunately, today there is no system of care for the elderly showing sufficient imagination and flexibility to permit full utilization of the manpower resources they represent. This is so even in countries in which the relative proportion of the aged is high. The services, facilities, and programs that do exist, even in our own technologically advanced society, assume a patronizing attitude that reflects the continuing underestimation of the elderly potential. The phrase "you can't teach an old dog new tricks" also needs to be critically reviewed. There is ample evidence that the elderly can master new subjects when they have the time and the enthusiasm. The increasing number of educational associations and the success of the French and British "University of the Third Age," catering to the elderly, is proof that the elderly are willing and able to learn.

Aging affects us all, personally and through our families. Although this book underlines the changes that occur with aging, and the majority of these are of a decremental nature, we must not give way to negative attitudes of gloom and despondency. "I did affirm to my readers in my young years that I was the happiest man I ever met and I reaffirm it at the age of ninety-one" (Arthur Rubenstein, 1980). The world-wide dramatic advances in science, technology, and social conditions foreshadow an era in which the elderly will comprise an increasing number of the population whose needs cannot be ignored. And, indeed, these advances have already significantly prolonged the average lifespan in prosperous as well as less economically advantaged countries. To meet the challenge of a growing elderly population we must try to become more informed about the nature of the aging process and its physiologic and pathologic consequences. We must keep a positive and optimistic approach and maintain continued high expectations that can enable us to achieve the goal of growing old successfully.

References

Beauvoir, S. de: *The Coming of Age*, 1st American ed., translated by Patrick O'Brien, Putman, New York, **1972.**

Bennett, N. G., and Garson, L. K.: Extraordinary longevity in the Soviet Union: Fact or Artifact. *The Gerontologist*, **26:**358–361, **1986.**

Bourliere, F.: *The Assessment of Biological Age in Man*, Public Health Papers, World Health Organization, Geneva, **1970.**

Brody, J. A.; Brock, D.B.; and Williams, T. F.: Trends in the health of the elderly population, *Ann. Rev. Pub. Health*, **8:**211–234, **1987.**

Coale, A. J., and Demeny, P.: *Regional Model Life Tables and Stable Populations*, 2nd ed., Academic Press, New York, **1983.**

Comfort, A.: *The Biology of Senescence*, 3rd ed., Elsevier, New York, **1979.**

Comfort, A.: *A Good Age*, Crown, New York, **1976.**

Cristofalo, V. J., and Balin, A. K.: Oxygen tension and vitamin E: Effects on cellular senescence. In Danon, D.; Shock, N. W.; and Marois, M. (eds.): *Aging: A Challenge to Science and Society*, Oxford University Press, Oxford, **1981.**

Directory and Yearbook, Government of India, Official Publications, New Delhi, **1981,** pp. 264–268.

Finch, C. E., and Schneider, E. L.: *Handbook of the Biology of Aging*, 2nd ed., Van Nostrand Reinhold, New York, **1985.**

Hande, H. V.: *Proceedings of the Eleventh Joint Conference of Central Councils of Health and Family Welfare*, New Delhi, Sept. 2–5, **1985.**

Hart, R. W., and Setlow, R. B.: Correlation between deoxyribonucleic acid excision-repair and life-span in a number of mammalian species. *Proc. Natl. Acad. Sci. USA*, **71:**2169–2173, **1974.**

Hayflick, L.: The limited *in vitro* lifetime of human diploid cell strains. *Exp. Cell. Res.*, **37:**614–636, **1965.**

Hendriksen, C.; Lund, E.; and Stomgard, E.: Consequences of assessment and intervention among elderly people, *Br. Med. J.* **289:**1522, **1984.**

Kane, R. A., and Kane, R. L.: *Assessing the Elderly*, Lexington Books, Lexington, MA, **1981.**

Kirkwood, T. B. C.: Comparative and evolutionary aspects of longevity. In Finch, C. E., and Schneider, E. L. (eds.): *Handbook of the Biology of Aging*, 2nd ed., Van Nostrand Reinhold, New York, **1985.**

Kohn, R. R.: Aging as a consequence of growth cessation. In Locke, M. (ed.): *Reproduction: Molecular, Subcellular and Cellular*, Academic Press, New York, **1965.**

Lansing, A. I.: A nongenic factor in the longevity of rotifers. *Ann. NY Acad. Sci.*, **57:**455–464, **1954.**

Leaf, A.: Long-lived populations: Extreme old age. *Am. Geriatr. Soc.*, **30:**485–487, **1982.**

Lints, F. A.: Insects. In Finch, C. E., and Schneider, E. L. (eds.): *Handbook of the Biology of Aging*, 2nd ed., Van Nostrand Reinhold, New York, **1985.**

Liu, R. K., and Walford, R. L.: Observations of the lifespans of several species of annual fishes and of the world's smallest fishes. *Exp. Gerontol.*, **5:**241–246, **1970.**

Maddox, G. L.: Growing old: Getting beyond the stereotypes. In Boyd, R. R., and Oakes, C. G. (eds.): *Foundations of Practical Gerontology*, Univ. of South Carolina Press, Columbia, **1969.**

Martin, G. M.; Ogburn, C. E.; and Sprague, C. A.: Effects of age on cell division capacity. In Danon, D.; Shock, N. W.; and Marois, M. (eds.): *Aging: A Challenge to Science and Society*, Oxford University Press, Oxford, **1981.**

Mazess, R. B., and Forman, S. H.: Longevity and age exaggeration in Vilcabamba, Ecuador. *J. Gerontol.*, **34:**94–98, **1979.**

McCay, C. M.: Chemical aspects of ageing and the effect of diet upon ageing. In Lansing, A. F. (ed.): *Cowdry's Problems of Ageing*, 3rd ed., Williams and Wilkins Co., Baltimore, **1952.**

McCay, C. M.; Pope, F.; and Lunsford, W.: Experimental prolongation of the life span. *Bull. NY Acad. Med.,* **32:**91–101, **1956.**

Medvedev, Z. A.: Caucasus and Altay longevity: A biological or social problem? *Gerontologist,* **14:**381–387, 1974.

Minot, C.: *The Problems of Age, Growth and Death: A Study of Cytomorphosis* (based on lectures at the Lowell Institute), Putman's, New York, **1908.**

Murray, M. A.: *My First Hundred Years,* W. Kimber, London, **1963.**

Rabin, D. L.: Waxing of the gray, waning of the green. In Committee on an Aging Society, Institute of Medicine and National Research Council. *America's Aging: Health in an Older Society,* National Academy Press, Washington, DC, **1985.**

Robertson, O. H., and Wexler, B. C.: Prolongation of the lifespan of Kokanee salmon (*Oncorhynkus nerka Kennerlyi*) by castration before beginning of gonad development. *Proc. Natl. Acad. Sci. USA,* **47:**609–621, **1961.**

Rowe, J. W., and Kahn, R. L.: Human aging: usual and successful. *Science,* **237:**143–149, **1987.**

Rubenstein, A.: *My Many Years,* 1st ed., Knopf, New York, **1980.**

Rubenstein, L. Z.; Josephson, K. R.; Wieland, G. D.; English, P. A.; Sayre, J. A.; and Kane, R. L.: Effectiveness of a geriatric evaluation unit: A randomized clinical trial. *N. Engl. J. Med.,* **311:**1664–1670, **1984.**

Rubenstein, L. Z.; Josephson, K. R.; Nichol-Seamons, M.; and Robbins, A. S.: Comprehensive health screening of well elderly adults: An analysis of a community program. *J. Gerontol.,* **41:**342–352, **1986.**

Rubenstein, L. Z.; Rhee L.; and Kane, R. L.: The role of geriatric assessment units in caring for the elderly. *J. Gerontol.,* **37:**513–521, **1982.**

Sacher, G.: Relation of lifespan to brain weight and body weight in mammals. In Wolstenholme, G. E. W., and O'Connor, M. (eds.): *The Lifespan of Animals,* Vol. 5, Little, Brown, Boston, **1959.**

Sacher, G.: Life table modification and life prolongation. In Finch, C. E., and Hayflick, K. (eds.): *Handbook of the Biology of Aging,* Van Nostrand Reinhold, New York, **1977.**

Salk, Y.: *The Survival of the Wisest,* Harper, New York, **1973.**

Sampson, A., and Sampson, S.: *The Oxford Book of Ages,* Oxford University Press, Oxford, **1985.**

Schneider, E. L.: A new approach to measuring biological age: Studies on human skin fibroblasts in tissue culture. In Danon, D.; Shock, N. W.; and Marois, M. (eds.): *Aging: A Challenge to Science and Society,* Oxford University Press, Oxford, **1981.**

Segall, P. E., and Timiras, P. S.: Patho-physiologic findings after chronic tryptophan deficiency in rats: A model for delayed growth and aging. *Mech. Ageing Dev.,* **5:**109–124, **1976.**

Segall, P. E.; Timiras, P. S.; and Walton, J. R.: Low tryptophan diets delay reproductive ageing. *Mech. Ageing Dev.,* **24:**245–252, **1983.**

Shock, N. W.: Discussion on mortality and measurement. In Strehler, B. L.; Ebert, J. D.; and Shock, N. W. (eds.): *The Biology of Aging: A Symposium.* Am. Inst. Biol. Sci., Washington, DC, **1960.**

Strehler, B. L.: *Time, Cells and Aging,* 2nd ed., Academic Press, New York, **1977.**

Williams, T. F.; Hill, J. G.; Fairbanks, M. E.; and Knox, K. G.: Appropriate placement of the chronically ill and aged. *JAMA,* **226:**1332–1335, **1973.**

CHAPTER

3 AGING AND DISEASE

Aging is usually considered to be a normal phenomenon that occurs in all members of a population. As defined in the previous chapter, it is associated with physiologic decline. It is also inevitably accompanied by increased incidence and severity of diseases, accidents, and stress. Deleterious factors, not lethal in themselves, may, from a very early age, gradually add to the physiologic decay and predispose the individual to functional losses or to specific diseases in later life. Death from "pure" old age is rare; rather, it may result "prematurely" from increased multiple pathology superimposed on homeostatic insufficiency.

It is difficult to isolate the effects of aging alone from those consequent to disease or to gradual degenerative changes that develop fully with the passage of time. Any demarcation among these three aspects can be only tentatively drawn at the present state of our knowledge. For example, it is reasonable to question whether the atheroma—the characteristic lesion of atherosclerosis—represents a degenerative process or a disease; in other words, whether it represents the consequences of age-related molecular changes in one or several of the arterial wall constituents, or the consequence of mechanical injury or of a virus. It has long been accepted, and with reason, that "old age is almost always combined with or masked by morbid processes." Certainly, late life is a period of increasing and multiple pathology during which it becomes progressively more difficult to distinguish conceptually between "normal" aging, which is universal, and specific diseases, which affect people differently.

The close association between aging and diseases affects the practical orientation of aging research (Johnson, 1985a). Some physiologists follow the traditional view that research in the area of aging should be aimed at specific functional and clinical entities rather than at aging as a whole. This approach, fundamentally pragmatic, envisions little chance of significantly influencing the overall aging process. By focusing on clarification of the etiopathogenesis and eventual treatment of a specific disease, the search for the immediate improvement of health and quality of life of the elderly is spotlighted. One example of such an approach is illustrated by the current interest in senile dementia of the Alzheimer type. Numerous gerontologists and scientists from various disciplines have rallied around the study of this disease: while the hope of conquering aging may seem too theoretical and far removed, the study of a specific disease projects a much more concrete image and a task achievable within a limited time.

In contrast, other gerontologists have argued that treatment and even cure of many diseases would prolong life by only a few years; for example, if cardiovascular diseases were cured overnight, the lifespan would be extended by about 5 years. Efforts, therefore, should be expended to elucidate the basic mechanisms of the aging process *per se*. Obviously, both research programs have merits and should be pursued simultaneously.

If we accept the view, presented in Chapter 2, that resistance to environmental stress declines with aging, then death can be attributed to any intervening accident or disease, however minor; in other words, the probability of dying from disease or injury would inevitably increase with the passage of time. In every organ, tissue, and in many cells, a time-dependent loss of structure, function, and chemistry proceeds slowly as the consequence of small, but accumulating, injuries (microinsults, according to Johnson, 1985b). For example, deterioration of skin elastin may result from bombardment by ultraviolet photons; degeneration of articular cartilage, from countless mechanical insults; opacification of the crystalline lens, from molecular injuries.

Indeed, it is when these small injuries act at the molecular level that the most significant consequences for aging may occur, such as the loss of genetic memory in the cell or the progressive cross-linking of collagen, the major structural protein of the body.

The diseases of the aged are properly the concern of those working in geriatrics rather than in gerontology (see definitions in Chapter 2). When we first considered the problem of diseases of the aged (Timiras, 1972), some selected aspects of the diseases were reviewed on the basis that studying the succession of events that finally culminate in functional failure and disease may uncover valuable clues concerning the more general process of aging. However, many excellent textbooks of geriatrics have been published in the interim, and the interested reader is referred to those (Brocklehurst, 1985; Cape *et al.*, 1983; Cassell and Walsh, 1984; Kane *et al.*, 1984; Pathy, 1985; Steinberg, 1983).

In this chapter, we shall first consider death-causing diseases and list some of the diseases related specifically to aging. Second, we shall discuss briefly the condition of "disuse" as a consequence of aging or disease, its impact on the rate of aging, and the possible influence of increased physical activity in delaying or alleviating the consequences of disuse and aging. Third, we shall present some examples in which disease has been used as a tool for inducing aging as illustrated in *in vivo* and *in vitro* models.

DEATH RATES THROUGHOUT THE LIFESPAN

If death is considered the end-point of aging (Chapter 1), information regarding the mechanisms underlying aging can be drawn from evaluation of the death rates of different populations. Death rate is expressed as the number of deaths in a given age interval divided by the number of individuals in that age interval. The resulting "age-specific death rate" may also be interpreted as the probability of death within a given age interval and a specific population (see Table 2–2). According to U.S. data, the probability of death within the next 24 hours or the next year is much greater at age 80 than at age 60. This increased probability of death with advancing age was reported for the first time in 1825 by the English actuary B. Gompertz, who demonstrated that in humans, the tendency to die increases exponentially with aging. That is, the older we get, the faster we get old! Data, from both human and animal populations, acquired since the last century show a remarkable similarity among mortality curves for different populations, whether the total lifespan is measured in days, as in *Drosophila*, or in years, as in humans (Johnson, 1985b; Jones, 1960). Regardless of the species, the death rate, as illustrated in Figure 3–1, increases exponentially until the population is exhausted. The consistency of this curve suggests that it represents one of the fundamental properties of living systems.

The reasons for the logarithmic increase in death rate with aging have not, so far, been adequately explained. It is particularly difficult to reconcile the physiologic decline, which progresses linearly with aging, with the increasing death rate, which progresses logarithmically. One suggested interpretation is that biologic systems have a certain built-in redundancy or functional reserve. A steady decline in function may proceed for many years without lowering the functional capacity below that required for homeostasis. Only when homeostatic needs can no longer be matched does failure of adaptive competence lead to disease and death (Johnson, 1985b).

Of interest is the fact that this logarithmic mortality continues even when severe public health problems are alleviated. For example, despite the progressive decline in infant and childhood mortality since the turn of the century, the tendency of the population to die during adulthood continued to double (in 1955) every 8.5 years (Jones, 1960). Under the current improved conditions of medical care, nutrition, and sanitation the rise in the death rate occurs at a later age, but once the curve has begun to rise, the doubling time of 8.5 years remains essentially unchanged. Of further interest is the observation that the increase is logarithmic in character in all countries whether the tendency to die is great, as in underdeveloped countries in which mortality rate is

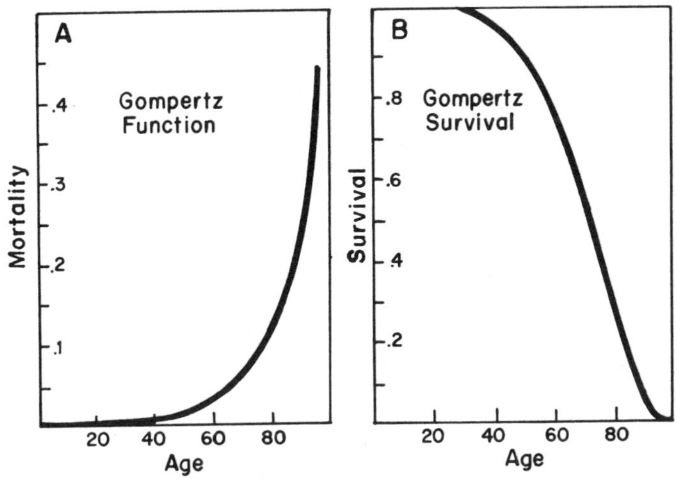

Figure 3–1. *Age-specific mortality rate and survival curves.*

A. Age-specific mortality rates for white males. *B*. Derived survival curve.

typically high, or slight, as in well-developed countries that have experienced a rapid reduction in death rate.

As illustrated in Figure 3–2 and already discussed in Chapter 2, comparison of age-specific death rate curves from one country to another indicates that the essential differences are manifested earlier rather than later in the lifespan. Thus, infancy and childhood disease experiences are very important to health at all ages of life; in other words, optimal development may be directly related to the length of the lifespan and to the physical and mental well-being not only of the adult, but also of the elderly.

DISEASES OF OLD AGE—CAUSES OF DEATH?

The relationship between the aging process and disease is also supported by demographic studies of diseases of old age. Deaths from major causes in the U.S. population are obtained from Vital Statistics and can be plotted as a function of age. Those for 1955 were graphed by Kohn (1963, 1978, 1985) and represent an often-quoted source of information. While the patterns of death have varied considerably from the beginning of the century to now, values for 1955 are not too different from today's and, therefore, are presented here (Figure 3–3). In 1900, and the early years of this century, the three major causes of death in this country were tuberculosis, pneumonia, and diarrhea-enteritis. By 1949, and persisting to today, the three major causes of death are cardiovascular diseases, cancer (neoplasms), and accidents (including those consequent to violence). The curve of all causes of death is a straight line after maturity. This demonstrates that the probability of dying increases exponentially with aging, as already discussed. The death rate due to accidents increases sharply in late adolescence and young adulthood; it then remains constant until about 70 years of age, when it starts to rise again. Aging-related diseases such as those related to cardiovascular pathology or cancer do not equally affect all individuals, hence the heterogeneity of these diseases. In addition, with increasing age, individuals are affected by several diseases simultaneously, and, consequently, death may be due to a multiplicity of causes rather than a single one.

The major causes of death by age in the United States show a close relationship to cardiovascular pathology, primarily atherosclerosis (responsible for heart, kidney, and brain pathology) and hypertension. While, in Figure 3–3, neoplasms are shown as the first cause of death, they currently, in fact, represent the second cause. For example, in 1984, the annual mortality rate per 100,000 individuals in the United States was 362 deaths due to cardiovascular disease, 189 due to malignant neoplasms, and only 19 due to pneumonia and influenza. However, even mortality from respiratory

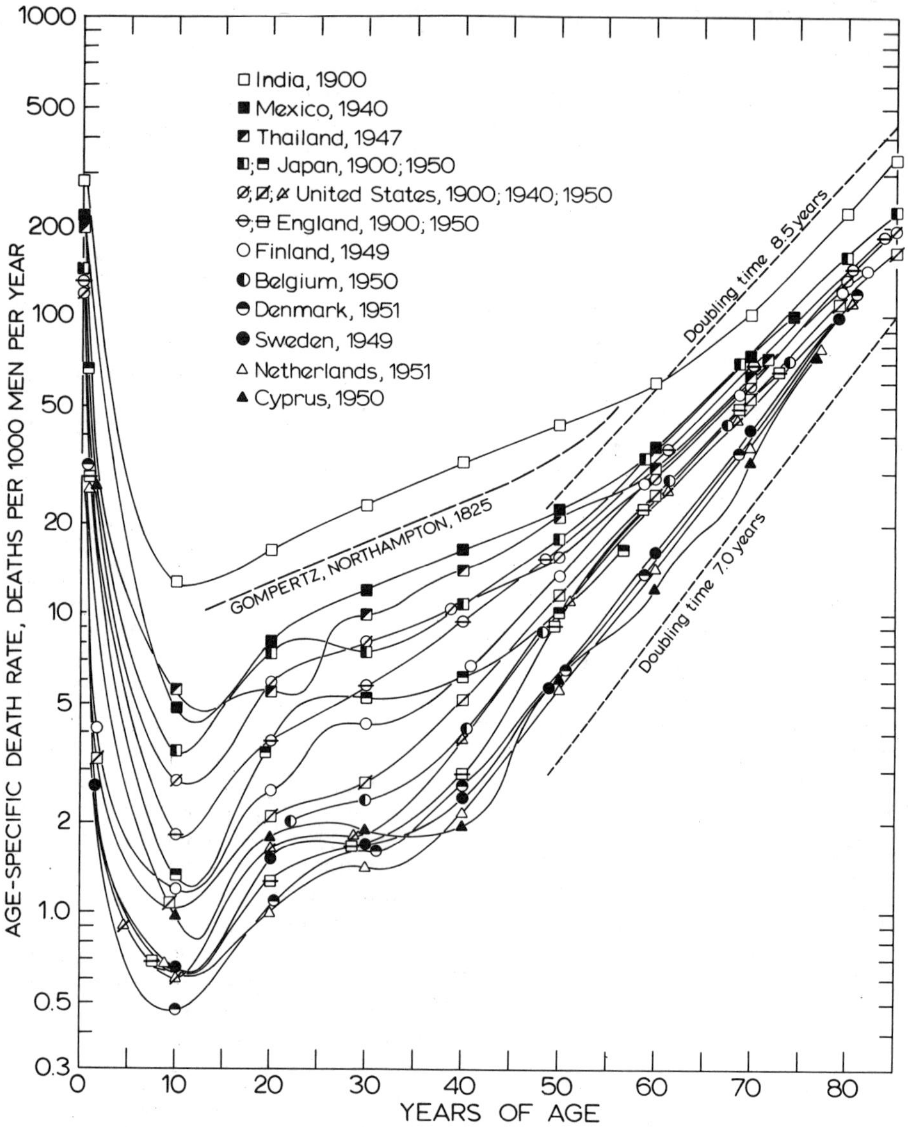

Figure 3–2. *Age-specific death rate in selected countries and years.*

The age-specific death rates are arranged on a logarithmic scale against age on a linear scale. Note that infant mortality rate is high in all nations, but higher in those countries characterized by low levels of socioeconomic development. Although mortality decreases in all nations throughout the childhood years, again, the poorer countries show a higher mortality. The graph illustrates strikingly that regardless of the reduction of mortality accomplished in infancy and childhood periods, the death rate demonstrates a consistent logarithmic rise with age, and curves plotted for each country begin to converge around the age of 60. Calculation of the death rate on this semilogarithmic scale indicates that for any selected age on the graph, the age-specific death rate doubles every 7 to 8.5 years, depending on which country is plotted. (From Jones, H.B. *A Special Consideration of the Aging Process, Disease, and Life Expectancy.* University of California Radiation Laboratory, Berkeley, 1955.)

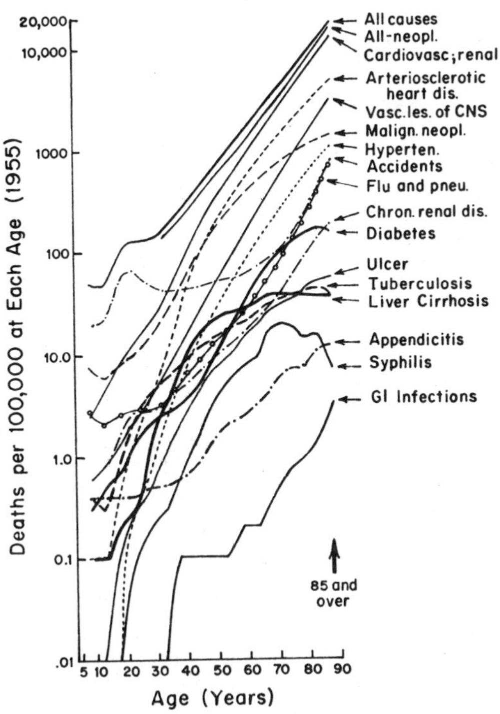

Figure 3–3. *Common causes of death by age in the United States.*

It is to be noted that life expectancy of adults would be increased by one to three years if malignant neoplasms could be cured (see curve for all causes minus neoplasms); by seven years if atherosclerosis were abolished; and by ten to eleven years if both neoplasms and atherosclerosis could be cured. (From Kohn, R.R.: Human aging and disease. *J. Chronic Dis., 16:*15–21, 1963.)

diseases, although considerably reduced now as compared to 1900, increases with aging.

Comparing the incidence of deaths due to cardiovascular diseases and malignant neoplasm, we find that at the age of 50 to 55 neoplasms are responsible for 20 to 30 percent of deaths in males and 30 percent in females while, at the same time, cardiovascular diseases are responsible for 50 percent of deaths in males and 40 percent in females. After 80 years of age, however, cancer mortality declines to less than 10 percent and cardiovascular mortality increases to 60 percent or more for both sexes.

It has been claimed that the life expectancy of adults would be extended by 1 to 3 years if malignant neoplasms were cured, by 5 to 7 years if atherosclerosis were prevented, and by approximately 10 years if both diseases were abolished. It is true that the spectacular advances in medicine in the last 100 years have been responsible in large part for the dramatic increase in the average lifespan, but further lengthening on this basis alone appears unlikely. Efforts, therefore, should be expended to elucidate the basic mechanisms, including the physiology of the aging process *per se*. An appreciation of these mechanisms is indispensable for a better understanding of the aging process. Without such an understanding, the etiopathology of the diseases of old age and their rational treatment cannot be achieved and the lifespan neither further improved nor prolonged.

RISK-FACTOR REDUCTION OR MEDICAL CARE: WHICH IS RESPONSIBLE FOR THE CURRENT DECLINE IN CARDIOVASCULAR DISEASE MORTALITY?

As will be discussed in detail in Chapter 17, one of the major life-threatening cardiovascular diseases involves atherosclerosis of the coronary arteries, that is, the arteries that supply blood to the heart. This disease, known as coronary heart disease (CHD) (or coronary artery disease or ischemic heart disease), leads to reduction of blood flow to the heart with resulting angina pectoris and myocardial infarction; it represents the major single cause of disability and death in the United States. CHD prevalence increases with age but is less in women than men until about 70 years of age, when it becomes the same in both sexes.

In the last 25 years the prevalence of this disease has declined significantly in all sectors of the adult population. For persons aged 35 to 74 years, the rate of mortality for CHD has fallen by 30 percent (Pell and Fayerweather, 1985); this fall is all the more remarkable because it occurred after a sustained period of rising death rates from this cause dating back to at least 1940. The recent decline in the United States is also striking, for it is larger than that observed in any other country (although we must not forget that the CHD incidence is also among the highest!). This decline in CHD morbidity and mortality may be ascribed to our better understanding of the nature of the disease itself and, hence, the availability of more effective preventive and therapeutic interventions. The most important factor in this decline appears to be the "improvement of the life-style," primarily, amelioration of the diet, increased physical exercise, and cessation of cigarette smoking. Clearly, we have been doing the "right things" with respect to improving the hygienic and dietary conditions of our life (Stamler, 1985).

The second factor is therapeutic improvement,

including: better control of hypertension, better medical care in hospital, and more widespread use of coronary bypass surgery and other methods of coronary revascularization.

It has been concluded from the available data that improved medical care probably made some contribution to the decline in mortality from CHD but that the major source of the decline has been a downward trend in the incidence of the disease. The latter has been brought about by our better understanding of both the underlying effect of age, in general, and the factors that influence the aging of the cardiovascular system, in particular.

Table 3–1. GENERAL CHARACTERISTICS OF DISEASE IN THE ELDERLY

Symptoms
Vague and subtle
Atypical
Unreported
Chronic versus acute
Multisystem disease
Altered response to treatment
Increased danger of iatrogenicity (medically induced morbidity and/or mortality)

Table 3–2. HOLISTIC VIEW OF THE ELDERLY

In geriatrics, it is necessary
to differentiate the aging process from disease
to correlate physical state with psychosocial environment

DISEASES OF OLD AGE—HOW THEY DIFFER

As remarked in an early text, geriatrics is "a reaction against the belief that, after the age of 65, a patient is too old to be clinically interesting and therapeutically rewarding" (Howell, 1970). Indeed, the diminished physiologic competence of old people led to selective vulnerability and impaired capacity for recovery and rehabilitation. As children are not just "little or young adults," the elderly are not just "old adults." They have many specific characteristics and concerns related to their physical and mental health. Of course, the wide range of individuality and variability makes many generalizations inappropriate; however, certain principles should be borne in mind when considering the clinical manifestations of disease in the elderly (Table 3–1).

First, knowledge of age-related physiologic changes should permit differentiation of the characteristics of the aging process from the signs and symptoms of disease. For example, dementia is not a normal, unavoidable consequence of aging and should be investigated as any other disease process instead of being attributed to "old age" (Chapter 9). Likewise, anemia is not a normal part of aging and a cause should be searched out. Indeed, one of the tasks of the geriatrician is to be able to differentiate aging from disease and to treat both as independent, but related entities.

Second, one of the challenges of geriatrics arises from the multiplicity of problems confronting the elderly. One cannot adequately treat disease without considering the psychologic, economic, and social situation of each individual (Table 3–2). This global, "holistic" view of the individual should be taken for all patients, of course, but it becomes crucial for the elderly, for whom loneliness, financial hardship, and social instability have enormous impacts on health and well-being. As mentioned previously and worth repeating, one of the main characteristics of the pathology of old age is the multiplicity of the diseases simultaneously affecting the same individual. Autopsy often reveals numerous lesions involving so many organs of the body that it is difficult to know which one was responsible for death. Thus, geriatric medicine is also complicated by the increased incidence of multiple disease processes with increasing age. The pathologist is often perplexed as to how the patient managed to live so long with such a "load" of diseases. This pathologic multiplicity is particularly evident in the 70-to-90-year group in contrast to the pathology of the 60-year-old, which reveals a limited number of lesions at autopsy.

The multiple pathology of the elderly poses many problems in diagnosis and treatment. Particularly crucial becomes the need for multiple therapeutic approaches and the danger associated with "polypharmacy" (Chapter 24). Due to their impaired homeostatic mechanisms, the elderly do not tolerate therapeutic mistakes as well as younger patients. Considerations of risk versus benefit, while important in all medical decisions, become crucial when dealing with elderly patients. Altered drug reac-

Table 3–3. COMMON FATAL DISEASES IN OLD AGE

GENERAL HOSPITAL (% AFFECTED)					GERIATRIC UNIT (% AFFECTED)		
	AGE					AGE	
DISEASE	65–69	70–74	75–79	80+	DISEASE	80–89	90+
Cancer	29	27	27	24	Atherosclerosis	21	30
Cardiovascular	25	25	32	36	Mycardial degeneration	19	10
Respiratory	14	12	13	10	Bronchopneumonia	17	25
Digestive	12	9	13	16	Cancer	10	7
Nervous system	11	9	8	6	Cerebral thrombosis	9	—
Renal tract	4	7	5	3	Chronic bronchitis	7	—
Other	5	1	2	5	Other*	16	28

*Senile dementia frequent in old age. Due to chronicity patients placed in long-term care facilities.

tions and interactions to commonly used drugs should be considered potential dangers lest they lead, together with the deceased physiologic competence and the multiple pathology, to the most serious of complications of medical treatment of the elderly, iatrogenic disease, that is, medically-induced disease (Chapter 24).

As shown in Table 3–3, a number of diseases are more frequent in old individuals than in young and are responsible for their death. A list of common fatal lesions in old individuals compiled from hospital records in the United States and other developed countries shows atherosclerosis (including hypertension and myocardial and cerebral vascular accidents) and cancer to be the diseases most related to old age. It should be noted that when the information is secured not only from general hospitals but specifically from geriatric units, the distribution of diseases is somewhat different, with atherosclerosis and dementia being the major causes of hospitalization and deaths and cancer a lesser cause, especially after 80 years of age. It may be mentioned here that after 60 years of age, hospitalization days per person per year increase dramatically from 2 days to 2 weeks (Figure 3–4), an increase that has a significant impact on the cost of medical care.

Of the many diseases that afflict the elderly, certain medical problems are clearly relegated to the older population while some overlap with those found in younger adults (Table 3–4). Diseases that are primarily limited to the elderly include osteoporosis, osteoarthritis, adenocarcinoma of the prostate, temporal arteritis, and polymyalgia rheumatica. Diseases associated with aging include adult-onset diabetes (non-insulin-dependent), Alzheimer's and Parkinson's diseases, neoplasm, emphysema, and hypertension. Some diseases in these first two groups will be discussed in the corresponding chapters as a comparison between "normal" aging versus disease. Examples of diseases associated with aging and with more clear-cut etiologies include septicemia, pneumonia, cirrhosis, nephritis, and diseases due to the advanced stage of atherosclerosis.

Another problem of the pathology of old age is the atypical fashion of disease presentation (Table 3–1). Sepsis without fever is common. Myocardial infarction may occur without chest pain and present either asymptomatically or with syncope or congestive heart failure. Even for such well-characterized diseases as thyrotoxicosis, appendicitis, peptic ulcer, and pneumonia, the senile patient often has atypical symptomatology. For example, pneumonia may present with a chief complaint of confusion but lack any history of cough. Characteristic of the elderly is that diseases tend to be chronic and debilitating rather than acute and self-limiting; symptomatology tends to be more subtle and vague. Thus, recognition and diagnosis of disease in the elderly require a high degree of alertness on the part of health-care providers.

The goal of treatment is likewise modified: frequently a cure is not the main objective, rather efforts should be shifted toward prevention and relief. Often the pri-

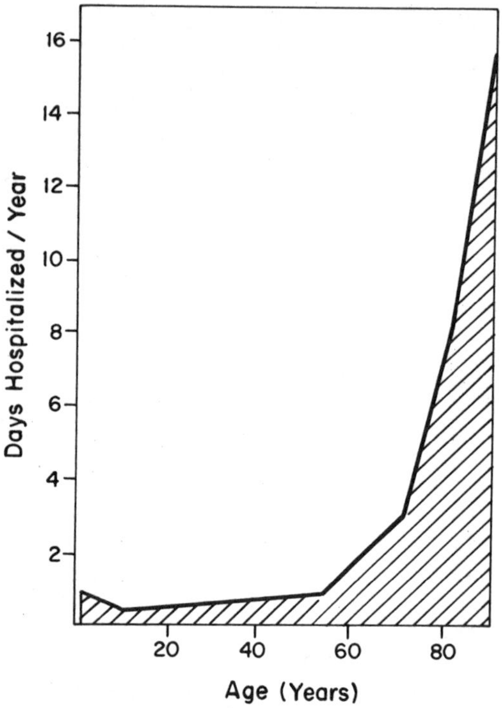

Figure 3–4. *Days spent in hospital according to age.*

Number of days hospitalized per year according to age increases after 55 years of age and increases precipitously after age 70.

Table 3–4. DISEASES OF THE ELDERLY

Limited to aging	
Osteoporosis	Prostatic adenocarcinoma
Osteoarthritis	Polymyalgia rheumatica
	Temporal arteritis
Associated with aging	
Known etiology	
Septicemia	Nephritis
Pneumonia	Cerebrovascular disease
Cirrhosis	Myocardial infarction
Unknown etiology	
Adult-onset diabetes (non-insulin-dependent)	Alzheimer's disease
	Parkinson's disease
Neoplasm	Emphysema
Hypertension	

mary goal is to maximize the ability of the elderly to function (see Chapter 24). Quality of life versus prolongation of life becomes a significant issue that creates medicolegal and ethical dilemmas that are heatedly debated but remain still largely unresolved.

Self-Awareness of Disease in the Elderly. It has been claimed that the elderly complain excessively about poor health, aches and pains, and a variety of symptoms. In fact, considering their multiple pathology, they do not complain enough. The reticence of old people to seek help from health care providers may be ascribed to several factors: (1) the often mistaken assumption that nothing can be done about the problem; (2) the fear of dreaded disease, i.e., cancer; (3) the lack of knowledge of what is normal aging; and (4) therefore, the failure to discriminate among a variety of deficits and disturbances, those due to "old age" from those due to disease.

To remedy some of these misconceptions, a vigorous educational campaign must be promoted. Such a campaign should include information on normal changes with age in various body functions, geared to the level of the particular audience and accompanied by brief descriptions of the diseases associated with aging, and should promote awareness of the many interventions possible to extend and improve the quality of life. Such a campaign should not be limited to geriatric centers; education of aging should be started in secondary schools in parallel with other programs (e.g., sex education) related to health and social issues.

DISUSE AND AGING

Many of the changes that accompany aging coincide closely with those associated with physical inactivity. Changes induced by bed rest as a consequence of disease may be superimposed on aging changes and further accelerate the aging process. Studies of long-term space travel have revealed that weightlessness in space also induces changes resembling those of aging and physical inactivity. The relationship between disuse (due to bed rest, insufficient exercise, or lack of gravity) and aging has some definite practical implications inasmuch as it permits us to envision that prevention and rehabilitation of the disuse phenomena may also ameliorate some of the deficits of old age. This association of disuse and aging is apparent at all functional levels. A brief list of the functions affected is presented in Table 3–5, where we have also noted the eventual beneficial effects of physical exercise programs. Only a few ex-

Table 3–5. ALTERATIONS OF PHYSIOLOGIC PARAMETERS IN AGING, PHYSICAL INACTIVITY, WEIGHTLESSNESS (IN SPACE) (POSSIBLY RESPONSIVE TO PHYSICAL ACTIVITY)

Reduced
Maximum oxygen consumption (Vo_2 max)
Resting and maximum cardiac output
Stroke volume
Sense of balance
Body water and sodium
Blood cell mass
Lean body mass
Glucose tolerance test
Sympathetic activity and neurotransmission
Thermoregulation
Immune responses
Increased
Systolic blood pressure and peripheral resistance
Vestibular sensitivity
Serum total cholesterol and triglycerides
Urinary nitrogen and creatinine
Bone calcium loss
Variable
Endocrine changes
Altered EEG
Altered sleep
Changes in specific senses

amples will be discussed here. Similar information has already been presented in Chapter 2 and more details will be presented in the chapters where we consider the aging of the respective systems. At the top of the list is a decrease in maximum oxygen consumption (Vo_2), which measures indirectly the ability of the organism to transport oxygen from the atmosphere to the tissues. This transport is significantly reduced with age (Astrand, 1960; Shepard, 1966) at the rate of about 1 percent per year (DeVries, 1970; Dehn and Bruce, 1972) and with bed rest (Saltin *et al.*, 1968; Birkhead *et al.*, 1964); in both cases, a program of physical activity slows down the decline (Bortz, 1980).

Vo_2 max depends on cardiac output, which also decreases with age and bed rest, especially as a result of decreased stroke volume (Chapter 19). Simultaneously, blood pressure increases with age and weightlessness. In all cases, both younger and older subjects are able to benefit from exercise. Studies of exercise and movement programs for elders have shown significant improvement in several joint movements and subjective perception of improved mobility and well-being. At all ages, "practice makes perfect." However, for the elderly more than for other age groups, activity programs must be tailored to the individual for optimal duration, frequency, and intensity as well as conditioning.

Although numerous investigations have been conducted to identify the best exercise regimen for each case, no particuar regimen has been conclusively devised so far. Nevertheless, some generalizations have emerged that can be profitably applied to many elderly subjects: depending on the health status of the subject, the exercise must be moderate and its duration, frequency, and intensity increased slowly; warmup and stretching exercises are recommended to guard against injuries. To profit from the exercise program not only physically but also psychologically, it is recommended to choose interesting and enjoyable physical activities, preferably involving group participation. The latter can also alleviate loneliness, one of the most devastating problems of the elderly. In relation to the potential psychologic and mental value of exercise, it should be noted that experiments in rats have shown that raising and maintaining the animals in an "enriched" environment with many stimuli increases brain weight and dendritic branching (Diamond *et al.*, 1977; Connor *et al.*, 1980). Likewise, an exercise program is capable of delaying the involutional changes seen with aging within the spinal cord and peripheral nerves (Vogt and Vogt, 1946; Retzloff and Fontaine, 1965). Thus, the common aphorism "use it or lose it" may have significant implications for the well-being of the elderly (Bortz, 1982). Clearly, physical inactivity is not the cause of aging nor does current evidence suggest that exercise might arrest the aging process (Fitzgerald, 1985). In fact, some investigators claim that strong exercise may stimulate the formation of free radicals and accelerate aging (Chapter 4). While it has not yet been possible to test the impact of exercise on longevity in humans, following a physically active life and other hygienic principles may allow us "to approach our true biogenetic potential for longevity" (Bortz, 1982).

INDUCTION OF DISEASE AS A TOOL FOR THE STUDY OF AGING

A cause-effect relationship between disease and aging has been variously explored, depending on the specific hypotheses entertained by different investigators. Most often, disease has been used to accelerate the onset and course of aging processes and, thereby, to test therapeutic and prophylactic measures that might prevent or slow down both disease and aging. Other attempts have focused on "segmental" aging, that is, induction of aging in a selected organ, tissue, or cell type to mimic specific aspects of aging. Examples of these experimental approaches include genetic manipulation, increased free-radical accumulation, inoculation of slow viruses, interference with nervous and endocrine functions, induction of wear-and-tear and stress, administration of mutagens and carcinogens, and so forth. As for the study of normal aging (see Chapter 2), the use of tissue or cells in culture has proven quite useful in inducing abnormal cellular aging and identifying causes, manifestations, and consequences of the abnormalities. A number of human diseases associated with premature or accelerated aging, the so-called progeria and progerialike syndromes, and some *in vivo* and *in vitro* models of aging illustrate the respective usefulness and shortcomings of clinical and experimental approaches, both *in vivo* and *in vitro*.

Human Diseases Associated with Accelerated Aging: Progeria and Progeroid Syndromes

Sporadic cases of syndromes having multiple characteristics of premature (early onset) or accelerated (rapid progression) aging occur in humans. It is unclear how far any of these syndromes can be regarded as a genuine acceleration of the timing mechanisms that determine senescence. They are apparently pleoitropic genetic defects, and when one of the major features is accelerated aging, they are designated as progeria. When accelerated aging is associated with other prevalent defects, they are called progerialike or progeroid or "segmental" syndromes; one example is Down's syndrome.

Progeria syndromes, however, do not quite duplicate all the pathophysiology of aging; each syndrome presents an acceleration of only some of the characteristics associated with normal aging. Progeria is described as being of two main types, infantile and adult. The infantile form (Hutchinson-Gilford syndrome) becomes apparent at a very early age and is associated with stunted growth, failure of sex maturation, and signs of aging, such as skin atrophy, hypertension, and severe atherosclerosis; death occurs in the twenties, usually consequent to coronary heart disease.

The adult form (Werner's syndrome) resembles more closely the changes associated with aging, with respect to both the affected individual's physical appearance and the disease pattern. The onset of this premature aging syndrome occurs between the ages of 20 and 30 years, and death ensues a few years from the onset, usually due to a cardiovascular accident.

Similarities and Differences Between Werner's Syndrome and Aging. Major features of Werner's syndrome include: shortness of stature; senile appearance; cataracts and graying of the hair beginning at 20 to 30 years; skin changes (i.e., tautness, atrophy or thickening, ulceration) designated as scleroderma; joint deformities, soft tissue calcifications, and osteoporosis; atrophy of muscles and connective tissue; early cessation of menstruation; increased incidence of neoplasmas. Most of these features occur in aging as well, but at a later age and in different degrees.

Among some of the major differences between Werner's syndrome and aging are: the type of inheritance—universal, multifactorial in aging and autosomal, recessive in Werner's; the high incidence of hypertension in aging, but not in Werner's; the presence of dementia and other CNS degenerative disorders in aging, but not in Werner's; the occurrence of soft tissue calcifications, uncommon in aging, but common in Werner's. These differences are sufficient to justify the statement that Werner's syndrome is not merely a process of premature or accelerated aging. Rather, it should be viewed as a "caricature" of aging (Epstein, 1985). Both Werner's and aging may represent the result of generalized metabolic processes or aberrations thereof. Indeed, the overlap between the two entities is not surprising inasmuch as the various tissues of the human organism have only a limited repertoire of reactions to genetic abnormalities and environmental insults (Salk *et al.*, 1985). Irrespective of similarities or differences, a study of the features of Werner's syndrome and aging will conceivably be useful in achieving an understanding of both.

Tissue culture studies of fibroblasts, in both infantile and adult syndromes, reveal a shortening of the cell replicating ability which has been interpreted as supportive of accelerated aging (Salk *et al.*, 1985). The etiology of the syndromes remains obscure, but among the several causes proposed, neuroendocrinologic dysfunction is supported by the stunted growth, failure of gonadal maturation, and diabetes, either singly or in combination.

Another example of a syndrome characterized by several symptoms including accelerated aging and premature death is Down's syndrome, or mongolism, which is due to trisomy at chromosome 21. The incidence of the syndrome is greatest among children born from mothers 40 years of age and older, and the genetic abnormality has therefore been related to aging processes involving the oocytes (Chapter 13). Although in 20 to 30 percent of cases the extra chromosome is contributed by the father, paternal age does not seem to have any significant effect on the incidence of the syndrome (Erickson, 1979).

Individuals affected by Down's syndrome may present somatic malformations, but the major deficit is represented by severe mental disability. Affected subjects, who live to reach 30 years of age and more, present many signs of accelerated aging, including senile dementia of the Alzheimer type (SDAT) superimposed on the mental retardation (Heston, 1982) (Chapter 9). Animal models have also been proposed for the study of Down's syndrome. The mouse is the animal of choice, for it is possible to introduce trisomy of chromosome 16 (Epstein *et al.*, 1985) and produce individuals with some phenotypic characteristics of Down's syndrome, such as cardiovascular defects, neurologic alterations, and retardation of brain maturation (de la Cruz and Oster-Granite, in press) as well as early aging (Brooksbank and Balazs, in press). Proposed as a good *in vitro* model to induce experimentally the premature aging of neurons is the transfer of the trisomy 21 from the fibroblast donor cells to neuroblastoma cells (Cole and Timiras, 1986).

EXPERIMENTALLY INDUCED AGING IN ANIMALS

Premature aging has been induced in a number of laboratory animals as well as in captive wild animals by various methods derived from the rationale of the different theories of aging, especially the neuroendocrinologic, immunologic, and free-radical theories. One of the favorite methods is to expose the animal to stress, that is, to excessive environmental (including physical, emotional, and social) demands. Stress will activate or interfere with all three regulatory systems, that is, will disturb neuroendocrine balance, alter immunologic competence and tolerance, and increase the production of free radicals (Chapter 12). Stress, produced by repeated disruption of conditioned responses in young adult dogs, leads to neurologic disturbances, EEG abnormalities resembling those of old animals, graying of the coat, muscular weakness, weight loss, and so forth (Frolkis, 1982). Stress or injection of cortisol to mimic adrencortical stimulation, in association with a high-lipid or high-cholesterol diet, accelerates atheroma formation in rabbits (Constantinides, 1965). High doses of vitamin D given along with calcium to rats precipitate calcification of the skin, heart, blood vessels, and other tissues usually susceptible to calcium deposits in old age (Selye *et al.*, 1961).

Other often-used methods to induce premature aging in animals involve administration of the appropriate antigens to induce autoimmune responses against sequestered proteins. This technique is employed, for example, in the experimental induction of multiple sclerosis. Still other interventions utilize inoculation of animals with viruses or viral particles (e.g., the so-called prions) to mimic some of the degenerative diseases of old age. One model, which resembles symptomatically and pathologically (e.g., accumulation of amyloid) human senile dementia of the Alzheimer type, is the disease "scrapie," which occurs in sheep, is caused by a slow virus, and can be reproduced in laboratory animals (Prusiner *et al.*, 1983; Carp *et al.*, 1984; Merz *et al.*, 1984). Attempts to isolate the virus or prions of senile dementia of the Alzheimer type and to induce the disease in laboratory animals are still unsuccessful.

Another condition caused by a retrovirus and often associated with senile dementia is the acquired immune deficiency syndrome

(AIDS) (see Chapter 8). As for SDAT, attempts to reproduce the neurologic symptoms (dementia) and neuropathology (e.g., brain atrophy, loss of neural cells, abnormal proteins) of AIDS in experimental animals (sheep, mice, primates) have so far been unsuccessful since only chimpanzees are infected with the virus, but the neural lesions are quite different from those of humans (Barnes, 1986). As in the case of progeria, none of the animal models exhibits all the symptoms and pathology of old age; each model only partially mimics the aging process of humans. The aging process of humans is complex and its mechanisms are difficult to isolate; therefore, mammals with aging processes resembling the human process are used for such studies. Humans and other primates take decades to age, and even the 2 to 3 years required in a short-lived mammal like the rat or mouse is a long, impractical period for experimentation and innovation. A major obstacle, then, to a better understanding of the complicated and lengthy processes governing mammalian aging and age-related pathology is the paucity of useful model systems wherein events can be accelerated and, hopefully, simplified. Moreover, within a model system, markers reflecting adequate indices of some segment of the aging or pathologic process must be found (Gibson *et al.*, 1978; Reff and Schneider, 1982). In this respect, *in vitro* models involving only a single group of cells in rigorously controlled conditions can be and are being widely and profitably utilized to study cellular and molecular aging.

IN VITRO MODELS FOR AGING

The most successful *in vitro* models are those utilized in the study of cancer, one of the major causes of death in the elderly, although not exclusively a disease of old age. Much cancer research is based on the reasonable premise that human cancer can be unraveled by studying carcinogenesis in animals. Indeed, cancer is a major age-related pathology, and the process of carcinogenesis may be studied both *in vivo* and *in vitro* because transformed (i.e., cancer) cells exhibit a set of known properties that can be readily selected for, assayed, and identified. During the last 70 years, since coal tar was shown to be carcinogenic to the skin of rabbits, many ways have been found to produce cancer in experimental animals (Cairns, 1981; Cairns and Logan, 1983; Logan and Cairns, 1982).

The many shortcomings of these models soon became apparent, such as deciding on the best models for human cancers and creating a cancer cell in which to study the early "initiation" and subsequent "promotion" steps of the carcinogenic process. Thus, established *in vitro* models for carcinogenesis (Kennedy *et al.*, 1980) and the related but more general process of mutagenesis (Ames *et al.*, 1973) have been instrumental in our understanding of oncogenes, their activation, and the resultant cancer. There are two essential differences between normal cells and cancer (tumor) cells; one is that the tumor cells have the capacity to divide forever—they are immortal and, thus, escape senescence; the other is that their growth is controlled abnormally. There is growing recognition that the development of tumors may be due as much to loss growth inhibition as to increased growth stimulation (Marx, 1986). In order to understand carcinogenesis, both growth inhibitory and stimulatory processes must be clarified. Indeed, natural carcinogenesis is a multistage process, involving, as a first step, clonal expansion and, as a second step, transformation into cancer cells.

Evidence for the multistep nature of carcinogenesis can be found in epidemiologic studies, such as those that show a relationship between the incidence of lung cancer and the frequency and duration of smoking. Another example of cervical carcinoma. The first visible step in the production of the cancer of the uterine cervix is, commonly, the appearance of an expanding clone of abnormal cells (cervical dysplasia). The clone generally regresses and disappears, but sometimes it gives rise to a still more abnormal family of cells (carcinoma *in situ*), and it is among these that the fully invasive cancer arises. The sequence then involves: (1) the release or liberation of cells from the physical (cell-to-cell interactions) and chemical (growth inhibitory factors) restraints of an organized epithelium (the uterine epithelium); (2) a relaxation of the rules of differentiation, which would oppose continuing cell division; and (3) exemption from the rule of finite lifespan (which regulates "normal" cells) (Chapter 2).

It is a great simplification to study these different steps, so to speak, "telescoped" in cultured cells, where the first step, that is, liberation from regional restraints *in situ*, has already achieved (Heldin and Westermark, 1984). Certain cell lines (e.g., the NIH line 3T3 mouse fibroblasts) are capable of taking up raw DNA and of being transformed to permanent tumorigenicity if the absorbed DNA is derived from animal or human tumors or tumorigenic cell lines. Since human DNA contains specific sequences not found in mouse DNA, it has been possible to isolate these human genes that are tumorigenic for 3T3 cells and, in part, presumably responsible for the cancers from which they were derived. The results of these experiments demonstrate dramatically that alteration of the genome is an essential step in the production of some cancers (Weinstein *et al.*, 1984). Other factors involved in tumorigenicity include a variety of mutagens capable of cell mutation and oncogenes capable of producing transformation by activation of specific genes through rearrangement, mutation, or viral infection. A number of cellular oncogenes have been described, such as *ras* and *myc*, originating in retrovirus and capable of inducing abnormal growth or cancer transformation or both (Marshall, 1984; Robertson, 1983).

Aging is a more general phenomenon than cancer and other pathologies, and we lack sufficiently specific markers to characterize the induction of aging processes in a model system. Because aging is complex, and different tissues may age and develop age-related pathology from multiple causes and at different times (see Chapter 2), induction of true aging in a whole animal may actually prove to be impossible. The limited "segmental" progeroid pathology discussed above and observed in all the known human syndromes manifesting some signs of accelerated aging (Martin, 1978) reinforces this point. The induction of a limited set of markers for aging or age-related pathology has become a more attainable goal (Gibson *et al.*, 1978; Reff and Schneider, 1982).

Table 3–6. *IN VIVO* MODELS FOR SENILE DEMENTIA ALZHEIMER TYPE (SDAT)

1. Spontaneous neuropathologic lesions
    - Senile plaques in brains of old dogs and monkeys
    - Abnormal filaments in old monkey brains
2. Experimentally induced neuropathologic SDAT-like lesions (cognitive impairment and behavioral changes)
    - Slow viruses (prions)
        - Senile plaques in selected mouse strains
        - Spongioform changes in sheep and other species
    - Aluminum
    - Microtubule disrupting agents (colchicine, taxol)
        - Accumulation of straight filaments
3. Surgical, electrical, or chemical lesions of SDAT-susceptible brain regions (cognitive impairment and behavioral changes)
    - Hippocampus
    - Basal nucleus of Meynert

IN VIVO AND *IN VITRO* MODELS FOR SENILE DEMENTIA OF THE ALZHEIMER TYPE

One example of such experimental studies is our current efforts to identify a model for SDAT. This is one of the degenerative diseases of the elderly most rapidly increasing in incidence. It has received considerable attention in the last few years and has stimulated the need to create models for its study. Attempts have been made to reproduce this condition, characterized by marked cognitive and behavioral abnormalities and specific pathology (see Chapter 9) utilizing *in vivo* and *in vitro* models.

The *in vivo* models include: spontaneously occurring neuropathologic lesions resembling (but not exactly reproducing) SDAT in several animal species (e.g., monkeys, dogs, rodents) (Ball *et al.*, 1983; Campbell *et al.*, 1980; Bartus *et al.*, 1982; Dean and Bartus, 1985; Zilles, 1985); induced lesions resembling those of SDAT through the inoculation of slow viruses (Prusiner, 1984; Fraser and McBridge, 1985) or the administration of specific substances such as aluminum (Crapper *et al.*, 1978; Petit *et al.*, 1980) or the induction of autoimmune reactions (Lal *et al.*, 1985); or lesioning specific brain areas related to memory and cognitive functions (Azmitia *et al.*, 1981; Arendash *et al.*, 1984; Gage *et al.*, 1984; Leventer and Hanin, 1985; Pepeu *et al.*, 1985; Spencer *et al.*, 1985) (Table 3–6). None of these models has proven satisfactory, especially with respect to reproducing the pathology of the disease, that is, the presence, in discrete brain areas, of neurofibrillary tangles of paired helical filaments (PHF) (Mann, 1985), neurotic plaques (Masters *et al.*, 1985), and vascular amyloid (Wong *et al.*, 1985).

It may be possible, however, to model certain aspects of neuronal senescence *in vitro* by utiliz-

Table 3–7. *IN VITRO* MODELS FOR SENILE DEMENTIA ALZHEIMER TYPE (SDAT)

1. Spontaneously occurring paired helical filaments (PHF) in cultured cortical human cells (Alzheimer brain extracts not necessary for PHF induction)
2. Experimentally induced SDAT-like lesions by addition to cultured neurons of:
   - Aluminum and microtubule-disrupting agents
     - Neurofibrillary tangles of straight filaments in cultured neurons from humans, rabbits, rats, and mice
   - Excitatory amino acids, glutamate, and/or aspartate
     - PHF in human cultured neurons
3. Addition to differentiated human teratocarcinoma neurons, individually or combined, of:
   - Aluminum, colchicine
     - Tangles of straight filaments
   - Doxorubicin
     - PHF reactive fibers and tangles

ing some specific markers, such as those of SDAT pathology. Indeed, segmental neuronal aging *in vitro* has been demonstrated in response to specific types of damage due to free radicals (Melhorn and Cole, 1985), hormones (Sapolsky *et al.*, 1985, 1986), or other toxins (Langston *et al.*, 1983; Moroni *et al.*, 1984). Current studies, utilizing human tumor cell lines (teratocarcinoma), have shown that several markers of SDAT can be induced in response to a number of agents, particularly doxorubicin, known to produce a marked axonopathy with neurofilamentous tangles, nuclear heterochromatization, and decreased transcription (Cole, 1986; Cole and Timiras, 1987). A summary of the *in vitro* studies is presented in Table 3–7. The results of these studies suggest that normal neuronal aging and age-related neuronal pathology may be viewed as a response to specific types of damage against the general background of responses of cells to stress.

At the systemic physiologic level, many investigators have noted an apparent relationship between stress and aging (Selye, 1950), hence the use of stress to induce aging in animals, as discussed above. However, despite some studies of generalized cellular response to stress, such as heat shock proteins (Napolitano *et al.*, 1985), the cellular response has been sadly neglected by most gerontologists and pathologists. The production *in vitro* of SDAT lesions in response to selected types of damage argues for its production *in vivo* by a similar damage (Cole *et al.*, 1985; Cole, 1986; Cole and Timiras, 1986). This damage or stress response may be conceptualized in the context of the general cellular stress response and has been applied to put SDAT pathology in a useful heuristic framework for further experimentation in SDAT material and in neuronal aging.

References

Ames, B. N.; Durston, W. E.; Yamasaki, E.; and Lee, F. D.: Carcinogens are mutagens: A simple test system combining liver homogenates for activation and bacteria for detection. *Proc. Natl. Acad. Sci. USA*, **70:**2281–2285, **1973.**

Arendash, G. W.; Strong, P. N.; and Mouton, P. R.: Intracerebral transplantation of cholinergic neurons in a new animal model for Alzheimer's disease. In Hutton, J. T., and Kenny, A. D. (eds.): *Senile Dementia of the Alzheimer Type,* Alan R. Liss, New York, **1984.**

Astrand, I.: Aerobic work capacity in men and women with special reference to age. *Acta Physiol. Scand.*, **49** (suppl.169):1–92, **1960.**

Azmitia, E.; Perlow, M.; Brennan, H.; and Lauder, J.: Fetal raphe and hippocampal transplants into adult and aged C57B1/6N mice: A preliminary immunocytochemical study. *Brain Res. Bull.*, 703–710, **1981.**

Ball, M. J.; MacGregor, J.; Fyfe, I. M.; Rapoport, S. I.; and London, E. D.: Paucity of morphological changes in the brains of ageing beagle dogs: Further evidence that Alzheimer lesions are unique for primate central nervous system. *Neurobiol. Ageing,* **4:**127–131, **1983.**

Barnes, D. M.: Neurosciences advance in basic and clinical realms. *Science,* **234:**1324–1326, **1986.**

Bartus, R. T.; Dean, R. L.; and Beer, B.: The cholinergic hypothesis of geriatric memory dysfunction. *Science,* **217:**408–417, **1982.**

Birkhead, N. C.; Haupt, G. J.; and Issekutz, B., Jr.: Circulatory and metabolic effects of different types of prolonged inactivity. *Am. J. Med. Sci.*, **247:**243, **1964.**

Bortz, W.: Effects of exercise on aging—Effect of aging on exercise. *J. Am. Geriatr. Soc.*, **28:**49–51, **1980.**

Bortz, W. M.: Disuse and aging. *JAMA,* **248:**1203–1208, **1982.**

Brocklehurst, J. C.: *Textbook of Geriatric Medicine and Gerontology,* Churchill Livingstone, Edinburgh, **1985.**

Brooksbank, B. W. L., and Balazs, R.: Development of the brain and aging in a common human aneuploidy, Down's syndrome. In Meisami, E., and Timiras, P. S. (eds.): *Handbook of Human Growth and Development Biology,* CRC Press, Boca Raton, FL, Vol. I, 1988.

Cairns, J.: The origin of human cancers. *Nature,* **289:**353:357, **1981.**

Cairns, J., and Logan, J.: Step by step into carcinogenesis. *Nature,* **304:**582–583, **1983.**

Campbell, B. A.; Krauter, E. E.; and Wallace, J. E.: Animal models and aging: Sensory-motor and cognitive function in the aged rat. In Stein, D. G. (ed.): *Psychobiology of Aging: Problems and Perspectives,* Elsevier, Amsterdam, **1980.**

Carp, R. I.; Merz, G. S.; and Wisniewski, H. M.: Transmission of unconventional slow virus diseases and the relevance to AD/SDAT transmission studies. In Wertheimer, J., and Marois, M. (eds.): *Senile Dementia: Outlook for the Future,* Alan R. Liss, New York, **1984.**

Cape, R. D. T.; Coe, R. M.; and Rossman, I. (eds.): *Fundamentals of Geriatric Medicine,* Raven Press, New York, **1983.**

Cassel, C. K., and Walsh, J. R. (eds.): *Geriatric Medicine,* Vols. I and II, Springer-Verlag, New York, **1984.**

Cole, G. M.: Induction of Alzheimer's amyloid protein in a cultured human cell line. Ph.D. thesis, **1986.**

Cole, G. M.; Wu, K.; and Timiras, P. S.: A culture model for age-related human neurofibrillary pathology. *Int. J. Dev. Neurosci.*, **3:**23–32, **1985.**

Cole, G. M., and Timiras, P. S.: Aging-related pathology in human neuroblastoma and teratocarcinoma cell lines. In Vernadakis, A.; Privat, A.; Lauder, J. M.; Timiras, P. S.; and Giacobini, E. (eds.): *Model Systems of Development and Aging of the Nervous System,* Martinus Nijhoff Publishing, Boston, MA, **1987.**

Connor, J. R.; Diamond, M. C.; and Johnson, R. E.: Ageing and environmental influences on two types of dendritic spines in the rat occipital cortex. *Exp. Neurol.*, **70**:371–379, **1980.**

Constantinides, P.: *Experimental Atherosclerosis*, Elsevier, Amsterdam, **1965.**

Crapper, D. R.; Karlik, S.; and DeBoni, U.: Aluminum and other metals in senile (Alzheimer) dementia. In *Alzheimer's disease: senile dementia and related disorders*. In Katzman, R. D., and Blick, K. L. (eds.): *Aging*, vol. 7, Raven Press, New York, **1978.**

Dean, R. L., and Bartus, R. Y.: Animal models of geriatric cognitive dysfunction: Evidence for an important cholinergic involvement. In Traber, J., and Gispen, W. E. (eds.): *Senile Dementia of the Alzheimer Type. Early Diagnosis, Neuropathology and Animal Models*, Springer-Verlag, Berlin, **1985.**

Dehn, M., and Bruce R.: Longitudinal variations in maximal oxygen uptake with age and activity. *J. Appl. Physiol.*, **33**:805–807, **1972.**

de la Cruz, F. F., and Oster-Granite, M. L.: Neural bases of mental retardation. In Meisami, E., and Timiras, P. S. (eds.): *Handbook of Human Growth and Developmental Biology*, CRC Press, Boca Raton, FL, Vol. I, 1988.

DeVries, H.: Physiological effects of an exercise training regimen upon men aged 52–88. *J. Gerontol.*, **25**:325–336, **1970.**

Diamond, M. C.; Johnson, R. E.; and Gold, M. W.: Changes in neuron and glia number in the young, adult and ageing rat occipital cortex. *Behav. Biol.*, **20**:409–418, **1977.**

Epstein, C. J.: Werner's syndrome and aging: A reappraisal. In Salk, D.; Fujiwara, Y.; and Martin, G. M. (eds.): *Werner's Syndrome and Human Aging*, Plenum Press, New York, **1985.**

Epstein, C. J.; Cox, D. R.; and Epstein, L. B.: Mouse trisomy 16: An animal model of human trisomy 21 (Down syndrome). *Ann. NY Acad. Sci. USA.*, **450**:157–168, **1985.**

Erickson, J. D.: Paternal age and Down syndrome. *Am. J. Hum. Genet.*, **31**:489–497, **1979.**

Fitzgerald, P. L.: Exercise for the elderly. *Med. Clin. North Am.*, **69**:189–195, **1985.**

Fraser, H., and McBride, P. A.: Parallels and contrasts between scrapie and dementia of Alzheimer type and ageing: Strategies and problems for experiments involving life span studies. In Traber, J., and Gispen, W. H. (eds.): *Senile Dementia of the Alzheimer Type. Early Diagnosis, Neuropathology and Animal Models*, Springer-Verlag, Berlin, **1985.**

Frolkis, V. V.: *Aging and Life-Prolonging Processes*, Springer-Verlag, New York, **1982.**

Gage, F.; Bjorkland, R.; Stenevi, U.; Dunnett, S.; and Kelly, P.: Intrahippocampal septal grafts ameliorate learning impairments in aged rats. *Science*, **225**:533–536, **1984.**

Gibson, D. C.; Adelman, R. C.; and Finch, C. E.: *Development of the Rodent as a Model System of Aging*, U.S. Government Printing Office, DHEW publication no. (NIH)79-161, **1978.**

Gompertz, B.: On the nature of the function expressive of the law of human mortality and on a new mode of determining life contingencies. *Phil. Trans. R. Soc. London*, **2**:513–585, **1825.**

Heldin, C- H., and Westermark, B.: Growth factors: Mechanism of action and relation to oncogenes. *Cell*, **37**:9–20, **1984.**

Heston, L. L.: Alzheimer's disease and Down's syndrome: Genetic evidence suggesting association. *Ann. NY Acad. Sci. USA.*, **396**:29–37, **1982.**

Howell, T. H.: *A Student's Guide to Geriatrics*, 2nd ed., Charles C Thomas, Springfield, IL, **1970.**

Johnson, H. A. (ed.): *Relations Between Normal Aging and Disease*, Aging, vol. 28, Raven Press, New York, **1985a.**

Johnson, H. A.: Is aging physiological or pathological? In Johnson, H. A. (ed.): *Relations Between Normal Aging and Disease*, Aging, vol. 28, Raven Press, New York, **1985b.**

Jones, H. B.: *A Special Consideration of the Aging Process, Disease and Life Expectancy*, University of California, Radiation Laboratory, Berkeley, **1955.**

Jones, H. B.: The relation of human health to age, place and time. In Birren, J. E. (ed.): *Handbook of Aging and the Individual*, University of Chicago Press, Chicago, **1960.**

Kane, R. L.; Ouslander, J. G.; and Abrass, I. B.: *Essentials of Clinical Geriatrics*, McGraw-Hill, New York, **1984.**

Kennedy, A. R.; Fop, M.; Murphy, G.; and Little, J. B.: Relationship between x-ray exposure and malignant transformation in C3H10T 1/2 cells. *Natl. Acad. Sci. USA.*, **77**:7262–7266, **1980.**

Kohn, R. R.: Human aging and disease. *J. Chronic. Dis.*, **16**:5–21, **1963.**

Kohn, R. R.: *Principles of Mammalian Aging*, 2nd ed., Prentice-Hall, Englewood Cliffs, NJ, **1978.**

Kohn, R. R.: Aging and aging-related diseases: Normal processes. In Johnson, H. A. (ed.): *Relations Between Normal Aging and Disease*. Aging, vol. 28, Raven Press, New York, **1985.**

Lal, H.; Forster, M. J.; and Nandy, K.: Immunologic factorsa related to cognitive/behavioral dysfunctions in aging. In Traber, J., and Gispen, W. H. (eds.): *Senile Dementia of the Alzheimer Type. Early Diagnosis, Neuropathology and Animal Models*, Springer-Verlag, Berlin, **1985.**

Langston, J. W.; Ballard, P.; Tetrud, J. W.; and Irwin, I.: Chronic Parkinson in humans due to a product of meperidine-analog synthesis. *Science*, **219**:979–981, **1983.**

Leventer, S. M., and Hanin, I.: AF64A cholinotoxicity: Functional aspects. In Traber, J., and Gispen, W. H. (eds.): *Senile Dementia of the Alzheimer Type. Early Diagnosis, Neuropathology and Animal Models*, Springer-Verlag, Berlin, **1985.**

Logan, J., and Cairns, J.: The secrets of cancer. *Nature*, **300**:104–105, **1982.**

Mann, D. M. A.: The neuropathology of Alzheimer's disease: A review with pathogenic, aetiological, and therapeutic considerations. *Mech. Ageing Dev.*, **31**:213–255, **1985.**

Marshall, C.: Functions of *ras* oncogenes. *Nature*, **310**:448, **1984.**

Martin, G. M.: Genetic syndromes in man with potential relevance to the pathobiology of aging. *Birth Defects* (original article series), **14**:5–39, **1978.**

Marx, J. L.: The yin and yang of cell growth control. *Science*, **232**:1093–1095, **1986.**

Masters, C. L.; Multhaup, G.; Simms, G.; Pottieser, R. N.; and Beyreuther: Neuronal origin of a cerebral amyloid: Neurofibrillary tangles of Alzheimer's disease contain the same protein as the amyloid of plaque cores and blood vessels. *EMBO J.*, **4**:2757–2763, **1985.**

Mehlhorn, R. W., and Cole, G. M.: The free radical theory of aging: A critical review. *Adv. Free Radical Biol. Med.*, **1**:165–223, **1985.**

Merz, P. A.; Rohwer, R. G.; Kascsak, R.; Wisniewski, H. M.; Somerville, R. A.; Gibbs, C. J.; and Gajdusek, D. C.: Infection-specific particle from the unconventional slow virus diseases. *Science*, **225**:437–440, **1984.**

Moroni, F.; Lombardi, G.; Monetti, G.; and Aldinio, C.: The exitotoxinquinolinic acid is present in the brain of several mammals and its cortical content increases during the aging process. *Neurosci. Lett.*, **47**:51–55, **1984.**

Napolitano, E. W.; Hutchinson, R. K.; and Liem, H.: Association of an endogenous heat shock protein (HSP70) with neuronal and non-neuronal cytoskeletal elements. *J. Cell Biol.*, **101**:30a, **1985.**

Pathy, M. S. J. (ed.): *Principles and Practice of Geriatric Medicine,* Wiley, Chichester (UK), **1985.**

Pell, S., and Fayerweather, W. E.: Trends in the incidence of myocardial infarction and in associated mortality and morbidity in a large employed population, 1957–1983. *N. Engl. J. Med.*, **312**:1005–1011, **1985.**

Pepeu, G.; Casamenti, F.; Bracco, L.; Ladinsky, H.; and Consolo, S.: Lesions of the nucleus basalis in the rat: Functional changes. In Traber, J., and Gispen, W. H. (eds.): *Senile Dementia of the Alzheimer Type. Early Diagnosis, Neuropathology and Animal Models,* Springer-Verlag, Berlin, **1985.**

Petit, T. L.; Biederman, G. B.; and McMullen, P. A.: Neurofibrillary degeneration, dendritic dying back and learning memory deficits after aluminum administration: implications for brain aging. *Exp. Neurol.*, **67**:152–162, **1980**

Prusiner, S. B.: Some speculations about prions, amyloid and Alzheimer's disease. *N. Engl. J. Med.*, **310**:661–663, **1984.**

Prusiner, S. B.; McKinley, M. P.; Bolton, D. C.; Cochran, S. P.; Bowman, K. A.; Groth, D. F.; and Bendheim, P. E.: Scrapie: A slow degenerative neurological disorder caused by prions. In Austin, L., and Jeffery, P. (eds.): *Molecular Aspects of Neurological Disorders,* Academic Press, New York, **1983.**

Reff, M. E., and Schneider, E. L.: *Biological Markers of Aging,* NIH publication no. 82-2221, **1982.**

Retzlaff, E., and Fontaine, J.: Functional and structural changes in motor neurons with age. In Welford, A. T., and Birren, J. E. (eds.): *Behavior Aging and the Nervous System,* Charles C Thomas, Springfield, IL, **1965.**

Robertson, M.: Paradox and paradigm: The message and meaning of *myc. Nature,* **306**:733–736, **1983.**

Salk, D.; Fujiwara, Y.; and Martin, G. M. (eds.): *Werner's Syndrome and Human Aging,* Plenum Press, New York, **1985.**

Saltin, B.; Blomquist, G.; and Mitchell, J. H.: Response to exercise after bedrest and after training: A longitudinal study of adaptive changes in oxygen transport and composition. *Circulation,* **33** (suppl. 7):1–78, **1968.**

Sapolsky, R. M.; Krey, L. C.; and McEwen, B. S.: Prolonged glucocorticoid exposure reduces hippocampal neuron number: Implications for aging. *J. Neurosci.*, **5**:1222–1227, **1985.**

Sapolsky, R. M.; Krey, L. C.; and McEwen, B. S.: The neuroendocrinology of stress and aging: The glucocorticoid cascade hypothesis. *Endocr. Rev.* **7**:284–301, **1986.**

Selye, H.: *Stress,* Acta, Montreal, **1950.**

Selye, H.: Stress and aging. *J. Am. Geriatr. Soc.*, **18**:669–680, **1970.**

Selye, H.; Gentile, G.; and Prioreschi, P.: Cutaneous molt induced by calciphylaxis in the rat. *Science,* **134**:1876–1877, **1961.**

Shephard, R. J.: World standards of cardiorespiratory performance. *Arch. Environ. Health,* **13**:664–672, **1966.**

Spencer, D. G.; Horvath, E.; Luiten, P.; Schuurman, T.; and Traber, J.: Novel approaches in the study of brain acetylcholine function: Neuropharmacology, neuroanatomy, and behavior. In Traber, J., and Gispen, W. H. (eds.): *Senile Dementia of the Alzheimer Type,* Springer-Verlag, Berlin, **1985.**

Stamler, J.: Coronary heart disease: Doing the "right things." *N. Engl. J. Med.*, **312**:1053–1055, **1985.**

Steinberg, F. U.: *Care of the Geriatric Patient,* Mosby, St. Louis, **1983.**

Timiras, P. S.: *Developmental Physiology and Aging,* Macmillan, New York, **1972.**

Vogt, C., and Vogt, O.: Aging of nerve cells. *Nature,* **158**:304–308, **1946.**

Weinstein, B. I.; Gattoni-Celli, S.; Kirschmeier, P.; Hsiao, W.; Horowitz, A.; and Jeffrey, A.: Cellular targets and host genes in multistage carcinogenesis. *Fed. Proc.*, **43**:2287–2294, **1984.**

Wong, C. W.; Quaranta, V.; and Glenner, G. G.: Neuritic plaques and cerebrovascular amyloid in Alzheimer disease are antigenetically related. *Proc. Natl. Acad. Sci. USA,* **82**:8729–8732, **1985.**

Zilles, K.: Morphological studies on brain structures of the NZB mouse: An animal model for the aging human brain? In Traber, J., and Gispen, W. H. (eds.): *Senile Dementia of the Alzheimer Type,* Springer-Verlag, Berlin, **1985.**

CHAPTER

4 THEORIES OF AGING

Ramesh Sharma

Define heterogeneity, phenotype

From even a cursory review, it emerges clearly that there are many theories of aging. The maximum lifespan potential is a constitutional feature of speciation subject to polygenic controls and to environmental influences. The enormous genetic heterogeneity that characterizes many species, particularly humans, and the complexity of environmental experiences create quantitative and qualitative variations of the senescent phenotype. Until now, no single theory has accounted for all phenotypes, although many have attempted to explain at least some of the major and most frequent aging phenomena. Inasmuch as all phenotypes result from an interaction between nature and nurture, an integrating view of these interactions may help in our endeavors toward a more fundamental understanding of aging. Thus, a most productive route to understanding the biology and pathology of aging (including the major aging-related diseases of humans) will be one that derives from a dissection of molecular, cellular, and systemic events. It is with this rationale in mind that the present chapter will examine the major theories of aging categorized as molecular, cellular, and systemic.

Molecular theories mainly assume that the lifespan of any species is governed by the genes interacting with environmental factors. Genetic information is stored in the genes (segments of nucleotides in DNA), is transcribed into RNA, and is subsequently translated into proteins. These proteins, either structural (e.g., collagen and keratin) or functional (e.g., enzymes and receptors), govern the form and function of organisms. Aging may result from changes in DNA template activity, which regulates the formation of the final cellular products.

Cellular theories include changes in cellular proteins (structural and functional) and other macromolecules that may occur as a function of age. These changes are produced with the passage of time under the influence of environmental factors (e.g., nutrition and stress) they may be chemical and/or morphologic and involve enzymes, hormones, age pigments, membrane permeability, macromolecule cross-linking, and changes in various cell organelles such as lysosomes and mitochondria.

Systemic theories ascribe aging of the entire organism to decrements in the function of a key system, such as the nervous, endocrine, and immune systems. Such decrements could be genetically programmed, as are the early developmental phases of the lifespan, or be the consequence of environmental insults. Alterations in the key system will generate changes throughout the entire organism.

Presented here is only a rapid survey of the major theories of aging some of which are discussed more completely in other chapters (see Chapters 7–9, 12, and 15).

MOLECULAR THEORIES

These theories originate with the concept that all individuals within a species have a similar length of life and that different species have different lifespans. For example, mayflies live only 1 day, houseflies 30 days, rats 3 years, dogs 12 years, horses 25 years, and humans 70 years (Comfort, 1979). It is presumed that there is some genetic program that determines the maximum lifespan for each species. Another argument for a genetic basis of aging is that (as well demonstrated in humans) the offspring of long-lived parents have a longer lifespan than those born from average-lived parents (Dublin, 1949). The average lifespan for females (approximately 78 years) is generally longer than for males (approximately 71 years) in most developed countries, like the United States, Sweden, and

Japan. This sex difference in lifespan is also observed in other groups of animals (Rockstein, 1974). An equally significant contribution to a genetic basis of aging is derived from the duration of the three phases of the lifespan—developmental, reproductive, and senescent. In most animals, the reproductive phase occupies a significant period in the lifespan followed by a postreproductive phase. In mammals, the time taken to reach reproductive maturity is correlated with maximum lifespan (Asdell, 1946; Kanungo, 1975) (see also Chapter 2). *Homo sapiens* and long-lived mammals take longer to reach reproductive maturity compared to other animals and continue to live after reproduction has ceased. Conversely, certain lower vertebrates (Pacific salmon, Atlantic eel, and lamprey) and invertebrates (octopus) die soon after their first reproduction as if reproduction might involve depletion of certain essential factors necessary for maintenance of later life. Expression of the genetic program that regulates the lifespan may be altered by various environmental factors. Some of the major molecular theories involve errors in this genetic program.

CODON RESTRICTION

All the genetic information stored in DNA directs the structure and function of the organism, although only part of the total DNA information is utilized by the cell at a given time. The information is transferred from DNA to messenger RNA (mRNA) by the process of transcription. The functional mRNA in eukaryotic cells is derived from excision of intervening sequences (introns) that are transcribed along and between information sequences (exons) by splicing. This mRNA is then translated into protein. The codon restriction theory of aging is based on the hypothesis that the fidelity or accuracy of translation, which depends on the cell ability to decode the triplet codons (three bases) in mRNA molecules, is impaired with aging (Strehler, 1977). The accurate reading of the codons is done by two main biomolecules: transfer RNAs (tRNAs) and aminoacyl-tRNA synthetases. Any change in these tRNAs and aminoacyl-tRNA synthetases may alter the rate of translation (decoding of the message).

There is experimental evidence for quantitative changes in the tRNAs and synthetases during development and aging. Ilan *et al.* (1970) have reported alterations in $tRNA^{tyr}$, $tRNA^{leu}$, and corresponding synthetases during the developmental period of the insect *Tenebrio molitor.* These quantitative alterations also occur in the isoacceptors of $tRNA^{arg}$ and $tRNA^{tyr}$ during aging of the free living nematode *Turbatrix aceti* (Reitz and Sanadi, 1972). Support for this theory has come from the findings of Hosbach and Kubli (1979), who demonstrated that tRNA isolated from 35-day-old *Drosophila melanogaster* cannot be aminoacylated as well as that of 5-day-old flies. The aminoacylating ability of some synthetases of old flies is only 50 percent that of the young flies. The fetal rat liver contains six isoacceptors for $tRNA^{tyr}$ compared to the adult liver, which has only three (Yang, 1971). A lower ability of tRNA aminoaceylation has been reported in hepatic parenchymal cells of old rats (Mays *et al.*, 1979).

Changes in tRNAs and aminoacyl-tRNA synthetases with aging occur in plant systems as well. Young and old tissues of soybean cotyledons differ from each other in the kinds of completely chargeable tRNA that are present. Moreover, old tissue extracts are not only deficient in certain aminoacylating abilities but possess factors that inhibit the charging of some tRNAs by extracts of young cotyledons (Bick and Strehler, 1972). Gene sequencing of rabbit β-globin shows a highly restricted use of the synonymous codons for various amino acids; only 39 of the 61 usable codons are used in the framing of the message (Efstradiadis *et al.*, 1977). Comparison of the isoaccepting species of $tRNA^{lys}$ from early and late human fibroblasts shows a smaller proportion of these species in senescent cells than in those from early passage cultures (Agris *et al.*, 1985).

As a result of differentiation, cells would lose their ability to translate genetic information. Despite a number of supportive observations, this theory, based on the view that sequential changes in the tRNAs and aminocyl-tRNA synthetases during lifespan may lead to the aging of an organism, needs further validation. It is still difficult to explain the basic cause(s) for the alterations with aging in these message-reading molecules and the implications of such changes in aging phenomena.

SOMATIC MUTATION

Alteration of the structure of the DNA molecule changes the genetic message and results in differences in protein structure that lead to physiologic deficits. This proposed theory was based on the report that rats exposed to limited irradiation died at a younger age than nonirradiated controls (Szilard, 1959). These considerations were extended to humans (Warren, 1956; Henshaw, 1957; Failla, 1960; Sacher, 1977) and included a higher incidence of neoplasia in irradiated individuals, suggesting that irradiation accelerates the aging process. According to this theory, exposure to radiation damages DNA with subsequent induction of mutations, which, in turn, lead to progressive loss of genes is postmitotic cells throughout the lifespan. The increased rate of mutation and loss of functional genes decrease the production of functional proteins and cause cell death at a critical level.

Support for this theory was provided by the observation that increased exposure to x-rays shortens life expectancy and increases chromosomal aberrations in parallel with increasing doses of x-rays (Stevenson and Curtis, 1961; Curtis, 1964). Older animals have a greater number of chromosomal abnormalities than younger, and in short-lived mice, the rate of development of abnormalities is more rapid than in long-lived ones. These data suggest that natural radiation also affects the aging process. However, contrasting evidence negates a causative role for somatic mutation in aging.

In some species, such as humans, the sex chromosomes of females are similar (XX) but those of males are different (XY), while in others the reverse is true. If radiation is a cause for aging, then one might expect a longer life for individuals with identical sex chromosomes. However, in most species, females generally live longer than males, irrespective of the chromosomal composition. Another example is the wasp, *Habrobracon,* in which males have either two sex chromosomes (diploid) or one (haploid). If both types of males are exposed to x-rays, the haploid male should die earlier than the diploid, but, in fact, this is not the case: both males have similar lifespans despite the greater resistance of the diploid male to ionizing radiation because of the larger number of repairable chromosomes (Clark and Rubin, 1961). Chemical substances that change DNA structure have no effect on lifespan (Curtis, 1966). Colchicine exposure of human fetal lung fibroblasts produces 60 percent tetraploid cells, which continue to divide (Thompson and Holliday, 1978) and have growth rate and lifespan similar to those of diploid cells. Diploid as well as tetraploid human skin fibroblasts likewise have similar lifespans (Hoehn *et al.,* 1975). The somatic mutation theory is further contradicted by studies of the effects of low-dose ionizing radiation on the lifespan of human fibroblasts *in vitro*; irradiation of early embryonic as well as postnatal cells may shorten, prolong, or have no effect on doubling potential and lifespan (Macieira Coelho *et al.,* 1977, 1978; Azzarone *et al.,* 1980).

Somatic mutations are no longer regarded as a probable cause of aging because the rate at which they occur in the absence of ionizing radiation is too low to account for overall age changes (Maynard-Smith, 1966). Furthermore, the primary lesions of aging are different from those of radiation (Walburg, 1975). Radiation acts primarily on dividing cell lines such as bone marrow stem cells, leukocytes, and gut epithelial cells, and its effects are observed after cell division. In contrast, effects of age are centered in cell lines that no longer divide, such as nerve and muscle cells.

Most cells have mechanisms for the repair of damaged DNA molecules (Hart and Setlow, 1974; Wheeler and Lett, 1974) and there is little evidence that DNA repair mechanisms decline in senescent animals (Tice, 1978); rather, these repair mechanisms appear more effective in long-lived species as compared to short-lived (Figure 4–1) (Hart and Setlow, 1974). The species-specific differences in the lifespan of animals could be attributed to the ability of animals to tolerate DNA damage rather than

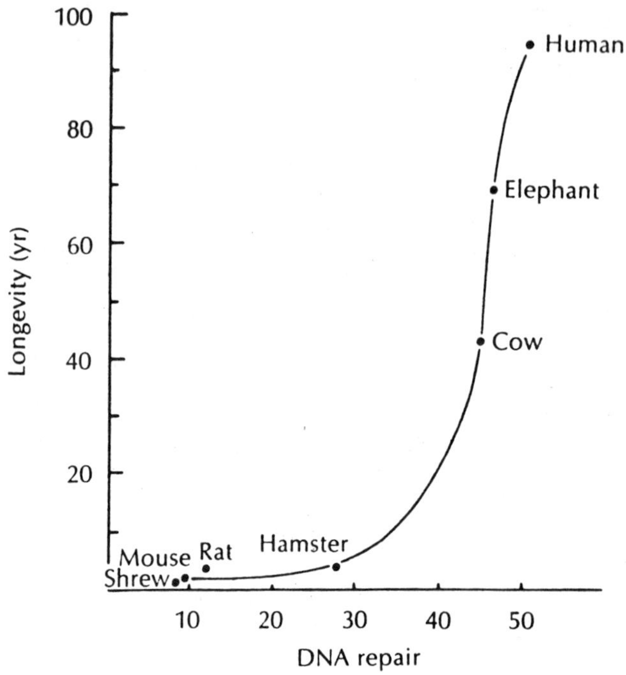

Figure 4–1. *Correlation between longevity and ability to repair DNA by replacement of thymine dimers following ultraviolet radiation in different mammals.* (From Sinex, F.M., In Finch, C.E.; Hayflick, L. (eds.): *Handbook of the Biology of Aging,* Van Nostrand Reinhold Co., New York, 1977.)

to repair. The presence of multiple copies of the same message coded within the DNA would offer protection to DNA damage. The number of repetitive genes for the major rRNA is 5 to 10 in bacteria, 100 to 130 in *Drosophila,* and 250 to 600 in vertebrates (Medvedev, 1972), suggesting a correlation between the number of repetitive genes and the lifespan of the species. Cutler (1973) reported that the average redundancy of transcribing mRNA in the brain was greater in humans than cows and greater in cows than mice. The higher the redundancy of transcribing mRNA, the longer is the lifespan. Based on available experimental evidence, radiation does not seem to play a major role in accelerating the aging process or in causing aging.

Error Theory

The form and function of organisms are governed by specific structural and functional proteins. Certain protein molecules, such as RNA polymerase and tRNA synthetases, are involved in the production of other proteins. Medvedev (1961) first advanced the concept that errors in the transmission of information through RNA to proteins may be responsible for cellular aging. This theory was extended to investigate which errors occurring in information transfer steps, such as transcription and translation, may cause accumulation of defective proteins and cause aging (Orgel, 1963; Medvedev, 1964). Errors such as the incorporation of wrong nucleotides into mRNA during transcription may change the triplet codons, or incorporation of wrong amino acids into protein during translation may change the amino acid sequence. Orgel (1973) further argued that production of functional proteins such as enzymes depends not only on the genetic information stored in DNA, but also on the protein synthetic machinery, and he pointed out that inaccuracy occurs in both protein and DNA syntheses (Figure 4–2). The initial error in proteins may be low, but it increases exponentially with the passage of time and may lead to an "error catastrophe" and ultimately death of the cell. The error accumulation can be expressed mathematically as $Et = Eo_{e\alpha t}$, where Eo is the initial error frequency, Et is the error frequency at time t, and α is a proportionality constant.

Evidence for the error theory is primar-

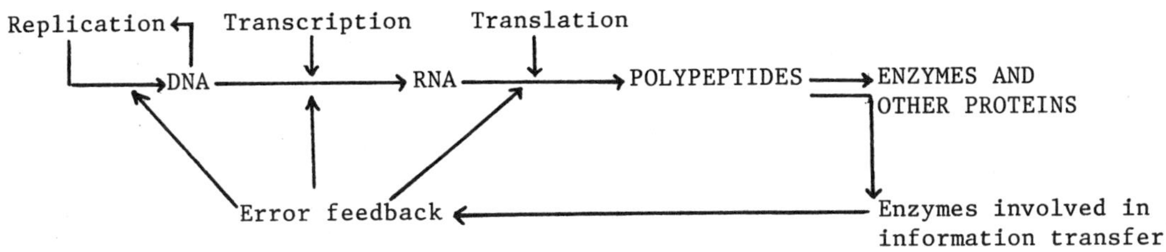

Figure 4–2. *Feedback of errors in protein synthesis during information transfer in biological systems.*

ily based on an experimentallv-induced error in fruitflies produced by feeding them with amino acid analogs. These flies have a shorter lifespan than normal (Harrison and Holliday, 1967). Much of the support for this theory comes from the work of Holliday and Tarrant (1972), who reported an increased accumulation of heat-labile glucose-6-phosphate dehydrogenase in old fibroblasts. These heat-labile enzymes in old fibroblasts also show an altered substrate specificity, indicating the presence of possible errors. Using immunologic techniques, the proportions of inactive lactate dehydrogenase (LDH) in human fibroblasts, isocitrate lyase in the nematode, and aldolase in mouse liver increase in old age (Lamb, 1977). Functionally altered enzymes are known to accumulate in various animal tissues with age (Gershon, 1979; Rothstein, 1979). The decrease in the functional activity of tissues with increasing age would be due to accumulation of such altered proteins. Some reports suggest that altered enzymes in old tissues are generated by conformational changes (Sharma and Rothstein, 1978; Sharma *et al.*, 1980).

Many reports contradict the occurrence of errors in protein that may cause aging. Kanungo and Gandhi (1972) could not detect any age-related differences in liver malate dehydrogenase (MDH) using immunologic preparations. Kinetic properties (K_m and K_i) and electrophoretic mobilities of rat hepatic cytoplasmic alanine aminotransferase (Patnaik and Kanungo, 1976) and aspartate aminotransferase (Sharma and Patnaik, 1982) do not reveal age-related differences. Studies of aldolase from mouse liver (Gershon and Gershon, 1973) and cytoplasmic superoxide dismutase (SOD) from liver, brain, and heart of rats and mice have not detected differences in antigenicity, K_m, K_i, and electrophoretic mobility between young and old animals (Reiss and Gershon, 1976a,b). The fidelity of protein synthesis, measured in human diploid skin fibroblasts *in vitro,* remains unchanged as a function of age (Goldstein *et al.*, 1985). Mitochondrial proteins do not reveal changes in molecular weight or isoelectric point in young and old *Drosophila* (Fleming *et al.*, 1986), even though significant quantitative changes do occur with age. The fidelity of synthesis of mitochondrial proteins would then be preserved throughout the lifespan of *Drosophila*. Thus, there are sufficient data to show that errors in fidelity of protein synthetic machinery do not occur with increasing age and, therefore, cannot be responsible for aging.

GENE REGULATION THEORY

This theory was proposed to explain the two important characteristics of the aging process: (1) the gradual decline in adaptability to the environment after attaining reproductive maturity; and (2) the approximately fixed lifespan for a species (Kanungo, 1975, 1980). According to this model (Figure 4–3), senescence may result from changes in the expression of genes after reproductive maturity is reached. Differentiation and growth would follow sequential activation and repression of certain genes that are unique for these phases. Sequential activation and repression of genes occur for various hemoglobin chains during the gestational period in humans (Zuckerlandl, 1965). The hemoglobin, a tetramer protein, consists of $\alpha_2\varepsilon_2$ chains in the fetus at the age of 1 to 2 months of gestation. The α chain remains the same, but the ε chain is re-

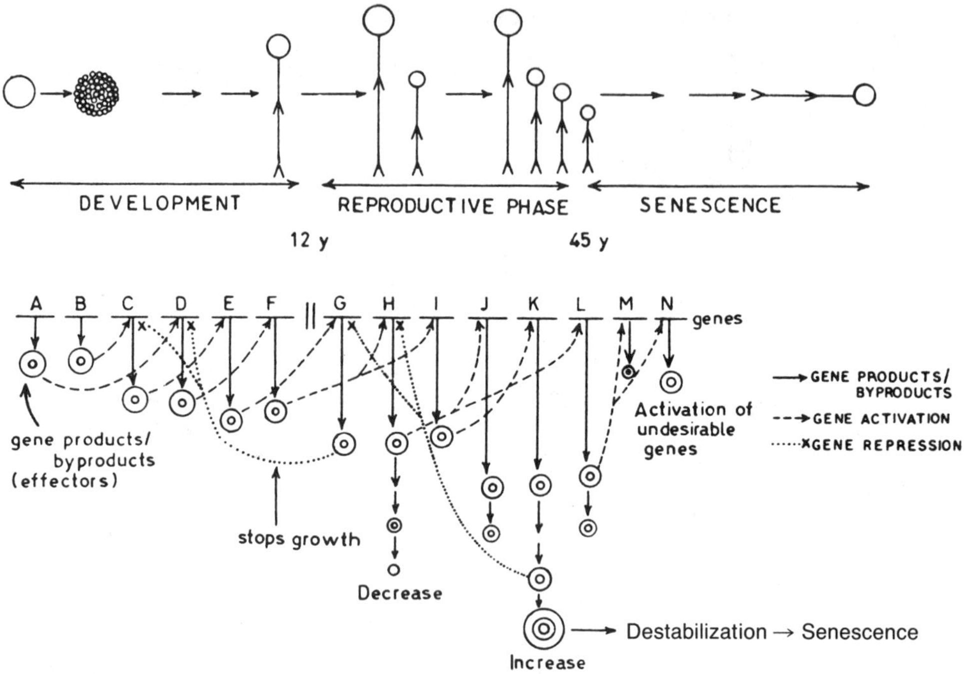

Figure 4–3. *Model for aging.*

(*Upper part.*) Various phases of the lifespan as development, reproduction and senescence. (*Lower part.*) The number of active genes for development (A to F) and reproductive (G to L) phases. No specific genes for senescence are visualized in this model. Development occurs by the sequential activation of genes (A to F); the product of gene A switching on gene B and so on. Some of the late development genes (E and F) switch on some unique genes (G and F) of early reproductive phase. The organism attains reproductive ability when required amounts of gene products are formed. Continued reproduction may cause depletion of certain factors necessary for the activity of certain essential genes. Switching off these genes may cause deterioration of some functions. It may also lead to accumulation of certain gene products beyond a certain level resulting in the activation of some undesirable genes (M and N), whose products may cause diseases, e.g., autoimmune diseases. The decline in physiological functions after certain periods of the reproductive phase may be due to destabilization of the function of the genes of the reproductive phase or adulthood. (From Kanungo, M.S.: *Biochemistry of Ageing*. Academic Press, London, 1980.)

placed by the γ chain in later phases of gestation. Just before birth, the γ chain is further replaced by the β chain, which gives rise to the adult hemoglobin ($\alpha_2\beta_2$). The synthesis of these chains is governed by different sets of genes. These genes are sequentially activated and repressed by certain factors during the development of the human fetus. Another example of the differential activation is lactate dehydrogenase (LDH) isoenzymes in different tissues during development (Markert and Ursprung, 1962). The proportion of M_4-LDH is significantly lower in the heart, brain, and skeletal muscle of old rats, and the gene responsible for synthesis of the M subunit would be somehow repressed in old age (Singh and Kanungo, 1968). Studies on rat hepatic alanine aminotransferase (AAT), a dimer having A and B subunits, have shown that the gene for A is more active in the early period of the lifespan and subsequently repressed, whereas the B subunit is activated in old age and the dimer is formed only by the B subunit (Patnaik and Kanungo, 1976). According to these studies, the sequential activation and repression of genes would not be restricted to development (Caplan and Ordahl, 1978), but would extend into adulthood and aging (Kanungo, 1980).

The genes responsible for the synthesis of various enzymes do not appear to undergo any change in their basic sequences during the lifespan. Rather, the observed changes in levels of enzymes may be due to alterations in the template activity of corresponding genes induced by various extrinsic and intrinsic factors. For example, the level and inducibility of many enzymes by hormones change in different tissues as a function of age without any sign of error incorporation into these molecules (Kanungo, 1980; Sharma and Patnaik, 1982, 1984, 1985). Modulating factors may either appear or disappear and/or their levels may change at different phases of the lifespan (Kanungo, 1980). The products or by-products of the genes responsible for differentiation and growth, on reaching critical levels, stimulate certain unique genes responsible for the reproductive phase. However, as a result of continued reproduction, certain factors may be depleted as they may not be replenished as fast as they disappear. Such factors may be of crucial importance for keeping certain genes expressed or repressed. They may also cause activation of undesirable genes and, thereby, lead to destabilization of expression of the unique genes that are required for reproduction—hence a gradual decline in reproductive rate with age. This model also predicts that should the organism be able to replenish the factors that become depleted owing to continued reproduction, the reproductive period and lifespan would be lengthened. This theory is supported by the data on the lifespan of mammals, particularly the reproductive phase, which has continuously lengthened with the progress of evolution (Cutler, 1975).

The lifespan of a species may be divided into three phases: developmental, reproductive, and senescent. Each phase has a characteristic duration, rate and regulatory mechanisms. The initiation, rate, and duration of developmental and reproductive phases depend on unique sets of genes that are sequentially activated and repressed. Human genetic diseases, such as progeria and progeroid syndromes, are in agreement with this sequence (Kanungo, 1980). Progeria is caused by the mutation of an autosomal gene. In this case, the newborn child appears normal and grows normally up to about 6 years; then the signs of aging, such as atherosclerosis, accumulation of lipofuscin, greying of hairs, and so forth, appear. Fibroblasts taken from a 10-year-old progeria patient do not show as many population doublings as those of a normal child of the same age. It appears that some genes responsible for normal development are altered to induce this condition. Perhaps the production of essential factors necessary for further development and growth is prevented by this mutation. The reproductive phase is not initiated owing to lack of switching on of the necessary genes during the later phases of development and growth. The lifespan is shortened following expression of the mutated gene. Another example is the sudden death of the female octopus, which lays eggs only once, broods them, reduces food intake, and dies soon after the hatching of the young (Wodinski, 1977). Removal of the two optic glands after spawning prevents brooding, and the octopus continues to eat and to grow and increases longevity. It appears quite obvious that certain factors are produced in the optic gland that are responsible for brooding and cessation of feeding followed by senescence and death. Egg laying may deplete certain factors, which may in turn cause the optic gland to produce a hormone that causes behavioral change. A similar phenomenon is observed in salmon and certain insects. Each species has a unique set of genes for development and reproduction. Their sequential activation or repression determines the duration of development and the onset of reproduction and is governed by the proper balance between various factors that are essential for maintenance of the reproductive phase. According to this model, no unique gene would be responsible for aging, nor is aging programmed, as are development and reproduction. Rather, normal aging would merely be a consequence of the organism attaining reproductive ability (irrespective of whether it reproduced).

CELLULAR THEORIES

These theories relate to the changes that occur in structural and functional elements of cells with the passage of time. They also concern the biomolecules after their synthesis is completed, suggesting that these changes impair the effectiveness of these molecules as a function of age.

WEAR AND TEAR

According to this theory, living organisms are like machines (Sacher, 1977); i.e., with repeated use, parts wear out, become defective, and the machinery finally fails to function. This assumption is not entirely appropriate: organisms have a mechanism by which they can repair their damages, whereas machines do not. The premise of this theory originates from the observation that the lifespan of poikilotherms is shortened by increasing the environmental temperature and prolonged by decreasing it; indeed, the metabolic rate of chemical reactions is increased by increasing temperatures, and the reverse is true for low temperatures. This phenomenon has been reported for fruitflies (Loeb and Northrup, 1917; Strehler, 1962) and rotifers (Fanestil and Barrows, 1965). The increased metabolic rate may shorten the lifespan by accelerating wear and tear. The lifespans of different animal species are inversely proportional to the basal metabolic rate (Sohal, 1976). Basal oxygen consumption rates of short-lived animals such as rats and mice are much higher than those of long-lived animals such as elephants and humans. Within the same species, however, it is difficult to correlate individual differences in lifespan with the metabolic rate.

AGE PIGMENTS

Accumulation of lipofuscin or age pigment is the most prominent age-associated change present in a variety of cell types from many organisms. It is predominantly deposited in nondividing cells such as neurons and cardiac myocytes (Figure 4–4) as a function of age (Strehler *et al.*, 1959; Brody and Vijayashanker, 1977; Miquel *et al.*, 1978). Lipofuscin accumulation has been reported in the cortex and hippocampus of humans (Friede, 1966), rhesus monkey (Brizzee *et al.*, 1974), and rat (Brizzee *et al.*, 1969; Brizzee and Ordy, 1979) as one of the common morphologic features associated with aging and has been correlated with the loss of neurons in old age. Lipofuscin is also deposited in dividing cells like liver (Essner and Novikoff, 1960), adrenal cortex (Szabo *et al.*, 1970), and testis (Miquel *et al.*, 1978). Its accumulation is also associated with the loss of cytoplasmic mass, mitrochondrial number, rough endoplasmic reticulum, and vacuolation of cytoplasm (Tonna, 1973). Indeed, lipofuscin accumulation may be a basic feature of cellular aging. The existence of a specific relationship between the rate of aging and lipofuscin accumulation was demonstrated in the housefly (Sohal and Donato, 1978). For example, the rate of lipofuscin deposition has been inversely correlated with the lifespan of many animals. The faster the rate of lipofuscin accumulation, the shorter will be the lifespan. The rate of lipofuscin deposition in the dog heart has been found to be approximately 5 times faster than in the human heart, a difference that roughly corresponds to the lifespan of these two species (Munnel and Getty, 1968).

The origin of age pigments is not clear, although it has been ascribed to morphologic and chemical causes. Lipofuscin would arise by a process of autophagocytosis involving lysosomes (Strehler, 1964; Samorajski *et al.*, 1965). A chemical hypothesis concerning the origin of lipofuscin suggests that it is an end-product of lipid peroxidation (Tappel, 1975). The cause for accumulation of age pigment remains to be explored. It is discussed in more detail in Chapter 5.

FREE-RADICAL THEORIES

The free-radical theory of aging postulates that free-radical reactions (modified by genetic and environmental factors) are involved in aging and age-related disorders (Harman, 1983, 1986). Free-radical reactions are ubiquitous in living organisms. These reactions arise upon exposure to ionizing radiations, from nonenzymatic and enzymatic reactions, particularly those of the energy-gaining processes such as reduc-

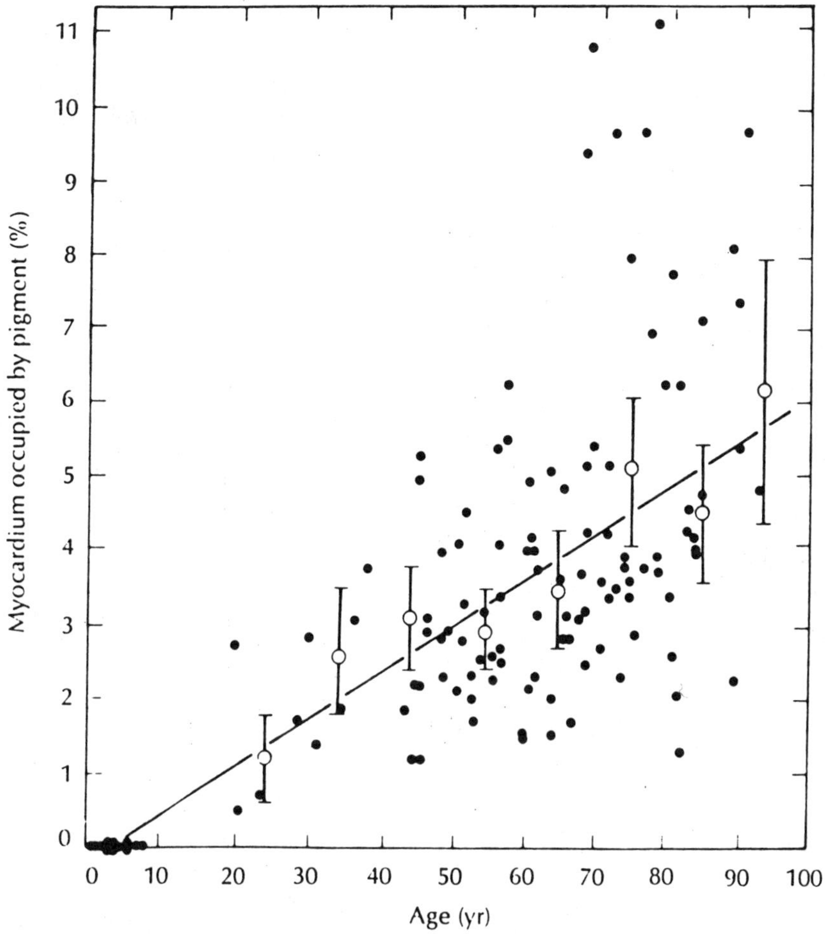

Figure 4–4. *Accumlation of lipofuscin as a function of age in human cardiac muscle.*

●, percentage of the myocardium occupied by pigment in individual cases; ○, means for 10-year periods; vertical bars represent standard errors of the means. Individual values are scattered but means represent a definite linear increase with age (From Strehler, B.L.; Mark, D.D.; Mildvan, A.S.; and Gee, M.V.: Rate and magnitude of age pigment accumulation in the human myocardium. *J. Gerontol.*, 14:430–39, 1959).

tion of O_2 to water (Harman, 1986). Free radicals are chemical compounds highly reactive owing to the presence of extra electrons in the outer orbit. These radicals include $O_2^{\cdot}$, $HO^{\cdot}$, $R^{\cdot}$ (any organic radical), $RO^{\cdot}$, and $RO_2^{\cdot}$ and participate in an interacting network of free-radical reactions going on continuously throughout the cells and tissues.

The deleterious effects of free-radical reactions can be repaired by the presence of antioxidants such as tocopherols (Harman, 1986), glutathione peroxidase (Flohe *et al.*, 1976), superoxide dismutases (Fridovich, 1977), elevated serum uric acid levels (Ames *et al.*, 1981), carotenes (Klebanoff, 1980), and DNA repair mechanisms (Hart *et al.*, 1979). Antioxidants that are known to inhibit free-radical reactions have been reported to prolong the lifespan of rotifers (Enesco and Verdone-Smith, 1980), *Turbatrix* (Epstein and Gershon, 1972), fruitflies (Miquel and Economos, 1979), and mice (Miquel and Economos, 1979). This theory predicts that overproduction of free radicals and/or reduction of their removal causes cell and molecular damage and ultimately aging of the organisms (Figure 4–5). This theory is presented in more detail in Chapter 7.

CROSS-LINKING THEORY

Many of the biologic macromolecules develop cross-linkages or bonds between identical molecules or with different molecules with the passage of time. These linkages alter the physical and chemical properties of these molecules (Bjorksten, 1968). Major support for this theory was provided by the work of Verzar (1963) on the extracellular fibrous protein collagen. Collagen is synthesized in all types of cells and is deposited extracellularly in all tissues. The structural unit of collagen is tropocollagen. It is a long (300 nm) and thin (1.5 nm in diameter) protein that consists of three coiled polypeptide subunits called α chains. Each α chain contains 1050 amino acid residues. The three chains wind around each other in a right-handed triple helix, which is held together by hydrogen bonds. The helix is rich in glycine, proline, and hydroxyproline amino acids. In collagen fibers, tropocollagen molecules pack together side by side and are stabilized by chemical cross-links between the chains. The mode of packing creates periodic striations in the structure of collagen fibers. The number of striations in the collagen of rat tail tendon and its thermal stability increase whereas solubility decreases with age (Figure 4–6). The increased cross-links in collagen would make it more insoluble with aging (Verzar, 1964). Cross-linking agents are produced during normal metabolism as charged groups. Such ionized groups are replaced in early life by normal metabolic processes, but accumulate in increasingly larger amounts in old age (Bjorksten, 1977). These groups react irreversibly with biomolecules like DNA and proteins and inactivate them, possibly reducing physiologic competence with aging (Verzar, 1964; Kohn, 1978). Increased cross-linking of aged collagen has been correlated with an increased rigidity of the cell membrane, a probable cause of the decreased potassium conductance of the membrane (Nagy, 1978) (Chapter 23). The higher intracellular potassium content

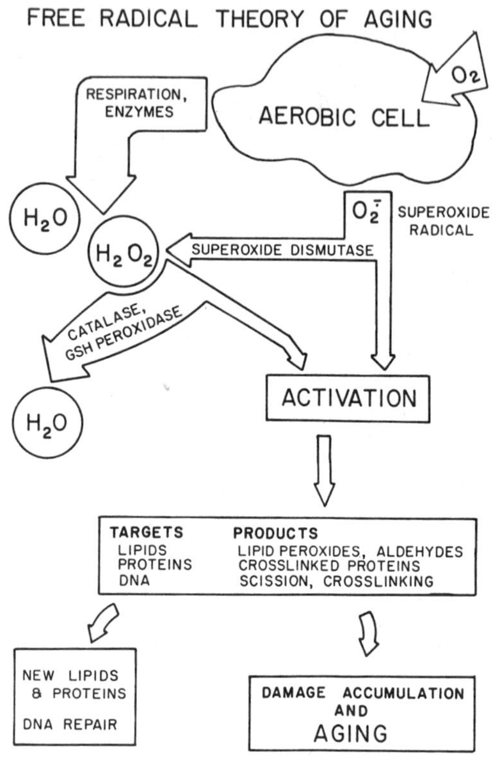

Figure 4–5. *Viewing this figure from top to bottom, oxygen, in the course of cell metabolism and via cell respiration and enzymes, gives rise to superoxide radicals and to peroxide molecules.*

Most free radicals are intercepted by three protective enzymes: superoxide dismutase (SOD), catalase, and glutathione peroxidase (GSH). The common by-product is water. Despite these protective mechanisms, products of free radical damage accumulate with time and such accumulation eventually results in impaired cell and organ function.

As shown in the lower center of this figure, lipids undergo peroxidation, proteins undergo crosslinking and DNA undergoes scission or crosslinking. All of these products impair normal cell function. Yet, at a young age and in the absence of disease or environmental noxious influences, repair enzymes are capable of containing this damage. In aging and under toxic conditions, damage is not repaired and may accumulate to compromise cell integrity, inducing aging and such diseases as cancer, atherosclerosis, and senile dementia. (Drawing by S. Oklund.)

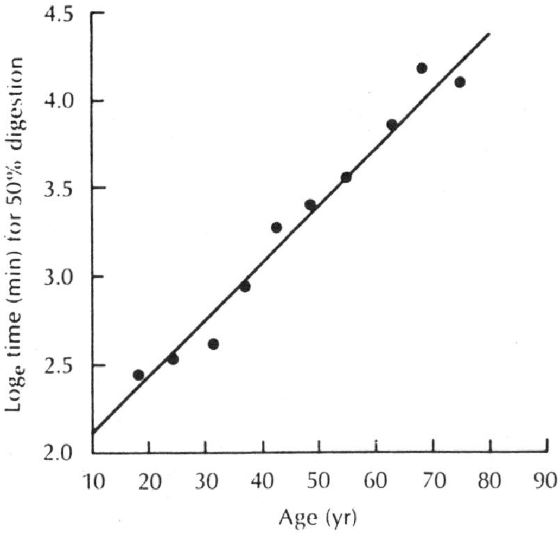

Figure 4–6. *Crosslinking of collagen.*

Collagenase digestion of human tendon collagen as a function of age. Straight line indicates increase in digestion time due to more crosslinks with age. (From Kohn, R.R.: *Principles of Mammalian Aging,* 2nd ed., Prentice-Hall, N.J., 1978.)

would in turn increase the intracellular ionic strength and lead to a decreased rate of transcription by chromatin and slowing down of protein synthesis (Nagy, 1978). Cross-links are present not only in extracellular collagen, but also in intracellular proteins (enzymes) as well as nucleic acids (DNA) (Bjorksten, 1977). The decrease in the extractability of chromosomal proteins from chromatin may be regarded as increased cross-linking with DNA (Hahn, 1970).

SYSTEM LEVEL THEORIES

Neuroendocrine Control Theory

According to Shock (1979), the overall performance of an animal is closely related to the effectiveness of a variety of control mechanisms that regulate the interplay between different organs and tissues. As discussed in Chapter 2, with aging, the effectiveness of homeostatic adjustments declines with consequent failure of adaptive mechanisms, and aging and death may be viewed as the result of this failure (Frolkis, 1982). Adaptation to stress, either external (from environmental stimuli) or internal (from emotional, hormonal, immunologic, and metabolic stimuli) depends on control mechanisms orchestrated by the nervous and endocrine system. The activity of several endocrine glands, thyroid, adrenals, gonads, is controlled directly by the pituitary gland and indirectly by the signals this endocrine gland receives from nervous centers, primarily the hypothalamus. For efficient adaptation, nervous and endocrine signals must be synchronized and responsive to the needs of the many functions they regulate (Timiras, 1978, 1980, 1983, 1985; Timiras *et al.,* 1982). However, with aging, some of the efficiency of the hypothalamo-pituitary signals is lost or altered (Everitt and Burgess, 1976), and this results in decreased function and increased pathology of most organs and tissue systems.

The neuroendocrine theory views aging as part of a lifespan program regulated by neural and hormonal signals (Figure 4–7). The program unfolds from fertilization through birth, childhood, adulthood, and finally, old age and death. According to this theory, command neurons in higher brain centers would act as "pacemakers" that regulate the "biologic clock" that governs development and aging. With the passage of time, aging changes may result from programmed deterioration or cessation of the programming that regulates homeostasis (Walker and Timiras, 1982). In either case, aging would be manifested through a slowing down or imbalance in the activity of the pacemaker neurons with consequent neurotransmitter and hormonal alterations and their repercussion on neural, muscular, and secretary functions. Such functional decrements are exemplified by involution of reproductive organs, loss of fertility, diminished muscular strength, lesser ability to recover from stress, and impairment of cardiovascular and respiratory activity.

Immunologic Theory

The immune system protects the individual from a variety of potentially harmful substances and organisms. Several organs, such as bone marrow, thymus, lymph

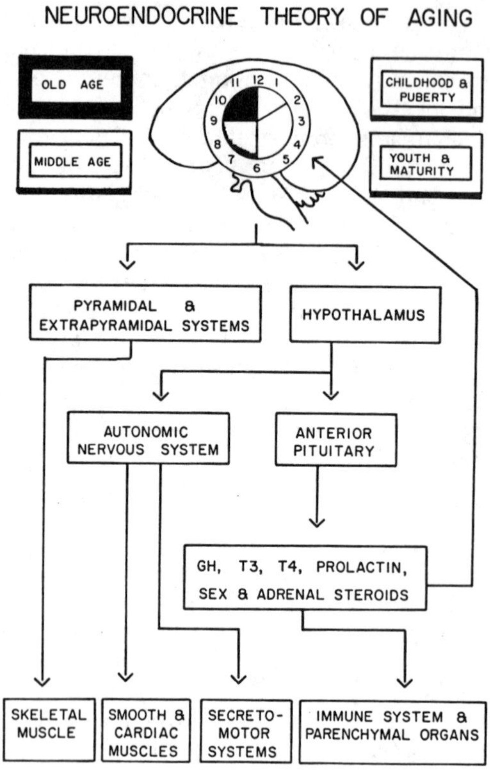

Figure 4–7. *The neuroendocrine theory views aging as part of a lifespan program regulated by neural and hormonal signals.*

The program unfolds, as shown at the top of the diagram, from fertilization through birth, childhood and puberty, youth and maturity, middle age and, finally, old age and death. "Command" neurons in higher brain centers would act as "pacemakers" that regulate the "biologic clock" governing development and aging.

As shown in the middle portion of the diagram, signals from these neurons would be relayed by neurotransmitters—acetylcholine, monamines and peptides—directly through the pyramidal and extrapyramidal systems to the skeletal muscles to regulate motor activity; or they would be relayed to the hypothalamus to stimulate autonomic and neuroendocrine neurons. Autonomic stimulation mediates the peripheral sympathetic and parasympathetic responses of the heart, smooth muscle, and exocrine glands. Hypothalamic hormones regulate the secretion of the anterior pituitary hormones and these, in turn, stimulate the peripheral endocrines to secret their respective hormones. As shown at the bottom of the diagram, several hormones—thyroid hormones, T4 and T3, adrenal and sex steroids, growth hormone (GH), and prolactin—act on specific receptors in target tissues and regulate metabolic, immunologic, reproductive, and adaptive functions necessary for the survival of the individual and the preservation of the species.

With time, aging changes may result from programmed deterioration or, alternatively, cessation of the programming that regulates homeostasis. In either case, aging would be manifested through a slowing down or imbalance in the activity of the pacemaker neurons with consequent neurotransmitter and hormonal alterations and their repercussion on neural, muscular, and secretory functions, e.g., involution of reproductive organs, loss of fertility, diminished muscular strength, lessened ability to recover from stress and impairment of secretory, cardiovascular, and respiratory activity. It is possible that programmed changes in the activity of genes are not confined to fertilization but may continue at late ages and are triggered by neural and hormonal influences. (Drawing by S. Oklund.)

---

nodes, and spleen, are involved in the production of immunologic responses directed toward the invading foreign (nonself) substances, called antigens. An antigen must either be a macromolecule or built up from macromolecules (i.e., viral particle). Most proteins and some polysaccharides and nucleic acids act as antigens. Two major types of cells are vital to an efficient immune response. One type is represented by the T-cell lymphocytes, matured in the thymus, and the other, the B-cell lymphocytes, stored in lymph nodes and spleen. T cells are responsible for cell-mediated immune responses that protect the body from pathogenic microorganisms, and also for rejecting foreign tissue grafts. The cytotoxic (killer) T cells destroy the antigen by direct attack on antigens. Subsets of T cells such as T helpers, T amplifiers, and T suppressors also influence immunologic cascade reactions by interacting with cytotoxic T cells and B lymphocytes. The B cells secrete antibodies (immunoglobulins) that bind to antigens and thereby help to destroy them. Competence of the immune system declines with aging (Figure 4–8). This decline has been attributed primarily to a reduced function of the thymus and T cells. The thymus begins to involute at adolescence and continues to atrophy throughout the lifespan. The active thymic epithelial cells produce a specific protein, called thymosin, which promotes T-cell maturation. With thymic involution, thymosin level declines, and this, in turn, diminishes the T cells' ability to destroy foreign substances (Kay, 1979, 1984). The ability of B lymphocytes to produce specific antibodies against antigens depends on T-cell function, which declines with the thymic involution and T-cell impairment. For these many reasons it has been proposed that the thymus gland may be the "clock" for immunologic aging (Kay, 1979). The probable cause of thymic involution is still not known. Another consequence of thymic involution in aging is the loss of immune tolerance, i.e., the ability to distinguish self from nonself. The autoimmune theory of aging (Blumenthal and Berns, 1964; Walford, 1969) proposes that aging results from the production of antibodies that react with normal cells of the body and destroy them. An age-related increase in autoimmune antibodies has been reported (Walford, 1969, 1974). Thus, aging would be the consequence of reduced immunologic surveillance and of increased autoantibody production (for more information see Chapter 8).

Hormonal influences on the immune system have long been known; for example, the involutionary actions of glucocorticoid hormones on the thymus and lymphatic system have been exploited successfully for the treatment of allergies and as immunosuppressant in organ transplantation. In addition, nervous influences also have been shown to regulate some aspects of the immune response. Thus, neuroendocrine and immunologic theories of aging may converge, or alterations in their function may articulate with each other to lead to aging changes. A neuroendocrine-immunomodulation of thymic aging has been demonstrated in experiments in which tumor (GH3) pituitary adenoma cells, which secrete both growth hormone and prolactin, can reconstitute thymic structure and improve T-cell production and function when implanted in old rats (Kelley *et al.*, 1986). The possibility of thymic rehabilitation in old age suggests that lymphoid cells in aged animals are not inherently defective, but, given the proper stimulus, can return to normal function.

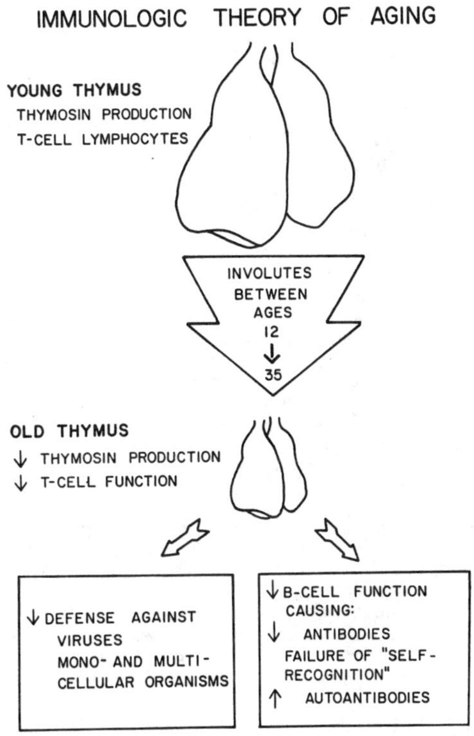

Figure 4–8. *Competence of the immune system declines with aging and immunologic involution may play an important role in the aging process and the induction of age-associated diseases.*

Decline in immunologic competence with aging has been attributed primarily to a reduced function of the thymus and T-cells. As shown in the middle portion of the diagram, the thymus begins to involute at adolescence and continues to atrophy throughout life; with thymic involution and declining thymosin production, T-cell activity and ability to fight foreign organisms diminishes. The ability of B-cell lymphocytes to produce specific antibodies against antigens depends also on T-cell function. This ability declines with thymic involution and T-cell impairment. Thus, as shown in the lower portion of the diagram, thymic insufficiency affects both T- and B-cell function and immunologic surveillance of foreign invaders is diminished. Another consequence of thymic involution with aging is the loss of immune tolerance, that is, the ability of distinguishing self from nonself. With aging, decreased tolerance and increased production of abnormal molecules induce the production of autoantibodies. These are directed against the individual's own tissues and cells, causing deterioration and destruction of the attacked organ, tissue, or cell, a condition that characterizes the so-called autoimmune diseases. (Drawings by S. Oklund.)

References

Agris, P. F.; Boak, A.; Basler, J. W.; Voorn, C. V.; Smith, C.; and Reichlin, M.: Analysis of cellular senescence through detection and assessment of RNAs and proteins important to gene expression: Transfer RNAs and autoimmune antigens. In Salk, D.; Fujiwara, Y.; and Martin, G. M. (eds.): *Werners Syndrome and Human Aging,* Plenum Press, New York, **1985.**

Ames, B. N.; Cathcart, R.; Schiviers, E.; and Hochstein, P.: Uric acid provides an antioxidant defense in humans against oxidant- and radical-caused aging and cancer: A hypothesis. *Proc. Natl. Acad. Sci. USA,* **78:**6852–6858, **1981.**

Asdell, S.: *Patterns of Mammalian Reproduction,* Comstock Publishing Co., Ithaca, New York, **1946.**

Azzarone, B.; Diatloff-Zito, C.; Billard, C.; and Macieira-Coelho, A.: Effect of low dose rate irradiation on the division potential of cells *in vitro.* VII. Human fibroblasts from young and adult donors. *In Vitro,* **16:**634–638, **1980.**

Bick, M. D., and Strehler, B.: Leucyl-tRNA synthetase activity in old cotyledons: Evidence on repressor accumulation. *Mech. Ageing Dev.,* **1:**33–42, **1972.**

Bjorksten, J.: The cross linkage theory of aging. *J. Am. Geriatr. Soc.,* **16:**408–427, **1968.**

Bjorksten, J.: Crosslinkage and the aging process. In Rockstein, M. (ed.): *Theoretical Aspects of Aging,* Academic Press, New York, **1977.**

Blumenthal, M. T., and Berns, A. W.: Autoimmunity and aging. In Strehler, B. L. (ed.): *Advances in Gerontological Research,* Academic Press, New York, **1964.**

Brizzee, K. P.; Cancilla, P. A.; Sherwood, N.; and Timiras, P. S.: The amount and distribution of pigments in neurons and glia of the cerebral cortex. *J. Gerontol.,* **24:**127–135, **1969.**

Brizzee, K. P., and Ordy, J. M.: Age pigments, cell loss and hippocampal function. *Mech. Ageing Dev.,* **9:**143–162, **1979.**

Brizzee, K. P.; Ordy, J. M.; and Kaack, B.: Early appearance and regional differences in intraneuronal and extraneuronal lipofuscin accumulation with age in the brain of a non human primate. *J. Gerontol.,* **29:**366–381, **1974.**

Brody, H., and Vijayashanker, N.: Anatomical changes in the nervous system. In Finch, C. E., and Hayflick, L. (eds.): *Handbook of the Biology of Aging,* Van Nostrand Reinhold, New York, **1977.**

Brody, H., and Vijayashanker, N.: Cell loss with aging. In Nandi, K., and Sherwin, I. (eds.): *The Aging Brain and Senile Dementia,* Plenum Press, New York, **1977.**

Caplan, A. I., and Ordahl, C. P.: Irreversible gene repression model for control of development. *Science,* **201:**120–130, **1978.**

Clark, A. M., and Rubin, M. A.: The modification by x-irradiation of the life span of haploids and diploids of the wasp, Habrobracon, sp. *Radiat. Res.,* **15:**244–253, **1961.**

Comfort, A.: *The Biology of Senescence,* 3rd ed., Elsevier, New York, **1979.**

Corsellis, J. A. N.: Neuronal loss in the aging brain. *Proc. 10th Intl. Congr. Gerontol.,* **1:**109–113, **1975.**

Curtis, H. J.: Cellular processes involved in aging. *Fed. Proc.,* **23:**662–667, **1964.**

Curtis, H. J.: *Biological Mechanisms of Aging,* Charles C Thomas, Springfield, IL, **1966.**

Cutler, R. G.: Redundancy of information content in the genome of mammalian species as a protective mechanism determining aging rate. *Mech. Ageing Dev.,* **2:**381–408, **1973.**

Cutler, R. G.: Evolution of human longevity and the genetic complexity governing aging rate. *Proc. Natl. Acad. Sci. USA,* **72:**4664–4668, **1975.**

Dilman, V. M.: The hypothalamic control of aging and age-associated pathology: The elevated mechanism of aging. In Everitt, A. V., and Burgess, J. M. (eds.): *Hypothalamus, Pituitary and Aging,* Charles C Thomas, Springfield, IL, **1976.**

Dublin, L. I.: *Length of Life: A Study of the Life Table,* Ronald Press, New York, **1949.**

Efstradiadis, A.; Kafatos, F.; and Maniatis, T.: The primary structure of rabbit β-globin mRNA as determined from cloned DNA. *Cell,* **10:**571–585, **1977.**

Enesco, H. E., and Verdone-Smith, C.: α-Tocopherol increases lifespan in the rotifer. *Philodina. Expl. Gerontol.,* **15:**335–338, **1980.**

Epstein, J., and Gershon, D.: Studies of aging in nematodes, IV. The effect of antioxidants on cellular damage and lifespan. *Mech. Ageing Dev.,* **1:**257–264, **1972.**

Essner, E., and Novikoff, A.: Human hepatocellular pigments and lysomes. *J. Ultra. Res.,* **3:**379–391, **1960.**

Everitt, A. V., and Burgess, J. A.: *Hypothalamus, Pituitary and Aging,* Charles C Thomas, Springfield, IL, **1976.**

Failla, G.: The aging process and somatic mutations. In Strehler, B. L. (ed.): *The Biology of Aging,* Am. Inst. Biol. Sci., Washington, DC, **1960.**

Fanestil, D. D., and Barrows, C. H. Jr.: Aging in the rotifer. *J. Gerontol.,* **20:**462–469, **1965.**

Finch, C. E., and Hayflick, L.: *Handbook of the Biology of Aging,* Van Nostrand, New York, **1977.**

Fleming, J. E.; Melnikoff, P. S.; Latter, G. T.; Chandra, D.; and Bensch, K. G.: Age dependent changes in the expression of Drosophila mitochondrial proteins. *Mech. Ageing Dev.,* **34:**63–72, **1986.**

Flohe, L.; Gunzies, W. A.; and Ladenstein, R.: Glutathion peroxidase. In Arias, I. M., and Jakoby, W. B. (eds.): *Glutathione: Metabolism and Function,* Raven Press, New York, **1976.**

Fridovich, I.: Oxygen radicals, hydrogen peroxide, and oxygen toxicity. In Pryor, W. A. (ed.): *Free Radicals in Biology,* Academic Press, New York, **1977.**

Friede, R. L.: *Topographic Brain Chemistry,* Academic Press, New York, **1966.**

Frolkis, V. V.: *Aging and Life-Prolonging Processes,* Springer-Verlag, New York, **1982.**

Gershon, D.: Current status of age related enzymes: Alternative mechanisms. *Mech. Ageing Dev.,* **9:**189–196, **1979.**

Gershon, H., and Gershon, D.: Inactive enzyme molecules in aging mice: Liver aldolase. *Proc. Natl. Acad. Sci. USA,* **70:**909–913, **1973.**

Goldstein, S.; Wojtyk, R. I.; Harley, C. B.; Pollard, J. W.; Chamberlain, J. W.; and Stanners, C. P.: Protein synthetic fidelity in aging human fibroblasts. In Salk, D.; Fujiwara, Y.; and Martin, G. M. (eds.): *Werners Syndrome and Human Aging,* Plenum Press, New York, **1985.**

Hahn, H. P. V.: The regulation of protein synthesis in the aging cell. *Exp. Gerontol.,* **5:**323–334, **1970.**

Harman, D.: Free-radical theory of aging: Consequences of mitochondrial aging. *Age,* **6:**86–94, **1983.**

Harman, D.: Free radical theory of aging: Role of free radicals in the organization and evolution of life, aging, and disease processes. In Johnson, J. E.; Walford, R.; Harman, D.; and Miquel, J. (eds.): *Free Radicals, Aging and Degenerative Diseases,* Alan R. Liss, New York, **1986.**

Harrison, B. J., and Holliday, R.: Senescence and the fidelity of protein synthesis in *Drosophila. Nature,* **213:**990–992, **1967.**

Hart, R. W.; D'Ambrosio, S. M.; Ng, K. J.; and Modak, S. P.: Longevity, stability and DNA repair. *Mech. Ageing Dev.,* **9:**203–223, **1979.**

Hart, R. W., and Setlow, R. B.: Correlation between deoxyribonucleic acid excision repair and lifespan in a number of mammalian species. *Proc. Natl. Acad. Sci. USA*, **71**:2169–2173, **1974.**

Henshaw, P. S.: Genetic transition as a determinant of physiologic and radiologic aging and other conditions. *Radiology*, **69**:30–36, **1957.**

Hoehn, H.; Bryant, E. M.; Johnston, P.; Norwood, T. H.; and Martin, G. M.: Nonselective isolation, stability and longevity of hybrids between normal human somatic cells. *Nature*, **258**:608–610, **1975.**

Holliday, R., and Tarrant, G. M.: Altered enzymes in aging human fibroblasts. *Nature*, **238**:26–30, **1972.**

Hosbach, M. A., and Kubli, E.: Transfer RNA in aging *Drosophila*: Extent of aminoacylation. *Mech. Ageing Dev.*, **10**:131–140, **1979.**

Ilan, J.; and Patel, N.: Mechanism of gene expression in *Tenebrio molitor. J. Biol. Chem.*, **245**:1275–1281, **1970.**

Kanungo, M. S.: A model for aging. *J. Theor. Biol.*, **53**:253–261, **1975.**

Kanungo, M. S.: *Biochemistry of Ageing*, Academic Press, London, **1980.**

Kanungo, M. S., and Gandhi, B. S.: Induction of malate dehydrogenese isoenzymes in livers of young and old rats. *Proc. Natl. Acad. Sci. USA*, **69**:2035–2038, **1972.**

Kay, M. M. B.: An overview of immune aging. *Mech. Ageing Dev.*, **9**:39–59, **1979.**

Kay, M. M. B.: Immunological aspects of aging: Early changes in thymic activity. *Mech. Ageing Dev.*, **28**: 193–218, **1984.**

Kelley, K. W.; Brief, S.; Westley, H. J.; Navakofski, J.; Bechtel, P. J.; Simon, J.; and Walker, E. B.: GH_3 pituitary ademoma cells can reverse thymic aging in rats. *Proc. Natl. Acad. Sci. USA*, **83**:5663–5667, **1986.**

Klebanoff, S. J.: Oxygen metabolism and the toxic properties of phagocytes. *Ann. Intern. Med.*, **93**:480–489, **1980.**

Kohn, R. R.: *Principles of Mammalian Aging*, 2nd ed., Prentice-Hall, Englewood Cliffs, NJ, **1978.**

Lamb, M. J.: *Biology of Aging*, John Wiley, New York, **1977.**

Loeb, J., and Northrup, J. H.: On the influence of food and temperature on the duration of life. *J. Biol. Chem*, **32**:103–121, **1917.**

Macieira-Coelho, A.; Diatloff, C.; Billard, C.; Borugeois, C. A.; and Malaise, E.: Effects of low dose rate ionizing radiation on the division potential of cells in vitro. III. Human lung fibroblasts. *Exp. Cell Res.*, **104**:215–221, **1977.**

Macieira-Coelho, A.; Diatloff, C.; Billard, M.; Fertil, B.; Malaise, E.; and Fries, D.: Effect of low dose rate irradiation on the division potential of cells in vitro. IV. Embryonic and adult human lung fibroblast-like cells: *J. Cell. Physiol.*, **95**:235–238, **1978.**

Markert, C. L., and Ursprung, H.: The ontogeny of isoenzyme pattens of lactate dehydrogenase in the mouse. *Dev. Biol.*, **5**:363–381, **1962.**

Maynard-Smith, J.: Theories of aging. In Krohn, P. L. (ed.): *Topics in Biology of Aging*, Interscience, New York, **1966.**

Mays, L. L.; Lawrence, A. E.; Ho, R. W.; and Ackley, S.: Age related changes in function of transfer ribonucleic acid of rat livers. *Fed. Proc.*, **38**:1984–1988, **1979.**

Medvedev, Z. A.: The molecular processes of aging. *Sowjet-Wiss Naturwiss, Beitr.*, **12**:1273–1280, **1961.**

Medvedev, Z. A.: The nucleic acids in development and aging. In Strehler, B. L. (ed.): *Advances in Gerontological Research*, Vol. 1, Academic Press, New York, **1964.**

Medvedev, Z. A.: Repetition of molecular-genetic information as a possible factor in evolutionary changes in lifespan. *Exp. Gerontol.*, **7**:227–238, **1972.**

Miquel, J., and Economos, A. C.: Favorable effects of the antioxidants sodium and magnesium thiazolidine carboxylate and the vitality and lifespan of *Drosophila* and mice. *Exp. Gerontol.*, **14**:279–285, **1979.**

Miquel, J.; Lundren, P. R.; and Johnson, J. E.: Spectrophotofluorometric and electron microscopic study of lipofuscin accumulation in the testes of aging mice. *J. Gerontol.*, **33**:5–19, **1978.**

Munnel, J., and Getty, R.: Rate of accumulation of cardiac lipofuscin in the aging canine. *J. Gerontol.*, **23**:154–158, **1968.**

Nagy, I. Z.: A membrane hypothesis of aging. *J. Theor. Biol.*, **75**:189–195, **1978.**

Orgel, L. A.: The maintenance of the accuracy of protein synthesis and its relevance to aging. *Proc. Natl. Acad. Sci. USA*, **49**:517–521. **1963.**

Orgel, L. A.: Aging of clones of mammalian cells. *Nature*, **243**:441–445, **1973.**

Patnaik, S. K., and Kanungo, M. S.: Soluble alanine aminotransferase of the liver of rats of various ages: Induction, characterization and changes in patterns. *Ind. J. Biochem. Biophys.*, **13**:117–124, **1976.**

Reiss, V., and Gershon, D.: Rat liver superoxide dismutase. Purification and age related modifications. *Eur. J. Biochem.*, **63**:617–623, **1976a.**

Reiss, V., and Gershon, D.: Comparison of cytoplasmic superoxide dismutase in liver, heart and brain of aging rats and mice. *Biochem. Biophys. Res. Commun.*, **73**:255–262, **1976b.**

Reitz, M. S., and Sanadi, D. R.: An aspect of translational control of protein synthesis in aging: Changes in the isoaccepting forms of tRNA in *Turbatrix aceti. Exp. Gerontol.*, **7**:119–129, **1972.**

Rockstein, M.: *Theoretical Aspects of Aging*, Academic Press, New York, **1974.**

Rothstein, M.: The formation of altered enzymes in aging animals. *Mech. Ageing Dev.*, **9**:197–202, **1979.**

Sacher, G. A.: Life table modification and life prolongation. In Finch, C. E., and Hayflick, L. (eds.): *Handbook of the Biology of Aging*, Van Nostrand Reinhold, New York, **1977.**

Samorajski, T.; Ordy, J.; and Keefe, J.: The fine structure of lipofuscin age pigment in the nervous system of aged mice. *J. Cell Biol.*, **26**:779–795, **1965.**

Sharma, H. K.; Prassanna, H. R.; and Rothstein, M.: Altered phosphoglycerate kinase in aging rats. *J. Biol. Chem.*, **255**:5043–5050, **1980.**

Sharma, H. K., and Rothstein, M.: Age-related changes in the properties of enolase from *Turbatrix aceti. Biochemistry*, **17**:2869–2876, **1978.**

Sharma, R., and Patnaik, S. K.: Properties of liver cytoplasmic asparate aminotransferase of rats of various ages. *Biochem. Int.*, **5**:561-566, **1982.**

Sharma, R., and Patnaik, S. K.: Regulation of citrate synthetase and phosphoenolpyruvate carboxykinase by hydrocortisone in the liver of aging rats. *Arch. Gerontol. Geriatr.*, **3**:167–174, **1984.**

Sharma, R., and Patnaik, S. K.: Age-depdendent response of aspartate aminotransferase isoenzymes to hydrocortisone in the brain of male rats. *Mol. Physiol.*, **7**:195–200, **1985.**

Shock, N. W.: Systems integration. In Finch, C. E., and Hayflick, L. (eds.): *Handbook of the Biology of Aging*, Van Nostrand, New York, **1977.**

Shock, N. W.: Systems Physiology and aging: Introduction. *Fed. Proc.*, **38**:161–162, **1979.**

Sinex, E. M.: The molecular genetics of aging. In Finch, C. E., and Hayflick, L. (eds.): *Handbook of the Biology of Aging*, Van Nostrand, New York, **1977.**

Singh, S. N., and Kanungo, M. S.: Alterations in lactate dehydrogenase of the brain, heart, skeletal muscle and liver of rats. *J. Biol. Chem.*, **243**:4526–4529, **1968.**

Sohal, R. S.: Metabolic rate and lifespan. In Cutler, R. G. (ed.): *Interdisciplinary Topics in Gerontology*, Vol.

9, Karger, Basel, **1976.**

Sohal, R. S., and Donato, H.: Effects of experimentally altered life spans on the accumulation of fluorescent age pigment in the housefly, *Musca domestica. Exp. Gerontol.,* **13:**335–341, **1978.**

Stevenson, K. G., and Curtis, H. J.: Chromosomal aberrations in irradiated and nitrogen mustard treated mice. *Radiat. Res.,* **15:**774–784, **1961.**

Strehler, B. L.: Further studies on the thermally induced aging of *Drosophila melanogaster. J. Gerontol.,* **17:**347–352, **1962.**

Strehler, B. L.: On the histochemistry and ultrastructure of age pigment. In Strehler, B. L. (ed.): *Advanced Gerontological Research,* Academic Press, New York, **1964.**

Strehler, B. L.: *Time Cells and Aging,* 2nd ed., Academic Press, New York, **1977.**

Strehler, B. L.; Mark, D. D.; Mildvan, A. S.; and Gee, M. V.: Rate and magnitude of age pigment accumulation in the human myocardiam. *J. Gerontol.,* **14:**430–439, **1959.**

Szabo, D.; Desinick, C.; Kros, I.; and Stark, E.: The ultrastructure of the aged rat zona fasiculata under various stressing procedures. *Exp. Gerontol.,* **5:**335–337, **1970.**

Szilard, L.: On the nature of the aging process. *Proc. Natl. Acad. Sci. USA,* **45:**30–45, **1959.**

Tappel, A.: Lipid peroxidation and fluorescent molecular damage to membranes. In Trumps, B., and Arstila, A. (eds.): *Pathology of Cell Membranes,* Academic Press, New York, **1975.**

Thompson, K. V. A., and Holliday, R.: The longevity of diploid and polyploid human fibroblasts: Evidence against somatic mutation theory of cellular aging. *Exp. Cell Res.,* **112:**281–287, **1978.**

Tice, R. R.: Aging and DNA repair capability. In Schneider, E. L. (ed.): *The Genetics of Aging,* Plenum Press, New York, **1978.**

Timiras, P. S.: Biological perspectives on aging: In search of a masterplan. *Am. Sci.,* **66:**605–613, **1978.**

Timiras, P. S.: Physiology of aging. In Mountcastle, V. B. (ed.): *Medical Physiology,* C. V. Mosby, St. Louis, **1980.**

Timiras, P. S.: Neuroendocrinology of aging: Retrospective, current, and prospective views. In Meites, J. (ed.): *Neuroendocrinology of Aging,* Plenum Press, New York, **1983.**

Timiras, P. S.: Physiology of aging: Brain and hormones set the pace of life. In Johnson, H. A. (ed.): *Relations Between Normal Aging and Disease,* Raven Press, New York, **1985.**

Timiras, P. S.; Choy, V. J.; and Hudson, D. B.: Neuroendocrine pacemaker for growth, development and aging. *Age Ageing,* **11:**73–88, **1982.**

Tonna, E. A.: An electron microscopic study of skeletal cell aging. II. The osteocyte. *Exp. Gerontol.,* **8:**9–16, **1973.**

Verzar, F.: *Lectures on Experimental Gerontology,* Charles C Thomas, Springfield, IL, **1963.**

Verzar, F.: Ageing of the collagen fiber. *Int. Rev. Connect. Tissue Res.,* **2:**245–299, **1964.**

Walburg, H. W., Jr.: Radiation-induced life shortening and premature aging. *Adv. Radiat. Biol.,* **5:**145–179, **1975.**

Walford, R. L.: *The Immunologic Theory of Aging,* Williams & Wilkins, Baltimore, **1969.**

Walford, R. L.: The immunologic theory of aging: Current status. *Fed. Proc.,* **33:**2020–2027, **1974.**

Walker, R. F., and Timiras, P. S.: Pacemaker insufficiency and the onset of aging. In Carpenter, D. (ed.): *Cellular Pacemakers,* vol. 2. John Wiley, New York, **1982.**

Warren, S.: Longevity and causes of death from irradiation in physicians. *JAMA,* **162:**464–468, **1956.**

Wheeler, K. T., and Lett, J. T.: On the possibility that DNA repair is related to age in nondividing cells. *Proc. Natl. Acad. Sci. USA,* **71:**1862–1865, **1974.**

Wodinski, J.: Hormonal inhibition of feeding and death in octopus: Control by optic gland secretion. *Science,* **198:**948–951, **1977.**

Yang, W. K.: Isoaccepting transfer RNAs in mammalian differentiated cells and tumor tissues. *Cancer Res.,* **31:**639–643, **1971.**

Zuckerlandl, E.: The evolution of hemoglobin. *Sci. Am.,* **212:**110–118, **1965.**

PART
II Molecular and Cellular Aging

CHAPTER
5 DEGENERATIVE CHANGES IN CELLS AND CELL DEATH

Although each cell type follows its own timetable of aging, some processes are shared by all cells or at least a large group of cells. A number of these common features will be summarized in this chapter with the caution, however, that it is practically impossible to separate age-related cellular changes from pathologic cellular changes associated with the diseases of old age. The ways in which cells, tissues, and organs, as well as whole organisms, respond to the innumerable noxious agents to which they are continually exposed are limited; consequently, similar structural, functional, and biochemical alterations may result from a myriad of causes related and unrelated to disease factors. In addition, the older individual will inevitably have been exposed to more diseases than the younger, and changes consequent to pathologic processes may be expected to be compounded with those due to physiologic aging.

Given these limitations, attempts have been made to identify in the aging process certain basic criteria that could be meaningfully applied at different levels of biologic organization. Thus, as already mentioned in Chapter 2, changes with aging may be qualified as *universal,* i.e., occurring in all members of the same species: as *intrinsic,* independent of environmental factors; as *progressive,* occurring gradually and cumulatively; and as *deleterious,* leading to decreased functional capacity and death (Strehler, 1977). This and similar classifications, although still controversial, offer, nevertheless, some useful guidelines for the selection of specific cells, tissues, and organisms as models for the study of aging.

In the present chapter, cellular aging will be discussed in terms of events specific to cellular aging and death. Irrespective of their cause, cellular and molecular changes often represent the final common pathway(s) of all degenerative alterations responsible for impairment and failure of cell function that are the consequence of cell injury in general. Severe alterations involved in the final stages of cell degeneration and resulting in cell loss are far easier to recognize than changes that, especially at their onset, are often too subtle to be analyzed by techniques presently available and, in many cases, only become manifest at advanced stages of aging.

Only a few specific cellular changes can be ascribed to aging *per se* according to the viability of tissues from old animals transplanted into young recipients. Exceptions are perhaps represented by the intracellular accumulation of the so-called "age pigments," verified by *in vivo* studies and the demonstration of the limited proliferative capability of cells cultured *in vitro,* the latter utilized as a model of cellular aging.

CELLULAR AGING

In complex organisms such as mammals, organs are formed by a variety of tissues, and tissues by a variety of cellular and extracellular elements, each aging at its own

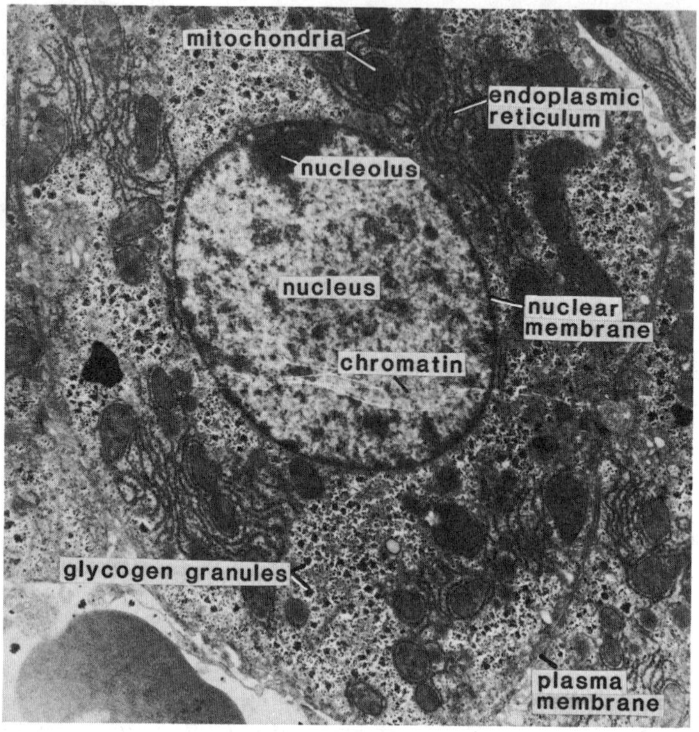

Figure 5–1. *Transmission electron micrograph of a mouse hepatocyte; overview of the major cell organelles. Mag. × 4900.* (Courtesy of Dr. M. Schliwa).

rate. At any given age and in any given tissue or organ, the degree of impairment varies with the cell type. In the nervous tissue, neurons do not divide after birth but undergo continuous and irreversible changes with age, whereas glial cells continue to divide throughout life. Within the cell, organelles age at different rates, and depending on the organelle, even a slight impairment may have crucial functional and biochemical repercussions on the entire cell. In the present section we shall review briefly the major cell constituents and their changes with aging.

Cellular Organization and Function. Since 1839 when Theodor Schwann first propounded the cell theory, the key to every biologic problem must ultimately be sought at the cellular and molecular level. Cells have undergone considerable specialization among higher animals, and no human cell can be called typical of all cells in the body. However, a composite model can be drawn showing the structures common to most cells in order to point out the shared anatomic features.

All cells have a membrane, a cytoplasm containing various organelles, and a nucleus (Figure 5–1). The *membrane* or *plasma membrane* surrounding the cell is approximately 100 Å thick and, like all membranes, it contains proteins and lipids. The ratio of these two major constituents, however, varies enormously: the inner mitochondrial membrane is 76% protein, whereas the myelin is 18% protein. The composition of lipids varies greatly among different membranes. The major structural unit is the phospholipid bilayer, with the hydrophobic fatty acid chains forming the interior of the membrane and the polar heads facing the surrounding watery surface. At physiologic temperatures, lipid (hydrocarbon) chains are relatively fluid and the bulk of lipids is in a liquid-crystalline state. This state, characterized by relatively higher fluidity, is to be distinguished from a gel phase in which lipid chains are rigid and closely packed with low fluidity. Carbohydrates, too, are an important constituent of many membranes.

The membrane is semipermeable and capable of active transport; that is, it allows some substances to pass through (e.g., potassium ions) but excludes other (e.g., sodium ions). Large molecules can gain entry to the interior of the cell, perhaps by passing through holes or pores, or can bind to receptor sites and stimulate cell activity. The cell surface also contains a number of molecular structures, cell-recognition sites, that sense or recognize external signals.

Other membranes that develop around the nucleus and the organelles within the cell have been given the name of *endoplasmic reticulum* (ER). These internal membranes are continuous with the plasma and nuclear membranes, furnishing a vastly increased and deeply invaginated surface area for exchanges within the fluid in which the cell is bathed. There are two types of ER: "rough," studded with ribosomes, and "smooth," without ribosomes. The rough ER participates in the synthesis of certain membrane and organelle proteins as well as the proteins to be secreted by the cell. The smooth ER is the site of the synthesis and metabolism of fatty acids and phospholoids.

The *Golgi apparatus*, a canalicular structure located in the cytoplasm near the nucleus, is the factory for the production or, more accurately, for the "packaging" of protein secreted by the cell and necessary to the production of membranes. The Golgi bodies are prominent in nervous and secretory cells. They may be involved in the transport of secretory products from the inside of the cell to the outside by the process of "exocytosis."

Within the cytoplasm, the most prominent organelles are the *mitochondria*. These are the "power plants" adapted to extract energy from the chemical bonds in the nutrients of the cell by oxidation. From each of these power plants, the yield of energy is made available to the energy-consuming processes of the cell, neatly stored in the phosphate bonds of the compound adenosine triphosphate (ATP). Each mitochondrion is a sausage-shaped membraneous structure about 150,000 Å long and 5000 Å in diameter, containing shelves or cristae. Stacked on these shelves and studding the exterior surface of the mitochondrion are packets of enzymes. These enzymes are involved in the transfer of electrons in biologic oxidations and in the synthesis of ATP through oxidative phosphorylation.

The *lysomes* are membrane-surrounded spherical vesicles in the cytoplasm. They contain a variety of degrading enzymes, such as acid hydrolases, which hydrolyze biopolymers (proteins, carbohydrate, and lipids) that are no longer needed. They also contain ribonucleases and deoxyribonucleases, which degrade RNA and DNA as well.

Granules attached to the endoplasmic reticulum are the *ribosomes*. Free ribosomes are also present in the cells. They are about 150 Å in diameter and are made of one layer and one small subunit. Sometimes three to five ribosomes are lumped together forming polyribosomes (polysomes). Ribosomes contain mostly ribonucleic acid (RNA) and proteins. They are the site of protein synthesis. Free ribosomes are involved in the synthesis of cytoplasmic proteins, whereas ER-bound ribosomes are involved in the synthesis of secretory and membrane/organelle bound proteins. These proteins are synthesized on the ribosomes using messenger RNAs transcribed from the DNA.

Different kinds of microtubules and microfilaments together form a flexible framework, the *cytoskeleton*. These protein structures give shape and form to the cell, are essential for cell motility and contractility, and facilitate intracellular communication or segregation. A third element of the cytoskeleton intracellular communication or segregation is *the microtrabecular network*, originally designated as the ground substance and now visualized as a network (under the high-resolution electron microscope).

Another type of membrane-surrounded organelle in the cytoplasm is the *peroxisome* or microbody—segregated within this structure are enzymes that form and use hydrogen peroxide (hence the name). Hydrogen peroxide, extremely toxic to the cell, is hydrolyzed by the enzyme catalase, which protects the cell from self-destruction by the action of peroxides.

A *nucleus*, present in all cells that divide, contains DNA responsible for the replication not only of proteins but also of the nucleic acids DNA and RNA. When the cell is in the resting stage, that is, in the process of growth between divisions, the chromatin (consisting of DNA, RNA, and specialized proteins) is diffusely distributed in the nucleus. The DNA thus makes maximum surface contact with other material in the nucleus from which it presumably pieces together the molecules of RNA and replicates itself. In preparation for cell division (by mitosis for all somatic cells, or by meiosis for the germ cells), the chromatin coils up tightly to form the *chromosomes*. The chromosomes, containing the genes, are the structures that carry a complete blueprint for all the heritable characteristics of the individual; a fixed number (diploid number) are present in each cell to be distributed equally to each daughter cell, except in the germ cells, where the number of chromosomes is halved (haploid number). The nucleus is surrounded by a nuclear membrane with pores. Inside the nucleus is the *nucleolus* rich in RNA, which is the site for assembly of ribosomes.

AGING CHANGES IN MEMBRANES

Microvilli, identifiable on the *cell surface* by scanning microscopy, are a common cellular feature. Their number increases with advancing age in specific cell types *in vivo* (e.g., glomerular podocytes) and in fibroblasts in later population doublings *in vitro* (Johnson, 1979; Kelly and Vogel, 1984). Such an increase is reduced by dietary restriction, a procedure that increases the lifespan of laboratory animals (Johnson and Barrows, 1980) (see Chapter 25). Cell surfaces are involved in several important functions such as cell-to-cell interaction, external signal reception, cell adhesion and motility, and maintenance of cell shape. Microvilli represent an extension of cell surface, especially important in increasing membrane transport and as a reserve for cell movement and division. Their increase with aging may be viewed as a compensatory attempt to correct, in part, decrements in cellular intercommunication leading to a diminished ability to maintain tissue, organ, and organism homeostasis, thereby precipitating aging, pathology and death (Johnson, 1984).

Age-related changes concern both *major membrane constituents*, lipids and proteins, as well as certain cytoskeletal elements that are membrane-bound. So far, emphasis in membrane research has been directed to the study of the lipid bilayer membrane fluidity and the effects of aging thereon. According to the "fluid mosaic model," membrane components are able to diffuse laterally in the plane of the membrane. This diffusion offers a potential mechanism for directed changes in the topography of specific membrane components, with proteins generally diffusing to a greater degree than lipids. Membrane fluidity is influenced by several factors, the most important being temperature, fatty acid unsaturation, cholesterol, and protein content. With aging, membrane lipids are susceptible to peroxidation and membrane fluidity is markedly altered by the increased presence of free radicals (Chapter 7).

Aging-associated changes in membrane composition, especially lipid components, vary depending on cell and membrane type, animal species, diet, exercise, hormones, antigens, mitogens, and so forth. For example, in myocardial mitochondrial membranes, although several phospholipids remain unchanged, cholesterol and cardiolipin are significantly increased in old (33 months) rats as compared to young (4 months) and variable changes in fatty acid composition lead to decreased unsaturation index, suggestive of decreased fluidity (Lewin and Timiras, 1984). Changes in *membrane fluidity* may induce alterations in cell responses involving excitability, transport, and responsiveness to endogenous and exogenous stimulation. As membrane receptors, proteins (and glycoproteins), move along the membrane lipid bilayer, they bind to ligands forming receptor-ligand complexes that aggregate in clusters, patches, or caps. The capacity for the formation and motility of receptor-ligand complexes seems to be diminished in aged individuals and in some forms of accelerated aging such as Down's syndrome (Naeim and Walford, 1980).

Membrane-Associated Cytoskeletal Structures. The affinity or relationship between plasma membrane and cytoskeleton appears to play an important role in the mobility and redistribution of receptor-ligand complexes. For example, in the process of receptor-ligand aggregations, cross-linked surface immunoglobulin becomes attached to actin (Flanagan and Koch, 1978), and this process is significantly lower in the aged (over 85 years. Another example is the implication of tubulin and "tau" microtubule-associated proteins in some aspects of the pathology of the aged brain. Tau proteins have been implicated in the pathology of senile dementia of the Alzheimer type (Chapter 9). These proteins appear associated with the formation of neurofibrillary tangles and neuritic plaques, where they are a major constituent of the paired helical filament and the intracellular amyloid fibrils (Chapter 9). Extensive phosphorylation of tau proteins favors cross-linking of tubulin to actin, whereas dephosphorylation inhibits it. In Alzheimer's disease abnormalities of tau protein could be due to the expression of the fetal form of protein in an attempt to regenerate the altered adult protein (Kosik *et al.*, 1986).

Cytoskeletal elements, by conveying information from cell membrane to intracellular components (Puck, 1977), play an important role in regulating several cell functions, including: response of lymphoid cells to mitogens (Chapter 8), chemotactic responsiveness of neutrofils, lipofuscin, lysosomal content, cell division (see Naeim and Walford, 1985). Alteration of these functions with aging suggests that disorganization of cytoskeletal structures may be a common denominator of some aging phenomena.

Other alterations with aging include lipofuscin accumulation (see below), peroxidation of intracellular membranes (Chapter 7), and alterations in enzymes (Chapter 6), physicochemical changes (leading to increased rigidity, decreased ion conductance), and reduced binding of several specific antigens such as histocompatibility antigens. These antigens are encoded by the major histocompatibility complex (MHC) genes; these receptors are transmembrane cell surface glycoproteins, which represent some of the best-studied surface markers of cells. They change quantitatively and qualitatively with aging, and these changes may be responsible for the increase in autoimmune diseases and other alterations of the immune system with aging (Chapter 8). MHC alleles influence maximum lifespan, DNA repair, free-radical scavengers, and some enzyme activity. They may also be involved in the genetic basis for aging.

AGING CHANGES IN CYTOPLASM

Data on age-related changes in the *endoplasmic reticulum* (ER), the site of protein and steroid synthesis (rough ER) and lipid metabolism (smooth ER), are conflicting. Such changes are important since several theories of aging are based on the fidelity of output of protein synthesis (Chapter 4). Biochemical studies show no or minimal change with aging, and the latter may be either increased or decreased. At the light microscope level, RNA-associated structures represented by the "Nissl bodies" decrease with aging in several cell types, especially those, like neurons, that do not divide after birth and persist throughout the lifespan.

The number of *mitochondria* is reduced with aging in neurons, presynaptic terminals of neuromuscular junction, liver and heart cells, and *in vitro* human fibroblasts. Mitochondrial size, on the other hand, is increased in some cells; this enlargement or "swelling" occurs not only in aging cells, but also in pathology and inadequately fixed cells. The latter is particularly true of the nervous system, where mitochondria often show vacuolations, perhaps due to hypoxia during fixation. Mitochondrial inclusions and changes in shape, perhaps the result of uncoupled respiration, may be the result of artifacts. Because of damage induced by free radicals originating as by-products of oxygen reduction during respiration (Chapter 7), disorganization of mitochondria has been considered the "Achilles' heel" of the aging cell (Fleming *et al.*, 1985). In the brain, the magnitude of tissue shrinkage during fixation depends on age, the shrinkage being more pronounced in tissues from young than old brains, probably because of the higher water content in the former (Haug, 1985). Tissue shrinkage would, undoubtedly, influence cell density as well as distribution and structure of organelles within the cell.

The *Golgi complex* is difficult to measure even with new techniques because it is not contained within a distinct boundary. It appears, however, to be increased in volume in some aging cells, such as rat cortical and vestibular neurons and fibroblasts.

Aging Changes in Nucleus

With advancing age, a number of alterations have been identified by electron microscopy *in vivo* and *in vitro*. They include: irregularities of shape and invagination, interpreted as consequent to reduced blood supply and cell metabolism; chromatin condensation, suggesting lowered functional activity; presence of inclusion bodies, particularly evident in pineal cells and neurons, perhaps related to alterations of intranuclear microtubules and microfilaments; increased number of nucleoli *in vivo* but decreased *in vitro*.

CELL INJURY AND CELL DEATH

The more our knowledge of cell complexity increases, the more we become aware of the difficulty of distinguishing between a normal and an abnormal cell and, even more so, between a normal adult and an aging cell. Formerly, it was considered an easy task to identify a living ameba: it withdrew from a noxious stimulus and, if it failed to withdraw, it was either sick or dead. Today, with current rapid advances in our knowledge in molecular structure, the line between health and injury, even in a simple organism such as the unicellular ameba, is being more finely drawn. Slight swelling of the mitochondria or minute increases in intracellular sodium levels have now become criteria for assessing injury or aging of a cell. Changes in cellular morphology represent only one aspect of cellular aging. Biochemical and functional changes consistently accompany, precede, or cause changes in structure.

If aging is a progressive alteration of structure and an impairment of function with time, then it becomes extremely difficult to differentiate cellular changes occurring with age from those due to injury. In both cases, morphologic changes underlie the functional disturbances that, if the injury is severe enough or the aging process sufficiently advanced, will lead to cellular death. In the present section, we shall briefly illustrate certain types of morphologic alterations in cells. Some aspects of cellular death must also be considered, but the causes of cellular aging and death have already been discussed in Chapter 4 with the theories of aging.

CELL DEGENERATION

Cellular degeneration or cellular infiltration usually refers to morphologic changes that are reversible. Yet, the same influences—injury or aging—that cause cellular degeneration or infiltration, applied over a longer period of time or to a more intense degree, ultimately lead to death of the cell, followed by the morphologic changes recognized as necrosis. In this sense, cellular degeneration and cellular death merely reflect two levels of severity of cell damage, the former compatible with recovery and the latter irreversible. Cellular degenerations and infiltrations have classically been subdivided into specific morphologic patterns based on the nature of the metabolite that accumulates within the cell. Some of the principal changes of this type are listed here; for more detail on this subject, the reader is referred to specialized textbooks of pathology.

CLOUDY SWELLING

Cloudy swelling, most frequently found in the renal tubular cells, hepatic cells, and cardiac muscle fibers, reflects a mild cellular alteration characterized by a slight edema (swelling) with granularity of the cytoplasm. It is ascribed to an increase in intracellular water localized specifically in the endoplasmic reticulum or the mitochondria and consequent to impairment of respiratory energy-releasing mechanisms. The loss of this energy presumably inhibits the cell in its continued excretion of sodium and water. Whether sodium is primarily affected and leads secondarily to increased intracellular water or whether changes in membrane permeability directly increase the passage of water has not yet been established. Edema is often preceded by a decrease in protein synthesis, but the relationship between this loss and edema of mitochondria and endoplasmic reticulum is not clear. A more severe form of intracellular edema is represented by "hydropic" or "vacuolar" degeneration, which is produced in the same way as cloudy swelling but implies a greater accumulation of water often accumulating in vacuoles and throughout the cytoplasm.

DEHYDRATION

Although edema represents a common correlate of cellular injury, a certain degree of dehydration occurs with age, as suggested by the shrunken appearance of skin in general and the "dried-up" appearance associated with senility. Water content decreases during the process of growth, from a total body water value of approximately 80 percent at birth to about 50 percent in the adult; however, further decrease of body water with advancing years occurs at a very slow rate. Indeed, some investigators claim that dehydration *per se* is not a characteristic of aging and that changes in body water with age involve a redistribution of water between extracellular and intracellular compartments rather than a net loss. Such a redistribution may be consequent to a number of factors related either to the cell population of the tissue considered (e.g., loss of cells, redistribution of cell population, replacement of specific cells with fibroblasts) or to shifts in water between intracellular and extracellular spaces (e.g., due to alterations in membrane permeability, ion distribution, energy required for transport). For example, in skeletal muscle of old rats, the extracellular fluid is nearly double that found in young and mature animals, whereas intracellular water and potassium remain relatively constant. In the case of heart, brain, and liver tissue of rats, little change occurs in the amount and composition of either extracellular or intracellular compartments. Conversely, chemical analysis of the kidney in both humans and rats indicates an increase in extracellular water and a considerable decrease in cell mass with age. There is, generally, a positive correlation between the decrease of protoplasmic units (e.g., loss of muscle fibers) and the increase in the proportion of extracellular water to total body water, and a negative correlation with the quantity of intracellular constituents (Andrew, 1968).

FATTY CHANGE

Fatty change (fatty deposition, fatty metamorphosis) refers to an abnormal accumulation of fat within cells (other than those of the adipose tissue) and represents a common response to a derangement of cellular metabolism. Often preceded by cloudy swelling, fatty change is indicative of severe cellular dysfunction, and although in itself it is a reversible alteration, it is often the harbinger of cell death.

In *fatty degeneration,* disturbances in intracellular utilization and mobilization of fat were formerly thought to induce fatty accumulation within the cell. *Fatty infiltrations* result from "systemic disturbances" that expose healthy cells to an excess of metabolites followed by injury to the cell and structural alterations. Consequently, fatty infiltration was assumed to result from "overloading" essentially healthy cells with excessive amounts of systemic fat. No previous cellular alterations appeared to be involved. The etiologic differences between degeneration and infiltration were also purported to be reflected in a differential regional distribution of the fat vacuoles within the cell—numerous small, perinuclear vacuoles characterizing the degenerative change, and solitary, large vacuoles, infiltration. Today, it has become clear that both processes reflect chemical and molecular derangements secondary to a wide variety of adverse influences within and without the cell; hence, the nonrestrictive term "fatty change" or "fatty metamorphosis" is preferred. Thus, the argument that fatty changes occurring in atherosclerotic lesions originate as a consequence of a primary alteration within the cells of the arterial wall, or are induced by infiltration of excess lipids circulating in the blood, can be resolved by accepting the view that both degenerative and infiltrative processes may be operative in the production of the atheroma (see Chapter 17).

The appearance of *fatty vacuoles,* whether small or large, represents an absolute increase in intracellular fat. Five possible mechanisms have been invoked to explain fat accumulation: increased transport of fat from the periphery to the liver; decreased mobilization from the liver; decreased cell utilization; increased liver cell synthesis of fat; and increased pinocytosis of chylomicrons from the gut. Normal fat metabolism depends on a continuous source of energy; therefore, any impairment of cellular respiration, either by damage of the mitochondria or by direct inactivation of respiratory enzymes, would diminish the activation and utilization of fatty acids. Lipids normally exist in the cell in two patterns: dispersed, micellar form (often not visible optically and not detected by the usual lipid stains) and visible droplets (characterized by specific staining reactions). The stability of the micellar form depends on the cellular content of the lipids and proteins that form lipoproteins, especially phospholipids, which seem to possess a significant stabilizing influence. Any imbalance in the concentration or quantity of these substances may transform invisible micellar fat into the visible globular form. Such an imbalance may occur when excess fat is brought to the cell, or is synthesized within the cell, when a deficiency of lipotropic factors results in inadequate synthesis of phospholipids, when the cell is poorly oxygenated and not enough energy is present to form ATP necessary for cell energy metabolism, or when cholesterol levels are increased. All these conditions, either singly or in association, may be found in aging cells and explain why fatty change is often one of the characteristic signs of the aged cell.

Stromal fatty infiltration, or fatty ingrowth, represents the accumulation of fat into connective tissue cells of the heart and pancreas, with transformation of these cells into adipose cells. As far as is known, these changes have no effect on cardiac or pancreatic function nor are they specifically associated with aging of these organs.

GLYCOGEN INFILTRATION (DEGENERATION)

Glycogen is normally present in all cells and is particularly abundant in muscle and liver cells. In certain conditions, abnormal amounts of glycogen accumulate within the cell producing microscopically visible vacuoles of glycogen within the cytoplasm or nuclei of the affected cells. Because these cells do not seem to be functionally damaged, and because cell death is not usually associated with such glycogen accumulation, this change is considered to represent a metabolic imbalance between glycogenesis and glycogenolysis; i.e., either excessive amounts of glucose produce abnormal amounts of glycogen or there is some derangement in the mechanisms for mobilization or utilization of glycogen stores, with consequent glycogen accumulation. Glycogen infiltrations are found chiefly in two disorders: diabetes mellitus and glycogen storage diseases (e.g., von Gierke's disease). In diabetes mellitus, glycogen vacuoles appear in liver and kidney cells and reflect the high levels of glucose in the blood and urine. To what extent diabetes mellitus can be considered a disease of aging is discussed elsewhere (see Chapter 16). In the glycogen storage diseases, the defect is one of mobilization, usually consequent to the inherited deficiency of an enzyme necessary for normal carbohydrate metabolism.

AGE PIGMENTS OR LIPOFUSCIN

The "age pigments," so called because of their accumulation in the cytoplasm of the cells with the passage of time, have been variously designated in the past as ceroid, chromolipoid, wear-and-tear pigment, yellow pigment, lipopigment, lipogene pigment, and senile pigment. "Lipofuscin" (lipo from the Greek: fat; "fuscin" from the Latin: dusky) is also employed interchangeably with "age pigments."

At the light microscope level, pigment is seen as yellow to brown round or oblong granules, diffused throughout the cytoplasm, in perinuclear clusters or polar aggregates. The latter types, which appear in older tissues, probably represent the more advanced forms. The characteristics of lipofuscin easily differentiate it from other cell components and inclusions, even though these characteristics vary among individuals according to the tissue and age of the subject.

Lysosomes and Lipofuscin. Lysosomes containing acid hydrolases are responsible for degrading polymeric deposits. Lipofuscin may derive from such deposits. Biochemical analyses of lipofuscin suggest that it is derived from a lipoprotein complex such as that found in cell membranes. Substances similar to lipofuscin can be produced by *in vitro* peroxidation of lipid and protein (see Chapter 7). No part of a cell is immortal; even in growing cells in which micromolecules and organelles are increasing, there is a constant degradation of membranes, proteins, and other constituents. Some of these molecules are nondegradable or cannot be degraded by the aged organelles and accumulate as undigested granules.

There are many explanations for the indigestibility of various materials, especially those of a lipoprotein nature. Lysosomes may be deficient in lipolytic enzymes, leaving many fatty substances undigested (De Duve, 1964). Possibly during digestion the peroxidation of fats, followed by copolymerization with protein, produces residues resistant to further degradation. Another source of slowly degraded material are the antibody-antigen complexes that form progressively with age. Any factor producing cell injury would seemingly activate the lysosomal system and control autodigestion. Thus, it becomes evident that any number of physical, chemical, or environmental agents could easily increase lipid deposition by simply overloading the variable capacities of the different cell populations to dispose of affected cellular structures. The extremely active cardiac muscle and nervous tissue accumulate a considerable amount of pigment during the life of an organism. The inadequacy of cells in disposing of these materials may have important functional consequences, for the cytoplasm is congested with residues capable of impairing the efficiency of its function, even though the effect may not be sufficient to jeopardize the life of the whole organism.

The presence of lipofuscin in aging organisms appears to be a phenomenon that is universal, phylogenetically, from Protozoa through Chordata, including man (Sohal, 1981). Indeed, the gradual accumulation of lipofuscin with age, first detected in nerve cells, was one of the earliest-recognized characteristics of this substance. Although lipofuscin has been found to accumulate in certain tissues, it is not found in others and displays a differential pattern of deposition within a given tissue. Indeed, age pigments seem to demonstrate certain cellular specificities. For example, the zona reticularis in the adrenal gland of the senile rat has five times more pigment than any other zone in that structure, whereas in the rat ovary, the pigment is localized exclusively in the perifollicular macrophages, not in the ovarian follicles (Reichel, 1968). Age pigments accumulate preferentially in the muscles of locomotion as opposed to those used to maintain posture (Kny, 1937). Given such cellular and regional differences within a single structure, and the fact that some tissues do not accumulate pigment at all, the assumption that age pigments are a homogeneous group of substances whose accumulation in different cells of the body results from the same processes in every case should perhaps be questioned.

The rate of lipofuscin deposition is consistent enough to render it a reliable index of chronologic age. Lipofuscin is scant or absent until age 10 in heart muscle and accumulates thereafter at a rate of 0.3 percent of the total heart volume per decade, or 0.6 percent of the intracellular volume per decade, independent of cardiac pathology or the presence or absence of heart failure (Chapter 4, Figure 4–4). Thus, the heart of a person living to be 90 years of age would be expected to have 6 to 7 percent of its intracellular volume occupied by age pigment (Strehler *et al.*, 1959).

It has been suggested that the formation of age pigments is caused, or at least influenced, both by extrinsic factors, such as drugs, hypoxia, vitamin E deficiency, and cirrhosis, and by intrinsic factors, which are essentially genetic. In this respect,

Strehler (1977) proposed that "rare and irreparable metabolic accidents beyond the genetic design gradually result in the accumulation of insoluble, nonfunctional, or noxious by-products of metabolism"—the so-called "clinker theory"—and he later postulated that lipofuscin formed because of a genetic omission rendering nondividing, nonreplaceable cells susceptible to slow deteriorative changes (stochastic senescence).

Yet, the evidence against generalized impairment of function in nondividing cells has been rather substantial, particularly with respect to human, rat, and mouse myocardia, which show no loss of ability to hypertrophy throughout adulthood despite increased deposition of age pigments. Even though pigment accumulation in neural cells is sufficient to displace the cell nucleus (see Chapter 9), whether this is an excessive accumulation of lipofuscin or whether the cell has degenerated from other causes and pigment masses formed as a result of such deterioration is not known. Batten's disease is a rare example of nerve cell degeneration associated with abnormal quantities of lipofuscin and can be distinguished from amaurotic familial idiocy by the characteristic accumulation of age pigments rather than the sphingolipids and brain atrophy of children so afflicted. It is plausible that the aggregations of lipofuscin characteristic of advanced age decrease cellular plasticity and, thus, interfere with the ability of the cell to maintain itself. Until precise methods are available to correlate the level of cellular function with the amount of lipofuscin present in a given tissue, however, the questions of whether the changes associated with age pigment accumulation are deleterious and whether they are causative or symptomatic remain unanswered. Without identification of the chemical nature of lipofuscin, any theories regarding the potential involvement of this pigment in aging can, at best, be considered only speculative. Nevertheless, the progressive increase of lipofuscin in the aging cell, and its association with pathologic processes characterized by accelerated aging, strongly suggest that the accumulation of these pigments is significant, if not integral, to the aging process and, as such, well justifies the amount of research to which it has been and continues to be subjected.

Properties of Lipofuscin Granules. One of the most consistent properties of lipofuscin is its autofluorescence in response to stimulation by visible or near-ultraviolet light. When viewed in the fluorescent microscope, it appears as a yellow, yellowish-green, and orange mass. Despite inherent differences in the composition of the granules from different specimens, the relative distribution of its three main constituents has been determined: lipid (19 to 51 percent), protein (30 to 50 percent), and acid hydrolysis-resistant residue (9 to 30 percent).

Analysis of the lipid component has demonstrated that phospholipids account for three-fourths of the lipids present (Ellender, 1981). Cholesterol and its derivatives, triglycerides, cephalins, lecithin, and sphingomyelin, comprise most of the specific lipids identified, with traces of fatty acids, sulfatides, and gangliosides.

Analysis of the protein fraction following acid hydrolysis has assigned a range of values for the amino acid composition (Hendley *et al.*, 1963a,b). Basically, the composition of the protein extracted from the pigment granules of cardiac muscle did not vary in composition or differ greatly from the amino acid composition of structural proteins isolated from a number of different biologic systems, including cell membranes. Therefore, the protein present would be a structural protein of a high lipid-binding capacity (Packer *et al.*, 1967). Enzymes in isolated lipofuscin granules and in intact tissues include acid phosphatase, alkaline phosphatase, esterase, β-glucuronidase, and succinic dehydrogenase, with differences perhaps (e.g., cathepsin, esterase, or acid phosphatase) in isolated granules with respect to both the types and the amount of enzymatic activity present.

Factors Affecting Pigment Deposition. Dietary factors affect the amount of lipofuscin present in cells. Nerve cells of vitamin E-deficient and senile rats contained significantly higher amounts of pigment (Wunscher and Kustner, 1967). The amount of unsaturated fat present in the diet, irrespective of protein and choline content, also influences lipofuscin deposition (Mason *et al.*, 1946) as does the presence of certain dietary additives, i.e., brown FK, a food coloring. These data agree well with data taken from human populations. It has been shown that the Japanese exhibit nearly twice the rate of pigment accumulation as corresponding American populations—a difference considered to be directly related to the unsaturated fat content of their diet (Strehler, 1977).

Environmental conditions specific to a given geographic location may influence the deposition of age pigments. Sheep grazing on mulga, a shrub indigenous to a certain area in Australia, exhibit a high lipofuscin content in the liver. The exact factor responsible for such an endemic response is still unknown (Winter, 1963).

The relationship between disease processes and abnormal lipofuscin deposition also has received considerable attention in recent years. It has been associated with hypoxia, cirrhosis, biliary cirrhosis as well as with intestinal malabsorption syndromes. Many vascular lesions, such as arterial plaques are similarly associated with abnormal amounts of lipofuscin (Chapter 17). Ceroid, a type of lipofuscin, is the only lipid constituent of arterial plaques that differs from circulating lipids in the plasma. The amount present seems to vary in direct proportion to the degree of intimal thickening in atherosclerotic alterations. Similarly, it has been found in pulmonary lipid emboli produced in choline-deficient rats.

AMYLOID

Amyloid is a generic term for proteinaceous fibrillar deposits with the properties of yellow to green birefringence in crossed polaroid illumination after staining with Congo red, a β-pleated sheet structure of the fibrils, and insolubility and resistance to enzymatic digestion (Glenner, 1980a,b). Amyloidosis or amyloid accumulation is not a single disease entity but a variety of different disease processes resulting in the deposition of specific fibrils (β-fibrillosis) from various proteins by several pathogenic mechanisms. Amyloidoses may occur in normal aging as well as in aging-associated diseases or in other debilitating diseases, for example, myeloma (primary systemic amyloidosis) produced by proteolytic cleavage of the N-terminal variable region of immunoglobulin light chain in phagocytic cells (Glenner *et al.*, 1971). In other systemic amyloidoses such as inflammatory amyloidosis, the amyloid fibrils derive from systemic amyloidotic protein or in familial amyloidotic polyneuropathy from a prealbumin variant or in hereditary Icelandic cerebrovascular amyloidosis from a trace serum variant (Ghiso *et al.*, 1986). In Alzheimer's disease three types of amyloid deposits have been recognized: intracellular neurofibrillary tangles, vascular amyloid, and plaque core amyloid (Glenner and Wong, 1984a,b) (see Chapter 10).

Deposition of amyloid has long been known to be present in degenerating tissues; however, controversy still exists regarding its origin and the mechanisms responsible for its deposition (Gorevic *et al.*, 1985). Amyloid may represent a heterogeneous composite that includes fragments of processed serum immunoglobulins and heterogeneous cells protein. Immunoglobulins, immune complexes, and nonimmunoglobulin molecules may be catabolized by phagocytes (microglial cells in the central nervous system) and the protein fragments degraded in lysosomes in a manner leading to the deposition of extracellular amyloid.

CELL DEATH AND NECROSIS

The terms "cell death" and "necrosis" are often used interchangeably, although they refer to quite different phenomena. As with the whole organism, cells die when their vital functions cease. Sometimes one particular vital activity comes to a halt before the others; e.g., the heart may continue to beat for a short time after respiration has ceased. Similarly, when cellular respiratory mechanisms are destroyed, synthetic activities may continue very briefly. This dissociation of vital functions at the cellular level makes it extremely difficult to be certain of the precise moment of cell death. "Although it is possible at certain stages to say of a cell that it is 'alive' or 'dead,' the transition period between these two stages is, as yet, ill-defined. It is not known which function or chemical reaction, when lost, is the first cause of irreversible damage to structural and metabolic integrity" (King *et al.*, 1959).

Necrosis, on the other hand, refers to distinct morphologic changes that permit recognition of the fact that the cell has died. Such morphologic changes occur only gradually; sudden cellular death, as occurs when cells are fixed in formalin, for example, is not associated with demonstrable alterations in cell morphology. Thus, the patient who dies suddenly of a myocardial infarction may show no cardiac morphologic alterations, at least as detectable by our present techniques. Had the patient survived 24 hours or longer, enzymatic changes would have ensued and eventually permitted recognition of the necrotic myocardium. The structural alterations of necrosis, then, are biochemically induced by enzymes of intra- and extracellular origin.

For example, even though the cell is deprived of oxygen, the glycogen processes continue to produce lactic acid, which accumulates and causes the intracellular pH to drop. The lowered pH activates lysosomal enzymes, and proteolytic digestion of the cell follows. Necrosis must also be distinguished from autolysis: in necrosis, cell death occurs while the organism is still alive, whereas in autolysis, cell death follows the death of the entire organism. Death of the entire organism is referred to as somatic death, which, for medicolegal purposes, is said to occur when cardiac function ceases. A number of events follow cessation of the heartbeat: cooling, stiffening of the body, clotting of the blood, discoloration of tissues, hemolysis of blood, and, finally, self-digestion or autolysis.

From a histologic point of view, several types of cell necrosis can be distinguished—coagulative, liquefactive, enzymatic, caseous, gangrenous, and fibrinoid—which all share the same general characteristics but differ in specific patterns and etiology. Perhaps the first definite morphologic indication of necrosis as revealed by the light microscope is represented by change in the nucleus, specifically, increased basophilia (black-blue pigmentation) and shrinkage of the nucleus, known as "pyknosis," with or without breakdown of the nuclear membrane. On the other hand, studies with the electron microscope identify the first lesion of cellular death as the deterioration of mitochondria, impairment of oxidative phosphorylation rather than as nuclear damage. The necrotic cells are either eliminated by enzymatic (lysosomal) dissolution and reabsorption or phagocytized by white blood cells.

Causes of Cell Death. All cells engage in four basic major activities: the production of energy needed for vital cell processes, synthesis of proteins (both enzymatic and structural), maintenance of the chemical and osmotic homeostasis of the cell, and reproduction. The ultimate causes of cell death must involve a derangement of these vital functions at the molecular level. Regrettably, in most instances, we can only guess at the manner in which aging adversely affects these functions. Several theories have been postulated to explain the cellular damage that occurs with the passage of time; however, the primary site of the lesion and its importance to survival remain to be established (Chapter 4).

TRANSPLANTATION STUDIES IN AGING

Surgical techniques and follow-up therapy of recipient patients have currently progressed to the extent that major restrictions to transplantation intervention are lack or scarcity of available organs rather than technologic limitations.

Some of the first experiments in which transplantation was used to investigate changes with aging were conducted in the 1950s: adrenocortical tissue from middle-aged rats (donors) was transplanted into young recipients, and these subsequently lived a little longer than control rats, with normal growth rates and reproductive performances (Geiringer, 1954, 1956). Although the lifespan of the recipient rats was slightly prolonged, it remained short of the maximal rat longevities obtained with other types of interventions such as dietary restriction (Chapter 25). Since then, many other experiments have confirmed that a large number of tissues—adrenal cortex, skin, pituitary, mammary epithelium, kidneys, blood stem cells—are capable of functioning normally well beyond donor lifespans when transplanted from an old donor to a young recipient (Harrison, 1985). Such transplantation procedures have opened several practical routes of interventions for replacement of diseased organs or deficient tissues; they have also served to validate or deny some theories of aging. For example, theories predicting that all tissues, and cells, age intrinsically, must be modified to recognize that, in many cases, tissues do not age as rapidly as the animal from which they come.

A major consideration in assessing the value of transplanted tissues is the ability to establish some functional criteria for identification of the transplanted tissues and their functional status. These may be at the organismic or tissue level, such as the color of hair produced by skin, the genotype of offspring produced by an ovary, the hemoglobin type produced by erythrocytes.

Other methods may utilize molecular

techniques, such as messenger RNA or DNA clones, embryonic nuclear transplantation. Utilizing the latter, for example, nuclei from embryonic cells were transferred into fertilized eggs, and normal mice were born with genetic markers characteristic of the transplanted nuclei (Illmensee and Hoppe, 1981). These results were obtained from embryonic nuclei, and it must yet be tested whether such products could also arise utilizing older or aged nuclei. Techniques are continuously being developed for transplants of vital organs (heart, kidney, liver, bone marrow) in humans. Well-defined measures are used to assure optimal matching histocompatibility (Chapter 8) and pre- and posttransplantation treatment that maximizes graft success and the individual's survival. These techniques should make possible long-term tissue transplantation between young and old donors. Another approach that shows promise is the use of cell cultured *in vitro* for use in *in vivo* transplants.

AGING UNDER GLASS; THE HUMAN FIBROBLAST

Tissue culture methods, "aging under glass," have potential value in transplantation but also are a valuable means of investigating developmental and aging phenomena (see also Chapter 3). By these techniques, control of milieu of the growing tissue or cell permits easier distinction of extrinsic and intrinsic factors in aging (Norwood and Smith, 1985). Several experiments have shown that somatic cell strains have a finite doubling potential *in vitro* and undergo aging and death even under optimal conditions of culture (Hayflick, 1977). Normal human fibroblasts, spindle-shaped cells most capable of sustained proliferation, derived from several embryonic organs, undergo a finite number of population doublings (approximately 50 doublings) after which the cultured cells degenerate and die. Once established in culture, the fibroblasts grow and multiply through successive passages: each time a culture has doubled in size, it is divided into two subcultures, each of which is allowed to double in size again; this process is repeated through a specified number of so-called doublings. Finally, the proliferative activity declines, the time required for the cells to double in number becomes longer, and this increased growth latency leads to complete failure of cell replication (Figure 5–2). This phenomenon is not caused by any deficiency or toxicity of the culture medium or methodologic artifact, but has been interpreted as a manifestation of intrinsic cellular senescence (Pool and Metter, 1984).

IMMORTALITY VERSUS MORTALITY OF CELLS

According to current views, most normal animal cells have a limited proliferative capacity when grown *in vitro*. Since the experiments of Carrel (1912), it was held that isolated cells maintained in culture were capable of unlimited proliferation—a view contradicted by current findings. The "immortality" of the fibroblasts claimed by Carrel in his studies of the heart of the chick embryo is now viewed as the result of a technical artifact. Two fundamental types of cells are now identified *in vitro*: according to the Tissue Culture Association, cell types can be distinguished according to their growth potential by the terms of "finite" or "continuous" used as prefixes to the general term of "cell line," which denotes a culture of multiple lineages arising from the subcultivation of a primary culture. Cells growing *in vitro* usually demonstrate a finite proliferative capacity and those with unlimited capacity for division are inevitably abnormal in one or more properties and most often resemble cancer cells (Rosengurt, 1986). The spontaneous occurrence of a transformed cell line with cells of unlimited growth *in vitro* is a rare event regardless of the species studied. The question of the mechanism(s) that limit the growth potential of fibroblasts remains unanswered, as well as that of the factors that stimulate growth potential. Molecular techniques utilizing viruses to study proliferative mechanisms may provide the needed information. For example, the temperature-sensitive strain of the tumor virus SV-40 can reinitiate DNA synthesis in senescent cells (Gorman and Cristofalo, 1982). It is not yet clear whether the limited *in vitro* proliferative potential of cultured cells is

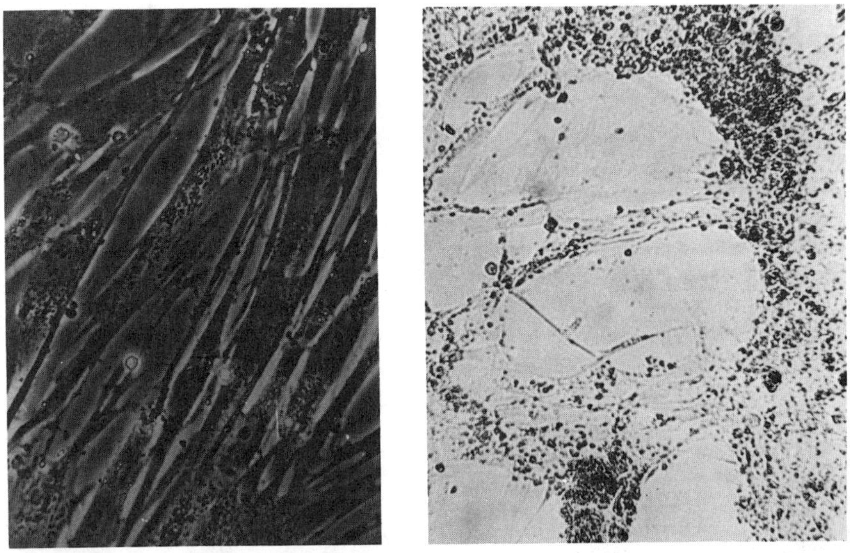

Figure 5–2. *Aging of human fibroblast* in vitro.

Phase contrast micrographs of the human diploid cell strain WI-38. *Left.* During active cell division. *Right.* At the end of its *in vitro* lifetime (after 50 doublings in cell culture). (Courtesy of Dr. L. Hayflick.)

determined by cell division rather than by calendar time (Roberts and Smith, 1980). Irrespective of its nature, the proliferative behavior and growth potential of cultured fibroblasts are influenced by a number of variables: medium composition (e.g., serum batch, nutrients), hormones (e.g., extension of cell lifespan by hydrocortisone), donor genotype (e.g., smaller number of doublings in some progeroid syndromes), tissue of origin (e.g., fibroblasts from lungs divide more rapidly than those from skin).

RELEVANCE TO CELLULAR AGING

Several studies have shown that the doubling capacity of cultured fibroblasts does vary with the age of the individual from whom the cells were taken, even though the cells appear biologically identical (Figure 5–3). For example, cells from lung tissue of adult humans reach the phase of declining mitotic activity and increasing degenerative changes after only 20 doublings, whereas cells from embryonic lung tissue undergo approximately 50 doublings before failure to proliferate (Martin *et al.*, 1970). A number of experimental approaches have corroborated the concept that the proliferative activity of cells is finite. Thus, in humans, cells taken from several tissues of normal individuals of different ages and of individuals affected by specific progeroid syndromes show that the replicative lifespan (as measured by the number of doublings of cultured human somatic cells): (1) is a function of the tissue of origin, e.g., fibroblasts from the skin showed the greatest number of doublings (30 to 45) and from the bone the smallest (1), with those from the muscle being intermediate (29 to 30 doublings); (2) is inversely related to the age of the donor; e.g., the number of doublings declines from approximately 45 between birth and 10 years of age to 30 by 80 to 90 years of age; and (3) is a function of the genotype of the donor; e.g., the number of cell doublings decreases to approximately 10 in Werner's syndrome (Chapter 3), as compared with the 40 doublings from normal individuals of the same age. Likewise in other types of progeria, the number of doublings is similarly reduced (Figure 5–4). However, in Down's syndrome, characterized also by accelerated segmental aging (e.g., accumulation of degenerative brain changes) (Chapters 9 and 10), and in diabetes mellitus, characterized by altered glucose transport (Chapter 16), contradictory results

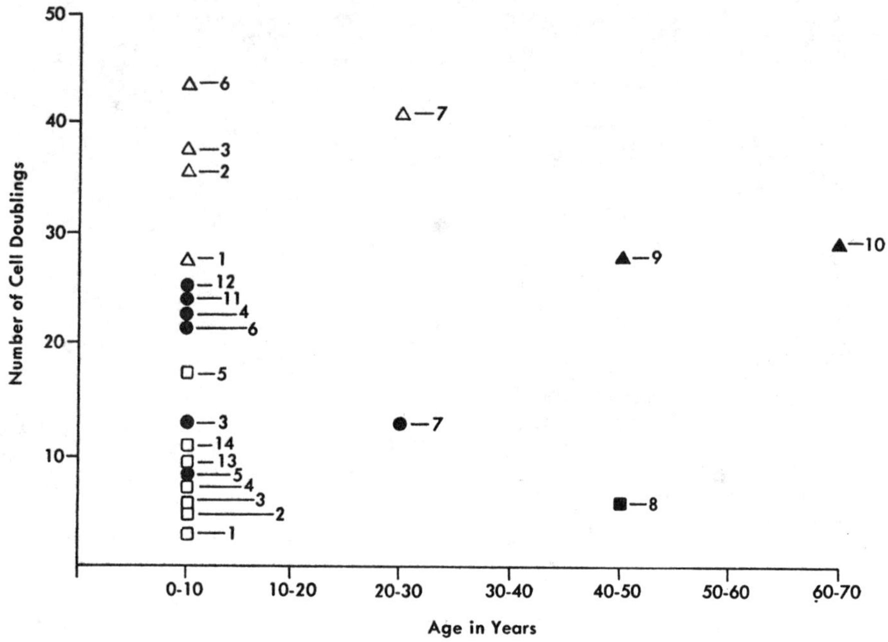

Figure 5–3. *Cumulative number of cell doublings achieved by human fibroblast cultures plotted as a function of the tissue of origin as well as the age of the donor.*

Open triangles, skin; *closed circles,* skeletal muscle; *open squares,* bone marrow spicules; *closed triangles,* testis (controls); *closed square,* testis (Werner's syndrome). The numbers to the right of each culture identify the patients. (From Martin, G.M.; Sprague, C.A.; and Epstein, C.J.: Replicative life-span of cultivated human cells: effects of donor's age, tissue, and genotype. Lab. Invest., *23:86–92, 1970.)*

seem to support or negate a reduced number of doublings.

If the capacity for cell division is taken as an index of cell function, then its loss can be extrapolated to indicate functional impairment with aging. *In vitro* aging is corroborated by numerous morphologic and biochemical alterations in human fibroblasts at or near the end of their proliferative lifespan; these have been extensively reviewed (Hayflick, 1977; Cristofalo *et al.*, 1985; Gracy *et al.*, 1985). Of particular significance are: (1) increasing heterogeneity of cell cycle activity; (2) increased number of lysosomes associated with the formation of autophagic vacuoles and residual bodies; (3) irregular lobation of nuclei; (4) swollen mitochondria, particularly the cristae; (5) abnormalities in the assembly of gap junctions.

Preliminary studies also suggest abnormal responses to external stimuli such as growth factors (e.g., insulin, mitogenic peptides). This altered responsiveness has been ascribed to a reduction of binding sites perhaps due to plasma membrane/cell surface abnormalities. Studies have focused on the membrane-associated glycoprotein fibronectin, which appears to be significantly reduced in the senescent fetal lung cultures (Vogel *et al.*, 1981).

It has been suggested that altered cell surface molecules may be of greater significance in aging *in vitro,* and eventually by extrapolation *in vivo,* than the decrements in proliferative capacity.

References

Andrew, W.: The fine structural and histochemical changes in ageing. In Bittar, E., and Bittar, N. (eds.): *The Biological Basis of Medicine,* Vol. 1, Academic Press, Inc., New York, **1968.**

Carrel, A.: On the permanent life of tissues outside of the organism. *J. Exp. Med.,* **15:**516–528, **1912.**

Christofalo, V. J.; Phillips, P. D.; and Brooks, K. M.: Cellular senescence: Factors modulating cell proliferation *in vitro.* In Woodhead, A. V.; Blackett, A. D.; and Hallaender, A. (eds.): *Molecular Biology of Ag-*

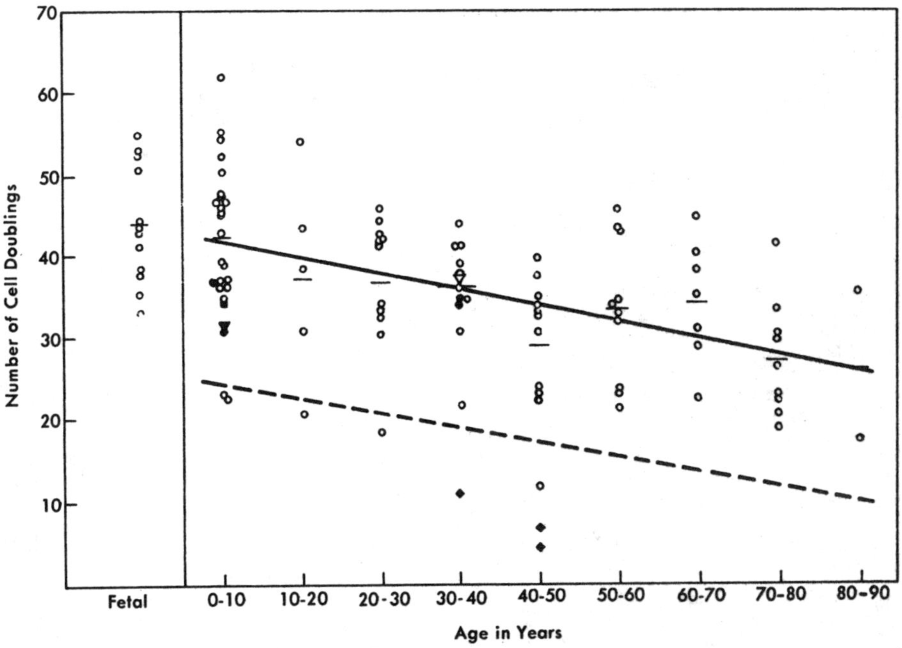

Figure 5–4. *Cumulative number of cell doublings achieved by human skin fibroblast cultures plotted as a function of the age of the donor.*

Open circles, control cultures; *closed diamonds,* Werner's syndrome homozygotes (Werner's syndrome is an autosomal recessively inherited disease characterized by a wide variety of striking degenerative features which have been referred to as a "caricature" of aging); *closed and open triangles,* two types (homo- and heterozygote) of progeria; *closed square,* Rothmund's disease (another recessively inherited disease which has sometimes been related to Werner's syndrome; *closed circles,* parallel cultures from the same donor. The mean for each group is indicated by a horizontal bar. The calculated linear regression line (solid line) for the control group is drawn between the 1st and 9th decades and has a regression coefficient of -0.20 ± 0.05 standard deviation cell doublings per year with correlation coefficient of -0.50. The dashed line is the lower 95% confidence limit for the regression line. In addition to Werner's syndrome, diagnoses for patients whose cultures fell below this line were: congenital heart disease, cystic fibrosis, diabetes mellitus, acute metabolic encephalopathy and carcinoma of the colon. (From Martin, G.M.; Sprague, C.A.; and Epstein, C.J.: Replicative life-span of cultivated human cells: effects of donor's age, tissue, and genotype. *Lab. Invest.,* 23:86–92, 1970.)

ing, Basic Life Sciences, Vol. 35, Plenum Press, New York, **1985.**

De Duve, C.: The lysosome. *Sci. Am.,* **208:**64–72, **1963.**

De Duve, C.: The lyosome: From cytases to lysosomes. *Fed. Proc.,* **23:**1045–1049, **1964.**

Ellender, M.: Chemical characterization of age pigments. In Sohal, R. S. (ed.): *Age Pigments,* Elsevier/North Holland, Amsterdam, **1981.**

Flanagan, J., and Koch, G. L. E.: Cross-linked surface Ig attaches to actin. *Nature,* **273:**278–281, **1978.**

Fleming, J. E.; Miquel, J.; and Bensch, K. G.: Age dependent changes in mitochondria. In Woodhead, A. V.; Blackett, A. D.; and Hollaender, A. (eds.): *Molecular Biology of Aging,* Basic Life Sciences, Vol. 35, Plenum Press, New York, **1985.**

Geiringer, E.: Homotransplantation as a method of gerontological research. *J. Gerontol.,* **9:**142–149, **1954.**

Geiringer, E.: Young rats with adult adrenal transplants: A physiologic study. *J. Gerontol.,* **11:**8–17, **1956.**

Ghiso, J.; Pons-Estel, B.; and Frangione, B.: Hereditary cerebral amyloid angiopathy: The amyloid fibrils contain a protein which is a variant of cystatin C, an inhibitor of lysosomal cysteine proteases. *Biochem. Biophys. Res. Commun.,* **136:**548–554, **1986.**

Glenner, G. G.: Amyloid deposits and amyloidosis. *N. Engl. J. Med.,* **302:**1283–1292, **1980a.**

Glenner, G. G.: Amyloid deposits and amyloidosis. *N. Engl. J. Med.,* **302:**1333–1343, **1980b.**

Glenner, G. G., and Wong, C. W.: Alzheimer's disease: Initial report of the purification and characterization of a novel cerebrovascular amyloid protein. *Biochem. Biophys. Res. Commun.,* **120:**885–890, **1984a.**

Glenner, G. G., and Wong, C. W.: Alzheimer's disease and Down's syndrome: Sharing of a unique cerebrovascular amyloid protein. *Biochem. Biophys. Res. Commun.,* **122:**1131–1135, **1984b.**

Glenner, G. G.; Ein, D.; Eanes, E. D.; Bladen, H. A.; Terry, W.; and Page, D. L.: Creation of "amyloid" fibrils from Bence Jones proteins *in vitro*. *Science*, **174:**712–714, **1971.**

Gorevic, P. D.; Elias, J.; and Peress, N.: Amyloid, immunopathology and aging. In Woodhead, A. D.; Blackett, A. D.; and Hollaender, A. (eds.): *Molecular Biology of Aging*, Basic Life Sciences, Vol. 35, Plenum Press, New York, **1985**.

Gorman, S. D., and Cristofalo, V. J.: Reinitiation of cellular DNA replication in senescent WI-38 cells by simian virus 40, *J. Cell Biol.*, **95:**21a, **1982.**

Gorman, S. D., and Cristofalo, V. J.: Evidence that senescent WI-38 cells are blocked in late G1. *In Vitro*, **20:**281, **1984.**

Gracy, R. W.; Chapman, M. L.; Cine, J. K.; Jahoni, M.; Tollefsbol, T. O.; and Yuksel, K. V.: Molecular basis of the accumulation of abnormal proteins in progeria and aging fibroblasts. In Woodhead, A. V.; Blackett, A. D.; and Hollaender, A. (eds.): *Molecular Biology of Aging*, Basic Life Sciences, Vol. 35, Plenum Press, New York, **1985.**

Harrison, D. E.: Cell and tissue transplantation: A means of studying the aging process. In Finch, C. E., and Schneider, E. L. (eds.): *Handbook of the Biology of Aging*, Van Nostrand Reinhold, New York, **1985.**

Haug, H.: Are neurons of the human cerebral cortex really lost during aging? A morphometric examination. In Traver, Y., and Gispen, W. H. (eds.) *Senile Dementia of the Alzheimer's Type. Early diagnosis, Neuropathology and Animal Models*, Springer-Verlag, New York, **1985.**

Hayflick, L.: The cellular basis for biological aging. In Finch, C. E., and Hayflick, L. (eds.): *Handbook of the Biology of Aging*, Van Nostrand Reinhold, New York, **1977.**

Hendley, D. D.; Mildvan, A. S.; Reporter, M. C.; and Strehler, B. L.: The properties of isolated human cardiac age pigment. I. Preparation and physical properties. *J. Gerontol.*, **18:**144–150, **1963a.**

Hendley, D. D.; Mildvan, A. S.; Reporter, M. C.; and Strehler, B. L.: The properties of isolated human cardiac age pigment. II. Chemical and enzymatic properties. *J. Gerontol.*, **18:**250–259, **1963b.**

Illmensee, K., and Hoppe, P. C.: Nuclear transplantation in *Mus musculus*: Developmental potential of nuclei from preimplantation embryos. *Cell*, **23:**9–18, **1981.**

Johnson, J. E., Jr.: Fine structure of IMR-90 cells in culture as examined by scanning and transmission electron microscopy. *Mech. Ageing Dev.*, **10:**405–443, **1979.**

Johnson, J. E., Jr., and Barrows, C. H.: Effects of age and dietary restriction on the kidney glomeruli of mice: Observations by scanning electron microscopy. *Anat. Rec.*, **196:**145, **1980.**

Johnson, J. E., Jr.: *In vivo* and *in vitro* comparisons of age-related fine structural changes in cell components. In Johnson, J. E., Jr. (ed.): *Aging and Cell Structure*, Vol. 2, Plenum Press, New York, **1984.**

Kelley, R. O., and Vogel, K. G.: The aging cell surface: Structural and biochemical alterations associated with progressive subcultivation of human diploid fibroblasts. In Johnson, J. E., Jr. (ed.): *Aging and Cell Structure*, Vol. 2, Plenum Press, New York, **1984.**

King, D. W.; Paulson, S. R.; Hannaford, B. S.; and Krebs, A. T.: Cell death. *Am. J. Pathol.*, **35:**369–381, **1959.**

Kny, W.: Uber die Verteilung des Lipofuscins in der Skeletmuskulatur in ihrer Beziehung zur Funktion. *Virchows Arch. (Pathol. Anat.)*, **299:**468–478, **1937.**

Kosik, K. S.; Joachim, C. L.; and Selkoe, D. J.: Microtubule-associated protein tau is a major antigenic component of paired helical filaments in Alzheimer's disease. *Proc. Natl. Acad. Sci. USA*, **83:**4044–4048, **1986.**

Lewin, M. D., and Timiras, P. S.: Lipid changes with aging in cardiac mitochondrial membranes. *Mech. Ageing Dev.*, **24:**343–351, **1984.**

Martin, G. M.; Sprague, C. A.; and Epstein, C. J.: Replicative life-span of cultivated human cells: Effects of donor's age, tissue, and genotype. *Lab.* Invest., **23:**86–92, **1970.**

Mason, K. E.; Dam, H.; and Granados, I.: Histological changes in adipose tissue of rats fed a vitamin E deficient diet high in cod liver oil. *Anat. Rec.*, **94:**265–288, **1946.**

Naeim, F., and Walford, R. L.: Disturbance of redistribution of surface membrane receptors on peripheral mononuclear cells of patients with Down's syndrome and of aged individuals. *J. Gerontol.*, **35:**650–655, **1980.**

Naeim, F., and Walford, R. L.: Aging and cell membrane complexes: The lipid bilayer, integral proteins and cytoskeleton. In Finch, C. E., and Schneider, E. L. (eds.): *Handbook of the Biology of Aging*, Van Nostrand Reinhold, New York, **1985.**

Norwood, T. H., and Smith, J. R.: The cultured fibroblast-like cell as a model for the study of aging. In Finch, C. H., and Schneider, E. L. (eds.): *Handbook of the Biology of Aging*, Vol. 2, Van Nostrand Reinhold, New York, **1985.**

Packer, L.; Deamer, D. W.; and Health, R. L.: Regulation and deterioration of structure in membranes, VI. Age pigments. In Strehler, B. L. (ed.): *Advances in Gerontological Research*, Vol. 2, Academic Press, New York, **1967.**

Pool, T. B., and Metter, J. D.: New concepts in regulation of the lifespan of human diploid fibroblasts *in vitro*. In Johnson, J. E., Jr. (ed.): *Aging and Cell Structure*, Vol. 2, Plenum Press, New York, **1984.**

Puck, T. T.: Cyclic AMP, the microtubule-microfilament system and cancer. *Proc. Natl. Acad. Sci. USA*, **74:**4491–4495, **1977.**

Reff, M. E.: RNA and protein metabolism. In Finch, C. E., and Schneider, L. (eds.): *Handbook of the Biology of Aging*, Van Nostrand Reinhold, New York, **1985.**

Reichel, W.: Lipofuscin pigment accumulation and distribution in five rat organs as a function of age. *J. Gerontol.*, **23:**145–153, **1968.**

Roberts, T. W., and Smith, J. R.: The proliferative potential of chick embryo fibroblasts: Population doubling vs. time in culture. *Cell Biol. Int. Rep.*, **4:**1057–1063, **1980.**

Rozengurt, E.: Early signs in the mitogenic response. *Science*, **234:**161–166, **1986.**

Sohal, R. S. (ed.): *Age Pigments*, Elsevier/North Holland, Amsterdam, **1981.**

Strehler, B. L.; Mark, D. D.; Mildvan, A. S.; and Gee, M. V.: Rate and magnitude of age pigment accumulation in the human myocardium. *J. Gerontol.*, **14:**430–439, **1959.**

Strehler, B. L.: *Time, Cells and Aging*, 2nd ed., Academic Press, New York, **1977.**

Vogel, K. G.; Kelley, R. O.; and Stewart, C.: Loss of organized fibronectin matrix from the surface of aging diploid fibroblasts (IMR-90). *Mech. Ageing Dev.*, **16:**295–302, **1981.**

Winter, H.: Distribution of environmental lipofuscinosis. *Aust. Vet. J.*, **39:**250–251, **1963.**

Wunscher, W., and Kustner, R.: Untersuchungen uber die mengenmassige Vertilung von Lipofuszin and Vitamin-E-mangel-Pigment in Nervenzellen von Ratten verschiedener Altersstufen. *Gerontologia*, **13:**153–164, **1967.**

CHAPTER

6 ENZYMATIC CHANGES DURING AGING

Ramesh Sharma

Enzymes are specific proteins that catalyze chemical reactions in biologic systems. Enzymatic studies were among the first biochemical changes demonstrated to occur during aging. Subsequently, a large literature has developed concerning changes in enzyme levels and has been well reviewed (Finch, 1972; Wilson, 1973, 1981; Kanungo, 1980). At present, this collected information is hard to correlate owing to the variability and contradictory nature of the reported results. Nevertheless, these studies have stimulated interest in aging research and for this reason they have benefited the field. One of the problems in obtaining consistent results is that the enzymes have been studied individually without relationship to others in a particular metabolic pathway. To study all the enzymes of one particular metabolic pathway would provide a complete profile of their biologic function during aging. In the present chapter, enzyme levels and changes in isoenzyme composition with aging are presented first and information thereon is summarized in corresponding tables. Following this, enzyme induction and kinetic changes during aging are described.

ENZYME LEVELS DURING AGING

It is difficult to draw from the current data (see Table 6–1) a unified pattern in enzymatic changes during aging. There is little consistency in the data from different workers. This is mainly owing to the different experimental procedures in measurement of enzyme activity and criteria for unit expression, such as per mg protein, per g wet weight of tissue, or per mg DNA. Moreover, animal strain and maintenance conditions also vary widely. Most enzyme assays have been performed with crude preparations, and results are related to wet weight and protein content, which themselves are subject to vary with age, sex, and strain. Most of the tissues analyzed consist of a heterogeneous cell population in which the changes in enzyme activity may not be similar or of the same magnitude in all cells.

Characteristics and Function of Enzymes. The most striking characteristics of all enzymes are their enormous catalytic power and specificity. They accelerate reactions by factors of 10^6 to 10^{12} as compared to uncatalyzed reactions. Enzymes are highly specific both in the reaction catalyzed and in their choice of reactants, called substrates. An enzyme usually catalyzes a single chemical reaction or a set of closely related reactions. The catalytic ability and specificity are determined by certain amino acid side chains of an enzyme molecule. These amino acids need not be adjacent to one another in the linear sequence of polypeptide and are brought into proximity, i.e., active site, by the folding of the primary sequence of amino acid residues. The binding of substrate to an enzyme usually involves formation of several types of noncovalent bonds: ionic, hydrogen, hydrophobic, and Van der Waals interactions. The active site of enzymes has an array of chemical groups that are precisely arranged so that the specific substrate can be more tightly bound than any other molecule.

Enzymes catalyze a wide variety of chemical reactions. Some, which catalyze oxidation/reduction, are grouped as *oxidoreductases*. Others, which catalyze transfer of different groups such as -CH3, PO4, NH3, etc., are termed *transferases*. *Hydrolases* catalyze hydrolytic reactions whereas *lyases* catalyze the addition of groups to double bonds, or vice versa. Isomerization reactions are catalyzed by *isomerases,* whereas *ligases* (synthetases) catalyze the condensation of two molecules coupled with the cleavage of a pyrophosphate bond of ATP or other triphosphates.

The activity of many enzymes is regulated. Their rate of synthesis, as well as their final concentration, is under genetic control and is influenced by small molecules such as hormones, substrates, and products of the metabolic pathways. Some enzymes are synthesized in an inactive precursor form and are activated at a suitable physiologic milieu. Another controlling mechanism is the covalent insertion of a small group on the en-

Table 6–1. CHANGES IN ENZYME LEVELS DURING AGING

ENZYME	ANIMAL	TISSUE	AGES STUDIED (MONTHS)	UNITS/MG	EFFECT OF AGE	REFERENCE
Oxidoreductases						
Cytochrome oxidase (T)	Mouse (M)	Liver	4,18,30	DNA; Protein	Decrease	Wilson, 1972
Glucose-6-phosphate dehydrogenase	Rat (M) (Sprague-Dawley)	Liver	3,24	Protein	Decrease	Wang and Mays, 1977
	Rat (M) (Fischer)	Liver	3,24	Protein	Increase	Wang and Mays, 1977
	Mouse (M)	Liver	4,18,30	DNA; Protein; Wet weight	Increase	Wilson, 1972
α-Glycerophosphate dehydrogenase (c)	Rat (F)	Liver	6,24	Protein	Decrease	Bulos *et al.*, 1971
Isocitrate dehydrogenase (c)	Rat (F)	Liver	6,10,13	Wet weight	Decrease	Webb and Bailey, 1975
Lactate dehydrogenase (c)	Rat (M)	Liver	6,21	DNA	Increase	Ross and Ely, 1954
	Rat (F)	Liver	12,24	Protein	No change	Schmuckler and Barrows, 1966
	Rat (F)	Liver	3,24	Wet weight	Decrease	Singh and Kanungo, 1968
	Mouse (M)	Liver	4,18,30	DNA; Protein; Wet weight	Increase	Wilson, 1972
	Mouse (F)	Liver	4,18,30	DNA; Protein; Wet weight	No change	Wilson, 1972
Malate dehydrogenase (c)	Rat (M)	Liver	2,18	DNA	Increase	Ross and Ely, 1954
	Rat (F)	Liver	6,21	Protein	Increase	Kanungo and Gandhi, 1972
	Rat (M)	Liver	1.5,8,24	Protein	Increase	Sharma and Patnaik, 1982b
Succinate dehydrogenase (T)	Rat (M)	Liver	6,21	Wet weight	No change	Ross and Ely, 1954
Glucose-6-phosphate dehydrogenase (c)	Mouse (F)	Brain	5,25	Wet weight	Increase	Wulf and Cutler, 1975
Lactate dehydrogenase (c)	Rat (F)	Brain	12,24	Protein	Decrease	Schmuckler and Barrows, 1967
	Rat (F)	Brain (CH)	3,10,13,24	Wet weight	Decrease	Singh and Kanungo, 1968
Malate dehydrogenase (c)	Rat (M)	Brain	1.5,8,24	Protein	Increase	Sharma and Patnaik, 1982b
Cytochrome oxidase (T)	Rat (F)	Kidney	13,27	Wet weight	Decrease	Barrows *et al.*, 1958
	Mouse (F)	Kidney	18,30	DNA; Protein; Wet weight	No change	Wilson and Franks, 1971
Glucose-6-phosphate dehydrogenase (C)	Mouse (M)	Kidney	6,18,30	DNA	Increase	Wilson and Franks, 1975
	Mouse (F)	Kidney	6,18,30	DNA	Decrease	Wilson and Franks, 1975
Lactate dehydrogenase (c)	Rat (F)	Kidney	12,24	Protein	No change	Schmuckler and Barrows, 1967
	Mouse (F)	Kidney	4,18,30	DNA; Protein; Wet weight	No change	Wilson and Franks, 1971
	Mouse (M)	Kidney	4,18,30	DNA; Protein; Wet weight	Increase	Wilson and Franks, 1971
Succinate dehydrogenase (c)	Rat (F)	Kidney	13,27	Wet weight	Decrease	Barrows *et al.*, 1958
	Rat (M)	Kidney	13,27	Wet weight	Decrease	Barrows *et al.*, 1958
Lactate dehydrogenase (c)	Rat (F)	Heart	12,24	Protein	No change	Schmuckler and Barrows, 1967
	Rat (F)	Heart	3,24	Wet weight	Decrease	Singh and Kanungo, 1968
Malate dehydrogenase (c)	Rat (F)	Heart	5,24	Wet weight	Decrease	Singh, 1973
Lactate dehydrogenase (c)	Rat (F)	Skeletal Muscle	3,30	Protein; Wet weight	Decrease	Schmuckler and Barrows, 1966
	Rat (F)	Skeletal Muscle	3,24	Wet weight	Decrease	Singh and Kanungo, 1968
Transferases						
Alanine aminotransferase (c,m)	Rat (F)	Liver	1.5,21	DNA; Protein	Decrease	Patnaik and Kanungo, 1976

Table 6–1. CHANGES IN ENZYME LEVELS DURING AGING (Continued)

ENZYME	ANIMAL	TISSUE	AGES STUDIED (MONTHS)	UNITS/MG	EFFECT OF AGE	REFERENCE
Aspartate aminotransferase (c)	Rat (M)	Liver	1.5,8,24	Protein	Increase up to 8 mo. then constant	Sharma and Patnaik, 1987
Aspartate aminotransferase (m)	Rat (M)	Liver	1.5,8,24	Protein	No change	Sharma and Patnaik, 1987
Collagen glucosyl transferase (T)	Rat (F)	Liver	3,8,14	Protein	Increase	Risteli and Kivirikko, 1976
Hexokinase (c)	Rat (M)	Liver	3,18	Protein	Decrease	Bartoc *et al.*, 1975
Phosphoenolpyruvate carboxykinase (c)	Rat (M)	Liver	1.5,8,24	Protein	Increase up to 8 mo. then decrease	Sharma and Patnaik, 1983
Phosphofructokinase (T)	Rat (F)	Liver	6,10,13	Wet weight	Increase	Webb and Bailey, 1975
Pyruvate kinase (c)	Rat (F)	Liver	6,10,13	Wet weight	Increase	Webb and Bailey, 1975
t-RNA methylase (c)	Mouse (M)	Liver	12,18,30	Protein	Decrease	Mays *et al.*, 1973
Tyrosine aminotransferase (c)	Rat (M)	Liver	1.5,19	Protein	No change	Ratha and Kanungo, 1977a
Tyrosine aminotransferase (m)	Rat (M)	Liver	9,19	Protein	Decrease	Ratha and Kanungo, 1977a
Aspartate aminotransferase (T)	Rat (–)	Brain	3,11,24	Protein	Increase	Oeriu, 1963
Aspartate aminotransferase (c)	Rat (M)	Brain (CH)	1.5,8,24	Protein	Increase	Sharma and Patnaik, 1985
Aspartate aminotransferase (m)	Rat (M)	Brain (CH)	1.5,8,24	Protein	Decrease	Sharma and Patnaik, 1985
Cholineacetyltransferase	Mouse (–)	Brain (Hipp)	8,24	Protein	Decrease	Vijayan, 1977
	Rat (M,F)	Brain (CH)	10,20	Protein	Decrease	James and Kanungo, 1978
Glutamic-pyruvic transaminase (T)	Rat (–)	Brain	3,11,24	Wet weight	Increase	Oeriu, 1963
Phosphoenolpyruvate Carboxykinase (c)	Rat (M)	Brain (CH)	1.5,8,24	Protein	Increase up to 8 mo. then decrease	Sharma and Patnaik, 1983
Pyruvate kinase (c)	Rat (M,F)	Brain (CH)	9,19	Protein	Decrease	Chainy and Kanungo, 1976
Pyruvate kinase (c)	Mouse (M)	Kidney	6,23	Protein	No change	Zorzoli and Li, 1967
	Rat (M)	Heart	9,19	Protein	No change	Chainy and Kanungo, 1978a
	Rat (F)	Heart	9,19	Protein	Decrease	Chainy and Kanungo, 1978a
	Rat (M)	Skeletal Muscle	9,19	Protein	Decrease	Chainy and Kanungo, 1978a
	Rat (F)	Skeletal Muscle	9,19	Protein	No change	Chainy and Kanungo, 1978a
Hydrolases						
Acid Phosphatase (T)	Rat (M)	Liver	6,21	Wet weight	No change	Ross and Ely, 1954
	Mouse (M,F)	Liver	4,18,30	DNA; Protein; Wet weight	Increase	Wilson, 1972
ATPase	Rat (M)	Liver	6,21	Wet weight	Increase	Ross and Ely, 1954
Fructose-1,6-diphosphatase (c)	Rat (M)	Liver	3,18	Protein	Decrease	Ross and Ely, 1954
Glucose-6-phosphatase	Rat (M)	Liver	6,10,13	Wet weight	Decrease	Singhal, 1967
	Mouse (M,F)	Liver	4,18,30	DNA; Protein; Wet weight	Decrease	Wilson, 1972
Lysyl hydroxylase (c)	Rat (F)	Liver	3,8,14	Protein	Decrease	Risteli and Kivirikko, 1976
Acetylcholinesterase	Rat (F)	Brain (CH)	2,6,16	Protein	Decrease	Moudgil and Kanungo, 1973
	Rat (M,F)	CH	10,20	DNA; Protein	Decrease	James and Kanungo, 1978
Cholinesterase	Rat (F)	CH	1.5,24	DNA; Protein	Decrease	Kaur and Kanungo, 1970
ATPase	Mouse (M,F)	Brain	4,28	DNA	Decrease	Hollander and Barrows, 1968
Glucose-6-phosphatase (T)	Rat (M)	Kidney	6,24	Protein	Increase	Grinna and Barber, 1972
	Mouse (F)	Kidney	4,18,30	DNA; Protein; Wet weight	Decrease	Wilson and Franks, 1971

Table 6–1. CHANGES IN ENZYME LEVELS DURING AGING (Continued)

ENZYME	ANIMAL	TISSUE	AGES STUDIED (MONTHS)	UNITS/MG	EFFECT OF AGE	REFERENCE
Acid phosphatase (T)	Rat (−)	Kidney	6,13,24	Protein	Decrease	Franklin, 1961
	Mouse (M)	Kidney	3,19	Wet weight	Decrease	Kurnick and Kernen, 1962
Acid DNase (T)	Rat (F)	Kidney	5,25	Protein nitrogen	Increase	Franklin, 1962
Alkaline DNase (T)	Rat (F)	Kidney	5,25	Protein nitrogen	Increase	Franklin, 1962
Alkaline phosphatase (T)	Mouse (M)	Kidney	4,18,30	DNA; Protein; Wet weight	Increase	Wilson and Franks, 1971
ATPase (T)	Rat (−)	Heart	5,20	Protein	No change	Honorati and Ermine, 1974
Cathepsin (T)	Rat (F)	Heart	3,12,24	Wet weight	Increase	Barrows and Roeder, 1961
ATPase (c)	Rat (M)	Skeletal Muscle	9,16,26	Wet weight	Decrease	Rockstein and Brandt, 1961
Lyases						
Aldolase (c)	Mouse (F)	Liver	3,31	Protein	Decrease	Gershon and Gershon, 1973
	Rat (M)	Liver	3,18	Protein	Decrease	Bartoc et al., 1975
	Rat (M)	Liver	2,24	Protein	No change	Anderson, 1976
ATP-citrate lyase	Rat (F)	Liver	6,10,13	Wet weight	Increase	Webb and Bailey, 1975
Ornithine decarboxylase	Rat (M)	Liver	2,12,30	Wet weight	Decrease	Ferioli et al., 1976
Citrate synthetase (m)	Rat (M)	Liver	1.5,8,24	Protein	Increase	Sharma and Patnaik, 1984
	Rat (M)	Brain	1.5,8,24	Protein	Increase	Sharma and Patnaik, 1984
Lygases						
Glutamine synthetase	Rat (F)	Liver	4.5,17	Protein	No change	Rao and Kanungo, 1972

c, cytoplasmic; m, mitochondrial; T, total; M, male; F, female; CH, cerebral hemispheres; Hipp, hippocampus.

zyme. A different kind of regulatory mechanism affects many reaction sequences where an enzyme that catalyzes the first step is inhibited by the end product. The extent to which an enzyme can increase the rate of a reaction depends on the activity of the enzyme, which is a function of the amount of active enzyme available and of the presence of substrates, cofactors, inhibitors, and activators. Changes in the levels or properties of these enzymes may alter the functional ability of an organism. Since enzymes are responsible for specific functions, the various phases of the lifespan of an organism, such as differentiation, development, and reproductive maturity, may depend on the activity of specific enzymes or their isoenzymes.

Some of the changes in enzyme levels due to differences in sex and strain are as follows: The activity of glucose-6-phosphate dehydrogenase increases in the kidney of aging male mouse whereas it decreases in the females (Wilson and Franks, 1971); that of lactate dehydrogenase increases in liver of aging male mice but does not change in females (Wilson, 1972); that of glycine-*n*-methyltransferase decreases in liver of aging mice but increases in the liver of aging rats (Mays *et al.*, 1973). In aging Sprague-Dawley rats, liver glucose-6-phosphate dehydrogenase activity is increased by half, but it is doubled in Fischer 344 rats (Wang and Mays, 1977). A 10-fold greater activity of L-glutamine D-fructose-6-phosphate aminotransferase was reported in the submandibular gland of female compared to male mice (Hosoi *et al.*, 1978). The activity of pyruvate kinase does not change in the heart of old male rats but it decreases in the same tissue of old females (Chainy and Kanungo, 1978a). Conversely, the same enzyme decreases in the skeletal muscle of old male rats whereas it remains unchanged in females.

Such variability in the data on enzyme level may also be due to the animal care and their physical activities. If older animals consumed more or less food than young ones or became more sedentary in old age, they would undergo differences in intermediary metabolism and hence variable enzyme levels (Rothstein, 1982). However, when animals are maintained under the same conditions, the variability in enzyme activity persists. This shows that enzymes are always subjected to varying degree of regulatory mechanisms depending on the food, environmental fluctuations, and hormonal and metabolic status of the animals.

Depending on the animal species, the activities of several enzymes decrease or increase or remain unchanged (Table 6–1). Even within each class, the activities of certain enzymes do not show a specific age-related pattern. There is not a single enzyme that shows consistent age-related changes in its activity in all species. However, alterations in the activities of various enzymes may affect the functional ability of organisms with age. The metabolic status of animals is coordinately regulated by a network of enzymes at different phases of the lifespan. Changes in the activities of certain lipogenic and gluconeogenic enzymes in rat liver have been reported at various ages, and lipogenic activity is diminished because of an age-dependent decline in nicotinamide-adenine dinuleotide (NADP)-malic enzyme and ATP-citrate lyase activity (Vitorca *et al.,* 1981). Enzymes of the oxaloacetate metabolism in the liver and brain of male rats of Wistar strain were studied as a function of age (Sharma and Patnaik, 1982a,b, 1985, 1986). The activities of cytoplasmic aspartate aminotransferase and malate dehydrogenase (gluconeogenic enzymes) are higher in these tissues in old rats and may be correlated with the higher involvement of the enzymes in the conversion of the oxaloacetate pool for gluconeogenesis in older rats.

The observed decrease in the levels of certain enzymes and the increase in others may be correlated with the decrease or increase in the template activity of the corresponding genes (Kanungo, 1980) and/or their internal regulation, depending on the need of metabolites as a function of age.

CHANGES IN ISOENZYME COMPOSITION

It is well known that during development, many proteins change from fetal to adult form. Differentiation and development occur because of sequential activation and repression of genes (Davidson and Britten, 1979). This is best exemplified by the shift of various chains of hemoglobin during the gestation period in humans (see Chapter 4).

Isoenzymes are enzymes performing the same function, but present in more than one molecular form within the same tissue or species. The best example is lactate dehydrogenase (LDH), a tetramer made of two different types of subunits called *M* (predominant form in skeletal muscle) and *H* (predominant in the heart). These two subunits are controlled by two separate genes. Various isoenzymes of lactate dehydrogenase are formed by combination of M and H subunits (M4, M3H, M2H2, MH3, and H4). Each isoenzyme is characteristic of individual tissue or cell population and is subject to different regulatory changes. Aerobic and gluconeogenic tissues contain mostly the *H* form, which is primarily concerned with the conversion of lactate to pyruvate. M-type LDH is predominantly found in anaerobic and glycolytic tissues, where it converts pyruvate to lactate (Markert and Ursprung, 1962). LDH isoenzymic composition is not only tissue specific, but also changes in the same tissue during development (Markert and Möller, 1959). The greater proportion of M4 isoenzyme is present in developing embryo of mammals as their metabolism is mostly anaerobic in nature. A shift toward H4 occurs as development proceeds. Contrary to this, a greater proportion of H4 isoenzyme is found in developing chick embryo, which grows in an aerobic milieu, and shows a shift toward M4 type during later stages of development.

These changes in the composition of isoenzymes are not restricted to development, but extend into adulthood and aging (Kanungo, 1980). The proportion of M4-LDH is considerably lower in the heart, skeletal muscle, and brain of older rats, with concomitant increase of H4-LDH in old age. The shift in isoenzymes of LDH has been correlated with the differing metabolic functions of the organisms as a function of age. The decrease in proportion of M4-LDH may cause a decrease in the ability of the tissue to cope with anaerobic conditions (Singh and Kanungo, 1968). Later work on pyruvate kinase, having four isoenzymes (PK1, 2, 3, and 4), shows that PK-4, the predominant form at birth, is replaced by PK3 after 14 days of postnatal life in the skeletal muscle of rats (Osterman *et al.,*

1973). Reiss and Rothstein (1975) reported a considerable alteration in the pattern of isoenzymes of isocitrate lyase in aged versus young nematodes, *Turbatrix aceti*. Further studies on cytoplasmic alanine aminotransferase (c-AAT) of the rat liver reveal that the phenomena of sequential changes do extend to old age (Patnaik and Kanungo, 1976). Young (5-week) rat liver has A type and adult (52-week) has both the isotypes (A and B) while old (100-week) has only the B isotype. Both subunits are under the control of two separate genes (Chen and Giblett, 1971). Genes for both the isotypes of hepatic c-AAT are sequentially activated and repressed at different phases of the lifespan in rats (Patnaik and Kanungo, 1976). Wang and Mays (1977) reported a quantitative difference in the mono-, di-, and tetrameric forms of glucose-6-phosphate dehydrogenase in the liver of young and old rats. The possible reason for such a shift in isoenzymes may be the regulatory changes in the activities of their corresponding genes, which may be brought about by certain endogenous factors according to a specific program (Kanungo, 1980).

ENZYME INDUCTION DURING AGING

Induction of enzymes is caused by several inducers or effectors, which may be either the substrate or a hormone or a metabolite or even an exogenous factor. This phenomenon is an adaptive process. The ability to initiate adaptive changes in the activity of many enzymes is impaired in old age (Adelman, 1975, 1981). The induction of enzymes by hormones during aging has been extensively reviewed (Pitot and Yatvin, 1973; Adelman, 1975; Dickerson and Basu, 1975; Kanungo, 1980). The magnitude of induction of many enzymes decreases with the increasing age of the animal. These enzymes are: tryptophan pyrrolase by tryptophan and estradiol (Haining and Correl, 1969; Patnaik and Sarangi, 1980), glucose-6-phosphatase, fructose-1, 6-diphosphatase, phosphoenolpyruvate carboxykinase by glucocorticoids (Singhal, 1967; Sharma and Patnaik, 1983), glucokinase by glucose (Adelman, 1970), malate dehydrogenase (MDH) (Kanungo and Gandhi, 1972; Sharma and Patnaik, 1982b), arginase (Rao and Kanungo, 1974), alanine aminotransferase (Patnaik and Kanungo, 1976), tyrosine aminotransferase (Ratha and Kanungo, 1977a), aspartate aminotransferase (AsAT) (Sharma and Patnaik, 1985, 1987), ornithine aminotransferase (Rahman and Peraino, 1973) of the rat liver by glucocorticoids; and phosphofructokinase and phosphohexose isomerase of the uterus (Singhal *et al.*, 1969), acetylcholinesterase (Moudgil and Kanungo, 1973), and pyruvate kinase (Chainy and Kanungo, 1978a) of the brain by sex steroids.

The degree of induction of glutamate synthetase (Rao and Kanungo, 1972) and creatine phosphokinase (Srivastava and Kanungo, 1980) increases with the increasing age of the rat. The lag period for the induction of certain enzymes, such as tyrosine aminotransferase by cold exposure (Finch *et al.*, 1969) and glucokinase by insulin (Adelman, 1970), increases in old age. However, the lag period for the induction of mitochondrial glycerophosphate dehydrogenase by thyroxine (Bulos *et al.*, 1972) and tyrosine aminotransferase by corticosteroids or insulin (Finch *et al.*, 1969) in the rat liver does not change with age. Age-related variations in the response of isoenzymes to hormones have been well studied. Cytoplasmic-MDH but not mitochondrial-MDH is inducible by cortisone and hydrocortisone in aged rats (Kanungo and Gandhi, 1972; Sharma and Patnaik, 1982b). Furthermore, cytoplasmic-AsAT is inducible in the liver and brain of rats of all the ages but mitochondrial AsAT remains unresponsive (Sharma and Patnaik, 1985, 1986).

The expression of age-related adaptive changes in enzyme induction has been categorized into four general patterns of response, as shown in Figure 6–1 (Adelman, 1975): (1) The response has an altered adaptive latent period or initiation time following stimulus without affecting the magnitude of induction; (2) the response shows a decrease or increase in the magnitude of induction with no change in the latent periods; (3) the response alters both the latent period and the magnitude of induction; and (4) age-related changes do not occur in the induction pattern.

The patterns of enzyme adaptation, as is

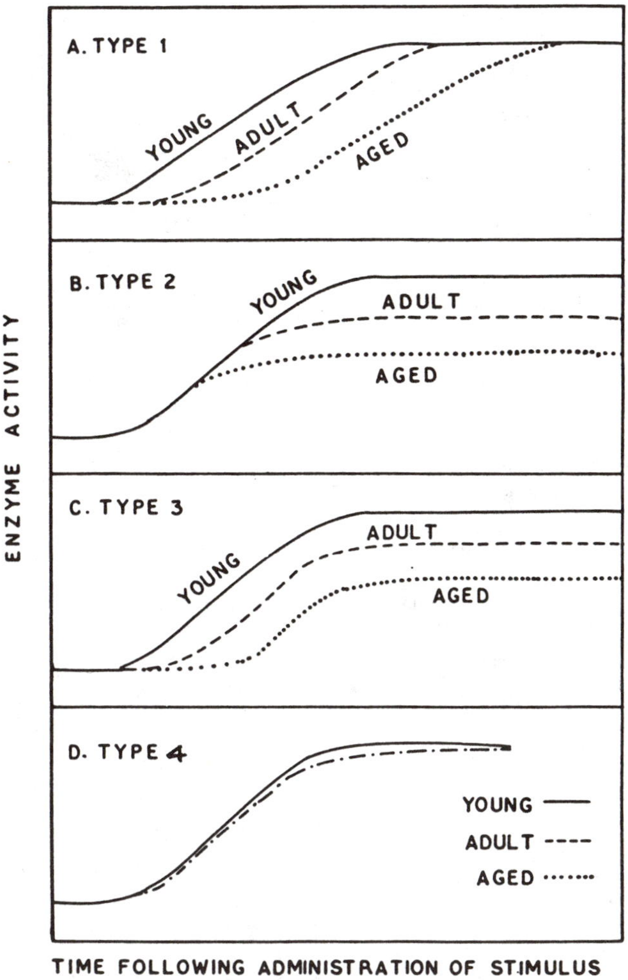

Figure 6–1. *Patterns of age-dependent enzyme adaptation.*

The expression of age-related adaptive changes in enzyme induction has been categorized into four general types (*A, B, C,* and *D*). Each type has been discussed in the text. (From Adelman, R.C.: In Parke, D.V. (ed.): *Enzyme Induction,* Plenum Press, New York, 1975.)

the case for normal enzyme levels, are also susceptible to considerable variation related to difference in species, strain, sex, and conditions of environmental maintenance and the physiologic state of the animals. In general, the magnitude of the response is decreased and the lag period is increased in old age (Table 6–2). Identical dosages of stimuli per unit of body weight elicit weaker biochemical responses in older animals, although the reverse is seen in a few cases (Gusseck, 1972). The degree of tissue responsiveness would be directly proportional to the amount of steroid hormones bound to specific receptors (Baxter and Forsham, 1972). Age-dependent impairment in responsiveness to the hormonal and other biochemical stimuli are dependent not only on receptor level, but also on the physicochemical properties of receptor molecules (Kalimi, 1984; Sharma and Timiras, 1987).

Hormonal Actions. The first step in the action of a hormone is the binding to a specific receptor, which is located on the cell surface or in the cytosol and/or nucleus of the target cells. Hormones act as the signaling molecules and are composed of several distinct classes of biologic compounds, such as glycoproteins, steroids, polypeptides, and modified amino acids. All hormones act via receptor proteins. The function of these specialized receptors is at two levels: (1) specific hormone recognition and (2) initiation of a series of cellular events leading to characteristic responses to the hormone. Hormone receptors reside at different cellular locations, depending on the hormone ligand. For example, receptors are on cell surface for polypeptide hormones, cytoplasm and/or nucleus for steroids, and nucleus for thy-

Table 6–2. ENZYME INDUCTION DURING AGING

ENZYME	ANIMAL (SEX)	TISSUE	AGES STUDIED (MONTHS)	EFFECTORS	MAGNITUDE OF RESPONSE*	REFERENCE
Acetylcholinesterase	Rat (M)	Brain (CH)	10,20	Estradiol & Testosterone	D	James and Kanungo, 1978
Adenylate cyclase	Rat (M,F)	Liver	3,12,24	Epinephrine	I	Kalish *et al.*, 1977
	Rat (M)	Fat cells	2,12,24	Epinephrine	D	Cooper and Gregerman, 1977
Alanine aminotransferase (c)	Rat (F)	Liver	7,21	Hydrocortisone	D	Patnaik and Kanungo, 1976
Alanine hydroxylase	Rat (F)	Liver	1.3,9.9,19.8	Phenobarbital	D	Kato and Takanaka, 1968
Alkaline phosphatase	Mouse (F)	Uterus	6,11,21	Estradiol	D	Holinka et al., 1977
Arginase	Rat (F)	Liver	2,17	Cortisone	NC	Rao and Kanungo, 1974
Aspartate aminotransferase (c)	Rat (M)	Liver; Brain (CH)	1.5,8,24	Hydrocortisone	D	Sharma and Patnaik, 1985, 1987
Choline acetyltransferase	Rat (M,F)	Brain (CH)	10,20	Testosterone	I	James and Kanungo, 1978
Fatty acid synthetase	Mouse (M)	Liver	1,8,18	Fatless diet	D	Eisenbach *et al.*, 1976
Fructose-1,6-diphosphatase	Rat (M)	Liver; Kidney	2,12,24	Hydrocortisone	D	Frolkis *et al.*, 1979
Glucokinase	Rat (M,F)	Liver	2,14,24	Glucose	NC	Adelman, 1970
Glucose-6-phosphatase	Rat (M)	Liver	1,6,12,15	Dexamethasone	D	Singhal, 1967
Glutamine synthetase	Rat (F)	Liver	2,18	Cortisone	D	Rao and Kanungo, 1972
α-Glycerophosphate dehydrogenase	Rat (F)	Liver	12,28	3,3,5-Triiodothyronine	NC	Bulos *et al.*, 1971, 1972
Malate dehydrogenase (c)	Rat (F)	Liver	3,18	Cortisone	D	Kanungo and Gandhi, 1972
	Rat (M)	Liver; Brain	1.5,8,24	Hydrocortisone	D	Sharma and Patnaik, 1982b
Ornithine aminotransferase	Rat (M,F)	Liver	1,2	High-casein diet	D	Rahman and Peraino, 1973
Phosphoenolpyruvate Carboxykinase	Rat (M)	Liver	1.5,8,24	Hydrocortisone	D	Sharma and Patnaik, 1983
Phosphofructokinase	Rat (M)	Prostate	1,3,12	Testosterone	D	Singhal, 1967
Pyruvate Kinase	Rat (M,F)	Brain (CH)	9.5,19.5	Estradiol	D	Chainy and Kanungo, 1976
Serine dehydratase	Rat (M)	Liver	1,12	High-protein diet	D	Rahman and Peraino, 1973
Tryptophan pyrrolase	Rabbit (F)	Liver	2,4,10	Fasting	D	Wu and Rosenthal, 1966
Tyrosine aminotransferase (c)	Rat (M)	Liver	9,19	Hydrocortisone	D	Ratha and Kanungo, 1977a
Tyrosine aminotransferase (m)	Rat (M)	Liver	9,19	Hydrocortisone	I	Ratha and Kanungo, 1977a

*Old values compared to young values.
I, increase; D, decrease; NC, no change; M, male; F, female; c, cytoplasmic isoenzyme; m, mitochondrial isoenzyme.

roid hormones. The effects of most peptide hormones that bind to cell surface-associated receptors are mediated by the generation of second messengers, which, in turn, activate various intracellular processes. In contrast, steroid hormones appear to exert their effects by the translocation of cytoplasmic steroid-receptor complexes to specific acceptor sites on the chromatin within the nucleus. The potential nuclear receptor sites for steroid-receptor complexes are specific and nonspecific DNA sequences, nuclear-associated proteins, and chromatin (DNA + proteins). The specific molecular mechanism by which nuclear-associated steroid-receptor complexes alter gene expression is unknown. Possibly, they alter the localized chromatin structure by modifying DNA structure and/or directly affecting RNA polymerase activity. It is possible that more than one mechanism operates in a particular target tissue. They may also elicit primary (short) and/or secondary (long-term) responses.

Hormone-mediated responses are controlled partly by binding to specific intracellular receptors and then by translocation of hormone-receptor complexes to nuclear acceptor sites (Yamamoto and Alberts, 1976). All of the molecular events in hormone actions subsequent to receptor binding are subject to alteration with age (Roth, 1981). The impairment in the magnitude of induction of various enzymes by hormones may be due to either decreased concentration of receptor binding sites or altered properties of receptors molecules as a function of age (Kanungo, 1980; Roth, 1981; Kalimi, 1984; Sharma and Timiras, 1987). It should be stressed here that hormones and their receptors are very important in the maintenance of overall adaptive response of enzymes at various phases of the lifespan. Changes in these molecules may lead to an altered synthesis of enzymes as a function of age, which may cause functional deterioration of organisms.

CHANGES IN THE KINETIC PROPERTIES OF ENZYMES

The hypothesis that proteins are altered during aging was proposed by Orgel (1963) and has been discussed in Chapter 4. The proposed concept was based on the assumption that faulty proteins would be formed as a function of age. The hypothesis creditably stimulated a great deal of work, both theoretical and practical (Gershon and Gershon, 1973; Gallant and Palmer, 1979; Kirkwood, 1980; Kanungo, 1980; Rothstein, 1982), to demonstrate whether or not old organisms would produce error-containing proteins. Search for errors was vigorously pursued by measuring in great detail the kinetic properties (K_m, K_i), molecular weight, electrophoretic mobility, heat stability, and antigenicity of various enzymes among different ages and species of animals. Such studies were useful for detecting changes in structural and functional aspects of enzymes present in old age. The initial evidence for altered enzyme properties emerged from the studies of Gershon and Gershon (1970) on isocitrate lyase from senescent free-living nematodes. Subsequent to this report, several enzymes were reported to be altered in old free-living nematode, *Turbatrix aceti*: isocitrate lyase (Reiss and Rothstein, 1975), phosphoglycerate kinase (Gupta and Rothstein, 1976a), enolase (Sharma *et al.*, 1976), and aldolase (Reznick and Gershon, 1977). Altered properties of superoxide dismutase (Reiss and Gershon, 1976) and phosphoglycerate kinase (Sharma *et al.*, 1980) were reported from liver and muscle of aged rats, respectively.

Subsequently, many enzymes have been purified and their kinetic properties reported to be unaltered with age. These enzymes are: acetylcholinesterase (Moudgil and Kanungo, 1973), pyruvate kinase (Chainy and Kanungo, 1978b) in brain; malate dehydrogenase (Kanungo and Gandhi, 1972), tyrosine aminotransferase (Ratha and Kanungo, 1977b), alanine aminotransferase (Patnaik and Kanungo, 1976), and aspartate aminotransferase (Sharma and Patnaik, 1982a) in liver of old rats. Triosephosphate isomerase from nematodes (Gupta and Rothstein, 1976b) and enolase from rat muscle and liver (Rothstein *et al.*, 1980) remain unaltered in aged animals.

For a few enzymes, there is still disagreement: mouse liver aldolase has been reported to be altered (Gershon and Gershon, 1973) or not altered (Petell and Lebherz, 1979; Burrows and Davison, 1980). Reiss and Gershon (1976) reported an altered superoxide dismutase in old rat liver, while the same enzyme appears unaltered in the liver of old mice and dogs (Burrows and Davison, 1980). Most molecular properties of enzymes remain unaltered with aging. This is true for properties such as molecular weight, K_m, K_i, and N- and C-terminal residues, number of sulfhydryl (-SH) groups, gel electrophoretic pattern, and immunodiffusion pattern (Rothstein, 1979, 1982; Kanungo, 1980). In some cases, however, differences have been reported for heat sensitivity and antigenic response. Heat sensitivity is generally altered in most enzymes studied, the old enzyme being less stable. Again the exceptions: nematode aldolase and phosphoglycerate kinase from rat muscle are more heat stable in old age (Rothstein, 1982), but nematode phosphoglycerate kinase does not differ in heat sensitivity (Gupta and Rothstein, 1976a). Thus, heat sensitivity acts as a tool to measure an altered enzyme but lacks uniformity.

In spite of some differences in the molecular properties of a few enzymes, there is enough evidence that negates the idea of errors in the proteins as a function of age. Most strikingly, there are no changes in young versus old enzymes using highly specific techniques of isoelectric focusing. Sequential changes and the possibilities of phosphorylation, acylation, esterification, and deamidation are hard to occur, otherwise they would have been detected by isoelectric focusing of enzymes. Moreover, if errors were made in transcription by RNA polymerase or during translation by tRNA synthetases, then all proteins would contain errors. Many proteins remain unaltered in old animals. Some enzymatic alterations in old animals may simply be due to a change in the shape of the molecules with no covalent modifications (Rothstein, 1982). Demchenko and Orlovska (1980) reported that aldolase A from young and old rabbit muscle differs in conformation. Gafni (1981) studied the properties of muscle glyceraldehyde-3-phosphate dehydrogenase from young and old rats. The old enzyme had lower specific activity and was more sensitive to heat without any detectable differences in amino acid composition, -SH groups, UV spectra, and sedimentation coefficient. Although there is no error in the protein synthetic machinery of old animals, it is after completion of synthesis that the altered enzymes may be produced by conformational changes. The apparent changes in the levels of enzymes and the shift in isoenzyme patterns express an adaptive response, coordinating with the intrinsic and extrinsic factors, of the hormonal and metabolic status of the animals as a function of age.

References

Adelman, R. C.: An age-dependent modification of enzyme regulation. *J. Biol. Chem.*, **245:**1032–1035, **1970.**

Adelman, R. C.: Patterns of age-dependent enzyme adaptation. In Parke, D. V. (ed.): *Enzyme Induction,* Plenum Press, New York, **1975.**

Adelman, R. C.: Enzyme adaptation during aging. In Florini, J. R. (ed.): *Handbook of Biochemistry of Aging,* CRC Press, Boca Raton, FL, **1981.**

Anderson, P. J.: The specific activity of aldolase in the livers of old and young rats. *Can. J. Biochem.* **54:**194–196, **1976.**

Barrows, C. H., and Roeder, L. M.: Effect of age on protein synthesis in rats. *J. Gerontol.*, **16:**321–325, **1961.**

Barrows, C. H.; Yiengst, M. J.; and Shock, N. W.: Senescence and metabolism of various tissues of rats. *J. Gerontol.*, **13:**351–355, **1958.**

Bartoc, R.; Bruhjis, R.; Klein, R.; Moldoveanu, E.; Oeriu, I.; and Oeriu, S.: Effect of age and -SH active groups on the activity of some enzymes involved in the carbohydrate metabolism. *Exp. Gerontol.*, **10:**161–164, **1975.**

Baxter, J. D., and Forsham, P. H.: Tissue effects of glucocorticoids. *Am. J. Med.*, **53:**573–589, **1972.**

Bulos, B.; Sacktor, B.; Grossman, I. W.; and Altman, N.: Thyroid control of mitochondrial α-glycerophosphate dehydrogenase in rat liver as a function of age. *J. Gerontol.*, **26:**13–19, **1971.**

Bulos, B.; Shukla, S.; and Sacktor, B.: Bioenergetic properties of mitochondria from flight muscle of aging blowflies. *Mech. Ageing Dev.*, **1:**227–231, **1972.**

Burrows, R. B., and Davison, P. F.: Comparison of specific activities of enzymes from young and old dogs and mice. *Mech. Ageing Dev.*, **13:**307–317, **1980.**

Chainy, G. B. N., and Kanungo, M. S.: Sex and age dependent response of pyruvate kinase of the brain of the rat to estradiol and testosterone. *Biochem. Biophys. Res. Commun.*, *72:*777–781, **1976.**

Chainy, G. B. N., and Kanungo, M. S.: Effects of estradiol and testosterone on the activity of pyruvate kinase of the cardiac and skeletal muscles of rats as a function of age and sex. *Biochim. Biophys. Acta,* **540:**65–72, **1978a.**

Chainy, G. B. N., and Kanungo, M. S.: Induction and properties of pyruvate kinase of the cerebral hemisphere of rats of various ages. *J. Neurochem.*, **30:**419–427, **1978b.**

Chen, S. H., and Giblett, E. R.: Polymorphism of soluble glutamic, pyruvic transaminase: A new genetic marker in man. *Science,* **173:**148–149, **1971.**

Cooper, B., and Gregerman, R. I.: Hormone sensitive fat cell adenylate cyclase in rat: Influence of growth, cell size, and aging. *J. Clin. Invest.*, **57:**161–168, **1977.**

Davidson, E. H., and Britten, R. J.: Regulation of gene expression: Possible role of repetitive sequences. *Science,* **204:**1052–1059, **1979.**

Demchenko, A. P., and Orlovska, N. N.: Age-dependent changes of protein structure. II. Conformational differences of aldolase of young and old rabbits. *Exp. Gerontol.*, **15:**619–627, **1980.**

Dickerson, J. W. T., and Basu, T. K.: In Parke, D. V. (ed.): *Enzyme Induction,* Plenum Press, New York, **1975.**

Eisenbach, L.; Shimron, F.; and Yagil, G.: The effect of age on the regulation of glucose-6-phosphate dehydrogenase in mouse liver. *Exp. Gerontol.*, **11:**63–71, **1976.**

Ferioli, M.; Ceroti, G.; and Comolli, R.: Changes in rat liver ornithine decarboxylase activity during aging and effect of simulation by dexamethasone. *Exp. Gerontol.*, **11:**153–156, **1976.**

Finch, C. E.: Enzyme activities, gene function and aging in mammals. *Exp. Gerontol.*, **7:**53–67, **1972.**

Finch, C. E.; Foster, J. R.; and Mirsky, A. E.: Aging and the regulation of cell activities during exposure to cold. *J. Gen. Physiol.*, **54:**690–712, **1969.**

Franklin, T. J.: Activity of liver and kidney acid phosphatase at different stages in the life span of the rat. *Biochem. J.*, **79:**34, **1961.**

Franklin, T. J.: The influence of age on the activity of some acid hydrolases in the rat liver and kidney. *Biochem. J.*, **82:**118–122, **1962.**

Frolkis, V. B.; Bezrukov, V. V.; and Muradian, Kh. K.: Hypothalamic-pituitary-adrenocortical regulation of induction of some enzymes of carbohydrate and amino acid metabolism in aging. *Exp. Gerontol.*, **14:**65–76, **1979.**

Gafni, A.: Purification and comparative study of glyceraldehyde-3-phosphate dehydrogenase from the muscles of young and old rats. *Biochemistry,* **20:**6035–6040, **1981.**

Gallant, J., and Palmer, L.: Error propagation in viable cells. *Mech. Ageing Dev.*, **10:**27–38, **1979.**

Gershon, H., and Gershon, D.: Detection of inactive enzyme molecules in aging organisms. *Nature,* **227:**1214–1217, **1970.**

Gershon, H., and Gershon, D.: Inactive enzyme molecules in aging mice: Liver aldolase. *Proc. Natl. Acad. Sci. USA,* **70:**909–913, **1973.**

Grinna, L. S., and Barber, A.: Age-related changes in membrane lipid content and enzyme activities. *Biochim. Biophys. Acta,* **288:**347–353, **1972.**

Gupta, S. K., and Rothstein, M.: Phosphoglycerate kinase from young and old *Turbatrix aceti. Arch. Biochem. Biophys.*, **445:**632–644, **1976a.**

Gupta, S. K., and Rothstein, M.: Triosephosphate isomerase from young and old *Turbatrix aceti. Arch. Biochem. Biophys.*, **174:**333–338, **1976b.**

Gusseck, D.: Endocrine mechanisms and aging. In Strehler, B. L. (ed.): *Advances in Gerontological Research,* Academic Press, New York, **1972.**

Haining, J. L., and Correl, W. W.: Turnover of tryptophan-induced tryptophan pyrrolase in rat liver as a function of age. *J. Gerontol.*, **24**:143–148, **1969**.

Holinka, C. F.; Hetland, M. D.; and Finch, C. E.: The response to a single dose of estradiol in the uterus of ovariectomized C57BL/6J mice during aging. *Biol. Reprod.*, **17**:262–264, **1977**.

Hollander, J., and Barrows, C. H., Jr.: Enzymatic studies in senescent rodent brains. *J. Gerontol.*, **23**:174–179, **1968**.

Honorati, M., and Ermini, M.: Myofibrillar and mitochondrial ATPase activity of red, white, diaphragmatic and cardiac muscle of young and old rats. *Experientia*, **30**:215–216, **1974**.

Hosoi, K.; Kobayashi, S.; and Ucha, T.: Sex difference in L-glutamine D-fructose-6-phosphate aminotransferase activity of mouse submandibular gland. *Biochim. Biophys. Acta*, **543**:283–292, **1978**.

James, T. C., and Kanungo, M. S.: Effect of sex steroids on choline acetyltransferase and acetylcholinesterase of cerebral hemisphere of male rats of various ages. *Biochim. Biophys. Acta*, **538**:205–211, **1978**.

Kalimi, M.: Glucocorticoid receptors: From development to aging. A review. *Mech. Ageing Dev.*, **24**:129–138, **1984**.

Kalish, M. I.; Katz, M. S.; Pineyro, M. A.; and Gregerman, R. I.: Epinephrine- and glucagon-sensitive adenylate cyclases of rat liver during aging. *Biochim. Biophys. Acta*, **483**:452–466, **1977**.

Kanungo, M. S.: *Biochemistry of Ageing*, Academic Press, London, **1980**.

Kanungo, M. S., and Gandhi, B. S.: Induction of malate dehydrogenase isoenzymes in livers of young and old rats. *Proc. Natl. Acad. Sci. USA*, **69**:2035–2038, **1972**.

Kato, R., and Takanaka, A.: Effect of phenobarbital on electron transport system, oxidation and reduction of drugs in liver microsomes of rats of different age. *J. Biochem.*, **63**:406–408, **1968**.

Kaur, G., and Kanungo, M. S.: Alterations in the activity and regulation of cholinesterase of the nervous tissue of rats of various ages. *Ind. J. Biochem. Biophys.*, **7**:122–125, **1970**.

Kirkwood, T. B. L.: Error propagation in intracellular transfer. *J. Theoret. Biol.*, **82**:363–382, **1980**.

Kurnick, N. B., and Kernen, R. L.: The effect of aging on the deoxyribose nuclease system, body and organ weight and cellular content. *J. Gerontol.*, **17**:245–253, **1962**.

Markert, C. L., and Möller, F.: Multiple forms of enzymes: tissue, ontogeny, and species specific patterns. *Proc. Natl. Acad. Sci. USA*, **45**:753–762, **1959**.

Markert, C. L., and Ursprung, H.: The ontogeny of bioenzyme patterns of lactate dehydrogenase in mouse. *Dev. Biol.*, **5**:363–381, **1962**.

Mays, L. I.: Borek, E.; and Finch, C. E.: Glycine n-methyl transferase is a regulatory enzyme which increases in aging animals. *Nature*, **243**:411–413, **1973**.

Moudgil, V. K., and Kanungo, M. S.: Effect of age on the rat on induction of acetylcholinesterase of the brain by 17β-estradiol. *Biochim. Biophys. Acta*, **329**:211–220, **1973**.

Oeriu, S.: Research on the relation between vitamin coenzymes in relation to the age of the animal and under the influence of certain substances proper to the organism. *Biokhimiia* (Rus), **28**:3–8, **1963**.

Orgel, L. E.: The maintenance of the accuracy of protein synthesis and its relevance to aging. *Proc. Natl. Acad. Sci. USA*, **49**:517–521, **1963**.

Osterman, J.; Fritz, P. J.; and Wuntch, T.: Pyruvate kinase isoenzymes from rat tissues. Developmental studies. *J. Biol. Chem.*, **248**:1011–1018, **1973**.

Patnaik, S. K., and Kanungo, M. S.: Soluble alanine aminotransferase of the liver of rats of various ages: Induction, characterization and changes in patterns. *Ind. J. Biochem. Biophys.*, **13**:117–124, **1976**.

Patnaik, S. K., and Sarangi, S.: Age-related response of tryptophan pyrrolase to 17β-estradiol in the liver of female rats. *J. Biochem.*, **87**:1249–1252, **1980**.

Petell, J. K., and Lebherz, G. L.: Properties and metabolism of fructose diphosphate aldolase in livers of old and young mice. *J. Biol. Chem.*, **254**:8179–8184, **1979**.

Pitot, H. C., and Yatvin, N. B.: Interrelationships of mammalian hormones and enzyme levels in vivo. *Physiol. Rev.*, **53**:228–325, **1973**.

Rahman, Y. E., and Peraino, C.: Effect of age on patterns of enzyme adaptation in male and female rats. *Exp. Gerontol.*, **8**:93–100, **1973**.

Rao, S. S., and Kanungo, M. S.: Induction of glutamine synthetase of the liver of young and old rats. *Mech. Ageing Dev.*, **1**:61–70, **1972**.

Rao, S. S., and Kanungo, M. S.: Age-dependent induction of arginase in the liver of rats. *Ind. J. Biochem. Biophys.*, **11**:208–212, **1974**.

Ratha, B. K., and Kanungo, M. S.: Induction of particulate and soluble isoenzymes of tyrosine aminotransferase by hydrocortisone in the liver of rats as a function of age. *Biochem. Biophys. Res. Commun.*, **76**:925–929, **1977a**.

Ratha, B. K., and Kanungo, M. S.: Alterations in tyrosine aminotransferase isoenzymes of liver of rats as a function of age. *Mech. Ageing Dev.*, **6**:431–439, **1977b**.

Reiss, U., and Gershon, D.: Rat liver superoxide dismutase. *Eur. J. Biochem.*, **63**:617–623, **1976**.

Reiss, U., and Rothstein, M.: Age-related changes in isocitrate lyase from the free-living nematode, *Turbatrix aceti*. *J. Biol. Chem.*, **250**:826–830, **1975**.

Reznick, A. Z., and Gershon, D.: Age-related alterations in purified fructose-1,6-diphosphate aldolase in the nematode *Turbatrix aceti*. *Mech. Ageing Dev.*, **6**:345–353, **1977**.

Risteli, J., and Kivirikko, K. I.: Intracellular enzymes of collagen biosynthesis in rat liver as a function of age and in hepatic injury induced by dimethylnitrosamine. *Biochem. J.*, **158**:361–367, **1976**.

Rockstein, M., and Brandt, K. F.: Changes in the phosphorus metabolism of the gastrocnemius muscle in aging white rats. *Proc. Soc. Exp. Biol. Med.*, **107**:377–380, **1961**.

Ross, M. H., and Ely, J. O.: Aging and enzyme activity. *J. Franklin Inst.*, **258**:63–66, **1954**.

Roth, G. S.: Changes in hormone receptors during adulthood and senescence. In Florini, J. R. (ed.): *Handbook of Biochemistry in Aging*, CRC Press, Boca Raton, FL, **1981**.

Rothstein, M.: Aging and alteration of enzymes: A review. *Mech. Ageing Dev.*, **4**:325–338, **1975**.

Rothstein, M.: The formation of altered enzymes in aging mammals. *Mech. Ageing Dev.*, **9**:197–202, **1979**.

Rothstein, M.: *Biochemical Approaches to Aging*, Academic Press, New York, **1982**.

Rothstein, M.; Coppens, M.; and Sharma, H. K.: Effect of aging on enolase from rat muscle, liver and heart. *Biochim. Biophys. Acta*, **614**:591–600, **1980**.

Schmuckler, M., and Barrows, C. H., Jr.: Age differences in lactic and malic dehydrogenase in the rat. *J. Gerontol.*, **21**:109–111, **1966**.

Schmuckler, M., and Barrows, C. H., Jr.: Effect of age on dehydrogenase heterogeneity in the rat. *J. Gerontol.*, **22**:8–13, **1967**.

Sharma, H. K.; Gupta, S. K.; and Rothstein, M.: Age-related alteration of enolase in the free-living nematode, *Turbatrix aceti*. *Arch. Biochem. Biophys.*, **174**:324–332, **1976**.

Sharma, H. K.; Prasanna, H. R.; and Rothstein, M.: Altered phosphoglycerate kinase in aging rats. *J. Biol. Chem.*, **255**:5043–5050, **1980**.

Sharma, H. K., and Rothstein, M.: Altered enolase in aged *Turbatrix aceti* results from conformational changes in the enzyme. *Proc. Natl. Acad. Sci. USA*, changes in the enzyme. *Proc. Natl. Acad. Sci. USA,* **77**:5865–5868, **1980.**

Sharma, R., and Patnaik, S. K.: Properties of liver cytoplasmic aspartate aminotransferase of rats of various ages. *Biochem. Int.,* **5**:561–566, **1982a.**

Sharma, R., and Patnaik, S. K.: Differential regulation of malate dehydrogenase isoenzymes by hydrocortisone in the liver and brain of aging rats. *Dev. Growth Differ.,* **24**:501–505, **1982b.**

Sharma, R., and Patnaik, S. K.: Induction of phosphoenolpyruvate carboxykinase by hydrocortisone in the liver and brain of rats as a function of age. *Biochem. Int.,* **7**:535–540, **1983.**

Sharma, R., and Patnaik, S. K.: Age-related response of citrate synthetase to hydrocortisone in the liver and brain of male rats. *Experientia,* **40**:97–98, **1984.**

Sharma, R., and Patnaik, S. K.: Age-dependent response of aspartate aminotransferase isoenzymes to hydrocortisone in the brain of male rats. *Mol. Physiol.,* **7**:195–200, **1985.**

Sharma, R., and Patnaik, S. K.: Regulation of aspartate aminotransferase isoenzymes in the liver of aging rats. *Arch. Gerontol. Geriatr.,* **6**:27–32, **1987.**

Sharma, R., and Timiras, P. S.: Regulatory changes in glucocorticoid receptors in the skeletal muscle of immature and mature male rats. *Mech. Ageing Dev.,* **37**:249–256, **1987.**

Singh, S. N.: Effect of age on the activity and citrate inhibition of malate dehydrogenase of the brain and heart of rats. *Experientia,* **29**:42–43, **1973.**

Singh, S. N., and Kanungo, M. S.: Alterations in lactate dehydrogenase of the brain, heart, skeletal muscle and liver of rats. *J. Biol. Chem.,* **243**:4526–4529, **1968.**

Singhal, R. L.: Effect of age on phosphofructokinase induction in rat prostate and seminal vesicle. *J. Gerontol.,* **22**:343–347, **1967.**

Singhal, R. L.: Effect of age on the induction of glucose-6-phosphatase and fructose-1,6-diphosphatase in rat liver. *J. Gerontol.,* **22**:77–88, **1967.**

Singhal, R. L.; Valadares, J. R. E.; and Ling, G. M.: Estrogenic regulation of uterine carbohydrate metabolism during senescence. *Am. J. Physiol.,* **217**:793–797, **1969.**

Srivastava, S. K., and Kanungo, M. S.: A comparative study of the inducibility of cardiac creatine phosphokinase by corticosteroids in rats of various ages. *Biochem. Med.,* **23**:64–69, **1980.**

Vijayan, N. K.: Cholinergic enzymes in the cerebellum of the senescent mouse. *Exp. Gerontol.,* **12**:7–11, **1977.**

Vitorca, J.; Satrustegui, J.; and Machado, A.: Metabolic implications of aging: changes in activities of key lipogenic and gluconeogenic enzymes in the aged rat liver. *Enzyme,* **26**:144–152, **1981.**

Wang, R., and Mays, L.: Opposite changes in rat liver glucose-6-phosphate dehydrogenase during aging in Sprague-Dawley and Fischer 344 male rats. *Exp. Gerontol.,* **12**:117–124, **1977.**

Webb, J., and Bailey, E.: Changes in the activities of some enzymes associated with hepatic lipogenesis in the rat from weaning to old age and the effect of sucrose feeding. *Int. J. Biochem.,* **6**:813–819, **1975.**

Wilson, P. D.: Enzyme patterns in young and old mouse liver and lungs. *Gerontologia,* **18**:36–54, **1972.**

Wilson, P. D.: Enzyme changes in aging mammals. *Gerontologia,* **19**:79–125, **1973.**

Wilson, P. D.: Enzyme levels in animals of various ages. In Florini, J. R. (ed.): *Handbook of Biochemistry in Aging,* CRC Press, Boca Raton, FL, **1981.**

Wilson, P. D., and Franks, L. M.: Enzyme patterns in young and old mouse kidneys. *Gerontologia,* **17**:16–32, **1971.**

Wilson, P. D., and Franks, L. M.: The effect of age on mitochondrial ultrastructure and enzymes, *Adv. Exp. Med. Biol.,* **53**:171–183, **1975.**

Wu, S. Y., and Rosenthal, H. L.: Induction of tryptophan pyrrolase activity in starving rabbits of different ages. *Proc. Soc. Exp. Biol. Med.,* **122**:414–417, **1966.**

Wulf, J., and Cutler, R.: Altered protein hypothesis of mammalian aging processes. I. Thermal stabilities of glucose-6-phosphate dehydrogenase in C57BL/6J mouse tissue. *Exp. Gerontol.,* **10**:101–117, **1975.**

Yamamoto, K., and Alberts, B. M.: Steroid receptors: elements for modulation of eukaryotic transcription. *Ann. Rev. Biochem,* **45**:721–746, **1976.**

Zorzoli, A., and Li, J. B.: Gluconeogenesis in mouse kidney cortex. Effect of age and fasting on glucose production and enzyme activities. *J. Gerontol.,* **22**:151–157, **1967.**

CHAPTER

7 OXYGEN RADICAL GENERATION AND PROTECTIVE SYSTEM

Assessment of Their Involvement in Aging

Rolf J. Mehlhorn

INTRODUCTION

An attractive alternative to programmed senescence in vertebrates is the notion that aging is due to wear-and-tear, similar to the all-too-familiar cause of the inevitable failure of mechanical devices like automobiles. Of course, biologic organisms, unlike cars, have the capacity to repair themselves, and hence the various formulations of wear-and-tear theories must contend with the question of why repair is incomplete (see also Chapter 4). A reasonable answer is that no repair system can be absolutely efficient, particularly if the damage is so random that macromolecules are altered in virtually limitless variety. One wear-and-tear theory, which embodies the characteristic of unpredictable molecular alterations, is the free radical theory of aging. It was proposed by Harman in 1956 as follows: "Aging results from the deleterious effects of free radicals produced in the course of cellular metabolism" (Harman, 1956). Growing evidence supports an involvement of free radicals in life-shortening diseases, although efforts to use predictions of the free radical theory to achieve increases in maximum lifespan extension have met with limited success, at best (Mehlhorn and Cole, 1985). The principal objective of this chapter is to critically assess the current status of the available evidence concerning free radical involvement in aging.

CHEMISTRY AND BIOCHEMISTRY

Free-Radical Chemistry

Free radicals are molecules, rarely occurring in nature, that contain one or more "unpaired" electrons, sometimes also referred to as "free spins." A free-radical molecule containing a single unpaired electron is frequently denoted by $R\cdot$, where the dot refers to the unpaired electron, e.g., the glutathionyl radical $GS\cdot$. Free radicals rarely arise naturally because of the familiar chemical principle that valence electrons in atoms form chemical bonds, each of which consists of an electron pair. Energy must be supplied to break chemical bonds, and usually, the resulting molecular fragments are free radicals. Once formed, these free radical fragments will combine rapidly with other free radical fragments, or with each other, to form nonradical products:

$$R\cdot + R'\cdot \longrightarrow R{:}R'$$

Hence, even if sufficient energy is available to break bonds, the proportion of free radicals among nonradicals is usually very low. Examples of reactive free radicals include the very reactive hydroxyl radical, OH· and moderately reactive alkyl radicals, which can result from the decomposition of lipid peroxides in biologic membranes.

Free radicals can pose a considerable hazard to biologic systems because of their unique chemistry. The most reactive radicals attack other molecules indiscriminately, often produce chain reactions, and sometimes cause cross-linking of molecules, including vital macromolecules like DNA and critically important enzymes. Some of the products of free radical chemistry are completely foreign to the repair or turnover enzymes of the cell. For example, when two proteins become cross-linked, the product of this reaction may be resistant to attack by proteolytic enzymes. Hence, the usual metabolic turnover processes may fail to degrade such cross-linked molecules to provide amino acids for the synthesis of new biomolecules. Cross-linked products can accumulate progressively in cells, as in the example of age pigments, which increase with age in the cells of animals (see Chapters 4 and 5).

OXYGEN

Oxygen in its ground state, i.e., ordinary gaseous oxygen, is a so-called triplet molecule, having two electrons with unpaired spins. Thus, ordinary oxygen can be thought of as a biradical. Oxygen is an example of a radical that is normally quite stable. However, in the presence of other free radicals, or in a collision with a molecule that is chemically very reducing, oxygen is often extremely reactive. When an oxygen molecule collides with another free radical, the favorable energetics of electron pairing imply that a new addition product, called a peroxyl radical, will readily be formed, and indeed this is the reason that free radical damage is greatly aggravated in the presence of oxygen. If oxygen reacts with some nonradical molecule that has a sufficiently reducing chemical potential, a one-electron transfer to oxygen can occur, resulting in O_2^-, the superoxide radical. In such an electron transfer reaction the energy that is required to break one bond is recovered in the formation of another bond. An example is the formation of superoxide radicals when molecular oxygen reacts with reduced flavins. However, fortunately for the evolution of biologic systems on earth, the energy of the bond that is formed when oxygen becomes superoxide is very weak, so that very few bonds can be broken in reactions with normal oxygen.

When oxygen reacts with another radical, the resulting peroxyl radical molecules are also reactive and will abstract hydrogen atoms from a variety of other molecules, leading to chain reactions and accumulation of hydroperoxides. Such free radical chain reactions are familiar to food chemists, occurring readily in fats to cause rancidity. The facile occurrence of analogous free radical chain reactions in biologic membranes, referred to as lipid peroxidation, is a major oxidative damage mechanism in cells.

The chemical products of free radical reactions involving oxygen are often quite reactive themselves, and this has earned many of them the designation of "active oxygen" molecules. Several active oxygen species are of interest in biologic damage processes. These include the hydroxyl radical, OH·, the superoxide radical, O_2^-, and the two nonradicals: singlet oxygen, $^1O_2$, and hydrogen peroxide, H_2O_2. The most reactive is the hydroxyl radical—virtually no biologic molecule is immune to its attack. Hence, organisms have evolved elaborate defenses to ensure that the hydroxyl radical arises as infrequently as possible. Singlet oxygen, which often arises during free radical reactions, is also reactive, although not as reactive as the hydroxyl radical.

Hydrogen peroxide is of interest as a potential damaging species because, in the presence of freely dissolved or loosely bound iron or copper, it can decompose to produce hydroxyl radicals. Because of the destructiveness of hydroxyl radicals, hydrogen peroxide decomposition could be a major source of biologic damage under conditions of iron or copper release from protein binding sites.

The superoxide radical is not very reactive chemically, but its lack of reactivity may be offset by the abundance of this radical species in aerobic biologic environments. It may exert its damaging effects by serving as a reductant for ferric ion, particularly when iron is sequestered within some proteins, thus releasing the ferrous iron into aqueous solution. Superoxide radicals react with each other to produce hydrogen peroxide. The fact that no organisms can survive life in air without the superoxide dismutase protective enzyme (or high concentrations of free manganese ions in one exceptional microorganism) provides compelling evidence that superoxide poses a great threat to aerobic cells.

ANTIOXIDANTS

Biologic systems have evolved a multiplicity of defenses against oxidative attack. Indeed, the discovery of one defensive substance, the enzyme superoxide dismutase (SOD), has played a pivotal role in the explosive expansion of our understanding of oxidative damage in recent years. We now know that a considerable variety of proteins and smaller molecules are involved in protecting the cell against the threat of free radical reactions. In addition, considerable energy expenditures are made by cells to repair such damage when the protective systems fail to intercept all the endogenous and exogenous free radical initiators. Some 40-odd enzymes are constantly repairing damaged DNA, and both lipids and proteins are being turned over continuously. Thus it seems that organisms pay dearly for the privilege of aerobic life.

Superoxide Dismutases (SODs). At least three different types of SODs are now known. In mammals a copper-zinc enzyme is found in cells, excluding the intramitochondrial matrix, which contains a manganese-containing enzyme. Concentrations of SODs in cells are relatively high; e.g., in spinach chloroplasts 0.24% of the total soluble protein is SOD.

Catalase. This enzyme decomposes hydrogen peroxide and oxidizes alcohols and other reduced organic molecules using H_2O_2 as a hydrogen acceptor. Catalase is located exclusively in the peroxisomes of most cells. It is also found in red cells. Some humans lack this enzyme altogether yet seem to suffer no adverse effects under normal circumstances, possibly because of the existence of another peroxide-decomposing enzyme (see below).

Glutathione Peroxidases. These enzymes also act on hydrogen peroxide but can also use organic hydroperoxides as electron acceptors. The most active form of this enzyme contains selenium and is found throughout the cell except for peroxisomes. A group of enzymes, the glutathione-S-transferases, reacts with organic hydroperoxides. Some 10 percent of the total soluble liver protein consists of these enzymes.

Vitamin E. This lipid-soluble vitamin is a phenolic antioxidant that functions by donating a hydrogen atom to lipid peroxyl radicals. The resulting vitamin E radical is relatively unreactive, and hence free radical chains arising in biologic membranes are terminated highly effectively by this antioxidant.

Uric Acid. A striking difference between the higher apes and other animals is their relatively long lifespan. This longevity and the attribute of a large brain, which accounts for a large fraction of the total oxygen consumption, may be partially the result of retention of the antioxidant uric acid, which is a product of purine metabolism. Two evolutionary alterations have led to high tissue concentrations of urate: loss of peroxisomal urate oxidase and active reabsorption of urate from the kidney. In model experiments urate is an effective antioxidant and singlet oxygen scavenger.

Ascorbic Acid. This popular vitamin is an effective aqueous antioxidant that can terminate free radical chain reactions by donating hydrogens. Ascorbate may also serve to protect membranes by donating hydrogens to vitamin E radicals, thus regenerating the lipid antioxidant. Ascorbate can act as a free radical initiator, however, because of its tendency to autoxidize, particularly at alkaline pH or in the presence of free iron.

Carotenes. β-Carotene is a potent quencher of singlet oxygen that acts by an energy transfer mechanism whereby the singlet-oxygen molecule is converted to the relatively harmless triplet-oxygen molecule, while the carotene molecule is promoted to its triplet state. Subsequently, the excited carotene releases its energy harmlessly as heat. In this reaction carotene acts catalytically, without being consumed in the reaction. Epidemiologically, carotenes, like vitamin E and selenium, are correlated with good health, including resistance to cancer.

CELLS, TISSUES, AND ANIMALS

Free Radicals in Aerobic Cells

Free radicals are produced in aerobic cells during normal oxidative metabolism (Chance *et al.*, 1979). Elaborate defensive systems wage a constant battle against active oxygen species in all aerobic organisms. A measure of the threat posed by oxygen radicals is that the antioxidant enzymes comprise a significant fraction of the total protein content of aerobic cells.

Most *oxygen consumption* in mammals occurs in their mitochondria. Although it is known that the mitochondrial respiratory chain operates as an array of enzymes that perform electron transfer reactions very similar to those occurring in free radical reactions, the structures of these enzymes ensure that no uncontrolled chemical reactions occur. In particular, no release of active oxygen molecules occurs from the site of oxygen binding—cytochrome oxidase. However, despite the tightly controlled flow of reducing equivalents through the respiratory chain, some leakage of reductants from mitochondria does occur at sites other than cytochrome oxidase, causing release of superoxide radicals into the cell. In addition, other organelles and some soluble enzymes appear to cause both univalent and divalent oxygen reduction. Estimates of hydrogen peroxide production from subcellular fractions are given in Table 7–1.

Cells of the immune system destroy invasive microorganisms by mechanisms involving active oxygen molecules. The destructive molecular species produced by immune system cells may sometimes contribute a substantial fraction of an animal's total oxidative damage burden. Of particular interest is the potential posed by these cells for amplifying the damage produced by free radicals. Increasing evidence shows that oxidative damage, particularly lipid peroxidation, generates chemotactic factors that attract leukocytes to an area of high free radical activity and that the

Table 7–1. SUBCELLULAR SOURCES OF HYDROGEN PEROXIDE*

ORGANELLE	FUNCTION	H_2O_2 PRODUCTION (% OF TOTAL)
Mitochondria	ATP production	15%
Peroxisomes	Divalent oxidations	35%
Endoplasmic reticulum	Mixed-function oxidations	45%
Cytosol	Xanthine oxidation	5%

*Source: Chance, B., Sies, H., and Boveris, A.: Hydrogen peroxide metabolism in mammalian organs. *Physiol. Rev.*, **59**:527–605, 1979.

resultant inflammatory process can lead to increases of free radical damage. Such processes are probably important factors in pulmonary damage associated with emphysema and pollutant exposure and in atherosclerosis (see Chapters 17 and 19).

It could be argued that the protective systems, as they have evolved in the higher species, are so effective that the accumulation of damage is negligible, and that aging arises from causes other than wear-and-tear. The gradual progress of the changes that occur with aging implies that highly sensitive assays of damage, coupled to sophisticated data analysis, will be required to demonstrate a net accumulation of free radical damage, consistent with a progressive and irreversible decline of viability.

A general scheme showing cellular sources and targets of free radicals is presented in Chapter 4 (Figure 4–5). This scheme identifies the major sources of superoxide radicals in the cell, protective systems that remove these radicals and their dismutation product, H_2O_2, and some potential means whereby these active oxygen species can become further activated for reaction with biologic target molecules. It also identifies major targets, reaction products, and pathways for repairing the damage. The fundamental precept of the free radical theory of aging is that some reaction targets are not repaired and damage gradually accumulates, thus compromising cellular integrity.

GENETIC DISORDERS

In principle, an analysis of genetic disorders, involving defects in antioxidant defenses, could resolve whether the free radical theory of aging is valid. Unfortunately, although several examples of human mutations in one or more of the protective enzymes or antioxidant vitamins are known, including individuals with reduced levels of catalase, glutathione (GSH), GSH peroxidase, or defective vitamin E absorption, none of these show signs of accelerated aging that can be clearly distinguished from pathology (Mehlhorn and Cole, 1985).

Conversely, several genetic syndromes that exhibit some features of accelerated aging, the so-called "segmental progeroid syndromes," exhibit damage that could be consistent with increased free radical damage (see also Chapter 3). These include Down's syndrome, ataxia telangiectasia, Cockayne's syndrome, and, possibly, Werner's syndrome, which exhibits genetic instability, yet has normal levels of SOD, GSH peroxidase, and radiation-induced repair. The molecular basis of these "geromimetic" diseases may involve accelerated rates of chromosome breakage, and the diseases frequently exhibit radiation sensitivity that suggests a high susceptibility to free radical damage.

Fanconi's anemia also exhibits characteristics of oxygen radical damage, but the pathology is so severe that death occurs in infancy or early childhood, and the only sign of an age-related effect is increased malignancy. Devastating genetic deficiencies of this type do not permit normal development, and frequently, disease-linked premature death precludes distinguishing symptoms of accelerated aging from pathology.

Down's syndrome is characterized by a 50 percent elevation of the copper-zinc SOD (Cu/Zn-SOD) above normal levels of this enzyme. This increased protection against superoxide radicals fails to confer antiaging benefits; indeed, some aspects of age-related pathology, notably senile dementia, are accelerated. There are conflicting reports concerning altered brain lipofuscin accumulation, an *in vivo* index of lipid peroxidation. *In vitro* lipid peroxidation appears to be accelerated. In patients with trisomy 21, red blood cells are abnormally sensitive to lysis in the presence of paraquat, a molecule that causes an increase in cellular superoxide production. Fibroblasts from trisomy 21 sufferers exhibit enhanced lipid peroxidation. The apparent increase in free radical damage under conditions of elevated Cu/Zn-SOD levels can be explained by a concurrent decrease in manganese SOD (Mn-SOD) levels in some tissues. In primates Mn-SOD is not found exclusively in mitochondria, but also occurs in nuclear and other cellular compartments. In some tissues Mn-SOD may account for more than 50 percent of the total SOD content. Hence, an increase in Mn-SOD in Down's syndrome might readily compensate for a de-

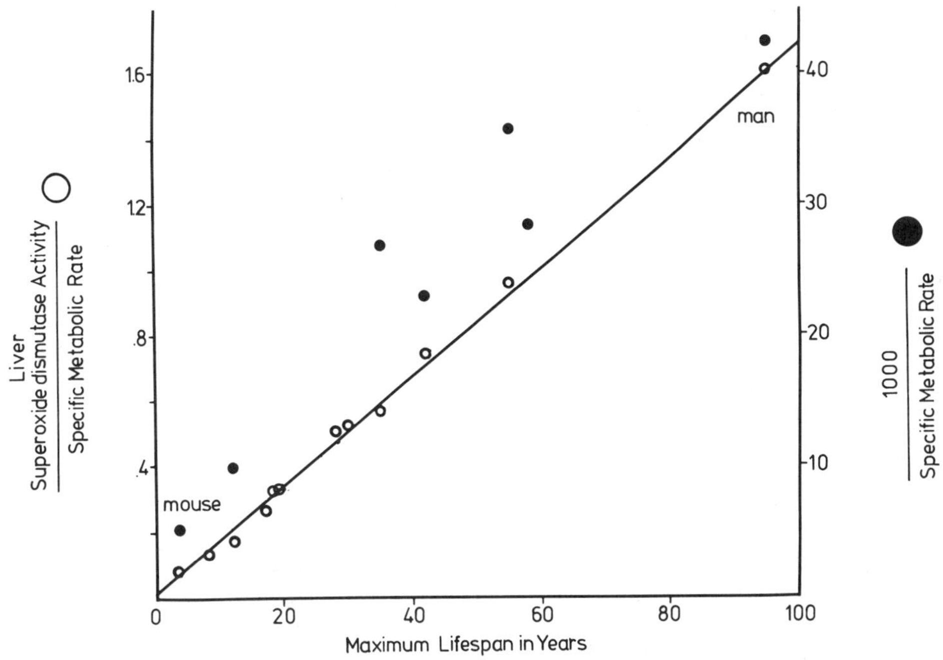

Figure 7–1. *Lifespans of 2 rodent and 12 primate species as a function of inverse metabolic rate, and the effect of multiplying by the liver SOD activity on the correlation.* (Adapted from tabulated data of Tolmasoff, *et al.*, 1980.)

crease in the copper-zinc enzyme, but it is not yet clear which tissues undergo such compensations. In patients with monosomy 21 ("21q- or anti-Down's syndrome"), cells possess only 50 percent of normal Cu/Zn-SOD but normal Mn-SOD. Although these patients suffer from developmental abnormalities and poor survival, there are no obvious signs of accelerated aging.

The difficulty of dissociating disease from aging has been a major obstacle in exploiting genetic analyses to resolve aging mechanisms. Nevertheless, the available genetic data suggest that biologic concentrations of catalase, vitamin E, glutathione, and glutathione peroxidase are probably not critical determinants of rates of aging, while levels of superoxide dismutase and the overall oxygen radical defensive capacity (viz., whole body radiation) may be important factors. Thus, the evidence can presently offer only modest support for the free radical theory of aging.

LIFESPANS AND METABOLIC RATE

To a first approximation, the specific metabolic rate of homeothermic species is inversely proportional to the maximum lifespan (Figure 7–1) (Tolmasoff *et al.*, 1980). This correlation can also be expressed as follows: the total oxygen consumption per unit weight is the same for all animals that attain their maximum lifespan. If one assumes that free radical production is proportional to the rate of aerobic metabolism, then the association between metabolic rates and lifespans can be rationalized in terms of the free radical theory of aging. The species that live longer than expected on the basis of their metabolic rates, e.g., *Homo sapiens,* appear to have improved antioxidant defenses, including higher concentrations of SOD and uric acid. The effect of SOD on maximum lifetime energy potential (LEP), a measure of the maximum attainable lifespan of an animal, corrected

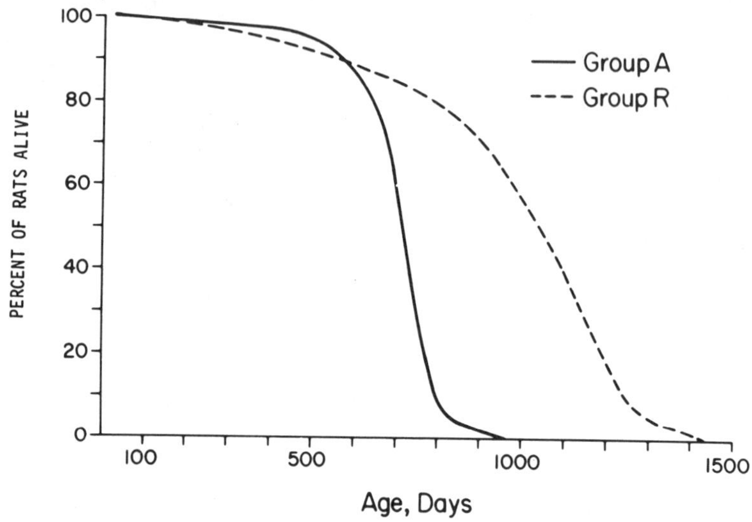

Figure 7–2. *Survival curves for* ad libitum-*fed (*group A*) and food-restricted (*group R*) SPF Fischer 344 rats.* (From Yu, *et al.*, 1982, reproduced with permission.)

for differences in specific metabolic rates, is shown in Figure 7–2.

In the brain, a direct correlation between superoxide dismutase and species lifespan has been found, while five other antioxidant factors showed no such correlation. Cutler and his collaborators have screened a number of antioxidants for their correlation with longevity in different species and have found that, in addition to SOD, serum carotenoids and vitamin E appear to correlate positively with longevity, while vitamins A and C are relatively uncorrelated. Glutathione, glutathione peroxidase, and glutathione-S-transferase seem to be negatively correlated with lifespans. The same group of investigators have also reported that the susceptibility of whole brain homogenates to autoxidation is an inverse function of species lifespan.

Correlative evidence for an association between metabolic rate and free radical processes has been obtained by direct detection of tissue free radicals with electron spin resonance (ESR) spectroscopy. ESR signals have magnitudes that correlate directly with metabolic rate and inversely with lifespan. Lipofuscin particles, which are products of free radical-mediated oxidative polymerization, sometimes contain ESR signals characteristic of metal-ion complexes. Some lipofuscin particles isolated from the human brain contain both copper and iron and exhibit free radical signals that increase progressively with age. Thus, cumulative free radical damage may occur with age, but further basic studies are required to establish the relationship of ESR signals to metabolically generated free radicals.

LIFESPAN MODIFICATION

Ideally one would like to test the free radical theory definitively by specifically manipulating the rate of free radical damage and demonstrating a corresponding effect on maximum lifespans. In principle, free radical damage is a function of both the rate of radical formation and the interception of these radicals by protective factors, either of which may be amenable to experimental control. (See Table 7–2.)

Effects of Ionizing Radiation and Chemical Mutagens. A straightforward example of free radical-mediated damage is radiation injury (see Chapter 4). However, there is no clear evidence that a slight increase in free radicals, imposed by low-level radiation, shortens lifespan. Rather, chronic radiation exposure causes a variety of cancers and other diseases. Similarly, chronic exposure

Table 7–2. STRATEGIES FOR INTERVENING IN THE AGING PROCESS BASED ON FREE RADICAL CAUSALITY ASSUMPTION

DECREASE FREE RADICAL STRESS	INCREASE PROTECTION
Stress	Antioxidant factor
Cigarettes	Vitamin C
Oxidized fats	Uric acid
Nuts infected with molds	Selenium
	Methionine
Some pickled vegetables	Vitamin E
	β-Carotene
Combustion products	
Asbestos fibers	
Immune effects	Transition metal control
Reduce infections	Zinc*
Speed wound healing	
Drugs	
Centrophenoxine/Gerovital*	
Allopurinol after ischemic episode	
Control body fat	
Low-fat diet	
Caloric restriction	

*Speculative

to mutagens (nitrogen mustards) does not appear to shorten lifespan, once the effects of increased disease incidence are taken into account. The implications of these studies for the free radical theory of aging are difficult to interpret, in part because of a lack of good aging parameter, which would facilitate discerning effects of disease from those of aging.

Caloric Restriction. The most dramatic lifespan extensions that have been achieved with dietary manipulations are increases in maximum lifespan of up to 50 percent that have been achieved by caloric restriction.

The efficacy of caloric restriction in prolonging lifespan (Figure 7–3) might suggest, at first, that there is a direct relationship between caloric intake and metabolic rate, and, hence, that such restriction lowers the rate of free radical production and damage. However, caloric restriction leads to lowered weight, and this must be taken into account. In studies with rats, when the effects of food restriction were analyzed in terms of both decreased body weights and metabolic rates, it was found that the specific metabolic rates of the smaller food-restricted animals were in fact greater than those of *ad libitum*-fed animals. The food-restricted animals lived longer than the controls, contrary to the expectation that specific metabolic rate is inversely related to the aging rate. Thus, at first sight the data on caloric restriction seem to contradict the free radical theory. Further progress in achieving a meaningful interpretation of the effects of caloric restriction may hinge on being able to relate metabolic rates to free radical fluxes.

Effects of Antioxidants. Studies with dietary antioxidants have shown that, although the mean lifespan is increased, there is no significant increase in the maximum lifespan, as would be expected if the aging rate had been altered (Mehlhorn and Cole, 1985). Side effects of antioxidants must also be considered, e.g., possible caloric restriction effects associated with foul-smelling food additives like 2-mercaptoethylamine. Another potential problem with dietary antioxidants in whole animals is a possible lack of specificity. For example, antioxidants are claimed to enhance immune function, and some quinone antioxidants, such as 2(3)-tert-butyl-4-hydroxy-anisole (BHA), induce the microsomal DT diaphorase and UDP-glucuronyl transferase systems and hence may accelerate the removal of potentially mutagenic chemicals that could affect aging by nonradical mechanisms. Two other synthetic antioxidants, BHT and ethoxyquin, have been shown to induce hepatic enzymes. Thus, increased lifespan that correlates with antioxidant feeding may be due to effects other than free radical quenching.

The accumulation of lipofuscin is increased with vitamin E deficiency and decreased with dietary antioxidants. However, there is as yet no convincing evidence that lipofuscin accumulation correlates with age-related cell loss. On the contrary, among the brain stem nuclei, the inferior olive has high lipofuscin levels and shows no age-related cell loss. Moreover, there are examples of cells that accumulate lipofuscin but do not exhibit a decline in function. This was illustrated by cell-sorting experiments with cultured fibroblasts, which separated populations of cells on the basis of fluorescence intensity and showed

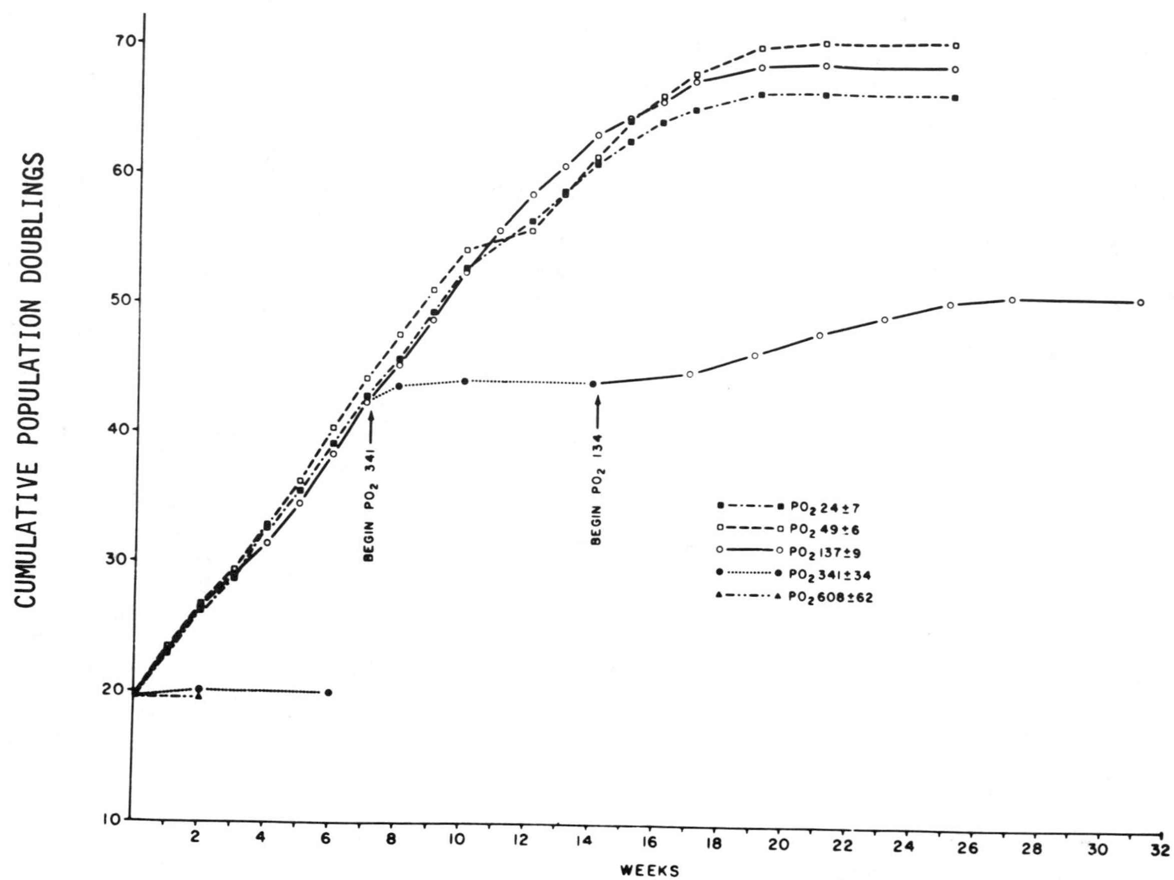

Figure 7–3. *The effect of oxygen tension on the number of cell doublings in culture of human diploid cells (WI-38), showing inhibition of the* in vitro *lifespans above but not below ambient (P_{O2} = 137 mm Hg) oxygen concentrations.* (From Balin, et al., 1977, reproduced with permission.)

that fluorescent cells suffered no loss of proliferative potential.

Thus, the evidence for antioxidant-mediated lifespan extension in vertebrates does not argue persuasively for a causal role of free radicals in aging. This fact is generally acknowledged by advocates of the free radical theory, who offer two general explanations that could sustain the basic concept: (1) the principal site of damage (e.g., mitochondrial DNA) is not protected by exogenous antioxidants, or (2) the endogenous defense system is regulated to maintain a fixed overall level of protection so that simple attempts to increase protection by some dietary manipulation fail owing to compensatory decreases in endogenous defenses ("compensatory downregulation").

Since the largest fraction of mammalian oxygen consumption occurs in mitochondria, free radical damage might occur primarily in these organelles and mitochondria could play a role as pacemakers. This hypothesis could explain some of the failures of the original free radical theory of aging. Excessive concentrations of the phenolic antioxidants could also react with mitochondrial electron transport components to impair mitochondrial metabolism. Such reactions could explain the futility of extending lifespan with antioxidants of this type.

Another explanation for the failure of antioxidants to confer substantial lifespan extension, "compensatory downregulation of endogenous antioxidant defenses," argues that when increased concentrations of exogenous antioxidants reduce the flux of radicals, the cell decreases its production of other defensive enzymes. However, the fact that lipofuscin accumulation can be reduced by feeding antioxidants in the absence of lifespan extension, and that tumor incidence can be reduced by feeding exogenous antioxidants, suggests that antioxidants can effectively reduce the rate of free radical damage in some tissues without undue compensatory downregulation.

***In Vitro* "Aging Models".** The doubling potential of cultured mammalian cells like fibroblasts has been perceived as a meaningful *in vitro* aging model because it correlates with species lifespan and with the age of the cell donor and is reduced by life-shortening genetic disorders in humans. To explore the possibility that the finite doubling potential of the cells is due to free radical damage, a number of investigators have varied the oxygen tension during cell growth and studied how this affected the doubling limit. No increase in the maximum number of doublings could be achieved by lowering the oxygen concentration below ambient levels, although increased oxygen concentrations curtailed both growth rates and the doubling number (Figure 7–4).

Cultured human fibroblasts can be transformed by treatment with SV40 virus to remove the limited growth potential; i.e., the transformed cells become "immortal." The transformed cells are aneuploid, genetically unstable, and, often, DNA repair-deficient. When these transformed cells are exposed to higher-than-ambient oxygen concentrations, they too are slowed in their growth rate. It has been shown that this oxygen-induced decline in growth rate is due to an inhibition of DNA replication, suggesting that the effect of high oxygen concentrations on growth rates is not necessarily related to free radical formation. In normal fibroblasts, oxygen also modulates growth and can affect the process of differentiation. A stimulating effect of low oxygen tension on fibroblast growth rate may serve a regulatory role in wound healing. These multiple effects of oxygen in fibroblasts underscore the ambiguities associated with interpreting experiments with the replicative limit model in terms of free radical damage alone.

Adrenocortical cells in long-term culture, grown on certain batches of 10 percent fetal bovine serum, are essentially completely deficient in both vitamin E and in selenium when not supplemented with these nutrients (Hornsby *et al.*, 1984). This has set the stage for analyzing effects of these antioxidants in determining the *in vitro* "lifespan" of these cells. Supplementation with either vitamin E or selenium protects the cells from the toxic effects of added cumene hydroperoxide, demonstrating the efficacy of these nutrients in ameliorating the effects of oxidative damage. However, the long-term growth of the cells is nearly identical in the absence or presence of these antioxidants, suggesting that oxidative damage is not a significant determinant of the doubling potential in adrenocortical cells. Alternatively, this experiment may indicate that rapid cell growth under optimal conditions enables cells to outpace the damaging effects of free radical chemistry and that damage only becomes apparent with cumulative radical damage when metabolically active cells have a limited capacity to divide.

The validity of the replicative limit model as an aging model is unclear (Bell, 1984); hence, negative evidence obtained with it should not necessarily be taken as an indictment of the free radical theory of aging. The central difficulty with the proliferative limit model lies in its questionable significance for *in vivo* aging. There is no solid evidence for a proliferative limit occurring during normal *in vivo* aging, and it seems likely that functional losses that precede the *in vitro* proliferative limit are responsible for aging.

Exercise. A promising experimental strategy for manipulating metabolic rates is exercise. The analysis of exercise effects requires that both the intensity of exercise and prior training be taken into account. Increased radical damage appears to occur with intensive exercise in untrained animals, and positive adaptations, conferring increased resistance to oxidative damage, are observed in endurance-trained animals.

Studies with intense physical activity in untrained rats have suggested an increase in free radical damage, e.g., increased lipid peroxidation products in liver and skeletal muscle homogenates and in mitochondrial fractions. Experiments with rats have shown that plasma glutathione disulfide increases significantly with intensive exercise and that vitamin E deficiency is associated with a marked decrease in endurance capacity, suggesting that lipid peroxidation may play a role in muscle fatigue upon exhaustion.

Rodents that have been exercise trained throughout life live longer than their sedentary counterparts, consistent with a positive effect of exercise training on mean lifespan. Although the mechanism of the lifespan extension is unresolved, it may involve caloric restriction, since exercised animals accumulate less body fat than sedentary animals. Endurance training appears to decrease the susceptibility of skeletal muscles to lipid peroxidation, consistent with an adaptive response of protective systems. Endurance training raises the activity of the enzyme glutathione reductase in both skeletal and cardiac muscles. This enzyme serves an antioxidant function by maintaining glutathione in its reduced state, thus enabling glutathione peroxidase to perform its function of hydroperoxide reduction. Exercise training markedly retards the appearance of high plasma glutathione disulfide concentrations during intensive exercise, supporting the notion that exercise training increases the capacity of an animal to maintain highly reduced glutathione levels for long periods of intensive activity.

SUSCEPTIBLE ORGANELLES, CELLS, AND TISSUES

Because the cell populations in different tissues are likely to vary in their redundancy, regenerative capacity, free radical production rates, antioxidant defenses, and DNA repair rates, some tissues may be particularly sensitive to free radical damage, and these could determine aging rates in the organism. For example, metabolically active, nondividing cells like the neurons could well be the most susceptible targets of oxidative damage. Indeed, there is a loss of neurons with age, but such loss appears to be species-specific and to be a function of the tissue location. The surprising durability of neuronal tissue despite its large oxygen utilization appears, at first sight, to be incompatible with free radical involvement in age-related functional declines. However, a large portion of the oxygen utilization is in axons and terminals that are physically removed from sensitive and nonrenewable targets like the nuclear genome. Moreover, neuronal mitochondria do not appear to produce superoxide radicals at a site that is a major source of these radicals in other cells. Finally, considerable cell redundancy may prevent functional deficits from becoming clinically significant. As a rule, more than 40 percent cell loss is required in a neuronal system before functional loss in the central nervous system is apparent.

Because mitochondria are dependent on the nuclear genome for many of their proteins and are sensitive to the cellular environment (ions, substrates) and even hormonal stimulation (viz., thyroid hormone effects on mitochondrial replication), it is difficult to confidently infer intrinsic mitochondrial damage from age-related mitochondrial dysfunction. However, mitochondrial dysfunction and depletion do occur in aging postmitotic cells and may prove to be a major factor in aging. Miquel and his colleagues have postulated that mitochondria are the "Achilles' heel" of postmitotic cells because mitochondrial DNA is not protected by a histone coat, is in close proximity to sites of oxygen radical production and lipid peroxidation, and is dependent on a possibly inadequate DNA repair system (Fleming *et al.*, 1982).

Systemic Effects

One of the most obvious characteristics of aging is the gradual decline of physiologic integrity, including the progressive loss of neurologic, immunologic, humoral, and metabolic function. Evidence for free radical involvement in all of these debilitating processes is growing. However, organelle and cellular redundancy and renewal may be able to compensate for the damage sufficiently to sustain function. Thus, the epithelia lining the digestive tract and skin, the blood cells, and the liver may be extensively damaged and yet regenerate on a regular basis. In these renewing cell populations, the principal danger of damage appears to be neoplastic transformation.

Because aging is characterized by an increased incidence of infectious diseases, one might expect immunosenescence to play a crucial role in physiologic aging (see Chapter 8). Declines in immune function begin relatively early and appear to be heavily dependent on thymic involution and selective T-cell aging. Immunologic declines can be, at least partially, reversed by thymic grafts or thymic hormone therapy, but complete restoration requires an additional young bone marrow graft.

Evidence for free radical involvement in immunosenescence is based on selective vulnerability of the immune system to radiation and other free radical-generating agents. T cells, which age more rapidly than B cells are reported to be more vulnerable to oxygen radicals and to accumulate more lipofuscin; treatment of aging mice with 2-mercaptoethanol delays the accumulation of T-cell lipofuscin and the decline of immune function with age and increases the mean lifespan.

The thymus may also be selectively vulnerable to free radical damage. The first age-related loss in size (thymic involution) can be ascribed to the loss of the most radiosensitive (cortical) lymphocytes. The medullary epithelial cells that secrete thymic hormones are heterogenous, and the early loss is again that of the most radiosensitive cells, which are active metabolically, require vitamin C for their secretory activity, and appear to accumulate intrinsically autofluorescent substances (age pigments). Although there are probably developmentally programmed cellular and hormonal controls of thymic involution, significant oxidative damage seems to be involved as well.

Many antioxidants are immune stimulants and will enhance immune function both *in vivo* and *in vitro* with both young and old cells. Part of this effect appears to be due to the maintenance of reduced sulfhydryl groups. Although antioxidant treatment can boost immune function at any age, it does not markedly reduce the rate of basic aging of the immune system.

Disease

Balin has emphasized the importance of separating the effects of specific life-extending treatments that may reduce the incidence of disease and hence most likely affect only mean lifespans from those that affect basic aging rates (Balin, 1982). As reviewed in the preceding sections, free radicals do not seem to determine maximum lifespan. However, mean lifespan is well correlated with the incidence of disease, and many diseases that shorten mean lifespans are aggravated by free radical processes (see, for example, Pryor, 1986).

Some of the support for free radical involvement in disease is outlined in the following sections.

Cancer. The process whereby a normal cell becomes transformed, i.e., whereby it assumes the uncontrolled growth characteristics of a cancer cell, seems to involve an alteration of the DNA, as shown by the fact that many chemicals that cause cancer in animals also cause mutations in microorganisms in the well-known Ames *Salmonella* revertant test. This test is often used as a predictor of risk for chemicals that are suspected to have carcinogenic potential.

The relationship between aging and cancer is complex; for example, neuroblastomas, many leukemias, and hormone-dependent tumors have radically different age patterns than most sarcomas and many carcinomas that rise with the second and fourth power of age, respectively. The incidence of most tumors, in a large variety of species, rises dramatically with age. This rise in cancer incidence with age may be attributed to several factors (Ebbesen, 1984): (1) Long-term carcinogen exposure increases the risk of initiation; e.g., lung cancer incidence reflects duration of smoking rather than chronological age. (2) The prolonged period required for one malignant cell to multiply and develop into a detectable tumor. (3) Aging itself increases the risk because of (a) a possible reduction in natural killer or other immune surveillance function, (b) an increase in the activation of procarcingogens, and (c) other factors, including demethylation-induced epigenetic instability and free radical-induced DNA damage.

The pathogenesis of neoplasia is thought to be a two-stage process: (1) initiation, produced by mutagenesis, abnormal differentiation, or viral infection, and (2) promotion, characterized by a prolonged latency allowing for the multiplication and evolution of initiated cells into a tumor. The process involves many variables, including tissue type, hormonal influence, proliferative rates, DNA repair capacity, environmental carcinogen exposure, viral infection, immune surveillance, and genotype (see also Chapter 3).

Work has progressed rapidly on the relationship between carcinogens and mutagens. Point mutations are implicated in the activation of ras oncogenes in human tumors, for example. However, for other oncogenes, for example, the myc family (e.g., Burkitt's lymphoma), there is a chromosomal translocation of the oncogene to an enhancer-amplified site, presumably activating oncogene expression. Epidemiologic evidence suggests that the point mutations may stem from a variety of environmental and intrinsic mutagens, including free radicals.

A number of potent chemical carcinogens, such as benzo[a]pyrene, form free radical derivatives in simple chemical systems and in isolated membranes of the endoplasmic reticulum. Some molecules are also converted to quinones by the cytochrome P-450 system, and these quinones can be substantially more toxic to cells (e.g., cultured fibroblasts) than their precursors. The mechanism of the quinone toxicity may be a catalytic reaction whereby the quinones undergo redox cycling with cellular electron donors and with molecular oxygen to produce superoxide radicals. For example, the quinones that result from the microsomal oxidation of benzo[a]pyrene are readily reduced by electron donors such as glutathione, NADH, and NADPH and by the DT diaphorase enzyme. As soon as the reduced quinol is formed, it reacts with molecular oxygen in one-electron transfer steps to form superoxide radicals. In the process of redox cycling, some semiquinone radical species can also react directly with cellular macromolecules, including DNA.

Gross genetic rearrangements, transpositions, and amplification appear to play a major role in the promotion process of carcinogenesis. It is quite probable that free radical damage is also involved in these processes. Since oxygen-derived radicals are capable of inducing mutations, and since they appear to have the capacity to cause chromosomal strand breakage, they should be able to participate in the gene rearrangements necessary to link a protooncogene with an enhancer element.

Current evidence that oxygen radicals

are involved in carcinogenesis includes the following:

1. Several genetic disorders with a high incidence of both chromosomal rearrangement and neoplasia, e.g., Fanconi's and Bloom's syndromes, appear to involve abnormally high oxygen radical-mediated damage. Unlike other syndromes predisposed to malignancy, Fanconi's anemia and Bloom's syndrome appear to have normal DNA repair capacity, but increased sensitivity to oxygen radical-generated damage.
2. Epidemiologic evidence suggests that dietary or endogenous factors rather than industrial products or environmental agents are responsible for the majority of human cancers (Doll and Peto, 1981; Totter, 1980). An involvement of lipid-peroxidation-linked oxygen radicals is supported by the implication of fat as a risk factor for many types of tumors and the inverse correlation of risk with dietary antioxidant intake (Ames, 1984). Other epidemiologic data show that high dietary intake of quinones or quinone precursors, which are capable of promoting free radical reactions, is attended by increased cancer incidence. Ionizing radiation also induces cancer in a dose-dependent manner. When cigarette smoke is trapped on glass wool, a large ESR signal can be observed and it seems quite plausible that this free radical component of cigarette smoke is a causative factor in its well-established link with cancer.
3. Oxygen-derived radicals are implicated in tumor promotion. Phorbol esters, the classical tumor promoters, produce extensive chromosomal damage and stimulate polymorphonuclear leukocytes to produce an abundance of superoxide and peroxides. Antipromoters such as retinoids and protease inhibitors inhibit oxygen radical production. DNA strand breakage correlates directly with promotional efficiency, and antipromotional ability correlates with inhibition of strand breaks. Promoter-induced chromosomal damage is inhibited by superoxide dismutase, but in some systems (lymphocytes) it is also inhibited by indomethacin and other inhibitors of prostaglandin synthetase that can produce unstable lipid peroxides and attendant oxygen radicals.

Phorbol esters have several other effects on cellular metabolism; in particular, they rapidly activate the protein kinase c pathway, a principal control point in the regulation of proliferation, and rapidly and reversibly induce many of the properties of the transformed phenotype. Hence, phorbol esters have a rapid and reversible short-term effect on cells that stimulates cell proliferation. They also generate free radical-mediated chromosomal damage, which may allow for an emergence of clones with activated oncogenes and a permanently malignant phenotype.

Phorbol esters are not the only promoters capable of producing oxygen radicals. In a recent review, Ames has assembled evidence that most promoters (e.g., phorbol esters, fat, TCDD, lead, cadmium, wounded tissue, asbestos, anthralin, peroxides, mezerein, telociden B, phenobarbitol, radiation, nitroso and nitro compounds, hydrazines, and polycyclic hydrocarbons) are also capable of generating oxygen radicals (Ames, 1984). While all of these agents have a multiplicity of other effects and there is, at present, no quantitative correlation between the efficiency of promotion and oxygen radical production, the qualitative correlation is striking. The evidence for a causal relation between oxygen radical production and promotion is also supported by the efficacy of antioxidants as anticarcinogens. In particular, vitamin E, selenium, glutathione, ascorbic acid, and β-carotene have proven effective in reducing tumor incidence.

Parkinson's Disease. Parkinson's disease is a strongly age-related pathology marked by a selective and progressive loss of pigmented catecholaminergic, particularly dopaminergic, neurons of the *substantia nigra* (see also Chapter 9). This loss, which may well be due to a selective vulnerability to oxidative damage, averages about 80 percent in autopsied patients, compared to only about a 40 percent loss seen in the oldest normal individuals. The current epidemiologic data suggest that Parkinson's disease is caused by some environmental agent(s) and reasonable candidates would be those producing excessive fluxes of oxygen radicals or other active oxygen species. Several investigators have speculated about possible oxidative mechanisms in the development of Parkinson's disease, including redox cycling of quinones derived from catecholamines and a role for hydrogen peroxide derived from monoamine oxidase.

Glutathione concentrations are low in human substantia nigra and almost absent from nigral tissue of patients who have succumbed to Parkinson's disease. Catalase and glutathione peroxidase have also been found to be abnormally low in patients with this disease. It is conceivable, however, that these reductions are the result of neuronal loss rather than decreases in cell-specific enzyme activities.

It has been claimed that brains of patients with Parkinson's disease contain abnormally high concentrations of iron. Since iron is normally sequestered in highly stable storage and binding proteins, it is conceivable that "free" iron may be present in these brains, which could catalyze hydroxyl radical formation in a Fenton-type of reaction.

An environmental neurotoxin like *N*-methyl-4-phenyl-1, 2, 3, 6-tetrahydropyridine, which selectively kills dopaminergic neurons, could displace dopamine from its storage vesicles (which are at acidic pH and therefore provide some protection against autoxidation) and thus drive an increased catecholamine autoxidation and an increased peroxide release from monoamine oxidase.

Thus, the evidence for free radical involvement in Parkinson's disease is suggestive, but further experiments are necessary before an unequivocal resolution of the mechanisms involved can be offered.

Autoimmune Disease. Because tolerance to self appears to require an active thymic role in the production of T suppressor cells as well as in the deletion of self-reactive clones, one might expect thymic involution and age-related immune dysregulation to result in an age-related increase in autoimmune disease. Further, the emergence of altered self antigens through persistent viral infection, posttranslational modifications, somatic mutation, or even postmaturational development of newly expressed genes could also bring about an increased number of autoimmune reactions with age (see Chapter 8).

Autoimmune phenomena like autoantibodies, glomerulonephritis, periarteritis, and probably some classes of senile amyloid increase with age. A major role of autoimmune pathology is played in the aging of some rodents, but not all strains and species seem to be affected. Hence, while some workers have hypothesized that autoimmunity is the major aging process and likened senescence to a chronic graft-versus-host reaction, the evidence is not consistent. In humans, most known or suspected autoimmune diseases, including rheumatoid arthritis, have a peak incidence in middle age, and it is difficult to assess the significance of autoimmune phenomena in human aging. Among rodents, in strains that are clearly autoimmune susceptible, such as NZB mice, antioxidant feeding has produced a delay in disease onset and lifespan extension. If autoimmunity is a major aging process and not a secondary pathology, then antioxidant feeding may be said to delay the accelerated aging that has been reported in NZB mice.

Several other diseases seem to involve free radicals in their etiology, including atherosclerosis, emphysema, arthritis, cirrhosis, and diabetes (Pryor, 1986).

INTERVENTIVE STRATEGIES

APPROACHES TOWARD ALTERING FREE RADICAL DAMAGE

Genetic analysis is one promising approach toward understanding how the expression of endogenous oxidative defenses is regulated, as illustrated by preliminary studies in yeast and by recent isolation of an oxygen-resistant Chinese hamster ovary cell line with elevated SOD, glutathione peroxidase, and catalase, which suggests the feasibility of similar analyses in mammalian cells.

The relationship between age and the enzymes that defend against free radical attack has attracted considerable interest but remains unresolved. As with other age-related biochemical and physiologic investigations, there are problems associated with species and tissue variability compounded by occasional conflicting reports from different laboratories. For example, in the rat brain, mitochondrial SOD is unchanged or increased with age, while CuSOD is unchanged or decreased. Rat brain cytosolic glutathione peroxidase is unchanged or decreased, mitochondrial glutathione peroxidase and reductase are increased, and both cytoplasmic and mitochondrial catalase are unchanged with age.

Because of the conflicting data and lack of corresponding information about metabolic rates and radical production, the interpretation of data on protective enzymes remains obscure, and further studies are needed to assess the significance of observed enzyme level changes.

LIFESPAN EXTENSION STRATEGIES BASED ON FREE RADICAL CONCEPTS

Even if free radicals are implicated only in life-shortening diseases, and do not make a contribution to the basic aging process, the general problems of the aged are so great that intervention in free radical-mediated damage is highly worthwhile. This section addresses some of the interventive measures that might be considered to reduce the incidence of free radical-potentiated diseases.

There is a growing awareness of the hazards of exogenous free radicals. These include cigarettes, oxidized fat, moldy nuts, pickled vegetables, burned meats, combustion products, and asbestos. Avoidance of these agents is likely to reduce the risk of the free radical-mediated diseases.

It is also feasible to reduce the impact of exogenous or metabolically generated radicals on cellular targets by ingesting antioxidants. Vitamin E, β-carotene, and BHT can protect against active oxygen species in the fatty tissues and in cell membranes. They are particularly effective in protecting against the harmful effects of certain drugs used in chemotherapy, which will kill cancer cells by free radical mechanisms.

Aqueous chemical reactions may be a more important free radical damage route than fatty tissue reactions. Unfortunately, there are no facile means to enhance the protection afforded by the water-soluble enzymes catalase and SOD. However, dietary selenium can be used to enhance glutathione peroxidase activity, although toxic overdoses are a concern. One can also consider vitamin C supplements, but this vitamin has the potential of acting as a pro- rather than an antioxidant in the presence of free transition metal ions. Uric acid is a water-soluble antioxidant factor that may confer benefits against singlet oxygen and may protect against the ravages of superoxide produced by xanthine oxidase. There may also be value in methionine supplementation to increase the biosynthesis of glutathione.

Since the immune system appears to do much of its work by exploiting the toxic properties of free radicals, another line of protection is to minimize activation of such free radical reactions. This can be achieved by avoiding infections, treating wounds promptly and effectively, using drugs to speed postoperative recovery, and using anti-inflammatory agents when appropriate.

Because of the possibility that transition metals may contribute substantially to free radical damage, it would be worthwhile to pursue strategies for minimizing their reactions. One suggestion that has been made is to use zinc supplementation as a strategy for displacing iron from binding sites that might otherwise be susceptible to reactions with iron or copper. This suggestion has to be regarded as highly speculative.

SUMMARY

The free radical theory of aging is faced with several serious difficulties that cast doubt on its validity as formulated. These include:

1. The failure of antioxidant therapy to significantly extend the maximum lifespan

of mammals. This failure is particularly troubling because the administration of antioxidants has clear-cut effects in reducing the extent of lipofuscin accumulation, a convincing demonstration that the antioxidants do protect some cellular targets susceptible to peroxidation. Antioxidant administration can also confer anticarcinogenic benefits, yet no significant maximum lifespan extension has been realized under these conditions.

2. The fact that the only effective strategy for lifespan extension, i.e., caloric restriction, has not been successfully correlated with metabolic rates or with rates of endogenous radical production, diminished oxidative damage, or enhanced protection.
3. The failure to demonstrate an expected oxygen concentration effect on the proliferative potential in the cultured cell aging model, assuming some relevance of this model to *in vivo* aging.

Acknowledgments: This work was supported by the National Institutes of Health (grant AG-04818).

References

Ames, B. N.: Dietary carcinogens and anticarcinogens. *Science,* **221:**1256–1264, **1984.**

Balin, A. K.: Testing the free radical theory of aging. In Adelman, R. C., and Roth, G. S. (eds.): *Testing the Theories of Aging,* CRC Press, Boca Raton, FL, **1982.**

Balin, A. K.; Goodman, D. B. P.; Rasmussen, H.; and Cristofalo. V. J.: The effect of oxygen and vitamin E on the lifespan of human diploid cells in vitro. *J. Cell Biol.,* **74:**58–67, **1977.**

Bell, E.: Cells may have escaped mortality, the price paid for fitness by multicellular organisms. In Scarpelli, D. G., and Migaki, G. (eds.): *Comparative Pathobiology of Major Age-related Diseases: Current Status and Research Frontiers,* Alan R. Liss, New York, **1984.**

Chance, B.; Sies, H.; and Boveris, A.: Hydrogen peroxide metabolism in mammalian organs. *Physiol. Rev.,* **59:**527–605, **1979.**

Doll, R., and Peto, R.: The causes of cancer-quantifiable estimates of avoidable risks of cancer in the United States today. *J. Natl. Cancer Inst.,* **66:**1190, **1981.**

Ebbesen, P.: Cancer and normal aging. *Mech. Ageing Dev.,* **25:**269–283, **1984.**

Fleming, J. E.; Miquel, J.; Cottrell, S. F.; Yengoyan, L. S.; and Economos, A. C.: Is cell aging caused by respiration-dependent injury to the mitochondrial genome? *Gerontology,* **28:**44–53, **1982.**

Harman, D.: Aging: A theory based on free radical and radiation chemistry. *J. Gerontol.,* **11:**298–300, **1956.**

Hornsby, P. J.; Aldern, K. A.; and Harris, S. E.: Adrenocortical cultures as model systems for investigating cellular aging. In Armstrong, D.; Sohal, R. S.; Cutler, R. G.; and Slater, T. S. (eds.): *Free Radicals in Molecular Biology, Aging, and Disease,* Raven Press, New York, **1984.**

Mehlhorn, R. J., and Cole, G.: The free radicals theory of aging: A critical review, *Adv. Free Radical Biol. Med.,* **1:**165–223, **1985.**

Pryor, W. A.: The free radical theory of aging revisited: A critique and a suggested disease-specific theory. In Butler, R. N.; Sprott, R. L.; Schneider, E. L.; and Warner, H. R. (eds.): *Modern Biological Theories of Aging,* Raven Press, New York, **1986.**

Tolmasoff, J. M.; Ono, T.; and Cutler, R. G.: Superoxide dismutase: Correlation with life-span and specific metabolic rate. *Proc. Natl. Acad. Sci. USA,* **77:**2777–2781, **1980.**

Totter, J. R.: Spontaneous cancer and its possible relationship to oxygen metabolism. *Proc. Natl. Acad. Sci. USA,* **77:**1763–1767, **1980.**

Yu, B. P.; Masoro, E. J.; Murata, I.; Bertrand, H. A.; and Lynd, F. T.: Life span study of SPF Fischer 344 male rats fed *ad libitum* or restricted diets: Longevity, growth, lean body mass and disease. *J. Gerontol.,* **37:**130–141, **1982.**

CHAPTER

8 AGING OF THE IMMUNE SYSTEM

Hal Sternberg

Perhaps the most dramatic and consequence-bearing age-related phenomenon is the decline in immunologic function with old age. Immune dysfunction, which is known to accompany aging, increases susceptibility to a number of disabling diseases having different etiologies. Despite great progress in pharmacologic and medical treatments, infectious diseases such as pneumonia and influenza (Galpin, 1981) rise exponentially after the age of 25, along with the increased incidence of cancer and autoimmune disease (Teller, 1972).

Immune function is dependent on a great number of different factors, such as major histocompatibility genes, hormonal, psychologic, and nutritional status, age, and prior history of antigenic exposure. As a result of these many variables, contradictory data exist regarding the aging of this function in humans. However, during the past decade much has been learned concerning the mechanism of immune reactions at a cellular and molecular level (Eisen, 1980; Hood *et al.*, 1984), and the recent progress on immunologic aging is the focus of this chapter.

Understanding the mechanisms of immune function and the influence of aging on immune function is not a simple matter. Immunologic reactions are often highly complex (Table 8–1) and require the participation of numerous humoral factors, cell types, tissues, and organs; therefore, it is difficult to present a simple, comprehensive, overview of the field. The present chapter will discuss age-related changes of the various components of the immune system. We begin with some background information concerning the immune system and an overview of the significance of age-related immune dysfunction. Thereafter, we will discuss age-related changes of the components of the immune system (from the thymus and thymic factors, to stem cells, lymphocytes, phagocytic cells, and natural killer cells), concluding with a brief summary and the possible reversibility of immunologic senescence.

SPECTRUM OF VITAL PROPERTIES AND ACTIVITIES

The immune system has the enormous task of recognizing that which is self from that which is nonself (or foreign). It must be diverse enough to defend against an almost unlimited variety of pathogenic microbes (viruses and bacteria) and sensitive enough to distinguish transformed cells (tumor cells) from normal cells. The specificity of the immune system toward potentially harmful foreign substances is indeed remarkable. This specificity guards against autoimmune reactions and allows for the detection of subtle changes that occur during tumorigenesis.

Age-related changes in immune function may have profound effects on susceptibility toward a variety of diseases of different etiologies, as well as influencing the ability to accept allogeneic transplants. Because breakdown in immune function with aging leading to increased autoantibody production and tissue degeneration could account for much age-related pathology, gerontologists have proposed that immune system failure may cause human aging (Walford, 1969), a proposal that has generated a great deal of interest and research in this area. Evidence does support the concept that aging of the immune system is rate limiting on the human lifespan, but cannot account for all manifestations of aging (collagen cross-linking, limited proliferative abilities of dividing cells, the accumulation of lipofuscin, and DNA damage in nondividing cells).

Table 8–1. COMPLEXITY OF THE IMMUNE SYSTEM AND IMMUNOLOGIC SENESCENCE

Components are multiple:
- organs and tissues
- cells
- secretory factors

Differential reactions depend on:
- immunogen (composition, route, dose, half-life)
- histocompatibility genes
- humoral, psychologic, and nutritional state
- prior antigenic history
- age

Immunologic senescence does not equally affect all components and activities of the immune system.

Differences in experimental approaches and subjective interpretation of data often lead to contradictory conclusions.

Table 8–2. MAJOR STRUCTURES OF THE IMMUNE SYSTEM

Bone marrow: Meshwork of connective tissue and stem cells contained within bone cavities. Stem cells are multipotent and differentiate into leukocytes and reticulocytes.

Lymph nodes: Glandlike structures, arranged in groups, interspersed throughout the lymphatic circulation. They consist of a fibrillar network where lymphocytes are organized, mature, and interact. They serve as sites where antigens are trapped and destroyed. Major lymphoid organs include adenoids, appendix, Peyer's patches, spleen, and tonsils.

Lymphatic vessels: Thin-walled vessels that direct the flow of lymph in a particular direction using valves. The lymph is pumped, upon muscle contraction and osmotic pressure, through the lymphatic system, into the lymphatic duct, and then into the large subclavian veins.

Reticuloendothelial system: Phagocytic cells contained in reticular tissues located in lymph nodes and liver.

Spleen: A relatively large lymphoid organ situated in the upper quadrant of the abdominal cavity. Like the thymus, it has a cortex and medulla. The cortex contains densely packed lymphocytes and germinal centers. The medulla has a variety of leukocytes and encapsulates the cortex (unlike other lymphoid tissues). Some regions are particularly rich in B lymphocytes and appear important for B-lymphocyte storage and activation.

Thymus: A lymphoid organ under the sternum that consists of a network of epithelial cells that secrete various polypeptide factors important for the maturation of thymocytes (which are also contained within the thymus) into T cells and immune function in general.

Complexity of the Immune System and Immunologic Senescence

Numerous components interact and participate in eliciting immune reactions (Table 8–2 and Figure 8–1). In addition to the organs and tissues listed in Table 8–2, many different cell types and secretory factors are involved. The cell types include B lymphocytes, T lymphocytes, monocytes, granulocytes, and natural killer cells (Figure 8–2), all of which are derived through bone marrow stem cell differentiation. The secretory factors include thymic factors and lymphokines (factors released by activated leukocytes that, in turn, stimulate other leukocytes), which, too, are critical in immune reactions.

The components that are involved in a particular reaction are not only dependent on the immunogen, but, as mentioned above, also dependent on histocompatibility genes and prior antigenic exposure. Another variable reflects the differences in methodology used in the experimental approaches, which may be responsible for differences of interpretation.

Not all components of the immune system may be equally affected by aging; a change in one component may not influence all immunologic reactions. For example, an age-related deficit in T-killer-cell activity may not influence the removal of an antigen that is normally destroyed by complement-mediated lysis or macrophage engulfment.

Immunologic Defense

Immunologic reactions can be triggered by an almost limitless number of substances called immunogens. These immunogens may or may not be associated with the surfaces of microorganisms. Among the substances that may be immunogenic and elicit an immune response are proteins, carbohydrates, lipids, or any combination of these. Immunogens that can induce antibody production and specifically bind to these antibodies are called antigens.

The generally accepted schema of a typical immune response is shown in Figure 8–1. A foreign substance (antigen) is first recognized by a macrophage that binds to the antigen. The macrophage presents the antigen to a T-helper cell and secretes the lymphokine, interleukin-1 (IL-1), that stimulates the T-helper cell. The activated T-helper cell, in turn, secretes the lymphokine interleukin-2 (IL-2), which stimulates cytotoxic T lymphocytes (T-killer). The T-

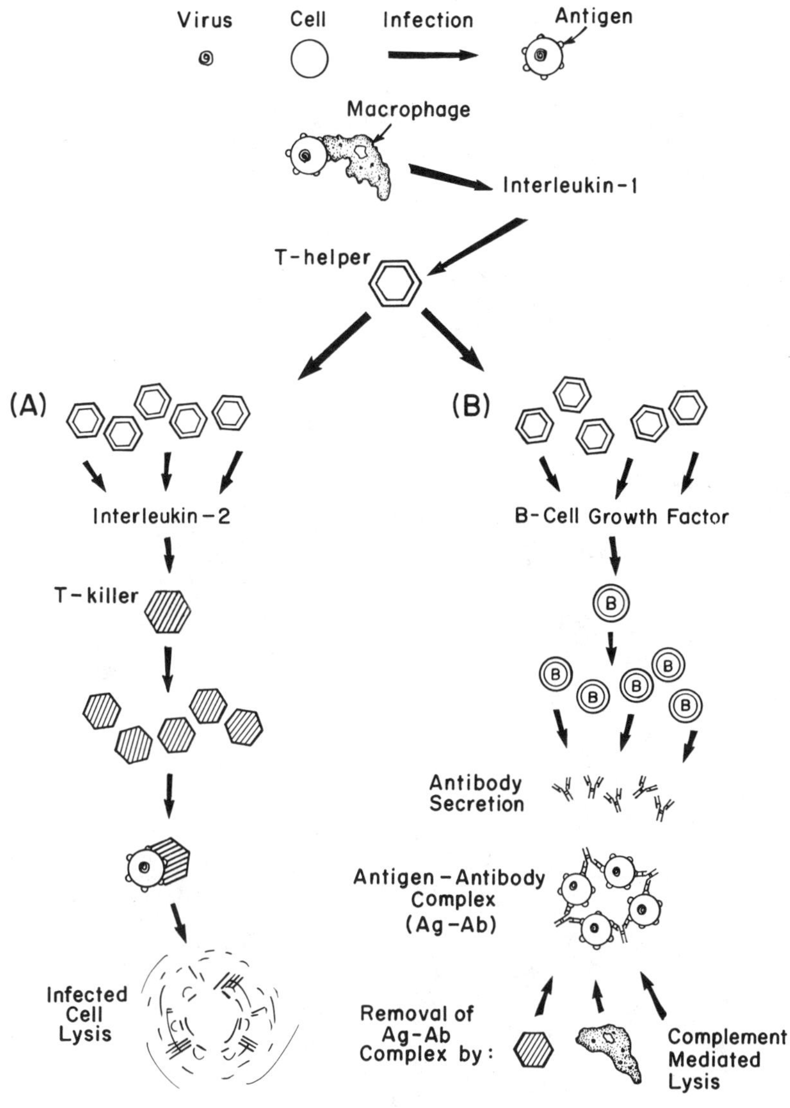

Figure 8–1. *Immune response to viral infection.*

(*Top.*) Cell infected by virus produces new surface antigen. This antigen is recognized by macrophage which produces IL-1. IL-1 stimulates T-helper cell proliferation. (*A*) Stimulated T-helper cells produces IL-2 which induces T-killer cell proliferation and lysis of antigen. (*B*) Some stimulated T-helper cells produce B-cell growth factors that promote B-cell proliferation and differentiation into mature antibody secreting plasma cells. Secreted antibodies complex with antigen. Ag-Ab complexes are removed by T-killer cells, macrophages, or complement-mediated lysis.

helper cell may also secrete B-cell growth factor that stimulates B lymphocytes to proliferate and secrete specific antibodies. Antibodies are structurally similar glycoproteins called immunoglobins that have a short half-life, on the order of days, and bind tightly to antigen. An antibody-coated antigen may be destroyed in various ways (listed in Table 8–3), depending on the antigen and class of immunoglobin (Ig) associated with it.

MAJOR HISTOCOMPATIBILITY GENES

Many of the mechanisms of immune function are encoded by a large gene cluster known as the

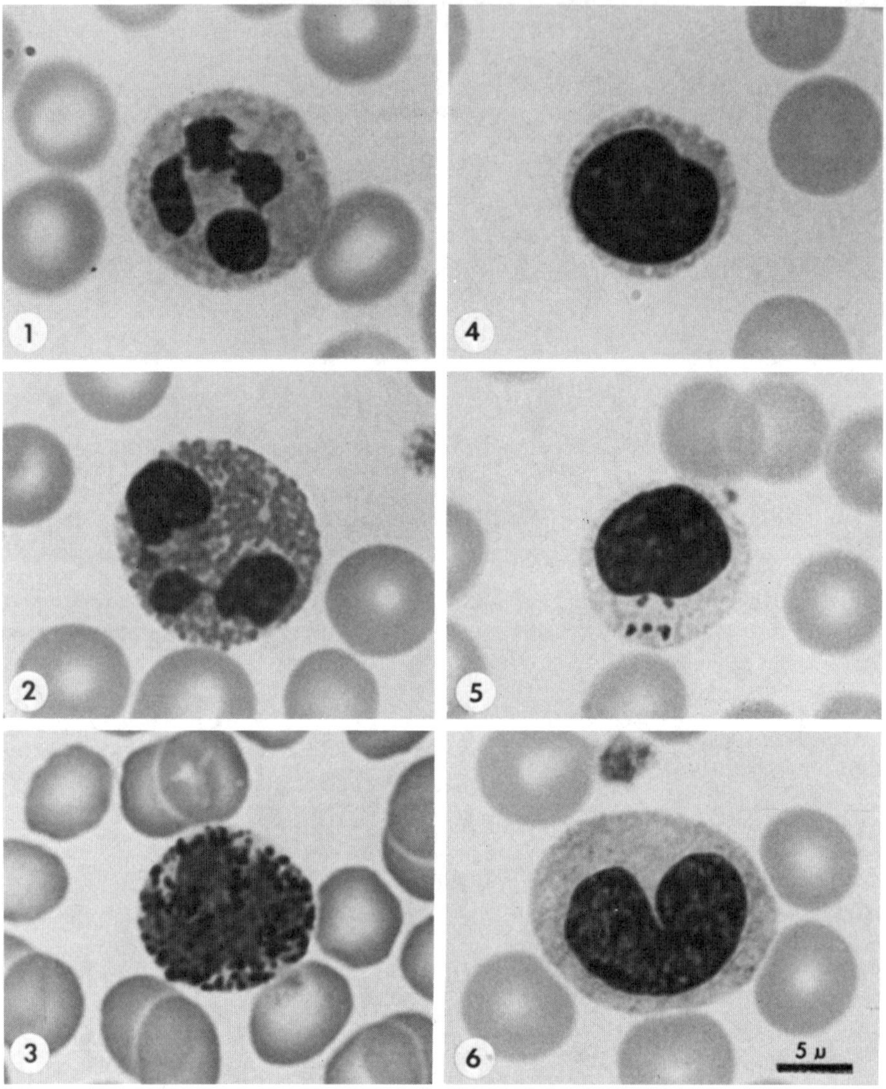

Figure 8–2. *Morphology of human leukocytes in Wright's stained smears of peripheral blood.*

(*1*) Polymorphonuclear neutrophil. Note: Multiple lobes of nucleus and very fine granules (lysosomes). (*2*) Polymorphonuclear eosinophil. Note: Nucleus is less lobated and granules (lysosomes) are larger and more regular. (*3*) Polymorphonuclear basophil. Note: Nucleus is not as markedly lobated; actually, it is cloverleaf in shape, but this is obscured by the large, coarse, and irregular granules (heparin and polyanionic histamine bound to a cationic protein). (*4*) Small lymphocyte. Note: Large nuclear:cytoplasmic ratio. Fate: Transforms into plasma cell (responsible for humoral antibodies) or into an heterogeneous population of cells (carrier of antibodies of the cellular immunity type, e.g., graft rejection, delayed hypersensitivity). (*5*) Medium lymphocyte. Note: Smaller nuclear:cytoplasmic ratio. A few coarse azurophilic granules can be distinguished in the cytoplasm. (*6*) Monocyte. Note: Characteristic indentation of nucleus and abundant cytoplasm that contains large numbers of fine azurophilic granules (lysosomes) giving the cytoplasm a "ground-glass" appearance. Fate: Transforms into macrophage upon entering connective tissue. (Courtesy of Dr. E. S. Evans.)

Table 8–3. POSSIBLE FATES OF ANTIBODY-COATED ANTIGEN

Phagocytic engulfment by neutrophils and/or macrophages
Lysis by cytotoxic T lymphocytes (T-killer cells)
Complement-mediated lysis

major histocompatibility complex (MHC). This "supergene" codes for a number of different products that play an important role in immunologic defense, such as complement levels, lymphocyte glycoprotein surface receptors, and lymphocyte ontogeny (Albert and Gotze, 1977). In humans, the loci of the MHC are called human leukocyte antigens (HLA). The HLA genes are in chromosome-6 of humans, while in mice the MHC is in loci designated H-2, within chromosome-17.

Susceptibility to disease is related in part to HLA alleles and resulting antigens (Dausset, 1977). Certain HLA alleles are correlated with a higher incidence of different diseases. For example, the HLA composition is an important component of susceptibility to such age-related diseases as rheumatoid arthritis, Graves' disease, multiple sclerosis, and diabetes, to name only a few.

The MHC may influence longevity. The percentage of women with the HLA-B8 allele declines with increasing age (Greenberg and Yunis, 1978), indicating that individuals with that allele have a shorter life expectancy than those having a different allele at that locus. A decreasing proportion with increasing age of HLA homozygous individuals suggests that HLA heterozygosity may be important for longer survival, particularly at the HLA-B8 locus. While it is clear that HLA genotype influences predisposition to age-related disease, how it does so is not clear. However, knowing the histocompatibility genes (haplotypes) and genetic predisposition for certain disorders enables taking special precautions to prevent them.

INFECTIOUS DISEASE: DEFENSE AGAINST MICROBES

Microorganisms reside in almost every corner of the environment, water, soil, and air. While some microbes are symbiotic with humans, others are pathogenic. To eliminate invading infectious agents there are *three lines of defense*. The first line is a physical barrier, such as the skin and mucous membranes lining the orifices. The second line of defense entails phagocytic digestion of invading agents by macrophages within various tissues. The third line of defense involves a humoral response toward the infectious agent. More specifically, the agent is destroyed by an immunologic reaction involving the binding of highly specific antibodies (that are secreted by mature B cells, plasma cells) to the antigenic components of the infectious agent.

Infectious diseases occur more frequently and are of greater consequence in the elderly. Some common infectious diseases include pneumonia, influenza, tuberculosis, meningitis, and urinary tract infections. The age-related rise in susceptibility to infections may be attributed to a decline in antibody production and/or decline in cell-mediated immunity.

With aging in humans, the level of circulating human antibodies begins to decline after sexual maturation. Perhaps the decline in serum levels is related to a decline in antibody responsiveness following antigen exposure. In fact, 10 times more antigen is required in old animals to induce maximal antibody responsiveness toward a primary antigen exposure (first time, in a lifetime, when exposed to a particular antigen) (Nordin and Makinodan, 1974). While data suggest that older animals have a lowered primary antibody response toward certain antigens, a substantial decline in the secondary antibody response (i.e., previously exposed) is less apparent.

With aging, immunologic protection against some antigenic agents changes: for example, certain antigens may be lost from the repertoire of antigens to which the immune system can elicit an appropriate antibody response. Although much of the research regarding antibody responsiveness toward antigens has been done using mice and dogs, similar changes in immune function may be a contributing factor toward the increase in susceptibility toward infections in old humans.

CELL-MEDIATED IMMUNITY (DELAYED-TYPE HYPERSENSITIVITY REACTIONS)

Delayed-type hypersensitivity (DTH) reactions have also been assessed as a function of aging. DTH reactions are triggered by an antigen that induces a cell-mediated response involving both T-cell and monocyte participation. More specifically, DTH reactions involve an interaction between the antigen and a particular T-helper-lymphocyte subset. The activated T-helper cells release lymphokines that both attract and stimulate macrophages and other leukocytes, resulting in localized tissue inflammation and nonspecific destruction of the antigen.

A variety of immunogens such as tuberculosis, streptokinase, and trichophyton have been used to demonstrate that DTH reactions are depressed with aging. Although some DTH reactions become depressed with aging (Gardner and Remington, 1977), others do not (Lvik and North, 1985). Therefore, the age-related decline in the ability of the immune system to perform certain delayed-type hypersensitivity reactions may result in heightened susceptibility toward only certain infectious diseases.

AUTOIMMUNE DISEASE

Autoimmune diseases are characterized by the production of antibodies and/or cytotoxic T lymphocytes toward self-antigens leading to dysfunction of the tissues attacked. A breakdown in the immune system ability to distinguish self from nonself can perceivably disrupt the function of every cell, tissue, and organ in the body. Not unexpectedly, there is a growing number of different diseases whose etiology has been related to an autoimmune reaction. Examples of autoimmune disorders that have been observed to be related to aging of humans are rheumatoid arthritis, autoimmune thyroiditis, lupus, and chronic hepatitis. Some of the common human autoimmune disorders where antibodies to self-antigens have been detected are listed in Table 8–4.

Table 8–4. AUTOIMMUNE DISORDERS

NAME OF DISORDER	TARGET TISSUE
Addison's disease	Adrenal gland
Agranulocytosis	Polymorphonuclear leukocytes
Allergic encephalitis	Brain
Episodic lymphopenia	T lymphocytes
Graves' disease	Thyroid gland (hyperactive)
Goodpasture's syndrome	Basement membranes (kidney glomerular and lung aveolar)
Hashimoto's thyroiditis	Thyroid gland (hypoactive)
Hemolytic anemia	Erythrocytes
Multiple sclerosis	Central and peripheral nervous system
Myasthenia gravis	Diaphragm muscle
Pemphigus vulgaris	Skin
Rheumatic fever	Heart muscle
Rheumatoid arthritis	Synovial membranes
Systemic lupus erythematosus	Multisystem (cellular constituents)
Thrombocytopenic purpura	Platelets

Interestingly, the risk of contracting certain autoimmune disorders has been correlated to histocompatibility genes. Thus, some individuals have a genetic predisposition to acquiring a variety of autoimmune disorders with advancing age.

Consistent with the theory that there is an age-related loss in the ability of the immune system to distinguish self from nonself, and the rise in autoimmune disorders, the levels of autoantibodies increase with aging in both mice and humans (Nandy and Bennett, 1983; Goidl *et al.*, 1983).

Tissue Grafts and Organ Transplants (Tolerance). Tissue and organ transplantation has become an increasingly popular therapeutic technique in the past decade because of advances in surgical techniques and equipment, as well as improved pharmacologic protocols. Eyes, kidneys, skin, bone marrow, and hearts are examples of organs that are commonly transplanted from allogeneic (genetically nonidentical individual of the same species) donors.

One major difficulty of surgical transplantation as a therapeutic treatment concerns immunologic rejection by the recipient of the allogeneic tissue. The more dissimilar the major histocompatibility antigens of grafted tissue are from the recipient, the greater the rejection. Therefore, in order to lessen the magnitude of rejection, surgeons attempt to match the histocompatibility antigens of the tissue donor to that of the recipient.

A number of immunosuppressive drugs, such as cyclophosphamide, fluorouracil, methotrexate, corticosteroids, and cyclosporine, improve the tolerance of allogeneic grafts. Unfortunately, many of these drugs have serious side effects. It has been reported that a factor present in early fetal calf thymus or serum can help induce immunologic tolerance (Czaplicki *et al.*, 1981). This work has not yet been repeated, but it seems increasingly promising that pharmacologic agents and regimens will soon become available that have limited side effects and allow tolerance of allogeneic grafts.

It is generally found that with aging there is a decline in the immunologic rejection of tissue grafts and consequently greater tolerance. Naturally, this is of great benefit to elderly individuals who can better tolerate grafted tissues and organs. Hence, not all age-related changes in immune function are necessarily deleterious, and some changes may be advantageous, such as reduced graft rejection.

TUMORS AND CANCER

An important function of the immune system is its role in preventing tumorigenic growth. Often associated with the development of neoplastic tissue are new (foreign) surface antigens that can potentially be distinguished and destroyed by the immune system. Immunologic reactions against tumor cells have been observed under experimental conditions. The components of the immune system implicated as playing a role in destroying tumor cells are activated macrophages, antibodies, complement, cytotoxic T cells, and natural killer cells. Despite the number of components and mechanisms by which tumor cells may be destroyed, some tumor cells may elude the immune system. One explanation for this is that some tumors may not express new, highly immunogenic, tumor-associated surface antigens. Thus, there is always a finite probability of contracting cancer even while immunologic competence is high.

With aging, there is a dramatic increase in the incidence of tumorigenesis, possibly due to age-related changes in some or all of the components of the immune system that are involved in destroying tumor cells. Some common cancers whose incidence is known to increase with aging include: breast, lung, prostate, stomach, pancreas, and leukemia.

Current cancer therapy involves various combinations of surgical removal, x-ray exposure, and chemotherapy. Many cancers can be eliminated by such regimes, but the side affects are often quite devastating. It is hoped that an understanding of immunologic senescence will provide an insight into cancer prevention and treatment.

LIFESPAN

Immunologic senescence has broad and profound manifestations and may influence:

- predisposition to various disorders of different etiology;
- ability to be treated with allografts;
- ability to distinguish self from nonself, causing the potential attack and disruption of nearly every cell.

Although it is well accepted that immunologic senescence is mostly responsible for the age-related increase in life-threatening diseases such as autoimmune disease, infectious disease, and cancer, it is not clear what role it may play in other disorders such as Alzheimer's disease and cardiovascular disease, whose incidence also rises with aging.

If aging of the immune system is a process that limits longevity, then delaying immunologic senescence would lengthen the lifespan. For example, treating mice with a substance (anti-I-J antibody) to prevent the normal age-related enhancement of T-suppressor cell activity and number significantly extended lifespan (Liu *et al.*, 1984). On the surface of T-suppressor cells are antigens that are encoded for by the I-J region of the H-2 gene complex in mice. In an attempt to reduce the age-related enhancement of T suppressor cell number, mice were treated on a weekly basis, from 18 months to death, with an anti-I-J antibody. This immunotherapy decreased T-suppressor activity and resulted in increased lifespan. An extension of lifespan was also observed upon treating mice with human dialyzable leukocyte extract, reported to enhance immune function. Although a slight increase in lifespan was observed, it was not as great as that found using the anti-I-J antibody.

Another example showed that treating adult mice, rats, or pigs with a thymic extract (three times per week for 2½ months), prepared from thymus tissue obtained during very early fetal development, dramatically lengthened the maximum lifespan of each species examined. In addition, the thymic extract treatment also prolonged the survival time of allogeneic and xenogeneic skin grafts (Czaplicki *et al.*, 1981) and reversed some age-related changes in thymic morphology. Finally, lifespan (of mice) has also been correlated to certain histocompatibility genes (Smith and Walford, 1977) and has been extended by splenectomy (Albright *et al.*, 1969) and calorie restriction (a means of delaying immunologic senescence (Weindruch *et al.*, 1982). In summary, evidence, not yet conclusive, indicates immunologic senescence affects lifespan. Because age-related immune dysfunction may be an important phenomenon limiting human lifespan, discerning which components of the immune system are influenced by aging is of great interest. Identification of these components that contribute to immunologic senescence may provide insight as to how to intervene and prevent the disorders that accompany it.

THYMUS AND THYMOSINS

The thymus is a lymphoid organ that is composed of epithelial cells, thymocytes, fat, and connective tissue. The organ is fully developed by the third month of gestation in humans. It reaches its maximum weight-to-body-weight ratio during neonatal life but continues to grow until puberty.

While histologic studies have shown that spleen and lymph nodes undergo relatively subtle changes with aging (fewer germinal centers), the thymus undergoes gross morphologic changes (Makinodan, 1977; Kay and Baker, 1979). After puberty, the thymus begins to involute and thymic weight declines dramatically (Boyd, 1932; Good and Gabrielson, 1964). The percentage of fat and connective tissue within the cortex and medulla of the thymus (which contains thymocytes and epithelial cells) increases. Before puberty about 20 percent of the medullary and cortical tissue is connective tissue and fat, but by age 40 about 80 percent of the tissue is composed of fat and connective tissue, with a corresponding decrease in thymocytes and epithelial cells. This intriguing, genetically programmed involutional event is thought to have a causal role in immunologic senescence.

Accompanying the morphologic changes of the thymus are changes in its biochemistry and physiologic function. The thymus has a network of epithelial cells that produce and secrete several polypeptide factors. Some of the better-characterized thymic factors that are produced by thymic epithelial cells include thymosin α-1, thymic humoral factor (THF), thymosin fraction-5 (TF-5), thymulin (facteur thymique serique, FTS), thymopoietin, thymic factor-X (TFX), and thymostimulin.

With aging, the number of cortical epithelial cells of the thymus remains unchanged, while the number of medullary epithelial cells diminishes (Haynes *et al.*, 1983). Consistent with this, the levels of thymosin α-1 progressively decline after age 20 (McClure *et al.*, 1982). Similar decreases have been found in human blood for other thymic-derived factors such as FTS and thymopoietin (Lewis *et al.*, 1978).

The thymic polypeptide factors appear to affect a variety of physiologic events. First, they are noted for their important role in regulating the maturation of pre-T lymphocytes (thymocytes), as monitored by the appearance of certain T-cell surface markers. In addition, the levels of thymic factors may regulate the production of lymphokines. Both thymosin fraction-5 (TF-5) and thymosin α-1 affect the *in vivo* production (in rodents) of both migration inhibitory factor (which blocks the migration of macrophages in culture) and interferons (class of proteins secreted by natural killer cells). TF-5 also influences interleukin-2 levels and colony-stimulating factor (which is produced in the spleen and whose levels do not decline with aging). Other possible physiologic roles of thymic factors are being investigated. For example, thymosins may influence the levels of endocrine hormones such as ACTH and LH, thereby affecting systems other than the immune system.

The age-related decline in the levels of thymic factors may contribute significantly to immune dysfunction (Zatz and Goldstein, 1985; Goldstein and Zatz, 1981). Administration of factors such as FTS, thymostimulin, thymopoietin, and thymosin α-1 reduces various aspects of age-related immune dysfunction. Also, when the thymus of old mice is replaced with the thymus of neonatal mice, the decline in the levels of brain-reactive autoantibodies suggests that thymic involution may aggravate age-related autoimmune disease and tissue degeneration (Nandy and Bennett, 1983).

Accumulating evidence that immunologic dysfunction is at least in part promoted by thymic involution and by the declining levels of thymic-derived factors (Lewis *et al.*, 1978; Kay, 1979) has promoted experimentation in human subjects. The thymic factors TF-5 and thymosin α-1 have been utilized in human clinical situations, and preliminary studies have revealed that they may be of some benefit. At present, a great scientific effort is directed to obtain large amounts of the various thymic factors, using recombinant DNA technology: thus the physiologic roles of these factors may be more thoroughly studied, in the hope they may be useful in treating human disorders.

AGING OF CELLULAR CONSTITUENTS

STEM CELLS

Stem cells comprise a multipotent dividing cell population residing primarily in bone marrow. They differentiate into erythrocytes and a variety of leukocytes such as T and B lymphocytes, monocytes, granulocytes, and so forth, which participate in immunologic reactions. Age-related changes in stem cell replication and/or differentiation would directly affect the population of cells that can partake in immunologic defense.

Proliferative Abilities. There is evidence both in support of and against a change in stem cell proliferative abilities with aging. Harrison *et al.* (1978) and others (Curtis and Tilley, 1971; Ogden and Micklem, 1976) have shown that stem cells have a limited capacity to divide, but this intrinsic capacity is not significantly affected by aging. In perhaps one of the most conclusive studies, mouse bone marrow cells of chromosomally marked young and old donors were serially transplanted together into young irradiated recipients (Harrison *et al.,* 1978). After five such serial transplantations of the marked cells into recipients, the stem cells of both the young and old donors ceased to divide. Prior to the fifth serial transplant, the stem cells from both the young and old donors continued to respond identically to stimulation by mitogens, phytohemagglutinin (PHA), or lipopolysaccharide. This study indicates that aging does not affect the capacity of stem cells to replicate but does suggest that stem cells have a limited intrinsic potential to divide. About five serial transplants were required to observe the limited proliferative potentials of these cells and thus would not be of consequence in a single, normal lifespan.

On the other hand, Sternberg has obtained evidence supporting an age-related change in stem cell proliferation kinetics (Sternberg *et al.,* 1977; Schneider *et al.,* 1979). Using the bromodeoxyuridine differential chromatid staining technique for *in vivo* analysis of cellular replication, it was found that the replication rates of stem cells within the bone marrow of old (24 month) rats were about 25 percent slower than those of younger (12 month) rats. Similar results were obtained using either male or female, Wistar or Fisher rats. In addition, preliminary experimentation indicates the same is true for mice, suggesting that this slowing down of cellular replication rates with aging is not sex, strain, or species specific and perhaps is a general phenomenon prevalent in all senescent mammals.

Bone marrow stem cells are by no means a homogeneous population of cells. In the study by Sternberg, discussed above, it was not established whether particular subsets of stem cells are affected by aging while others are not. For example, it is quite plausible that only the replication rates of the erythrocyte lineage are affected by aging while all leukocyte lineages are unperturbed. One cannot conclude that immune function would necessarily be affected by slower average replication rates of the heterogeneous population of stem cells. Nevertheless, the study does indicate that at least certain lineages of stem cell differentiation must be affected by aging, and stem cells in general are not beyond being affected by age despite the fact they may have the potential to proliferate normally (when transplanted from old into young serially) four times greater than the duration of a normal lifespan.

Perhaps this age-related decline in replication rates is a measure of an extrinsic environmentally induced phenomenon that is partly or wholly reversible. This is not inconsistent with Harrison's studies, which suggest that stem cells do not undergo intrinsic changes with aging. While bone marrow stem cells may divide more slowly in older animals owing to extrinsic (environmental) factors, their intrinsic capacity or potential to divide (i.e., when exposed to an environment such as that found in young animals) is not appreciably affected by aging.

Lifespan and Turnover Rate of Differentiated Stem Cells. Differentiated stem cells (lymphocytes, granulocytes, erythrocytes, and monocytes) have varying lifespans before they are removed from the circulation by macrophages. Cell types having the longer lifespan, and consequently the slower turnover rate, show the greatest age-related decline in function. A possible regulatory mechanism controlling the lifespan of differentiated stem cells may be the slow progressive appearance of a membrane component that is recognized by an IgG autoantibody. Such a mechanism has been demonstrated for the removal of red blood cells (Kay, 1985). The attachment of enough IgG to the specific membrane glycopeptide (62 kD) signals the engulfment and removal of "aged" RBC cells.

It is still unclear whether a similar mechanism regulates the lifespan and turnover rate of other differentiated stem cells. However, it seems likely that certain progressive changes in membrane composition will signal removal of other differentiated stem cells as well. Although still untested, it is possible that the age-related decline in cellular replication rates of stem cells is due to a decline in the progressive appearance of membrane signals, leading to slower turnover rates. It would be interesting to determine whether the progressive appearance of the RBC glycopeptide is influenced by organismic aging.

While little is known about the turnover of differentiated stem cells in general, further understanding of the mechanism of RBC removal and turnover may elucidate the mechanism controlling the removal and turnover of other differentiated stem cells. (See also Chapter 19.)

Effect of Aging on the Role of Stem Cells in Immunologic Reactions. There is evidence that the aging thymus induces changes in stem cells that result in lowered antibody production toward antigen. However, these changes are reversible (Harrison *et al.*, 1977; Farrar *et al.*, 1974). Antibody responsiveness toward the antigen sheep red blood cells declines with aging, but this decline is reversible. Indeed, stem cells from old donors, transplanted into young irradiated recipients, do not show a decline of antibody responsiveness with aging. Moreover, if the young irradiated recipients are also thymectomized, stem cells transplanted from old animals show a decline in antibody production, similar to that of old. This suggests that the thymus of young animals is important in reversing the age-related changes that have occurred in stem cells from old animals, and that thymic involution may play a major role in immunologic senescence.

Stem Cell Differentiation Pattern. It is becoming clear that with aging, not only do stem cell replication rates decline, but regulation of stem cell differentiation is altered (Gorczynski *et al.*, 1983; Gorczynski *et al.*, 1984). Although these changes may be extrinsically induced and reversible (Harrison *et al.*, 1977), they may be of serious consequence to an aging organism.

Stem cell differentiation is regulated by a variety of thymus-derived factors, such as thymosin and thymic factor-X, as well as the lymphokine interleukin-3 and colony-stimulating factor. With the possible exception of colony-stimulating factor, the serum levels of these polypeptide factors decline with aging (Zatz and Goldstein, 1985). These decreasing hormonal factors also influence the pattern of bone marrow stem cell differentiation. Hormonally-induced changes in stem cell differentiation patterns are believed to cause shifts in the numbers of certain progenitor cells and in the recognition repertoires of lymphocytes (Gorczynski *et al.*, 1983; Manheimer *et al.*, 1984). Such shifts would account for much of the data concerning immunologic senescence and are consistent with observations that the immunologic response of older individuals toward certain antigens differs from that of younger individuals. Though some immunologic reactions are not influenced by shifts in the pattern of bone marrow stem cell differentiation, others are, with a consequent increased susceptibility to cancer, autoimmune disease, and infectious disease.

T Lymphocytes

T lymphocytes are a heterogenous class of cells presently classified on the basis of their activities and surface membrane components (antigens). The three general classes of T lymphocytes are T-killer (Tk), T-helper (Th), and T-suppressor (Ts) cells. Tk lymphocytes (also called cytolytic or cytotoxic T lymphocytes) are effector cells that possess cytolytic activities, Ts lymphocytes are regulator cells that suppress Tk-cell activities, while Th lymphocytes are regulator cells that can stimulate Tk- or B-cell activities.

The proliferation and differentiation of T-cell progenitors (thymocytes) into mature T lymphocytes are dependent in part on various thymus-derived factors, such as thymosin and thymopoietin. With this in mind, one might expect that age-related involution of the thymus and the decline in the production of thymic factors (Zatz and Goldstein, 1985) would influence T-lymphocyte differentiation and activities. Consistent with this, numerous investigators have demonstrated age-related changes regarding the numbers and activities of various T-lymphocyte subpopulations.

Changes in Responsiveness to Mitogens with Aging. Certain populations of T lymphocytes can be stimulated to divide in culture upon exposure to various mitogens. Numerous studies have demonstrated that mitogenic stimulation of T cells is influenced by aging. For example, mitogenic stimulation by phytohemagglutinin (PHA) of cells from rodents (Kaplan and Garvey, 1981; Averill and Wolf, 1985) or humans (Gillis *et al.*, 1981; Schwab *et al.*, 1985) declines with increasing donor age. Similarly, studies with the mitogen, concanavalin A (con A), which possibly stimulates a different population of T cells than PHA, show a decline in proliferation of cells from rodents (Kaplan and Garvey, 1981) and humans (Gillis *et al.*, 1981) with increasing donor age, a decline also induced by other mitogens (TPA and pokeweed) including mitogenic monoclonal antibodies. While the decline in mitogenic responsiveness of T lymphocytes has been well demonstrated, the causes, direction, and magnitude of the age-related changes are still obscure. The decrease with aging of interleukin-2 (IL-2) (Thoman and Weigle, 1982; Miller, 1984), a T-cell growth factor, may contribute to the decline in T-lymphocyte proliferation, perhaps because of a decreased responsiveness of T cells to IL-2 or a decrease in the proportion of responsive T cells (Miller, 1984).

Interestingly, mitogenic responsiveness of T lymphocytes from an involuted thymus (of older humans) is greater than that observed from a younger thymus (Baroni *et al.*, 1983). The age-related enhancement of mitogenic responsiveness of thymic T cells may be related to the increase in the proportion of OKT3$^+$T lymphocytes, which have the T3-membrane antigen. Cells with this antigen are known to be more sensitive to mitogens, so an increase in prevalence of this subpopulation may account for the overall increase in mitogenic responsiveness of thymic T cells with aging. However, the unchanged or decreased OKT3$^+$ subpopulation in blood may account for the age-related decline in mitogenic activity of peripheral blood T lymphocytes (Jensen *et al.*, 1986).

Although one might predict that the age-related decline in thymic hormones, which have activities promoting T-cell growth and maturation, would lead to an increase in undifferentiated T cells (O'Leary *et al.*, 1983), no convincing evidence supports such a claim (as monitored by the prevalence of certain membrane antigens whose appearance is dependent on T-cell maturation) (Jensen *et al.*, 1986). This adds some confusion regarding the role (if any) of thymic involution on T-cell proliferation and maturation. Perhaps other factors may compensate for the loss of thymic hormones with age.

Cytotoxic Activity (T-Killer Cells). The cytotoxic activity of T lymphocytes appears to be depressed with aging (Zharhary *et al.*, 1984; Nordin and Collins, 1983; Gorczynski *et al.*, 1983). In particular, the T lymphocytes of elderly subjects display a reduced activity against allogeneic cells (Zharhary *et al.*, 1984). This decline may be due to an age-related decrease in the *numbers* of alloantigen-specific T cells possessing cytotoxic activity. Aged mice were found to have one-tenth the number of alloantigen-specific precursor cells compared to young (Nordin and Collins, 1983), which may account for the lowered cytotoxic activity against allogeneic cells.

Contrary reports state that the cytotoxic response toward allogeneic cells (spleen or tumor) is not affected by aging (Fitzgerald and Bennett, 1983). Apparently, the cytotoxic response against alloantigens is dependent on the experimental method employed.

In addition to the reported decline in alloreactivity with aging, the heterogeneity of alloantigens recognized by cytotoxic T cells declines as well (Gorczynski *et al.*, 1983), probably because of the reduced prevalence of certain subpopulations of T cells that have receptors for alloantigens. Such changes in T-cell recognition repertoire are thought to arise from changes in the regulation of differentiation of bone marrow stem cells (Gorczynski *et al.*, 1984b). The age-related change in stem cell differentiation pattern may result in a decline in both the heterogeneity of alloantigen-specific cytotoxic T cells and the reactivity of T cells toward alloantigens. Moreover, it may be a major reason for the increased tolerance of elderly individuals for allogeneic tissue and organ grafts. There is also an age-related decline in cytolytic activity toward both syngeneic tumor cells and parental strain

Define syngeneic

spleen cells, which agrees with the known rise in cancer incidence. In conclusion, fundamental changes in the pattern of stem cell differentiation may largely contribute toward the age-related decline in T-killer-cell activity, resulting in greater tolerance to allogeneic tissue transplants and higher tumor incidence.

Suppressor Activity of T Lymphocytes (T-Suppressor Cells). Suppressor activity of T lymphocytes appears to rise with aging in mice (Goidl *et al.*, 1983; Liu *et al.*, 1982) but may or may not rise in humans. Heightened T-suppressor-cell activity due to an increased proportion of T-suppressor cells may contribute to the age-related decline in immunologic reactivity toward alloantigens (Gupta and Good, 1978) and may also account for the increase in tolerance of allografts and tumor growth with aging. In addition, increased suppressor cell activity may contribute to the age-related decline in T-cell-mediated delayed-type hypersensitivity (DTH) reactions. DTH reactions are often elicited in response to infectious agents, and a stronger suppression of such immunologic reactions may increase the predisposition toward infections.

Suppressor cells are identified on the basis of their activity and of their membrane markers, such as I-J and Ly23 in mice (humans possess similar markers, i.e., T5). The proportion of cells having these markers increases with aging (Perry *et al.*, 1978). Treatment of mice with anti-I-J alloantiserum enhances resistance to syngeneic tumor growth, suggesting that the high incidence of tumors with aging may be due in part to heightened suppressor activities.

Most studies of age-related increases in suppressor cell activity were performed using mice. Humans are exempt from a similar age-related change; in fact, suppressor activity has been observed to decline in humans (Ceuppens and Goodwin, 1982). Consistent with this, the proliferative response of splenic suppressor cells toward certain allogeneic H-2 antigens is lowered in mice as well (Gottesman *et al.*, 1984). Apparently, the effect of aging on T-suppressor activity is complex. Numerous fundamental changes in the subset proportions and attributes of T-suppressor cells arise with aging.

Suppressor T cells, stimulated by antigen in old mice, are effective in inducing tolerance only when transplanted in old syngeneic recipients, but not young recipients (Hausman *et al.*, 1985). Similarly, suppressor cells that become stimulated in young mice are more active in inducing tolerance when transplanted into young syngeneic recipients. Perhaps a coordinated change in the pattern of differentiation of stem cells results in different subsets of suppressor cells that are active in immune reactions with aging.

Helper Activity of the T Lymphocytes (T-Helper Cells). T-helper cells are a class of lymphocytes that help enhance the activity of either T-killer cells or B cells toward antigen. T-helper cells release (1) IL-2, which stimulates T-killer-cell activity, or (2) B-cell growth factor and B-cell differentiating factor, which stimulate B cells.

T-helper cells may recognize and interact with B cells by two types of mechanisms. Some T-helper cells, called Th-1 cells, can recognize and bind to epitopes (specific sites) on antigens that are associated with immunoglobin receptor molecules on B cells. Others, such as Th-2 cells, may activate B cells after recognizing specific regions of antigen-associated B-cell membrane immunoglobins. Unlike Th-1 cells, the Th-2 cells do not bind directly to the antigen.

Several studies report an age-related decline in T-helper-cell activity (Callard and Basten, 1978; Frasca *et al.*, 1982). Such a decline may be related to the observed decrease in the number of Th-1 and Th-2 cells with aging (Doria *et al.*, 1980) but can be restored by *in vivo* administration of thymosin α-1. Thymosin administration may induce the maturation and proliferation of pre-T-helper cells, suggesting that the age-related decline in T-helper activity is due to the age-associated thymic involution and decline in thymic hormones such as thymosin α-1. Moreover, the decline in T-helper-cell regulator activity may promote immune dysfunction by diminished activation of T-killer cells and antibody-producing B cells.

AIDS. T-helper cells appear to be implicated in the acquired immunodeficiency syndrome (AIDS), a disease that is on the rise. This disease has been found to be caused by a retrovirus (containing RNA genetic material) called HTLV-3. The virus, which can be transferred by blood or seminal fluids, infects certain T-helper lymphocytes that possess a surface antigen designated T-4. Individuals diagnosed as having AIDS have defects in various aspects of cell-mediated immunity, including immunosurveillance of tumorigenic tissue. The disease results in death due to infections or cancer (Kaposi's sarcoma). The susceptibility to AIDS does not appear to be related to age, sex, or race, but is correlated highly with sexual behavior, intravenous drug use, and frequency of blood transfusions. While a cure is being searched, prevention of the disease is already being implemented. Careful blood donor screening, the elimination of sharing needles for intravenous injections, and careful selection of sexual partners may eradicate this dreadful disease.

PHAGOCYTIC CELLS: MACROPHAGES

Macrophages are derived from stem cells along the monocyte lineage. Monocytes are smaller than macrophages, circulate in the blood, infiltrate various tissues, and differentiate into mature macrophages that can play a variety of roles in immunologic responses. These include: nonspecific phagocytosis of an antigen, specific phagocytosis of an antibody-tagged antigen, and degradation of the contents of the phagocytic vesicle by lysosomal enzymes after fusion with lysosomes (Figure 8–3). The macrophage, which characteristically can adhere tightly to glass surfaces, appears to be the first leukocyte to recognize and bind to antigen and to present the antigenic epitope (in association with certain membrane-attached class II, HLA gene products) to T-helpers. In addition, macrophages can secrete lymphokines, such as IL-1, that modulate lymphocyte activity and immunologic responsiveness. To maximize T- and B-cell participation in immune responses it is necessary to expose these lymphocytes to antigen-pulsed macrophages. Macrophages exposed to antigen are very powerful enhancers of T- and B-cell proliferation and activity. However, not all macrophages are identical; some bind antigen, present it to T-helper cells, and are powerful inducers of T-lymphocyte proliferation, while others do not.

Lysosomal and Phagocytic Activity. The activity of lysosomal enzymes, such as β-glucuronidase, acid phosphatase, and cathepsin-D, becomes significantly elevated with aging (Tyan, 1981). Since lysosomal degradation of antigen and antigen-associated material follows phagocytosis, a rise in phagocytic activity might be expected. In contrast, phagocytic activity remains unchanged with aging or may be slightly depressed (Bongrand *et al.*, 1984; Vetvicka *et al.*, 1985). For instance, the phagocytic activity of human polymorphonuclear cells, granulocytes and monocytes, declines with aging (Bongrand *et al.*, 1984). It is unclear why lysosomal enzymes may become more prevalent with age, while phagocytic activity declines.

It is possible that the phagocytic cells are not turned over as quickly with aging and that the average age of these leukocytes increases with aging, as has been suggested for B cells (Tyan, 1977; Mosier *et al.*, 1977). Consistent with this, the membrane components and fluidity of phagocytes appear to be affected by aging (Vetvicka *et al.*, 1983), as might be expected if turnover rates were slower (Kay, 1985). Older phagocytic cells may accumulate lysosomal enzymes and have slightly lowered phagocytic activity.

Although age-related changes in lysosomal enzymes and phagocytic activity do appear relatively small, they may contribute to increased incidence of infectious disease.

Antigen Presentation. Antigen presentation by macrophages can be monitored by observing the effects on respondent lymphocytes. The amount of antigen necessary to evoke a vigorous immune response may be lowered several hundred times if antigen-presenting accessory cells such as macrophages are employed. The Ia molecule is a surface protein on antigen-presenting macrophages (coded for by the I region of the H-2 complex), which interacts with antigen. The Ia-antigen complex is recognized by and stimulates T-helper cells, which in turn will activate T- and B-effector cells. The proportion of the Ia^+ subpopulation of macrophages appears to rise with aging (Doria *et al.*, 1983). Because this subpopu-

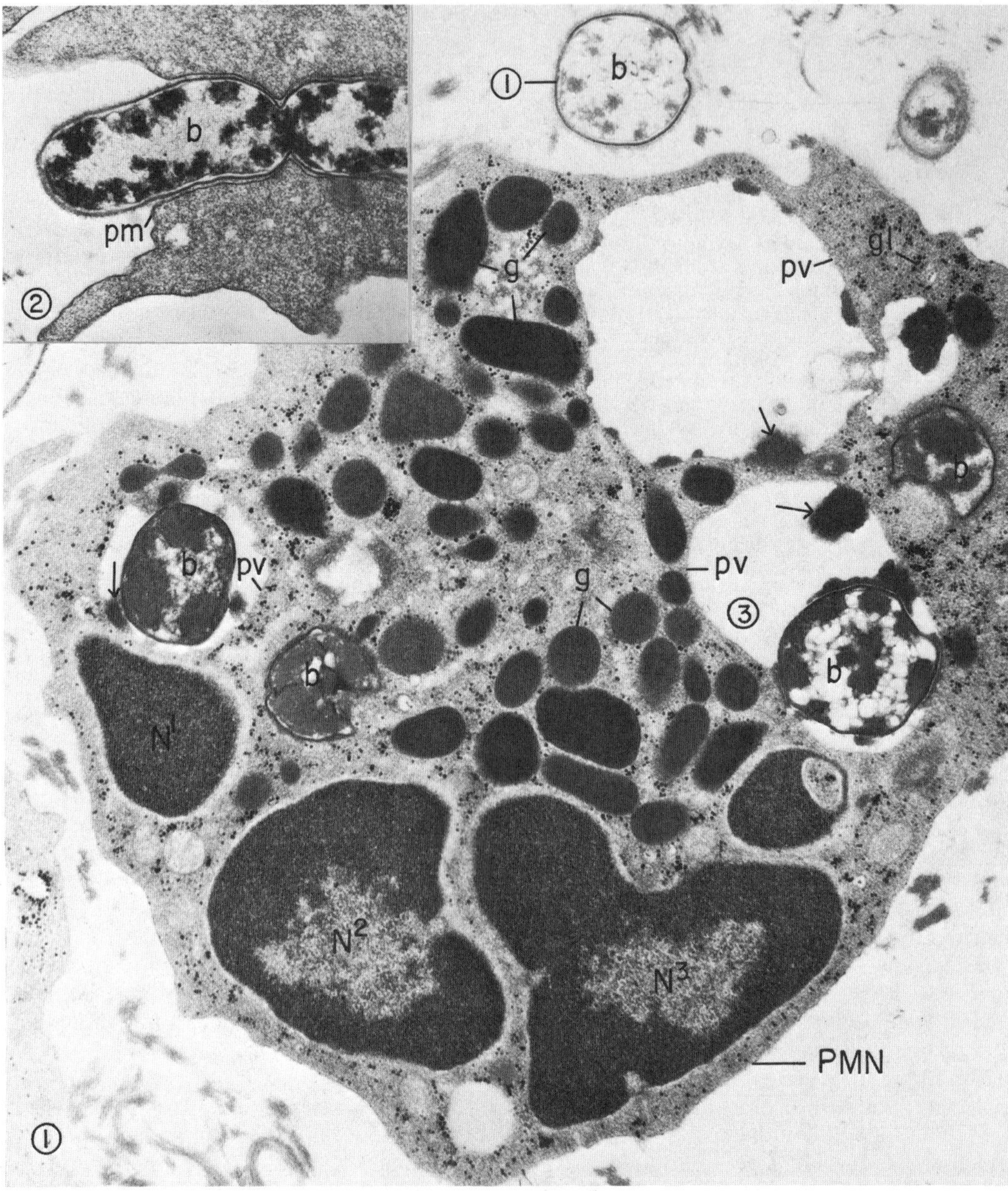

Figure 8–3. *Electron micrographs illustrating the various stages in the phagocytosis of bacteria by a highly specialized blood cell, the neutrophilic polymorphonuclear leukocyte (PMN).*

Note that the section cuts through three lobes of its multilobulated nucleus (N_1–N_3). Numerous granules (g) of several sizes, shapes, and densities fill the cytoplasm. Particles of glycogen (gl), which provides the energy for phagocytosis, can be seen scattered throughout the cytoplasm. The events of phagocytosis proceed as follows: (*1*) the cell approaches the external bacterium (b); (*2*) the bacterium (b) is engulfed and internalized by invagination of the cell's plasma membrane (pm), as shown in the insert (upper left), and (*3*) upon ingestion, the contents of the granules are discharged (arrows) into the digestive or phagocytic vacuole (pv). It has been demonstrated that these granules store antibacterial agents and lysosomal enzymes until they are needed to kill and digest microorganisms, a process that can occur within two minutes. (Courtesy of Dr. D. F. Bainton.)

lation is important for antigen presentation, increased antigen presentation activity by macrophages is expected with aging, as shown by some (Matsumoto *et al.*, 1982) but not by all (Vetvicka *et al.*, 1985). Further, this increase may be specific for only certain antigens.

The changes in macrophage subpopulation proportions that may be responsible for a slight enhancement in macrophage activity might improve protection against certain infectious agents. For example, protection against *Listeria monocytogenes* is heightened in aging mice, local and systemic infections are better prevented by nonspecifically activated macrophages of older mice, and peritoneal macrophages from older mice display improved suppression of bacteria grown *in vitro* (Matsumoto *et al.*, 1982).

In conclusion, evidence suggests that under some circumstances, immunologic protection provided by macrophages may be superior in older than younger subjects, but inferior in others. The possible influence of antigen-presenting macrophages on the recognition repertoires of B cells (Gorczynski *et al.*, 1984a) suggests that age-related changes are highly selective, coordinated, and perhaps quite purposeful.

NATURAL KILLER CELLS

Natural killer (Nk) cells are derived from bone marrow stem cells and are considered to be a subpopulation of lymphocytes. They have a number of morphologic and biochemical features in common with T lymphocytes, such as the presence of certain surface antigens and their responsiveness to lymphokines, which suggests Nk cells may arise from a T-lymphocyte lineage.

Nk cells possess cytolytic activity against tumorigenic cells, as well as virus-infected cells without previous sensitization (unlike T-killer cells). They are important for immunologic surveillance of neoplastic tissue, they mediate antibody responses, and they also affect hematopoiesis.

Comparison of the number of Nk precursor cells in the spleens of old and young mice (Fitzgerald and Bennett, 1983; Saxena *et al.*, 1984) shows fewer precursor cells in old mouse spleens, and in fact as few as one-half that of young (Fitzgerald and Bennett, 1983). The decreased number of Nk precursor cells with aging may be important in the age-related rise in tumorigenesis.

Does aging affect the cytolytic activity of Nk cells in humans? Some investigators could find no change in the ability of human Nk cells to lyse a variety of tumor cell lines (*in vitro*) (Adler and Nagel, 1981), while others, using mice, have detected a depression in Nk activity with aging (Albright and Albright, 1983; Fitzgerald and Bennett, 1983; Saxena *et al.*, 1984). The cytolytic activity of Nk cells from spleens of older mice can be increased, using Il-2, to a greater extent than that of young (Saxena *et al.*, 1984). Because the spleens of old mice contain fewer lymphokine-respondent Nk cells, the total Nk activity is still less than that of young, a deficit perhaps dependent on age-related changes in bone marrow effector cells (Fitzgerald and Bennett, 1983).

The activity of Nk cells can be modulated not only by lymphokines, but also by other environmental conditions, such as the lipoprotein composition of blood. The presence of certain lipoproteins can influence the binding of Nk cells to the target tissue *in vitro*; some lipoproteins depress the binding of Nk cells from aged donors more than from young (Antonaci *et al.*, 1984). Although target binding of Nk cells is affected by lipoproteins, lytic activity of attached Nk cells is not. Thus blood lipoproteins may contribute to the age-related decline in Nk cells activity and an enhanced risk of tumors.

B LYMPHOCYTES AND ANTIBODY PRODUCTION

Mature B cells, which are derived from bone marrow stem cells, secrete specific antibodies (Figure 8–4) and participate in the so-called humoral immunity. Antibody-antigen complexes that result from the secretion of antibodies into blood may trigger various events. For instance, the complex may induce complement-mediated lysis, T-lymphocyte cytolytic activity, and/or phagocytic activity of neutrophils or macro-

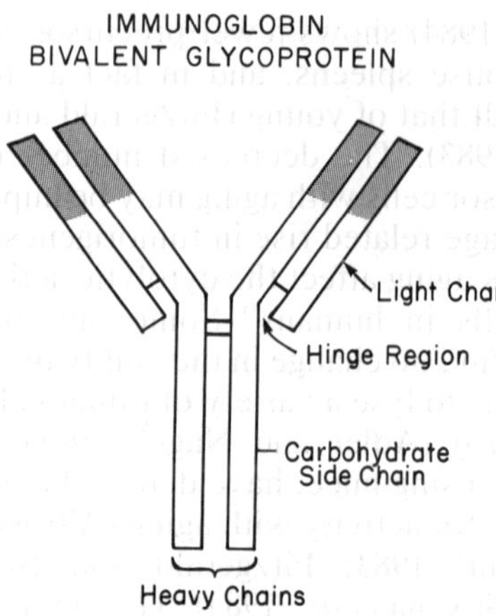

Figure 8–4. *The structure of a typical bivalent antibody, an antigen-specific glycoprotein (immunoglobulin).*

Two identical heavy polypeptide chains and two identical light chains are associated by disulfide bonds (as illustrated). The 5 major types of Ig heavy chains distinguish the 5 major classes of Ig molecules (IgA, D, E, G, M). Although the various types of heavy chains are structurally similar they are not identical, which accounts for their functional differences. IgA—found in exocrine secretions, more stable to aberant conditions. IgD—a receptor on B-cell membranes. IgE—binds mast cells, contributes to allergic reactions. IgM—a multivalent pentamer, secreted in a primary immune response, can stimulate complement mediated lysis and macrophage engulfment. IgG—the most abundant Ig in blood, stimulates complement-mediated lysis and macrophage engulfment. The antigen binding specificity of all immunoglobins is contained in the shaded region (as depicted), which is near the amino terminus and has a highly variable amino acid sequence.

phages, and result in the destruction or removal of the invading, antibody-tagged antigen. Both the class of Ig associated with the antigen and its binding pattern dictate the mechanism of antigen removal.

B-cell antibody production is dependent on prior antigenic history, duration and dose of antigen exposure, and, usually, T-cell participation. The great diversity of specific antibodies secreted in response to a wide variety of antigens is generated in B-lymphocytes through chromosomal rearrangements among genes that code for antibody structure (Tonegawa, 1985). Available evidence suggests a general decline in the ability of B cells to produce and secrete specific antibodies with aging (Mason-Smith, 1976; Mosier *et al.*, 1977; Zharhary and Klinman, 1983). After serial treatment with a T-cell-independent antigen (pneumococcal polysaccharide type III) B-cell antibody production was lower in old mice than in young (Mason-Smith, 1976). The antigen used induces the production of the IgM class of Ig, the predominant Ig secreted in older animals. Usually IgM is secreted during a primary response; the more mature B cells secrete IgG. The age-related decline in antibody production to this T-cell-independent antigen may be due to the B-cell subset failing to differentiate into mature IgG-producing cells (Mosier *et al.*, 1977). Not only does antibody production decline upon stimulation with T-cell-independent antigens, but it also declines in response to T-cell-dependent antigen (Zharhary and Klinman, 1983).

Some contrasting evidence suggests B-cell antibody production and subpopulation numbers do not change with aging. At the clonal level (using limiting dilution analysis) the number of mouse splenic B cells, respondent to a particular viral antigen (PR 8 influenza virus), is unchanged with aging (Zharhary and Klinman, 1984). However, overall antibody responses by B cells decline with aging (Zharhary and Klinman, 1983; Gorczynski *et al.*, 1983; Whistler and Newhouse, 1985). Such a decline may be ascribed to a shift in the subpopulations of B lymphocytes (changing their recognition repertoires) in parallel with changes in the pattern of stem cell differentiation.

Consistent with this, limiting dilution analysis has revealed an age-related decline in the population of certain antigen-specific B lymphocytes as well as a decline in the population of B lymphocytes that are respondent to the mitogen lipopolysaccharide (Gorczynski *et al.*, 1984a).

In summary, only certain subpopulations of B cells are influenced by aging. Thus, the administration of only certain antigens results in a lowered antibody response.

Mitogenic Responsiveness. B-cell mitogenic responsiveness is dependent on various factors, such as, the type of mitogen utilized, the animal species or strain, and the experimental approach of the investigators. Hence, investigators reach diverging conclusions: some investigators have detected a decline in B-cell mitogenic responsiveness toward plant lectins (Price and Makinodan, 1972; Hollingsworth and Evans, 1983; Whistler and Newhouse, 1985); others have not (Kay, 1979).

Interestingly, restoration of the age-related decline in B-cell proliferative responsiveness toward activated monocytes was possible by increasing the levels of IL-1 and/or IL-2 to which lymphyocytes were exposed (Whistler and Newhouse, 1985), however, not without considerable variation from individual to individual.

A possible mechanism for changes in B-cell activity may involve an age-related shift in the proportion of B-cell subpopulations, arising during shifts in bone marrow stem cell differentiation, that are responsive to certain mitogens (Zharhary and Klinman, 1983; Manheimer *et al.*, 1984).

B-Cell Number and Population Size

B lymphocytes are a heterogenous class of cells that differ in their maturational state, surface components, and mechanism by which their activity is regulated. An age-related change in B-cell maturation and/or subpopulation proportions may influence the humoral response and susceptibility to disease.

Despite reports of lowered B-cell mitogenic responsiveness and maturation with aging, the bone marrow of older mice possesses greater numbers of mature B cells than that of young controls (Tyan, 1977). On the other hand, the number of circulating B cells does not appear to change with age, while the ratio of B cells to T cells increases owing to a decline in T-cell number.

How can the greater numbers of mature B cells in bone marrow be reconciled with reports of lowered maturational development of B-cells with aging (Mosier *et al.*, 1977)? Perhaps, turnover rates of mature B cells decline with aging. If fewer cells are removed from the circulation, and if proliferative rates are only moderately slowed with aging, B cells may accumulate in bone marrow. Consistent with this view are reports of fewer germinal centers in lymphatic follicles with aging, as one might expect if there is a reduced need for new cells due to slower turnover rates. It has been observed that cell types having longer life-spans and slower turnover rates demonstrate the greatest age-related decline in function.

IS AGE-RELATED IMMUNE DYSFUNCTION REVERSIBLE?

The components and activities of the immune system are selectively affected by aging (Table 8–5). This selectivity leads to the questions of which and to what extent these changes are reversible.

Considerable evidence supports the proposition that age-related immune dysfunction can be at least partially reversed. Thymic factors such as thymopoietin (Weksler *et al.*, 1978), thymic fraction-5 (Goldstein *et al.*, 1983), and thymosin α-1 (McClure *et al.*, 1982), as well as lymphokines IL-1, IL-2, and γ-interferon (Saxena *et al.*, 1984; Zatz and Goldstein, 1985; Whistler and Newhouse, 1985), can restore various parameters of age-related immune dysfunction. Other treatments, e.g., 2-mercaptoethanol, levamisole, and synthetic polynucleotides, may also delay immune senescence. This provides great optimism for the potential of delaying age-related immune dysfunction in humans.

On the other hand, there are also data suggesting that delaying human immunologic senescence is not a simple matter. The involution of the thymus and subsequent decrease in thymic hormone levels are well-accepted factors in immunologic aging. Yet, the implantation of a thymus from a young mouse into an older thymectomized, syngeneic mouse does not provide prolonged improvement in immune function, as might have been predicted (Hirokawa *et al.*, 1976). Similarly, a close correlation is lacking between thymic involution and a reduction in serum thymic hormones. Such observations indicate that immunologic aging is not solely dependent on thymic involution, and that multiple independent events regulate immune senescence.

An explanation for the relative ineffectiveness of thymic transplants is that the signal that might trigger thymic involution is still active and reinitiates thymic involution of the transplant. It is likely that such a signal is derived from the nervous system, and thymic involution may be a result of specific neuronal cell loss and alterations. Neural signals regulate development and aging of specific systems such as the reproductive system, suggesting that such a

Table 8–5. IMMUNOLOGIC SENESCENCE

	Secretory Factors	
Thymus	Thymosin α-1 Facteur thymique serique Thymopoietin →	Decline Secretory factors
	Stem Cell Differentiation	
	influenced by:	
Bone marrow	Thymosin Thymic factor X → Colony stimulating factor Interleukin-3	Decline T-helper-cell proportion Alloantigen-specific Tk Natural-killer-cell number
		Increase Ts cell proportion B-cell/T-cell ratio
		Shift B-cell characteristics Antibody production
Consequences		Increase Tissue graft tolerance Cancer incidence Autoimmune disease Infectious disease

mechanism may induce aging of the immune system as well (Barnes, 1987).

Other data emphasize the difficulty of reversing or delaying human immune senescence. For example, old mice implanted with young bone marrow cells did not undergo improvement of immunologic function for extended durations (Hirokawa *et al.*, 1976). The internal environment within older animals may be "hostile" to young cells so that the young cells rapidly acquire the properties of the old. Only after the environmental factors capable of inducing in the older animals a youthful environment are identified, will implantations of young thymic tissue or bone marrow be effective in substantially delaying immune senescence.

There still remains a great deal to be learned concerning the mechanisms of immunologic aging, and while it may not be currently possible to delay, prevent, or reverse human immunologic senescence, continuing advances in immunology, and immunologic aging in particular, will guide us toward successful interventions in improving and prolonging life.

References

Adler, W. H., and Nagel, J. E.: Studies of immune function in a human population. In Segre, D., and Smith, L. (eds.): *Immunological Aspects of Aging*, Marcel Dekker, Inc., New York, **1981.**

Albert, E., and Gotze, D.: The major histocompatibility system in man. In Gotze, D. (ed.): *The Major Histocompatibility System in Man and Animals*, Springer-Verlag, New York, **1977.**

Albright, J. F.; Makinodan, T.; and Deitchman, J. W.: Presence of life-shortening factors in spleens of aged mice of long lifespan and extension of life expectancy by splenectomy. *Exp. Gerontol.*, **4**:267–276, **1969.**

Albright, J. W., and Albright, J. F.: Age-associated impairment of natural killer activity. *Proc. Natl. Acad. Sci. USA*, **80**(20)6371–6375, **1983.**

Antonaci, S.; Jirillo, E.; Ventura, M. I.; Garofalo, A. R.; and Bonomo, L.: Lipoprotein-induced inhibition of plaque-forming cells generation and natural killer cell frequency in aged donors. *Ann. Immunol. (Paris)*, **135c**(2):241–249, **1984.**

Averill, L. E., and Wolf, N. S.: The decline in murine splenic PHA and LPS responsiveness with age is primarily due to an intrinsic mechanism. *J. Immunol.*, **134**(6):3859–3863, **1985.**

Barnes, D. M.: Neuroimmunology sits on broad research base. *Science*, **237**:1568–1569, **1987.**

Baroni, C. D.; Valtieri, M.; Stoppacciaro, A.; Ruco, L. P.; Uccini, S.; and Ricci, C.: The human thymus in ageing: Histologic involution paralleled by increased mitogen response and by enrichment of OKT3+ lymphocytes. *Immunology*, **50**(4)4:519–528, **1983.**

Bongrand, P.; Bartolin, R.; Bouvenot, G.; Arnaud, C.; Delboy, C.; and Depieds, R.: Effect of age on different receptors and functions of phagocytic cells. *J. Clin. Lab. Immunol.*, **15**(1):45–50, **1984.**

Boyd, E.: The weight of the thymus gland in health and disease. *Am. J. Dis. Child.*, **43**:1162–1214, **1932.**

Callard, R. E., and Basten, A.: Immune function in aged mice. IV. Loss of T-cell and B-cell function in thymus dependent antibody responses. *Eur. J. Immunol.*, **8**(8):552–558, **1978.**

Ceuppens, J. L., and Goodwin, J. S.: Regulation of immunoglobin production in pokeweed mitogen-stimulated cultures of lymphocytes from young and old adults. *J. Immunol.*, **128**(6):2429–2434, **1982.**

Curtis, H. J., and Tiley, J.: The lifespan of dividing mammalian cells *in vivo*. *J. Gerontol.*, **26:**1–7, **1971.**

Czaplicki, J.; Blonska, B.; Klementys, A.; Klementys, K.; Kaluzewski, B.; and Pawlikowski, M.: The effects of blood sera from calf fetuses in various periods of fetal life on skin allograft survival time in mice and on human lymphocyte proliferation in vitro. *Thymus*, **3:**17–24, **1981.**

Dausset, J.: HLA complex in human biology in the light of associations with disease, *Transplant Proc.*, **9**(1):523–529, **1977.**

Doria, G.; D'Agostaro, G.; and Garavini, M.: Age-dependent changes in B-cell reactivity and T cell-T cell interaction in the *in vitro* antibody response. *Cell. Immunol.*, **53**(1):195–206, **1980.**

Doria, G.; Frasca, D.; and Adorini, L.: Immunoregulation of antibody response in aging. In Y. Yamamura and Tada, T. (eds.): *Progress in Immunology V*, Academic Press, Tokyo Japan, **1983,** 1549–1561.

Eisen, H. N.: *Immunology*, 2nd ed., Harper & Row, Philadelphia, **1980.**

Farrar, J. J.; Loughman, B. E.; and Nordin, A. A.: Lymphopoietic potential of bone marrow stem cells from aged mice: Comparison of the cellular constituents of bone marrow from young and aged mice. *J. Immunol.*, **112:**1244–1249, **1974.**

Fitzgerald, P. A., and Bennett, M.: Aging of natural and acquired immunity of mice. I. Decreased natural killer cell function and hybrid resistance. *Cancer Invest.*, **1**(1):15–24, **1983.**

Fitzgerald, P. A., and Bennett, M.: Aging of natural and acquired immunity of mice. II. Decreased T cell responses to syngeneic tumor cells and parental-strain spleen cells. *Cancer Invest.*, **1**(2):139–149, **1983.**

Frasca, D.; Garavini, M.; and Doria, G.: Recovery of T-cell functions in aged mice injected with synthetic thymosin-alpha-1. *Cell. Immunol.*, **72**(2):384–391, **1982.**

Galpin, J.: Immunity and microbial diseases. In Kay, M. M. B., and Makinodan, T. (eds.): *Handbook of Immunology in Aging*, CRC Press, Boca Raton, FL, **1981.**

Gardner, I. D., and Remington, J. S.: Age-related decline in resistance of mice to infection with intracellular pathogens. *Infect. Immunol.*, **16**(2):593–598, **1977.**

Gillis, S.; Kozak, R.; Durante, M.; and Weksler, M. E.: Immunological studies of aging: Decreased production of T-cell growth factor by lymphocytes from aged humans. *J. Clin. Invest.*, **67**(4):937–942, **1981.**

Goidl, E. A.; Choy, J. W.; Gibbons, J. J.; Weksler, M. E.; Thorbecke, G. J.; and Siskind, G. W.: Production of auto-antiidiotypic antibody during the normal immune response. VII. Analysis of the cellular basis for the increased auto-antiidiotype antibody production by aged mice. *J. Exp. Med.*, **157**(5):1635–1645, **1983.**

Goldstein, A. L., and Zatz, M. M.: Thymosin and aging. In Segre, D., and Smith, L. (eds.): *Immunological Aspects of Aging*, Dekker Publishing Co., New York, **1981.**

Goldstein, A. L.; Low, T. L. K.; Hall, N.; Naylor, P. H.; and Zatz, M. M.: Thymosin: Can it retard aging by boosting the immune capacity? In Regelson, W., and Sinex, F. M. (eds.): *Intervention in the Aging Process. Part A: Quantitation, Epidemiology and Clinical Research*, Alan R. Liss, New York, **1983.**

Good, R. A., and Gabrielson, A. B. (eds.): *Thymus in Immunobiology*, Hoeber-Harper, New York, **1964.**

Gorczynski, R. M.; Kennedy, M.; and MacRae, S.: Alteration in lymphocyte recognition repertoire during aging. II. Changes in expressed T-cell receptor repertoire in aged mice and the persistence of that change after transplantation to a new differentiative environment. *Cell. Immunol.*, **75**(2):226–241, **1983.**

Gorczynski, R. M.; Chang, M. P.; Kennedy, M.; MacRae, S.; Benting, K.; and Price, G. B.: Alterations in lymphocyte recognition repertoire during aging. I. Analysis of changes in immune response potential of B-lymphocytes from nonimmunized aged mice, and the role of accessary cells in the expression of that potential. *Immunopharmacology*, **7**(3–4):179–194, **1984a.**

Gorczynski, R. M.; Kennedy, M.; and MacRae, S.: Altered lymphocyte recognition repertoire during aging. III. Changes in MHC restriction patterns in parental T-lymphocytes and diminution in T-suppressor function. *Immunology*, **52**(4):611–620, **1984b.**

Gottesman, S. R.; Walford, R. L.; and Thorbecke, G. J.: Proliferative and cytotoxic immune functions in aging mice. II. Decreased generation of specific suppressor T-cells in alloreactive cultures. *J. Immunol.*, **133**(4):1782–1787, **1984.**

Greenberg, L. J., and Yunis, E. J.: Genetic control of autoimmune disease and immune responsiveness and the relationship to aging. In Bergsma, D., and Harrison, D. E. (eds.): *Genetics Effects on Aging*, Alan R. Liss, New York, **1978.**

Gupta, S., and Good, R. A.: Subpopulations of human T lymphocytes. X. Alterations in T, B, third population cells and T-cells with receptors for immunoglobin M(Tu) or G(Ty) in ageing humans, *J. Immunol*, **122**(4):1214–1219, **1978.**

Harrison, D. E.; Astle, C. M.; and Doubleday, J. W.: Stem cell lines from old immunodeficient donors give normal responses in young recipients. *J. Immunol.*, **118**(4):1223–1227, **1977.**

Harrison, D. E.; Astle, C. M.; and Delaittre, J. A.: Loss of proliferative capacity in immunohemopoietic stem cells caused by serial transplantation rather than ageing. *J. Exp. Med.*, **147**(5):1526–1531, **1978.**

Hausman, P. B.; Goidl, E. A.; Siskind, G. W.; and Weksler, M. E.: Immunological studies of aging. XI. Age-related changes in idiotype repertoire of suppressor T-cells stimulated during tolerance induction. *J. Immunol.*, **134**(6):3802–3807, **1985.**

Haynes, B. F.; Shimizu, K.; and Eisenbarth, G. S.: Identification of human and rodent thymic epithelium using tetanus toxin and monoclonal antibody A2B5. *J. Clin. Invest.*, **71**(1):9–14, **1983.**

Hirokawa, K.; Albright, J. W.; and Makinodan, T.: Restoration of impaired immune functions in aging animals. I. Effect of syngeneic thymus and bone marrow grafts. *Clin. Immunol. Immunopathol.*, **5**(3)371–376, **1976.**

Hollingsworth, M. A., and Evans, D. L.: Changes in spleen cell proliferative responses and resistance to syngeneic tumor challenge in aging NBR rats. *Mech. Ageing Dev.*, **22**(3–4):321–333, **1983.**

Hood, L. E.; Weissman, I. L.; Wood, W. B.; and Wilson, J. H.: *Immunology*, 2nd ed., The Benjamin/Cummings Publishing Company Inc., Menlo Park, CA, **1984.**

Jensen, T. L.; Hallgren, H. M.; Yasmineh, W. G.; and O'Leary, J. J.: Do immature T cells accumulate in advanced age. *Mech. Ageing Dev.*, **33:**237–245, **1986.**

Kaplan, P. J., and Garvey, J. S.: Age-related changes in responsiveness of various rat tissue lymphocytes to mitogens. *Immunol. Lett.*, **3**(6):357–363, **1981.**

Kay, M. M. B.: Immune system: Expression and regulation of cellular aging. In Bergener, M.; Ermini, M.; and Stahelin, H. B. (eds.): *Thresholds in Aging*, Academic Press, London, **1985.**

Kay, M. M. B.: An overview of immune aging. *Mech. Ageing Dev.*, **9:**39–59, **1979.**

Kay, M. M. B., and Baker, L. S.: Cell changes associated with declining immune function in aging series. In Cherkin, A.; Finch, C. E.; Kharasch, N.; Makinodan, T.; Scott, F. L.; and Strehler, B. S. (eds.): *Physiology and Cell Biology of Aging*, Raven Press, New York, **1979.**

Lewis, V. M.; Twomey, J. J.; Bealmar, P.; Goldstein,

G.; and Good, R. A.: Age, thymic involution, and circulating thymic hormone activity. *J. Clin. Endocr. Metab.*, **47**:145–150, **1978.**

Liu, J. J.; Segre, M.; and Segre, D.: Changes in suppressor, helper and B-cell functions in aging mice. *Cell Immunol.*, **66**:372–382, **1982.**

Liu, J. J.; Segre, D.; Gelberg, H. B.; Fudenberg, H. H.; Tsang, K. Y.; Khansari, N.; Waltenbaugh, C. R.; and Segre, M.: Effects of long-term treatment of mice with anti-I-J. monoclonal antibody and dialyzable leukocyte extract on immune function of lifespan. *Mech. Ageing Dev.*, **27**:359–372, **1984.**

Lvik, M., and North, R. J.: Effect of aging on antimicrobial immunity: Old mice display a normal capacity for generating protective T-cells and immunologic memory in response to infection with *Listeria monocytogenes*. *J. Immunol.*, **135**(5):3479–3486, **1985.**

Makinodan, T.: Immunity and aging. In Finch, C. E., and Hayflick, L. (eds.): *Handbook of the Biology of Aging*, Van Nostrand Reinhold, New York, **1977.**

Manheimer, A. J.; Victor-Kobrin, C.; Stein, K. E.; and Bona, C. A.: Antimmunoglobin antibodies. V. Age-dependent variation of clones stimulated by polysaccharide TI-2 antigens in 129 and MRL mice spontaneously producing anti-gamma-globulin antibodies. *J. Immunol.*, **133**(2):562–568, **1984.**

Mason-Smith, A.: The effects of age on the immune response to type III pneumococcal polysaccharide (SIII) and bacterial lipopolysaccharide (LPS) in BALB/c, SJL/J and C3H mice. *J. Immunol.*, **116**(2):469–474, **1976.**

Matsumoto, T.; Miake, S.; Mitsuyama, M.; Takeya, K.; and Nomoto, K.: Enhanced resistance to *Listeria monocytogenes* due to non-specifically activated macrophages in aged mice. *J. Clin. Lab. Immunol.*, **8**(1):51–54, **1982.**

McClure, J. E.; Lameris, N.; Wara, D. W.; and Goldstein, A. L.: Immunochemical studies on thymosin: radioimmunoassay of thymosin alpha-1. *J. Immunol.*, **128**(1):368–375, **1982.**

Miller, R. A.: Age-associated decline in precursor frequency for different T-cell mediated reactions, with preservation of helper or cytotoxic effect per percursor cell. *J. Immunol.*, **132**:63–68, **1984.**

Mosier, D. E.; Mond, J. T.; and Goldings, E. A.: The ontogeny of thymic independent antibody responses *in vitro* in normal mice and mice with an x-linked B-cell defect. *J. Immunol.*, **119**(6):1874–1878, **1977.**

Nandy, K., and Bennett, M.: Immune manipulations and brain reactive antibody formation in aging mice. *Mech. Ageing Dev.*, **22**:3–4, **1983.**

Nordin, A. A., and Makinodan, T.: Humoral immunity in aging. *Fed. Proc.*, **33**:2033–2035, **1974.**

Nordin, A. A., and Collins, G. D.: Limiting dilution analysis of alloreactive cytotoxic precursor cells in aging mice. *J. Immunol.*, **131**(5):2215–2218, **1983.**

Ogden, D. A., and Micklem, H. S.: The fate of serially transplanted bone marrow cell population from young and old donors. *Transplantation*, **22**(3):287–293, **1976.**

O'Leary, J. J.; Jackola, D. R.; Hallgren, H. M.; Abbasnezhad, M.; and Yasmineh, W.: Evidence for a less differentiated subpopulation of lymphocytes in advanced age. *Mech. Ageing Dev.*, **21**:109–120, **1983.**

Perry, L. L.; McClusky, R. T.; Benaceraff, B.; and Green, M. I.: Enhanced syngeneic tumor destruction by *in vivo* inhibition of suppressor cells using anti-I. J. alloantiserum. *Am. J. Pathol.*, **92**(2):491–506, **1978.**

Price, G. B., and Makinodan, T.: Immunologic deficiencies in senescence. 1. Characterization of intrinsic deficiencies. *J. Immunol.*, **108**:403–412, **1972.**

Saxena, R. K.; Saxena, Q. B.; and Adler, W. H.: Interleukin-2-induced activation of natural killer activity in spleen cells from old and young mice. *Immunology*, **51**(4):719–726, **1984.**

Schwab, R.; Hausman, P. B.; Rinnooy-Kan, E.; and Weksler, M. E.: Immunological studies of ageing. X. Impaired T lymphocytes and normal monocyte response from elderly humans to the mitogenic antibodies OKT3 and Leu4. *Immunology*, **55**(4):677–684, **1985.**

Schneider, E. L.; Sternberg, H.; Tice, R.; Senula, G.; Kram, D.; Smith, G.; and Bynum, G.: Cellular replication and aging. *Mech. Ageing Dev.*, **9**:313–324, **1979.**

Smith, G. S., and Walford, R. L.: Influence of the main histocompatibility complex in aging in mice. *Nature*, **46**:727–729, **1977.**

Sternberg, H.; Senula, G.; and Schneider, E. L.: The effect of age on cellular replication rates. *Gerontological Society* (Abstract), San Francisco, **1977.**

Teller, M. N.: Interrelationships among aging, immunity and cancer. In Sigel, M. M., and Good, R. A. (eds.): *Tolerance, Autoimmunity and Aging*, Charles C Thomas, Springfield, IL, **1972.**

Thoman, M. L., and Weigle, W. O.: Cell mediated immunity in aged mice: An underlying lesion in IL-2. Synthesis. *J. Immunol.*, **128**:2358–2361, **1982.**

Tonegawa, S.: The molecules of the immune system. *Sci. Am.*, **253**:122–131, **1985.**

Tyan, M. L.: Age-related decrease in mouse T-cell progenitors. *J. Immunol.*, **118**:846–851, **1977.**

Tyan, M. L.: Marrow stem cells during development and aging. In Kay, M. M. B., and Makinodan, T. (eds.): *Handbook of Immunology in Aging*, CRC Press, Boca Raton, FL, **1981.**

Vetvicka, V.; Fornusek, L.; Tlaskalova, H.; Sima, P.; and Pospisil, M.: Some properties and functions of macrophages during ontogeny. *Dev. Comp. Immunol.*, **7**:747–748, **1983.**

Vetvicka, V.; Tlaskalova-Hogenova, H.; and Pospisil, M.: Impaired antigen presenting function of macrophages from aged mice. *Immunol. Invest.*, **14**(2):105–114, **1985.**

Walford, R. L.: *The Immunological Theory of Aging*, Munksgaard, Copenhagen, **1969.**

Weindruch, R. H.; Kristie, J. A.; Naeim, H.; Mullen, B. G.; and Walford, R. L.: Influence on weaning-initiated dietary restriction on responses to T-cell mitogens and on splenic T cell levels in a long-lived F1-hybrid mouse strain. *Exp. Gerontol.*, **17**:49–64, **1982.**

Weksler, M. E.; Innes, J. B.; and Goldstein, G. J.: Immunological studies of aging. IV. The contribution of thymic involution to the immune deficiencies of aging mice and reversal with thymopoietin. *Exp. Med.*, **148**(4):996–1006, **1978.**

Whistler, R. L., and Newhouse, Y. G.: Immunosenescence of the human B-cell system: Impaired activation/proliferation in response to autologous monocytes pulsed with *Staph.* protein A and the effects of interleukins 1 and 2 compared to interferon. *Lymphokine Res.*, **4**(4):331–337, **1985.**

Zatz, M. M., and Goldstein, A. L.: Thymosins, lymphokines and the immunology of aging. *Gerontology*, **31**:263–277, **1985.**

Zharhary, D.; Segev, Y.; and Gershon, H. E.: T-cell cytoxicity and ageing: Differing cause of reduced response in individual mice. *Mech. Ageing Dev.*, **25**(1–2):129–140, **1984.**

Zharhary, D., and Klinman, N. R.: Antigen responsiveness of the mature and generative B cell populations of aged mice. *J. Exp. Med.*, **157**(4):1300–1308, **1983.**

Zharhary, D., and Klinman, N. R.: B-cell repertoire diversity to PR8 influenza virus does not decrease with age. *J. Immunol.*, **133**:2285–2287, **1984.**

PART
III Systemic and Organismic Aging

CHAPTER
9 AGING OF THE NERVOUS SYSTEM

Structural and Biochemical Changes

The study of the human nervous system, its development, adult state, and aging, and its alterations with disease, remains one of the most challenging and intriguing issues of our time. Despite increasing and rapid advances in our knowledge, we still have few direct answers to our many questions concerning the activities of the nervous system. Therefore, studies of the aging nervous system may provide valuable information on both aging processes and nervous functions. From comparison of the aging brain, with and without neurologic and psychiatric diseases of old age, emerge differences in the morphologic, biochemical, and functional nature of the normal and diseased states. These differences provide criteria to distinguish between the two. We shall, therefore, emphasize the normal aging of the nervous system while also using data from age-related disorders for comparisons.

Locations, mechanisms, and consequences of changes with aging within the nervous system, both central and peripheral, are summarized in Table 9–1. Aging changes are multiple and involve all organizational levels (Figure 9–1).

At the structural level, aging affects neurons and glial cells, their number and branching, as well as the synapse—a key site for the reception and transmission of the nervous impulse.

At the chemical level, aging modulates the metabolism, turnover, and receptors of several neurotransmitters, substances carrying or transmitting the neural signal at the synapse, as well as cellular metabolic processes. Aging also affects the membranes, both plasma and intracellular membranes, where lipid peroxidation and protein cross-linking accumulate, perhaps owing to the continuing action of free radicals (Chapter 7). Biochemical alterations of neural membranes impair excitability, fluidity, and transport. Equally important may be nuclear alterations in which DNA damage and failure of DNA repair may be reflected in disturbed protein synthesis.

At the functional level, aging influences electrical activity (spontaneous and evoked) or influences motor and sensory functions or cognitive and affective processes.

Consequences of aging may result in disturbances within the nervous system and in the organism as a whole. They involve motor and sensory decrements, alterations in sleep and EEG, memory impairment, and increased frequency and severity of neurologic and psychiatric disorders. In view of the key role of the nervous system in regulating all body functions, any impairment of its function will impact on the aging of the entire organism, particularly the efficacy of homeostatic adjustments to the environment.

STRUCTURAL CHANGES

BRAIN WEIGHT

With aging, brain weight decreases of between 6 and 11% have been reported in hu-

Table 9–1. CHANGES WITH AGING IN THE NERVOUS SYSTEM

Locations
Regional selectivity
Neuronal loss/gliosis
Reduced dendrites and dendritic spines
Synaptic susceptibility
Vascular lesions
Mechanisms
Neurotransmitter imbalance
Membrane alterations
Metabolic disturbances
Intra/intercellular degeneration
Consequences
Sensory and motor decrements
Sleep alterations and EEG changes
Memory impairment
Increased neurologic and psychiatric pathology
Impaired homeostasis

mans (Figure 9–2) although some claim such a decrease does not occur in mentally normal older individuals. This is in marked contrast with the reduction reported in many, but not all, demented individuals (Terry, 1982; Duara *et al.*, 1985; Haug, 1985) (Figure 9–3). Similarly, the brain volume, as measured by ventricular and sulcal dimensions at autopsy or by imaging techniques in the living, remains essentially unchanged in normal aged individuals. Most demented patients exhibit a marked enlargement of the ventricles with reduced cortical volume (Figure 9–4). Experimental animals vary, with rats showing no changes with aging, whereas dogs and monkeys demonstrate cerebral atrophy.

NEURONAL CELL LOSS

Because of the heterogeneity of nervous structures, aging affects the various portions of the nervous system differentially. One striking example of this diversity involves neuronal loss. In the normally aging human brain, loss of neurons is limited to discrete areas. The number of glial cells, however, increases with aging in most areas, and this increase, or gliosis, may represent a compensatory response not only to the limited neuronal loss, but also to neuronal impairment. Indeed, with aging, neurons undergo degenerative changes manifested by decreased number of dendrites and dendritic spines, the sites where transmission occurs, by disturbances of synaptic function and neurotransmission, and by intra- and intercellular accumulation of functionally inactive substances such as lipofuscin, melanin, and abnormal neurofibrillary and amyloid proteins. Synaptic alterations may be ascribed to dendritic defects or losses, alterations at the pre- and postsynaptic structures of neurotransmitter synthesis, release, or binding. Another compartment affected by aging is the cerebral vascular system, which undergoes the same atherosclerotic changes that involve the entire arterial vasculature; these atherosclerotic lesions commence at an early age, progress with age, and profoundly influence the neural tissue, which has a critical dependence on oxygen and glucose for normal metabolism and function.

Cells of the Nervous System. Cells of the nervous system include neurons and glial and endothelial cells. Neurons have long been regarded as the primary functional cells of the nervous system, although glial cells are five times more numerous. Neural structure varies with respect to the cell body and branches. The latter include the dendrites, which extend from the cell body and arborize, and a longer extension, the axon. Communication between cells is through synapses located in specific structures, spines and knobs, and is composed of the presynaptic membrane, a cleft, and a postsynaptic membrane. Present in the spines or knobs are vesicles or granules containing the synaptic transmitter synthesized in the cell. The axons may be surrounded by a specialized membrane, myelin, or may be unmyelinated. The myelinated fibers transmit the nerve impulse more rapidly than do the nonmyelinated ones.

Gial cells comprise astrocytes, which have end feet that surround blood vessels in the CNS; oligodendrocytes involved in myelin formation; and microglia, scavenger cells, which are part of the immune system. While the astrocytes have independent functions, they also interact to function as a neuronal-glial unit in such vital actions as memory, metabolism, and neural transmission.

Endothelial cells of cerebral capillaries form tight junctions that do not permit the passage of substances that pass through the junctions between endothelial cells in other tissues. In addition, cerebral capillaries are surrounded by the end feet of astrocytes. Both these special features of cerebral capillaries hinder the exchanges between plasma and brain interstitial fluid across capillary walls and represent the anatomic basis for the concept of a functional blood-brain barrier. This so-called barrier essentially protects the brain from endogenous metabolites and exogenous toxins and drugs in the blood and prevents neurotransmitters escaping into the general circulation.

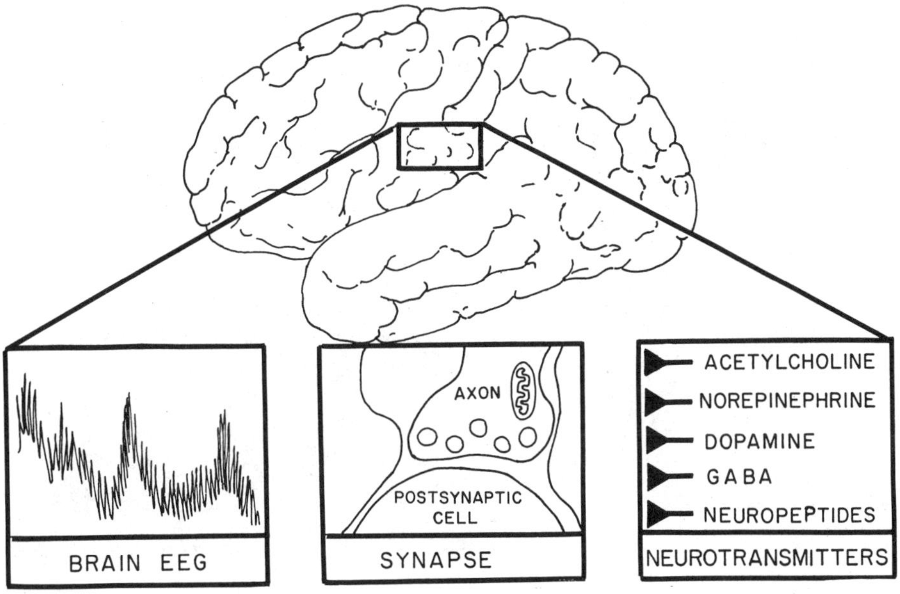

Figure 9–1. *Diagram of electrophysiological (brain EEG), functional (synapse), and chemical (neurotransmitters) sites for changes in the brain with aging.* (Drawing by S. Oklund.)

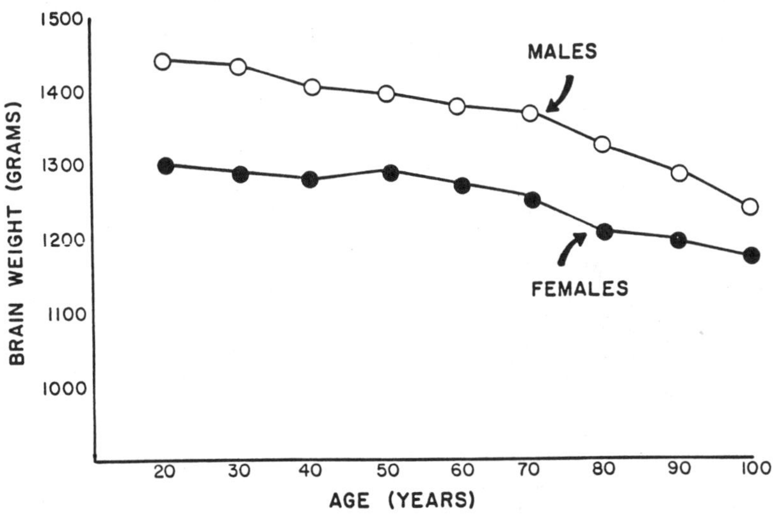

Figure 9–2. *Changes in brain weight with aging in human males and females.*

The number of neurons is established at birth in humans and at various pre- or postnatal ages in other animal species. Once they have differentiated, neurons lose the capacity to divide and, when lost, cannot be replaced. Because of the potentially significant consequences of such neuronal loss on the activity of the nervous system over time, neuronal number and its eventual changes with aging have been extensively investigated. Results of these studies, while not always concordant, show a moderate and regionally circumscribed neuronal loss throughout the lifespan (Brizzee, 1985; Duara *et al.*, 1985; Cole, 1985; Haug, 1985; Vernadakis, 1985). For example, neurons may be lost at the rate of 1 percent per year in the cerebral cortex but at a faster rate in the basal ganglia and cerebellum, tentatively related to the progressive deteriora-

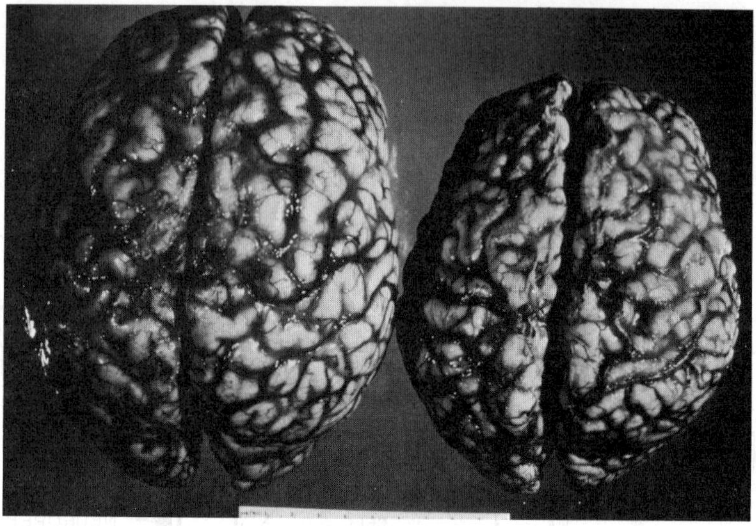

Figure 9–3. *Differences in size of normal (*left*) and Alzheimer's (*right*) brain.* (Courtesy of Dr. L.S. Forno).

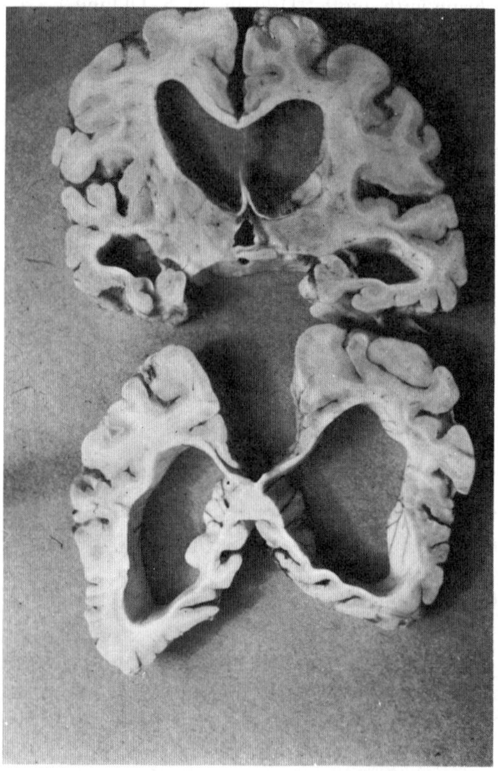

Figure 9–4. *Difference in size of ventricles of normal (*upper*) and Alzheimer (*lower*) brain.* (Courtesy of L. S. Forno).

tion of motor control in the elderly. In the locus ceruleus rich in catecholaminergic neurons, there is, after 60 years of age, a marked (40 percent) decrease in cell number, which has been related to a number of functional decrements such as alterations of sleep pattern in the elderly ascribed to catecholaminergic deficits, (Brody, 1978). Another area that seems to undergo significant neuronal loss is the nucleus basalis of Meynert, located in proximity of the amygdala, and of particular significance as it is thought to provide the primary cholinergic input to the cerebral cortex (Butcher and Woolf, 1986). Neuronal loss in this area is severe in individuals affected by senile dementia of the Alzheimer type but may not occur in normal elderly persons (Whitehouse *et al.*, 1982; Bondareff, 1986). In the spinal cord, the number of motor neurons remains unchanged until 60 years of age, after which a significant decrease (as much as 50 percent) occurs at late ages (Brizzee, 1985).

Cell number in experimental animals decreases slightly with aging, depending on the area considered, the type of cell, and the animal species. For example, in the cerebral cortex of rats, the number of neurons remains unchanged with aging. The glial cells, astrocytes and oligodendrocytes, increase in number. Microglia are unchanged

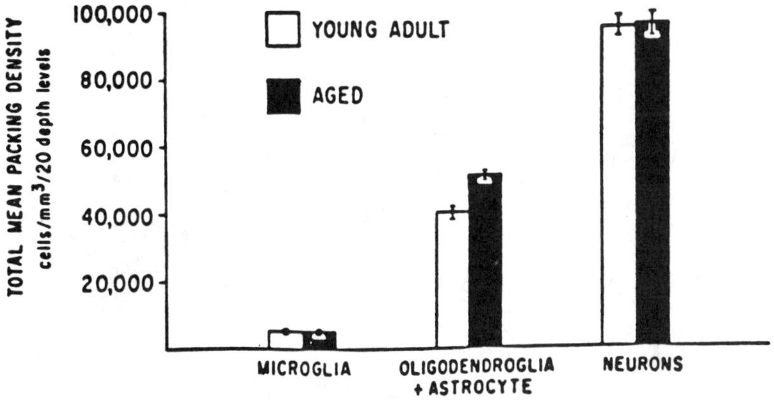

Figure 9–5. *Mean values for packing density for total depth of cortex for neurons, combined oligodendroglia and astrocyte population, and microglia population in young adult (109 to 113 days) and aged (763 to 972 days) male rats of the Long-Evans strain.*

Number of cells of each type is indicated by height of vertical bars and bracketed lines represent standard deviation. (From Brizzee, K.R.; Sherwood, N.; and Timiras, P.S.: A comparison of cell populations at various depth levels in cerebral cortex of young adult and aged Long-Evans rats. *J. Gerontol.*, *23*, 289–298, 1968.)

(Brizzee *et al.*, 1968) (Figure 9–5). Reduced numbers of neurons have been reported in discrete brain areas of aged monkeys, guinea pigs, rats, and mice (Brizzee, 1985), but when these animals are studied throughout the lifespan, a major reduction in cell number often occurs at young rather than old ages (Diamond *et al.*, 1978; Diamond, 1986).

Overall, neuronal loss with aging in humans and experimental animals seems to be restricted to specific CNS structures and to be associated in animal brains, and possibly in human brains, with an increase in glial cell number. The relatively mild cell loss reported in normal aging contrasts with the severe cell reduction reported in several diseases of the nervous system associated with aging, such as senile dementia of the Alzheimer type and Parkinson's disease, or genetic abnormalities, such as Down's syndrome with impaired mental function and precocious aging.

DENDRITIC LOSS WITH AGING

A reduction in the number of dendrites—the many processes that extend out from the cell body and arborize extensively—and of the dendritic spines—sites of synapses between axons and dendrites—has been reported in studies of normal aging. For example, the cortex of a young individual shows large pyramidal cells with abundant dendrites and dendritic spines. A corresponding zone, in an old individual, shows quite striking loss of dendrites and spines. Since dendrites undergo a certain degree of renewal continuously, it has been suggested that the denudation of the neurons, that is, the reduced number of dendrites, may not be a true loss, but rather, a slowing down of the renewal process. When the loss of dendrites is viewed in a network of neurons, then the consequences of diminished connectivity become apparent (Scheibel *et al.*, 1975; Scheibel and Tomiyasu, 1978) (Figure 9–6). In normal aging with continued environmental stimulation dendritic loss may be minimal, absent, or even supplemented with a degree of dendritic outgrowth; in senile dementia of the Alzheimer type (SDAT) and more so in presenile dementia, the dendritic loss is severe and progressive. With the loss of dendrites, there is also a loss of synapses, neurotransmission is reduced, and communication within and without the nervous system is impaired.

SYNAPTIC CHANGES WITH AGING

Even though generally quite moderate, alterations in the axon, the neuronal exten-

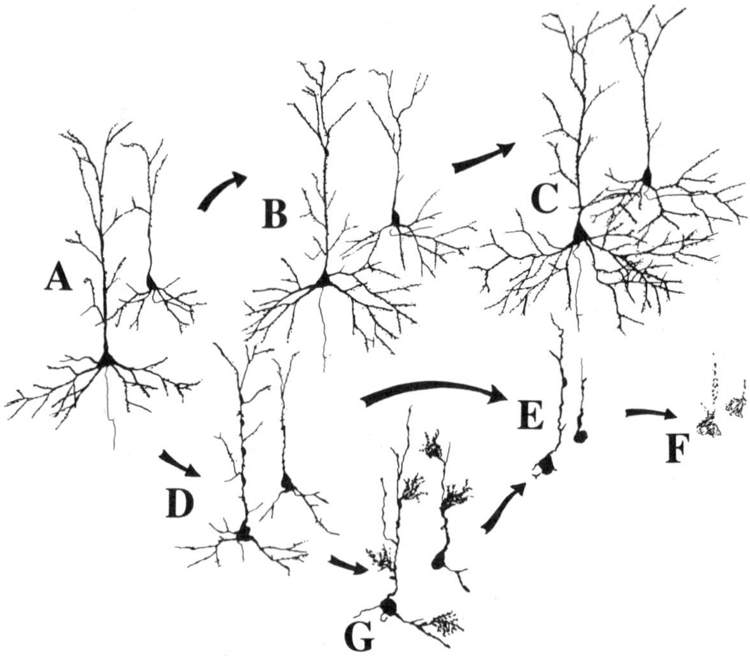

Figure 9–6. *Semi-schematized drawing summarizing the changes that may occur in pyramidal neurons of the aging human cerebral cortex.*

Sequence *A, B, C,* follows the changes that may occur in the normal aging cortex under the effects of continued physical and/or cognitive "challenge" and in the probable presence of continuing small amounts of neuronal loss. Increasing dendritic growth, especially in the peripheral portions of the basilar dendrites, reflects dendritic response to optimal cortical 'loading,' as well as presumed supplementary growth to fill neuropil space left by dendrite systems of those neurons that die.

Sequence *A, D, E, F,* epitomizes the progressive degenerative changes that characterize Senile Dementia of Alzheimer (SDAT), and includes progressive loss of dendritic spines and dendritic branches culminating in death of the cell. Basilar dendrite loss precedes loss of the apical shaft.

Sequence *A, D, G, E, F,* represents a unique pattern of deterioration of the dendrite tree found only in the familial type of Prensenile Dementia of Alzheimer. During the period of dendritic degeneration, bursts of spine-rich dendrites in clusters appear along the surface of the dying dendrite shafts. Such changes have been seen in neocortex, archicortex (hippocampus), and cerebellar cortex. The cause and/or mechanisms of these eruptive attempts at regrowth, even as the neurons are in a degenerative phase, are unknown. (Courtesy of Dr. A. B. Scheibel).

sion that carries impulses to the effector target cell, may contribute to the disruption of neural circuitry with aging. In the aging central nervous system, demyelination has been variably reported, as well as axonal swelling and changes in the number of neurofilaments and neurotubules. Changes in the neural cytoskeleton occurring with aging and repercussions therefrom on neuronal function are discussed in relation to disruption of neurofilaments, neurofibrillary tangles, particularly evident in the dementias (see Chapter 10). The decreased number of synapses in discrete areas of the aging brain may coincide with the corresponding loss of dendrites and dendritic spines. Apart from axonal changes, alterations in synaptic components—membrane, vesicles, and granules—have been variably reported. In addition, the "reactive synaptogenesis" or axonal sprouting that follows the loss of a neuron is slowed down with aging (Cotman and Holets, 1985). Such reactive synaptogenesis represents a compensatory reaction to neuronal loss or damage and is characterized by an increase in the number of synaptic contacts provided by the nearby neurons. Such a compensation would be less efficient in the old brain.

Within the cytoplasm, the Golgi apparatus and mitochondria are seen at times as dilated and fragmented (Mervis, 1981). The Nissl material is decreased, as well as the amount of RNA. The membranes of various other organelles and the nucleus may show infolding and distortion. The neurofibrillary tangles and neuritic plaques are found in the normal aging, but in much higher numbers in some diseases of the aged nervous system, such as senile dementia of the Alzheimer type and in some genetic diseases such as Down's syndrome. (See Chapter 10.)

ACCUMULATION OF LIPOFUSCIN

Another aspect of neural aging is accumulation of the age pigment, lipofuscin. Lipofuscin is a by-product of lipid peroxidation with both a protein and lipid component (see Chapter 5). It accumulates with aging in CNS cells, both neurons and glial cells, where it follows a regional distribution. Lipofuscin can be visualized as autofluorescent material *in vitro* or *in vivo* (Figure 9–7) as well as with the electron microscope as dark granules, either scattered in the cytoplasm or clustered around the nucleus (Figures 9–8, 9–9) (Brizzee *et al.*, 1969). The functional significance of lipofuscin is unclear; however, the consensus is that it is formed during the intracellular process of autophagia or self-digestion. The claim that lipofuscin accumulation interferes with intracellular function has not been substantiated.

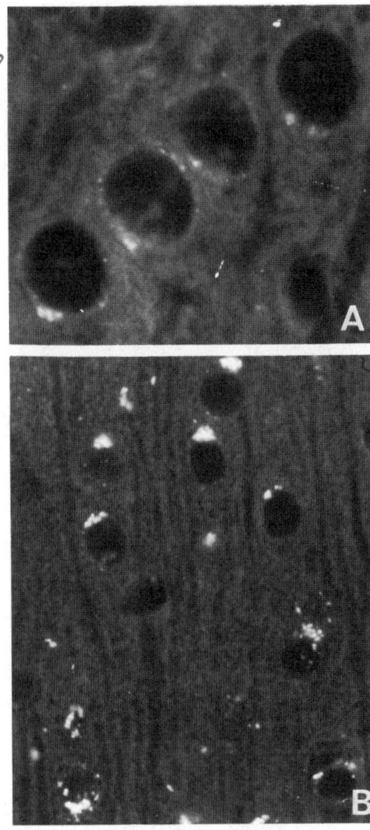

Figure 9–7. *Photomicrograph of unstained sections under blue light fluorescence illustrating lipofuscin pigment in neuron somata in cerebral cortex of male Long-Evans rats.*

A. Young adults (1D9–113 days), magnification 40×; *B*. aged rats (763 to 972 days), magnification 17× (From Brizzee, K. R.; Cancilla, P. A.; Sherwood, N.: and Timiras, P. S.: The amount and distribution of pigments in neurons and glia of the cerebral cortex. Autofluorescence and ultrastructural studies. *J. Gerontol., 24:*127–135, 1969.)

Lipofuscin Brain Distribution and Cell Activity. The proposal that the more active the cell, the less chance for lipofuscin accumulation is attractive. The plausibility of this idea is demonstrated in the time sequence of pigmentation of the cranial nerve nuclei of the guinea pig in which the less active mesencephalic nucleus of the trigeminal nerve shows earlier pigmentation than the more active somatic motor nuclei (Wilcox, 1959). The continually active cochlear nucleus and the dorsal motor nucleus of the vagus nerve and, perhaps, the Edinger-Westphal nucleus, exhibiting no pigment in old animals, have been cited as extreme and convincing examples of this hypothesis. Intracellularly, the pigment follows a sequential distribution that seems to be age-related as well: thus, lipofuscin pigments appear first as diffuse granules, then as perinuclear clusters, and finally as aggregates at the axon hillock and principal dendrites. Certain drugs, such as centrophenoxine, have been shown to reduce production of lipofuscin pigments, possibly by stimulating the activity of antioxidant enzymes. Experiments in centrophenoxine-treated animals and a few clinical trials have shown some improvement in certain behavioral tests: however, whether this is due to the action of the drug in reducing brain lipofuscin or to some secondary independent action (such as body weight loss) is not known (Nandy *et al.*, 1978).

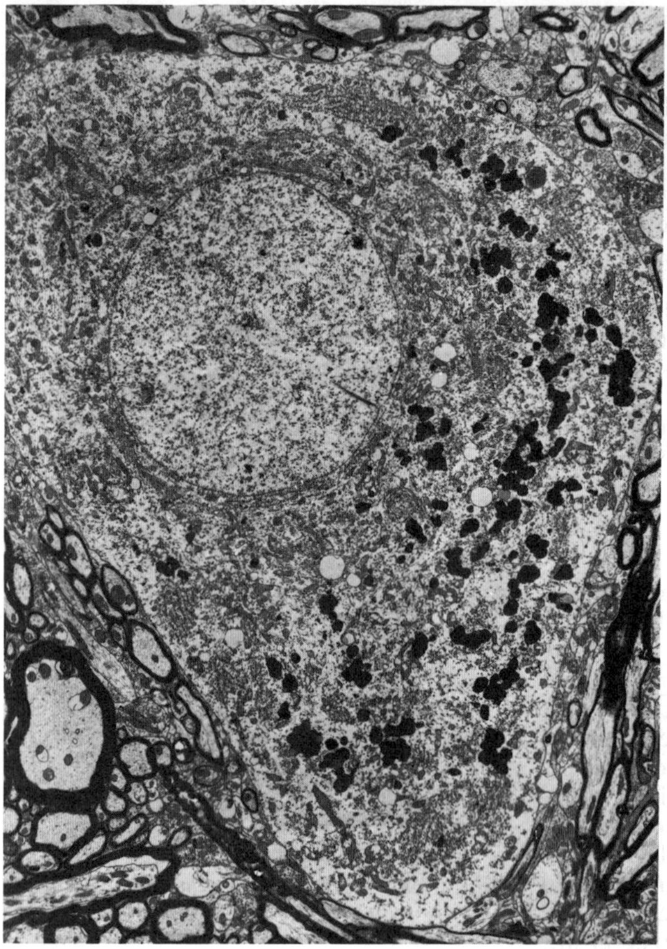

Figure 9–8. *A neuron from the cerebral cortex of a 605-day-old male Long-Evans rat.*

There are numerous dense bodies (lipofuscin) irregularly distributed in the perikaryon. Magnification 1800× (From Brizzee, K. R.; Cancilla, P. A.; Sherwood, N.; and Timiras, P. S.: The amount and distribution of pigments in neurons and glia of the cerebral cortex. Autofluorescence and ultrastructural studies. *J. Gerontol.*, *24*:127–135, 1969.)

NEUROFIBRILLARY TANGLES AND NEURITIC PLAQUES

Neurofibrillary tangles consist of intraneuronal tangled masses of fibrous elements, often flame-shaped bundles, coursing the entire cell body (Figure 9–10). They are present in normal aging, frequently found in the hippocampus, but their accumulation in the cortex and other brain areas is one of the pathologic hallmarks of senile dementia of the Alzheimer type (SDAT) (Iqbal *et al.*, 1982). In SDAT, tangles are in greatest number in the associative areas of the cortex, and their distribution is consistent with a primary toxin/infection spread through the olfactory system (Pearson *et al.*, 1985). Their density has also been correlated with the severity of the dementia, of the cell loss, and of the cholinergic deficits (Jacobs and Butcher, 1986).

Under the electron microscope, each fiber consists of a pair of filaments wound around each other to form a paired helical filament (PHF) (Terry, 1963). Chemically, PHF are highly insoluble and their precise protein composition is currently unknown. However, they react with monoclonal antibodies specific for neurofilament proteins or for microtubule-associated proteins. Since both neurofilaments and microtubules are normal constituents of the cytoskeleton, the immunologic reactivity of PHF supports the hypothesis that several cytoskeletal proteins are linked in the formation of these abnormal, helical filaments. Which proteins make up the core-

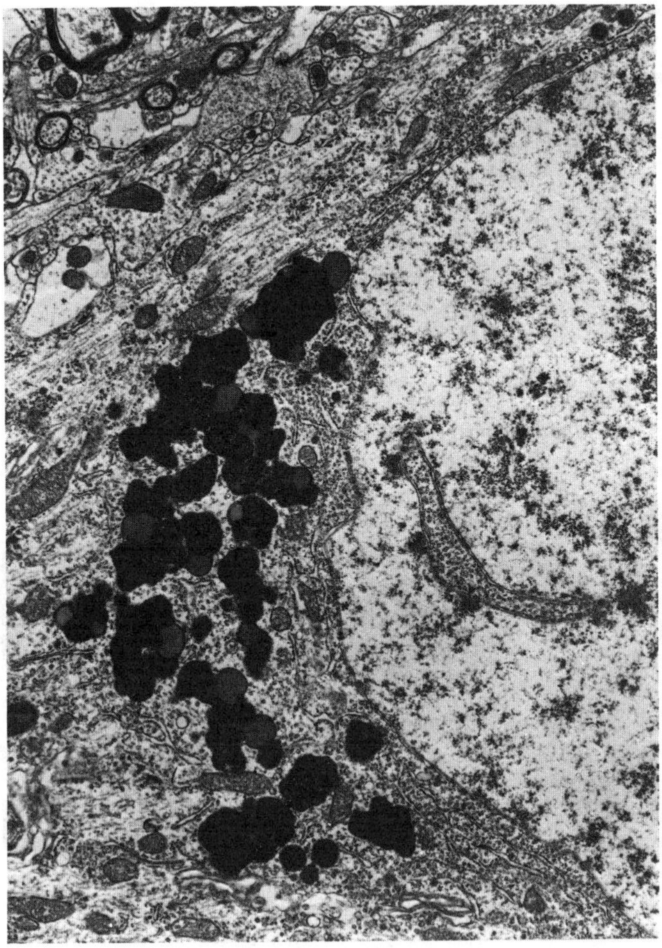

Figure 9–9. *A portion of a neuron from the cerebral cortex of a 605-day-old male Long-Evans rat.*

The lipofuscin granules are clustered at one pole of the nucleus. Magnification 7500× (From Brizzee, K. R.; Cancilla, P. A.; Sherwood, N.; and Timiras, P. S.: The amount and distribution of pigments in neurons and glia of the cerebral cortex. Autofluorescence and ultrastructural studies. *J. Gerontol., 24:*127–35, 1969.)

twisted filament and whether novel abnormal proteins are present are still unknown.

The neuritic plaques are situated extracellularly. Extremely rare in normal aging, they are abundant in SDAT, where they are found in the frontal, temporal, and occipital lobes and the hippocampus. Their distribution is similar to that of the neurofibrillary tangles, and the two structures are often found in close proximity. Typically, the plaque consists of a central core of amyloid surrounded by coarse, silver-stained fibers represented at the electron microscope by many dystrophic neurites (axon segments) with degenerated mitochondria, synaptic complexes, and dense bodies (Figure 9–11). Glial and microglial cells react to the plaque and accumulate about the abnormal nerve cell processes. One view is that the development of the plaque proceeds first from abnormalities of the neural processes to the deposition of amyloid and, only later, to reactive proliferation. Another view is that the primary alteration arises at the level of the brain capillaries and that amyloid or a precursor substance of blood origin leaks from the capillaries and diffuses into the cerebral tissue where it accumulates, leading to destruction of neurons and glial cells and plaque formation (Scheibel *et al.*, 1986).

The origin and nature of amyloid are discussed in Chapter 5. Possible stimuli to plaque formation include: (1) amyloid from a vascular source; (2) other blood toxins leaking from amyloid damaged or otherwise compromised vessels; (3) PHF production at nerve terminals and cell body tangles; (4)

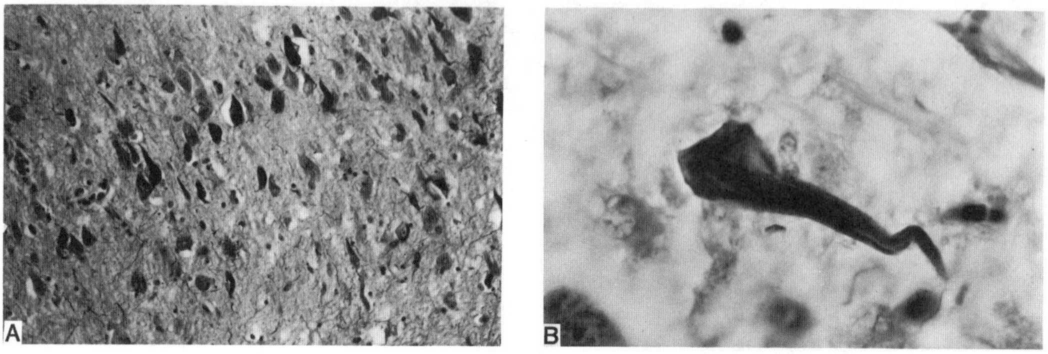

Figure 9–10. A. *Hippocampus, pyramidal layer (*low magnification*), neurofibrillary tangles accumulate in neuronal bodies and stain very darkly.* B. *Neurofibrillary tangle (*high power*) showing characteristic flame-shape.* (Courtesy of Dr. L. S. Forno).

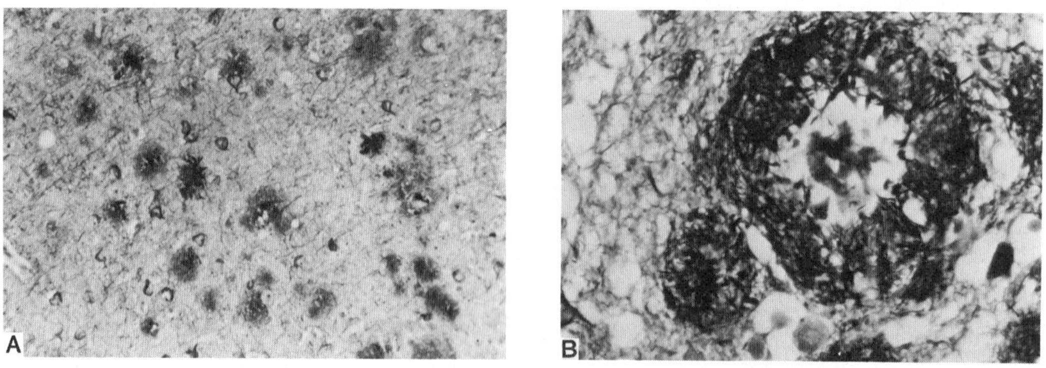

Figure 9–11. A. *Frontal cortex, silent area, presence of neuritic plaques, large, and neurofibrillary tangles, small (*low power*).* B. *Neuritic plaque (*high power*).* (Courtesy of Dr. L. S. Forno).

other damage to cell body or all terminals, for example from free radicals (see Chapter 7); and (5) infection by slow virus. The chemical composition of the plaque amyloid substance is not fully known but appears to consist of fibrous proteins, some with large molecular weights similar to that of immunoglobulins. Amyloid accumulates with aging in many tissues (e.g., heart, pancreas) besides brain, where it is found not only in the plaques but also around blood vessels (hence the blood-borne view of its origin) of the meninges and brain, and in the pituitary gland. The major protein of the plaque amyloid would be identical to the protein in vascular amyloid with an N-terminal sequence unrelated to any known sequenced protein (Glenner and Wong, 1984a,b; Masters *et al.,* 1985). Immunoglobulin and other serum proteins found in amyloid extracts may represent minor contaminants of neuritic plaques readily released by appropriate reactions without solubilizing the amyloid core. In the mammalian slow viral models for SDAT, such as scrapie, neuritic plaque-like structures contain amyloid cores that appear to be identical to or closely associated with the slow viral infectious agent; therefore, the identity of this viral-induced amyloid with the amyloid of the Alzheimer's plaque has served as a basis for the slow virus hypothesis of SDAT etiology (Prusiner, 1984). Several groups have reported on molecular cloning of the amyloid plaque core protein (APC) precursor gene from the brain. APC precursor is reported to be located on chromosome 21 and closely linked to restriction fragment polymorphic markers for familial Alzheimer's disease (Tanzi *et al.,* 1987).

The complete sequence for the precursor codes for approximately 80Kd protein with a membrane spanning region which includes most of the fragment found in amyloid plaque fibrils (Kang *et al.,* 1987). Further, in sporadic Alzheimer's disease, three cases have been reported to contain a duplication of a small region of chromosome 21 including the APC precursor gene (Delabar *et al.,* 1987). An apparently central role for the APC precursor gene in SDAT emphasizes the critical need for a culture model to examine the expression and processing of this protein.

CIRCULATORY CHANGES IN AGING

Vascular changes accompany the morphologic alterations we have described. These changes include atherosclerotic lesions common throughout the arterial vascular system. One of the consequences of atherosclerosis is the production of infarcts—areas of dying tissue and scar formation following interruption of circulation due to obstruction or rupture of blood vessels. The occurrence of multiple infarcts leads to progressive destruction of brain tissue, which may be responsible for a form of senile dementia, properly called "multiple-infarct senile dementia," contrasted with Alzheimer's dementia (Chapter 10). The cerebral capillaries are much more permeable at birth than in adulthood, and the blood-brain barrier develops during the early years of life. This barrier is a functional concept based on specific mechanisms of exchange across the cerebral capillaries different from all other vascular beds. This peculiar type of exchange permits only a few substances to enter the nervous tissue—hence the term "barrier"—and, thus, serves a protective function. The efficiency of the blood-brain barrier increases with age during early development. With aging and disease the blood-brain barrier may again become permeable at least to selected substances and the passage of blood-borne substances may represent one of the causes of such dementias as those of the Alzheimer type. Studies of the structure of cerebral capillaries at progressive ages reveal an increase in the capillary wall thickness in old rats and a decrease in capillary mitochondrial content in old monkeys. Although direct evidence for increased permeability of blood-brain barrier as the primary pathogenic factor in Alzheimer's disease is still lacking, defects of the blood-brain barrier may represent a common pathogenic mechanism linking many different risk factors (Mortimer and Hutton, 1985).

BIOCHEMICAL CHANGES

NEUROTRANSMISSION AND BRAIN PLASTICITY

Information processing in the nervous system involves neurons "talking" to each other or with target cells; therefore, research in synaptic transmission, central to neurobiology, is central to our understanding of the aging of the nervous system. As we know, the nervous system is modifiabale or "plastic," capable of adapting to environmental changes or to changes within the organism itself and of controlling its responses accordingly. Neural plasticity depends largely on the ability of synapses to modify their function when required—in terms of neurotransmission—or their number—in terms of replacement. Neuronal plasticity is maximal during development; whether it continues throughout aging and to what extent it remains efficient in old age is still not known, although we are aware of decrements (Will *et al.,* 1985).

One of the most-studied aspects of aging of the nervous system involves neurotransmitter changes at the synapse, including neurotransmitter turnover, release, and binding (Giacobini, 1982; Rogers and Bloom, 1985; Samorajski and Persson, 1985). Chemically, transmitters may be amines, amino acids, or peptides (Table 9–2). Of these, some may be viewed as classic, our knowledge of them extending back 70 years; they are: acetylcholine, the catecholamines, norepinephrine, epinephrine, and dopamine, and serotonin. More recently others have been associated with neurotransmission; these are certain of the amino acids, such as glycine and glutamate, and GABA. Of the most recent candidates, the peptides, more than 50 have been identified as "putative," that is, "probable" neurotransmitters; of these a few of the more extensively studied are enke-

Table 9–2. NEUROTRANSMITTERS AND MODULATORS IN THE NERVOUS SYSTEM

AMINES	AMINO ACIDS	PEPTIDES
Acetylcholine	Glutamate	Enkephalin
Catecholamines	Aspartate	Cholecystokinin
Norepinephrine	Glycine	Substance P
Epinephrine	GABA*	VIP*
Dopamine	Taurine	Somatostatin
Serotonin*	Histamine	TRH* and others

*Serotonine, 5-hydroxytryptamine, or 5-HT; GABA, γ-amino butyric acid; VIP, vasoactive intestinal polypeptide; TRH, thyrotropin-stimulating hormone.

phalin, substance P, and the neurohormone thyrotropin-releasing hormone (TRH). Some brain peptides, such as cholecystokinin and somatostatin, are also found in the gastrointestinal tract. Different transmitters—usually a classic neurotransmitter and a peptide—may coexist within the same neuron. Such "coexistence," resulting in "co-utilization" of several transmitters, vastly expands the potential diversity of synaptic communications. Indeed, the peptide often "modulates" or "modifies" the action of the classic neurotransmitter. For example, serotonin coexists with substance P and TRH in neurons of the rat medulla and spinal cord where the three neurotransmitters collaborate to induce motor and behavioral responses. In another example, the presence of cholecystokinin in a population of dopamine neurons in the rat mesencephalon has been extrapolated to suggest that the combination of the two neurotransmitters is relevant to our understanding and treatment of some mental disorders such as schizophrenia in humans.

A consequence of synaptic diversification is the increased complexity of neuronal communication and the need for a fine tuning of all chemical messengers, transmitters, and their modulators. Neurotransmitters have stimulatory or inhibitory actions, and, most important to the function of the nervous system, these actions must remain in balance. With aging, owing to the multiplicity of chemical messengers released by the neurons, alterations in function are more likely a consequence of imbalance among neurotransmitters rather than a consequence of a global alteration of single neurotransmitters. Such imbalance could involve the classic neurotransmitters—for which evidence is already available—or the sustaining peptides, or both.

Chemical Clasification of Synapses. Many synapses are classified according to the neurotransmitter released at this site. Examples of currently recognized synaptic transmitters include acetylcholine (ACh), norepinephrine (NE), serotonin (5-hydroxytryptamine), and γ-aminobutyrate (GABA), and the synapses are named accordingly. Briefly summarized are their synthesis, storage, release, postsynaptic interactions, and inactivation (Figure 9–12).

Cholinergic Synapse. Choline is the precursor of the transmitter ACh through the actions of the synthesizing enzyme choline acetyltransferase (CAT). ACh is free in the cytoplasm of the prejunctional axonal ending as well as contained in vesicles. Current concepts are that the release of cytoplasmic ACh initiates transmembrane events. Several distinct pre- and postsynaptic ACh receptors have been described. Receptor-bound ACh is inactivated by the enzyme acetylcholinesterase (AChE).

Adrenergic Synapse. NE's precursor is tyrosine, and the enzymes involved in synthesis are tyrosine hydroxylase (TH), dopa decarboxylase (DOD), and dopamine-β-hydroxylase (DBH). The primary degradating enzyme is mitochondrial monamine oxidase (MAO). NE is stored in vesicles. Once released, transynaptic degradation is initiated by catechol-0-methyltransferase (COMT). Currently four types of adrenergic receptors have been identified, both pre- and postsyaptic. Released NE not degraded by COMT may be taken up by the presynaptic neuron.

Serotonergic Synapse. The precursor of serotonin is tryptophan, and the important synthesizing enzyme is tryptophan hydroxylase (TrH); the degrading enzyme is MAO. Several different types of cell surface receptors are known.

Gabanergic Synapse. GABA is formed in the GABA-shunt pathway of the Krebs cycle. It is formed by the action of glutamic acid decarboxylase (GAD) from glutamate and is metabolized by deamination. Two receptors for GABA have been identifed in the central nervous system.

In the human brain, age differences in neurotransmitters, their synthesizing and degrading enzymes, and receptors are still fragmentary, tentative, and highly incomplete. The levels and activity of neurotransmitters and enzymes decline in many brain regions during normal aging. The respective receptor may or may not respond reciprocally to the neurotransmitter changes by increasing number and/or affin-

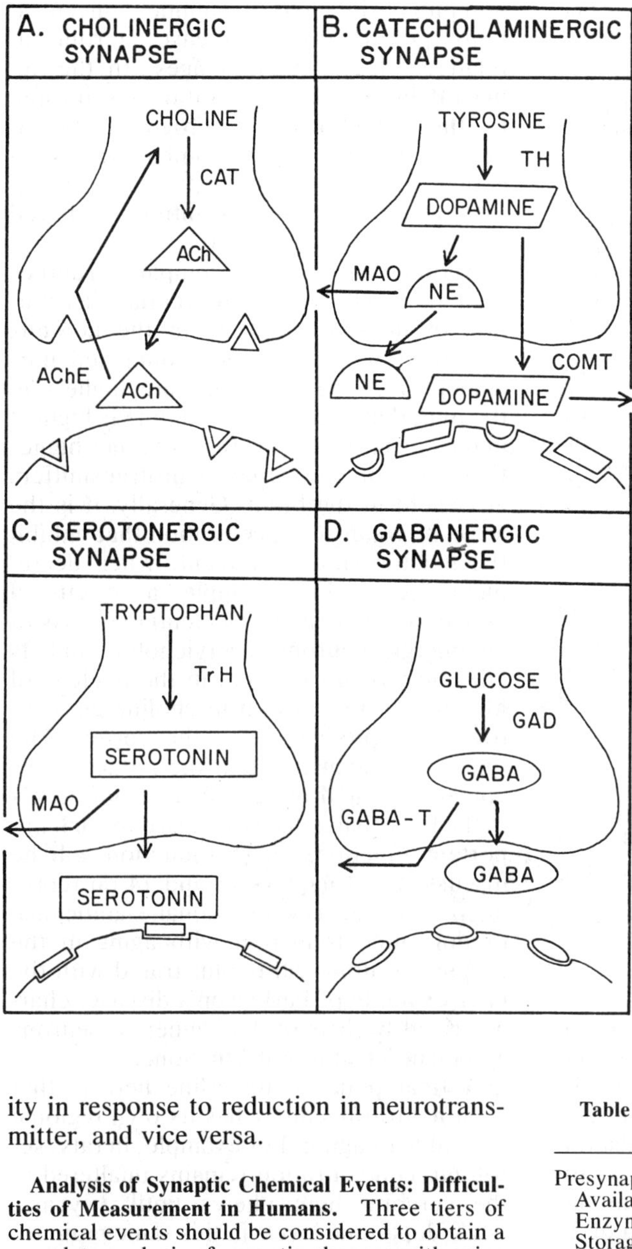

Figure 9–12. *Diagrams of established CNS synapses illustrating presynaptic synthesis, storage and metabolism, synaptic release, and postsynaptic binding.* (Drawing by S. Oklund.)

ity in response to reduction in neurotransmitter, and vice versa.

Analysis of Synaptic Chemical Events: Difficulties of Measurement in Humans. Three tiers of chemical events should be considered to obtain a complete analysis of synaptic changes with aging (Table 9–3): they should include the study of the following:

- presynaptic events, comprising availability of precursors, enzymatic synthesis, and degradation of transmitters, their storage in the cell or their release in the synaptic space, transmitter, reuptake, and ionic regulation;
- transynaptic events, comprising free neurotransmitters and enzymes for their degradation;
- postsynaptic events, comprising receptor binding, enzymatic degradation, ionic regulation, and induction of second messenger.

Table 9–3. MAJOR CHEMICAL EVENTS AT THE SYNAPSE

Presynaptic
Availability of precursors
Enzymatic synthesis and degradation
Storage or release
Transmitter reuptake
Ionic regulation
Transynaptic
Free neurotransmitter
Enzymatic degradation
Postsynaptic
Receptor binding
Enzymatic degradation
Ionic regulation
Second messenger

Unfortunately, in humans, information is limited to the measurement of the neurotransmitters and their metabolites in urine, blood, and cerebrospinal fluid and, more recently, to the use of labeled probes and imaging devices. The majority of these methods show how remote and indirect the sampling is from the involved central nervous system area. An alternative approach is to use pharmacologic agonists and antagonists of the transmitter under study. Under all conditions, it is difficult to control the clinical setting and/or accurately measure subtle changes in physiologic status. The intricacies of the synaptic complex make it currently impossible to develop a coherent description of the changes with aging in synaptic function, except in instances of pathologic events. Clearly, the current situation suggests that much is to be gained by the use of animal models from which to obtain information of the cellular and molecular mechanisms of synaptic function. Even in animals, the information on aging is still scarce and needs to be pursued vigorously.

A large number of neurotransmitters and modulators—as many as 200—are currently under investigation. If we consider that they are continually operative in signal transmission, we can appreciate how continuing demands from the environment and the necessity to maintain homeostasis may lead to disruption, so to speak "desynchronization," of neurotransmitter signals and thereby impairment of the function of the nervous system.

NEUROTRANSMITTER IMBALANCE

Neurotransmitter imbalance in old age may result from relatively minor, but consistent, changes in several neurotransmitters. The concentrations of serotonin, norepinephrine, and dopamine were measured in discrete brain regions of the rat brain from birth until 3 years of age, quite an old age for the rat with a median lifespan of 24 months (Timiras *et al.*, 1982, 1983, 1984). We omit here, for brevity, the early age-related changes, despite their significance for development, and compare the 6-month-old adult rat with rats at the old ages of 2 and 3 years. The data for the cerebral hemispheres, the hypothalamus, and the corpus striatum are presented in Figure 9–13. Overall, two major changes emerge: serotonin concentrations remain unchanged until very old age, when they increase, and norepinephrine and dopamine concentrations progressively decrease starting at relatively less advanced ages. In the aging rat brain, then, the ratio of serotonin to the catecholamines progressively increases. For the resulting imbalance to become functionally manifest it is sufficient that only one neurotransmitter be altered rather than an overall shift.

Another aspect of this comparison agrees with the well-known differential distribution of neurotransmitters in the nervous system. For example, serotonin and norepinephrine concentrations are highest in the hypothalamus, and dopamine is highest in the corpus striatum, 10 to 12 times higher than any of the other neurotransmitters anywhere in the brain. Generally, it is the areas of greatest concentration that exhibit the most severe decrement, when decrements occur. For example, as discussed above, in Alzheimer's dementia the loss of cholinergic neurons, acetylcholine and its enzymes, is most severe in the nucleus of Meynert, a region rich in cholinergic neurons with projections to the cortex. The functional significance of the reduced norepinephrine and increased serotonin levels in the hypothalamus with regard to such important functions as reproduction will be discussed in Chapters 13 and 14 on reproductive aging. The functional significance of dopamine reduction with aging in the corpus striatum will be illustrated with the later example of Parkinson's disease, characterized by loss of dopaminergic neurons and disorder of motor function.

A final point to underline here is that each neurotransmitter has its own regional timetable of aging. For example, in rats, serotonin concentration remains unaltered in the cerebral hemispheres until 3 years, while dopamine levels in this same brain region are reduced at 1 year of age (Timiras *et al.*, 1984). It is this differential rate of aging that may be responsible for creating an early neurotransmitter imbalance, well before significant decrements in each transmitter can be detected.

A detailed analysis of the cholinergic system in the nucleus of Meynert—one of the brain areas preferentially affected in SDAT—shows a marked decrease in presynaptic choline acetyltransferase activity

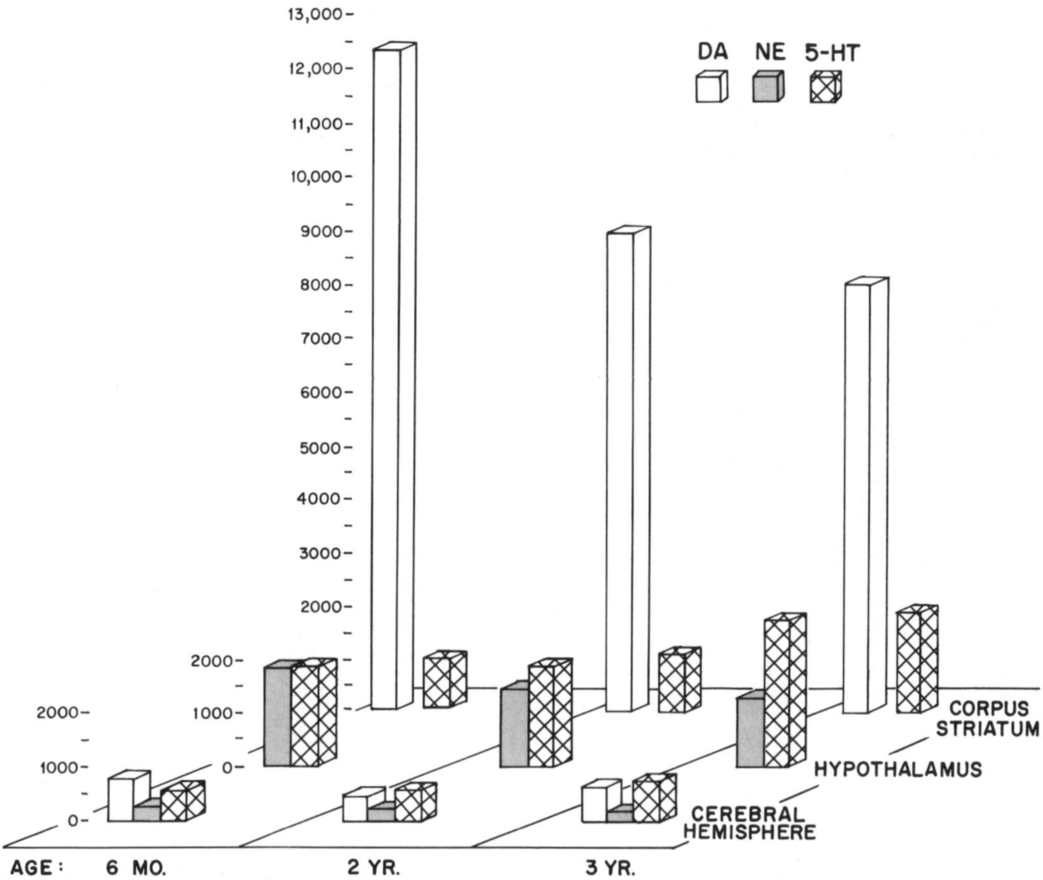

Figure 9–13. *Regional neurotransmitter changes with aging.*

Dopamine (DA), norepinephrine (NE), and serotonin (5-HT) have different patterns of aging in different brain areas. While little change occurs with aging in any of the neurotransmitters in the cerebral hemispheres, norepinephrine in the hypothalamus and dopamine in the corpus striatum decrease and serotonin increases.

and in the number of presynaptic receptors, but no change in the number of postsynaptic receptors (Figure 9–14). The presynaptic receptors, decreased in number with aging, normally function to regulate the release of acetylcholine in the presynaptic neuron. The postsynaptic receptors, which remain unchanged with aging, normally facilitate excitation of the postsynaptic neuron (Coyle, 1983).

From these studies, it appears that, in Alzheimer's patients, the lesion is primarily presynaptic (Nordberg *et al.*, 1982). These experiments suggest new agents for treatment. Administration of the acetylcholine precursor, choline or lecithin, has proven disappointing, as have the acetylcholinestrase inhibitors that act as the receptor. It is possible that agonists that enhance postsynaptic excitation may be effective, as well as antagonists for presynaptic receptors, which would prevent acetylcholine from inhibiting its own release, that is, disrupt its own negative feedback.

Although these results illustrate a pathologic condition rather than normal aging, they suggest that involvement at the synapse may occur at different levels; interventions, likewise, may be operative at different levels. Failure of a treatment at one level in the system does not preclude the success of intervention at another.

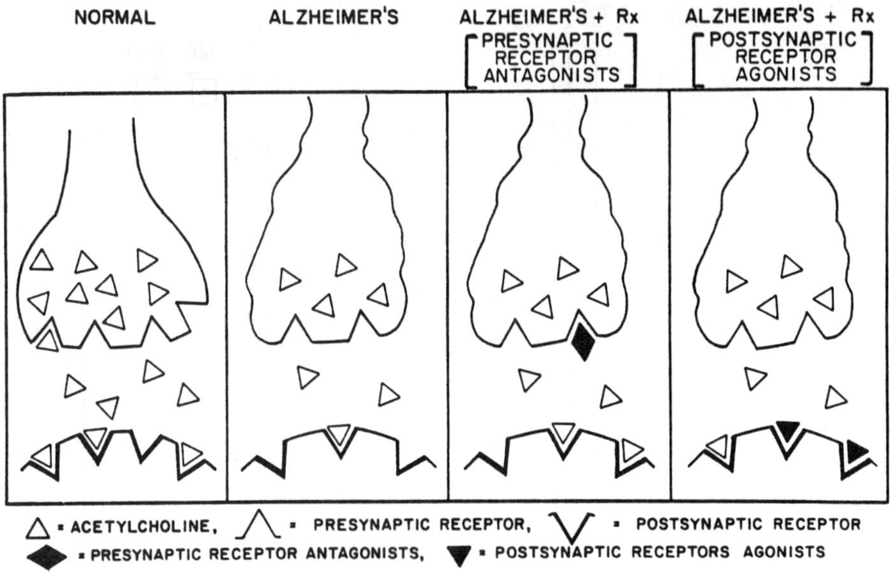

Figure 9–14. *Cholinergic synaptic changes with disease (SDAT), and treatment with presynaptic receptor antagonist or postsynaptic receptor agonist.*

Reduction in synthesis and release of ACh can be ameliorated by drugs that either prevent presynaptic re-uptake, provide more acetylcholine at synapse, or bind to and stimulate postsynaptic receptors. (Drawing by S. Oklund.)

AGING OF DOPAMINERGIC SYSTEMS AND PARKINSON'S DISEASE

Another system that undergoes changes with normal aging and with aging-associated diseases is the dopaminergic system. Dopamine, once considered an intermediary in the formation of norepinephrine, is now recognized as a distinct neurotransmitter. It is present throughout the brain, but its levels vary significantly from region to region. Currently four major dopaminergic pathways are recognized; the most prominent originates in the substantia nigra and extends to the corpus striatum (including the caudate nucleus and putamen), both structures of the so-called extrapyramidal system; the other dopaminergic pathways involve the limbic system, the hypothalamus, and the cortex (Table 9–4).

Table 9–4. DOPAMINERGIC PATHWAYS

Pathway	Function
Substantia nigra to corpus striatum	Regulates control of motor function from cortex
Substantia nigra to nucleus accumbens	Controls locomotion (forward movement)
Limbic system	Regulates emotion, behavior (sexual and aggressive)
Hypothalamus	Regulates endocrine releasing and inhibiting hormones
Neocortex	Regulates locomotor activity

Major Dopaminergic Pathways. The nigral-striatal pathway participates in central control of motor functions. Dopamine released at the caudate nucleus inhibits the stimulatory (cholinergic? glutaminergic?) input from the motor cortex. In the caudate, a balance is established between the inhibitory and excitatory control of motor activity. A deficit of dopamine results in rigor and tremor, whereas an increase of dopamine or a decrease of the excitatory input results in writhing movements, as in chorea. Similar to the striatum and also involved in motor control is the nucleus accumbens in the septal region, which controls locomotion (particularly forward movement). Within the limbic system other dopaminergic fibers synapse and mediate emotionality, sexual and aggressive behavior, and some neuroendocrine regulation. In the hypothalamus, a rich dopaminergic network regulates various endocrine releasing and inhibitory hormones. This dopaminergic activity will be discussed when the endocrine system is presented.

A less well-developed neocortical system is apparently activated by stress. Lesions of the sys-

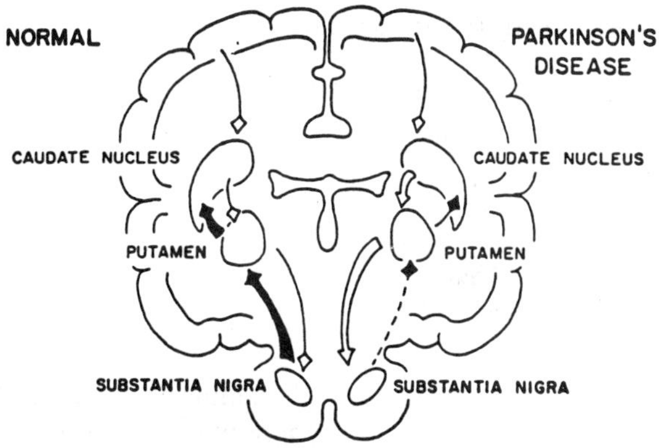

Figure 9–15. *Dopaminergic nigral-striatal pathway in the normal (*left dark arrow*) and in Parkinsonism (*right dashed line*).*

In Parkinsonism, dopaminergic neurons of the substantia nigra are lost, reducing dopamine (*right-dashed line*) to putamen-caudate (striatum) and subsequent control of cortical stimulatory effects. Increased excitatory transmission to extrapyramidal system (broad open arrow) is associated with tremor and rigor. (Drawing by S. Oklund).

tem induce locomotor hyperactivity and inability to suppress behavioral "stereotypic responses." These responses can be blocked by drugs that act as dopamine inhibitors. Uncontrolled stimulation of dopamine receptors would have, on the one hand, a euphoric action but, on the other hand, a psychotic action, perhaps involved in manic and schizophrenic syndromes.

With normal aging, dopamine content decreases, particularly in the corpus striatum, probably as a consequence of the loss of dopaminergic neurons (Figure 9–15). This decrease could explain some of the motor disorders of the elderly, such as the mincing gait and the tremors (see also Chapter 10). When these alterations become more pronounced and are associated with other, progressively more severe motor decrements and other neurologic and clinical manifestations, they are categorized as part of Parkinson's disease or parkinsonism (Haldick-Smith, 1985). This disorder involves rigidity, tremor, and akinesia (or loss of motor function). It is largely a progressive disease of the elderly; about 60 percent of those affected are age 70 or above. In parkinsonism, the dopaminergic neurons projecting to the caudate nucleus and putamen degenerate owing to reduced stimulation from the damaged substantia nigra. This damage is characterized by loss of neurons (perhaps due to the presence of free radicals, discussed in Chapter 7), gliosis, and the presence of specific inclusions, the so-called Lewy bodies (i.e., hyaline inclusions in neurons) (Figure 9–16) (Forno, 1982; Goldman *et al.,* 1983). Biochemical analysis shows a definite loss of dopamine in these regions.

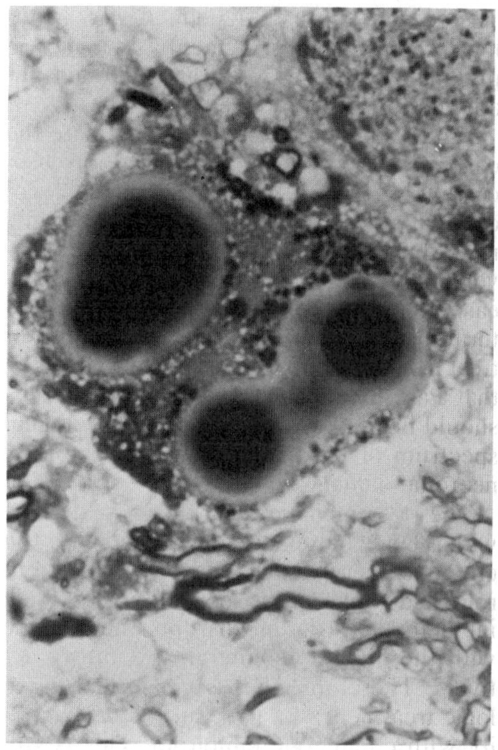

Figure 9–16. *Lewy bodies, intraneuronal cytoplasmic inclusions.*

The dense core is composed of apparently random, tightly packed aggregations of filaments, vesicular profiles, and poorly resolved granular material containing neurofilament antigens. These bodies are found in substantia nigra as well as in other CNS regions (Courtesy of Dr. L. S. Forno).

Table 9–5. DOPAMINE REPLACEMENT TECHNIQUES

Substantia nigra → Caudate
↑
Brain

Administration L-Dopa → Circulation L-Dopa → L-Dopa/dopamine

Brain
↑
Transplanted adrenal medullary tissue

Lewy bodies may be found in normal aging, but their incidence is much greater not only in Parkinson's but also in SDAT patients (Boller, 1985). There is an overlap in pathology between Parkinson's and Alzheimer's diseases (Goldman *et al.*, 1983). The prevalence of Alzheimer-type histologic changes and of dementia is higher in parkinsonians than in an age-matched unaffected population (Chen and Yase, 1985).

While motor abnormalities dominate the clinical picture of Parkinson's disease, current replacement therapy with levodihydroxyphenylalanine (L-Dopa), permits more patients to live long enough to develop more advanced features of the disease, that is loss of memory, dementia, postural instability, which are very difficult to treat (Lees, 1985). It has been suggested that Parkinson's and Alzheimer's diseases should be viewed as two poles of a clinical spectrum of which the common feature is neuronal damage.

The treatment of Parkinson's disease with L-Dopa has emerged as a model for the effective therapy of aging-associated neurologic disorders. The loss of dopaminergic input to the striatum disrupts the balance with the mainly cholinergic excitatory activity. Therefore, the original pharmacologic treatment was to reduce neural activity with cholinergic inhibitors. This is still used as an adjunct to replacement therapy with L-Dopa. The relative success of the therapy for parkinsonism is encouraging to pharmacologic intervention in other types of neurologic and psychiatric diseases of old age. Even though the treatment may not provide a "cure," it might ameliorate some of the more disturbing symptoms. Thus, while most of the neurologic and psychiatric diseases of old age may not as yet be "curable," they certainly are "treatable" and must be treated.

In parkinsonism, dopamine replacement is possible by the oral administration of L-Dopa, natural precursor of dopamine (Table 9–5). Unlike dopamine, L-Dopa is capable of passing through the blood-brain barrier. This is a rare instance when the administration of the neurotransmitter precursor is beneficial; however, this is not without its drawbacks. These are neurologic, and general, side effects and there is a gradual loss of effectiveness. The latter is probably due to continuing loss of dopaminergic neurons and reduction of the decarboxylase enzyme, which transforms L-Dopa into dopamine. It is at this late stage of the disease that other treatments such as the administration of bromocryptine, a dopamine agonist, may produce beneficial effects.

Replacement of dopamine has also been accomplished in humans by transplantation of medullary tissue from the adrenal glands to the substantia nigra in the brain. In the few patients who have undergone such transplantation, the individuals' own adrenal tissue was transplanted. However, a heterograft could be envisioned, since the blood-brain barrier protects the brain from invasion by immune cells and, thus, prevents graft rejection. Although the patients with such transplants still require L-Dopa to improve motor function, the dose of L-Dopa is reduced, a sign that the transplanted cells do secrete dopamine.

SMOKING AND PARKINSON'S DISEASE

While smoking is positively associated with a number of common diseases, there are some rarer diseases for which negative association has been noted. One such disease is parkinsonism, which is less common in smokers than nonsmokers according to several epidemiologic studies (Godwin-Austen *et al.,* 1982). The reason for this negative association is unclear; it is interesting to mention that in experimental animals (rats), nicotine, the major tobacco alkoloid, stimulates or increases brain dopamine and serotonin levels (Dominiak *et al.,* 1984). In the search for alternate or improved therapy for Parkinson's disease, a viable therapeutic alternative might be nicotine.

Drug-Induced Parkinson's Disease. A contaminant, 1-methyl-4-phenyl-1,2,3,6-tetrahydropyridine (MPTP), of illegally synthesized heroin acts specifically to induce a motor-deficit syndrome in experimental animals (mice, rabbits, monkeys) similar to Parkinson's disease in humans. In young animals, the syndrome is only incompletely produced, whereas in old animals the neuropathology and behavior of Parkinson's disease are completely reproduced. Older neurons appear more vulnerable to MPTP, either because of lowered ability to recover from toxic damage or because the damage is cumulative with other damage that has occurred over time (Lewin, 1986). A variety of environmental agents and/or stress may be involved in inducing other CNS degenerative diseases, such as senile dementia of the Alzheimer type, in which age is a key factor (see Chapter 10). This MPTP drug model is particularly useful in transplantation studies.

Transplant techniques have been derived from animal studies (Gage *et al.,* 1983, 1984). Basic techniques of neural transplantation have long been within the repertoire of the neuroscientist but only since the 1970s have they been systematically applied to the mammalian CNS. Transplants have shown promise in studying the development of various visual and olfactory centers by transplantation to novel locations in the brain, the reestablishment of endocrine function by fetal transplants into hypothalamic nuclei, and the repair of damaged functions by transplants of homologous fetal tissues in the hippocampus, nigrostriatal system, spinal cord, and autonomic ganglia (Sladek and Gash, 1984). While still a young field, such work has opened a fertile new area of investigation (Harrison, 1985).

METABOLIC CHANGES

In addition to neurotransmitters, other chemical constituents of the central nervous system are known to change with aging. A number of these are listed in Table 9–6.

Table 9–6. POSSIBLE TARGETS OF AGING CHANGES IN THE CENTRAL NERVOUS SYSTEM

Total water	Carbohydrates
Extra- and intracellular spaces	Circulation
Lipids	Energy metabolism
DNA, RNA, and protein	Oxygen uptake and glucose utilization
Amino acids	Blood-brain barrier

From clinical and experimental data, some generalizations can be drawn: changes are specific to discrete regions and structures; they follow differential timetables; and they differ according to the constituent considered. Because of the lack of consistent studies in humans during normal aging, only a few of these constituents will be discussed here. A good model of regional, age, and constituent specificity is presented by some amino acids that act as putative neurotransmitters. For example, of the excitatory amino acids, glutamic acid declines with aging in the cerebral cortex and brainstem of the rat, but not in the cerebellum and spinal cord (Timiras *et al.,* 1973). Glycine and GABA, inhibitory amino acids, increase with age in the cerebral cortex, cerebellum, and brainstem, but remain unchanged in the spinal cord. These observations are supportive of an imbalance among neurotransmitters with aging. Other changes with normal aging include:

- decreased water content of the brain (as of most other organs);
- alterations in extra- and intracellular spaces while electrolyte distribution remains essentially unchanged;
- regional decrease in protein content and synthesis (perhaps related to learning and memory impairments); increase in complexity of RNA molecules; and either an increase (perhaps related to gliosis) or no change in DNA content;
- decreased lipid synthesis, primarily decreased synthesis of membrane phospholipids due to increased variation in the structure of lipid substrates rather than to reduction of synthesizing enzyme activity or concentration of substrates; changes in membrane lipids would alter membrane fluidity and, in turn, nerve conduction and receptor binding;
- circulatory changes characterized by a progressive reduction in cerebral blood flow and a corresponding decrease in oxygen uptake, glucose utilization, and, consequently, energy metabolism.

Several parameters of cerebral energy metabolism such as cerebral blood flow, oxygen consumption, and glucose metabolism (cerebral metabolic rate) have been studied in humans and experimental animals utilizing tracers, autoradiography, computed tomography (CT) scans, positron emission tomography (PET), and magnetic resonance imaging (MRI). In general, changes are not marked and vary with the animal species, the brain area considered, the ambient sensory state, and the health of the subject. In particular, the sensory state (visual, auditory, proprioceptive, and so forth) in normal individuals seems to influence cerebral metabolism. Among the many studies conducted in humans, cerebral energy metabolism declines with age when age-related pathology is also reported; however, in a few studies the decline occurs in the absence of pathology. Studies in aged rats show little decline in energy metabolism, and when it occurs, it is primarily in sensory-related areas. Aged dogs, showing more neuropathologic changes with age, have significant reduction of glucose metabolism, especially in sensory related structures and the frontal and temporal cortices (Duara *et al.*, 1985).

References

Boller, F.: Parkinson's disease and Alzheimer's disease: Are they associated? In Hutton, J. T., and Kenny, A. D. (eds.): *Senile Dementia of the Alzheimer Type*, Neurology and Neurobiology, Vol. 18, Alan R. Liss, New York, **1985.**

Bondareff, W.: Neuropathology of nucleus basalis and locus ceruleus in Alzheimer's disease. In Scheibel, A. B.; Wechsler, A. F.; and Brazier, M. A. B. (eds.): *The Biological Substrates of Alzheimer's Disease*, Academic Press, New York, **1986.**

Brizzee, K. R.: Neuron aging and neuron pathology. In Johnson, H. A. (ed.): *Relations Between Normal Aging and Disease*, Raven Press, New York, **1985.**

Brizzee, K. R.; Cancilla, P. A.; Sherwood, N.; and Timiras, P. S.: The amount and distribution of pigments in neurons and glia of the cerebral cortex. Autofluorescence and ultrastructural studies. *J. Gerontol.*, **24:**127–135, **1969.**

Brizzee, K. R.; Sherwood, N.; and Timiras, P. S.: A comparison of cell populations at various depth levels in cerebral cortex of young adult and aged Long-Evans rats. *J. Gerontol.*, **23:**289–298, **1968.**

Brody, H.: Cell counts in cerebral cortex and brainstem. In Katzman, R.; Terry, R. D.; and Bick, K. L. (eds.): *Alzheimer's Disease: Senile Dementia and Related Disorders*, Aging, Vol. 28, Raven Press, New York, **1978.**

Butcher, L. L., and Woolf, N. J.: Central cholinergic systems: Synopsis of anatomy and overview of physiology. In Scheibel, A. B.; Wechsler, A. F.; and Brazier, M. A. B. (eds.): *The Biological Substrates of Alzheimer's Disease*, Academic Press, New York, **1986.**

Chen, K., and Yase, Y.: Parkinsonism-dementia, neurofibrillary tangles, and trace elements in the Western Pacific. In Hutton, J. T., and Kenny, A. D. (eds.): *Senile Dementia of the Alzheimer Type*, Neurology and Neurobiology, Vol, 18, Alan R. Liss, New York, **1985.**

Cole, G.: Neuropathology of ageing. In Pathy, M. S. J. (ed.): *Principles and Practice of Geriatric Medicine*, John Wiley & Sons, New York, **1985.**

Cotman, C. W., and Holets, V. R.: Structural changes at synapses with age: Plasticity and regeneration. In Finch, C. E., and Schneider, E. L. (eds.): *Handbook of the Biology of Aging*, Van Nostrand Reinhold, New York, **1985.**

Coyle, J. T.: Alzheimer's disease: A disorder of cortical cholinergic innervation. *Science*, **219:**1194–1190, **1983.**

Delabar, J. M.; Goldgaber, D.; Lamour, Y.; Nicole, A.; Huret, J. L.; deGrouchy, J.; Brown, P.; Gajdusek, D. C.; and Sinet, P. M.: Beta amyloid gene duplication in Alzheimer's disease and karyotypically normal Down syndrome, *Science*, **235:**1390–1392, **1987.**

Diamond, M. C.; Johnson, R. E.; and Gold, M. W.: Changes in neuron and glia number in the young adult and ageing rat occipital cortex. *Behav. Biol.*, **20:**409–418, **1977.**

Diamond, M. D.: Aging and environmental influences on the rat forebrain. In Scheibel, A. B.; Wechsler, A. F.; and Brazier, M. A. B. (eds.): *The Biological Substrates of Alzheimer's Disease*, Academic Press, New York, **1986.**

Dominiak, P.; Kees, F.; and Grobecker, H.: Changes in peripheral and central catecholaminergic and serotoninergic neurons of rats after acute and subacute administration of nicotine, *Klin. Wochenschr.*, **62:**76–80, **1984.**

Duara, R.; London, E. D.; and Rapoport, S. I.: Changes in structure and energy metabolism of the aging brain. In Finch, C. E., and Schneider, E. L. (eds.): *Handbook of the Biology of Aging*, Van Nostrand Reinhold, New York, **1985.**

Forno, L. S.: Pathology of Parkinson's disease. In *Movement Disorders*, Neurology 2, Butterworth, London, **1982.**

Gajdusek, D. C.: Chronic dementia caused by small unconventional viruses apparently containing no nucleic acid. In Scheibel, A. B.; Wechsler, A. F.; and Brazier, M. A. B. (eds.): *The Biological Substrates of Alzheimer's Disease*, Academic Press, New York, **1986.**

Gage, F. H.; Dunnett, S. B.; Stenevi, U.; and Bjorklund, A.: Aged rats: Recovery of motor impairments by intrastriatal nigral grafts. *Science*, **221:**996–998, **1983.**

Gage, F. H.; Bjorklund, A.; Stenevi, U.; Dunnett, S. B.; and Kelly, P. A.: Intrahippocampal septal grafts ameliorate learning impairments in aged rats. *Science*, **225:**533–536, **1984.**

Giacobini, E.: Cellular and molecular mechanisms of aging of the nervous system: Toward a unified theory of neuronal aging. In Giacobini, E.; Filogamo, G.; Giacobini, G.; and Vernadakis, A. (eds.): *The Aging Brain: Cellular and Molecular Mechanisms of Aging in the Nervous System*, Aging, Vol. 20, Raven Press, New York, **1982.**

Glenner, G. G., and Wong, C. W.: Alzheimer's disease: Initial report of the purification and characterization of a novel cerebrovascular amyloid protein. *Biochem. Biophys. Res. Commun.*, **120:**885–890, **1984a.**

Glenner, G. G., and Wong, C. W.: Alzheimer's disease and Down's syndrome: Sharing of a unique cerebrovascular amyloid protein. *Biochem. Biophys. Res. Commun.*, **122:**1131–1135, **1984b.**

Goldman, J. E.; Yew, S.; Chiu, F. C.; and Peress, N. S.: Lewy bodies of Parkinson's disease contain neurofilament antigens. *Science*, **221:**1082–1086, **1983.**

Godwin-Austen, R. B.; Lee, P. N.; Marmot, M. G.; and Stern, G. M.: Smoking and Parkinson's disease. *J. Neurol. Neurosurg. Psychiatry*, **45:**557–581, **1982.**

Haldick-Smith, M.: Parkinson's disease. In Pathy, M. S. J. (ed.): *Principles and Practice of Geriatric Medicine*, John Wiley & Sons, New York, **1985.**

Harrison, D. E.: Cell and tissue transplantation: A means of studying the aging process. In Finch, C. E., and Schneider, E. L. (eds.) *Handbook of the Biology of Aging*, Van Nostrand Reinhold, New York, **1985.**

Haug, H.: Are neurons of the human cerebral cortex really lost during aging? A morphometric examination. In Traber, Y., and Gispen, W. H. (eds.): *Senile Dementia of the Alzheimer's Type. Early Diagnosis, Neuropathology and Animal Models*, Springer-Verlag, New York, **1985.**

Iqbal, K.; Grundke-Iqbal, I.; Merz, P. A.; and Wisniewski, H. M.: Age-associated neurofibrillary changes. In Giacobini, E.; Filogamo, G.; Giacobini, G.; and Vernadakis, A. (eds.): *The Aging Brain: Cellular and Molecular Mechanisms of Aging in the Nervous System*, Aging, Vol. 20, Raven Press, New York, **1982.**

Jacobs, R. W., and Butcher, L. L.: Pathology of the basal forebrain in Alzheimer's disease and other dementias. In Scheibel, A. B.; Wechsler, A. F.; and Brazier, M. A. B. (eds.): *The Biological Substrates of Alzheimer's Disease*, Academic Press, New York, **1986.**

Kang, J.; Lemaire, H. G.; Unterbeck, A.; Salbaum, J. M.; Masters, C. L.; Grzeschik, K. H.; Multhaup, G.; Beyreuther, K.; and Muller-Hill, B.: The precursor of Alzheimer's disease amyloid A4 protein resembles a cell-surface receptor, *Nature*, **325:**733–736, **1987.**

Lees, A. J.: Cognitive deficits in Parkinson's disease. In Traver, J., and Gispen, W. H. (eds.): *Senile Dementia of the Alzheimer's Type. Early Diagnosis, Neuropathology and Animal Models*, Springer-Verlag, New York, **1985.**

Lewin, R.: Age factors loom in Parkinson research, *Science*, **234:**1200–1201, **1987.**

Masters, C. L.; Multhaup, G.; Simms, G.; Pottgieser, J.; Martins, R. N.; and Beyreuther, K.: Neuronal origin of a cerebral amyloid: Neurofibrillary tangles of Alzheimer's disease contain the same protein as the amyloid of plaque cores and blood vessels. *EMBO J.*, **4:**2757–2763, **1985.**

Mervis, R.: Cytomorphological alterations in the aging animal brain with emphasis on Golgi studies. In Johnson, J. E. (ed.): *Aging and Cell Structure*, Plenum Press, New York, **1981.**

Mortimer, J. A., and Hutton, J. T.: Epidemiology and etiology of Alzheimer's disease. In Hutton, J. T., and Kenny, A. D. (eds.): *Senile Dementia of the Alzheimer Type*, Neurology and Neurobiology, Vol. 18, Alan R. Liss, New York, **1985.**

Nandy, K.; Baste, C.; and Schneider, F. H.: Further studies on the effects of centrophenoxine on lipofuscin pigment in neuroblastoma cells in culture: An electron microscopic study. *Exp. Gerontol.*, **13:**311–322, **1978.**

Nordberg, A.; Adolfsson, R.; Marcusson, J.; and Winblad, B.: Cholinergic receptors in the hippocampus in normal aging and dementia of Alzheimer type. In Giacobini, E.; Filogamo, G.; Giacobini, G.; and Vernadakis, A. (eds.): *The Aging Brain: Cellular and Molecular Mechanisms of Aging in the Nervous System*, Aging, Vol. 20, Raven Press, New York, **1982.**

Pearson, R. C. A.; Esiri, M. M.; Hiorns, R. W.; Wilcock, G. K.; and Powell, T. S.: Anatomical correlates of the distribution of the pathological change in the neocortex in Alzheimer's disease. *Proc. Natl. Acad. Sci. USA*, **82:**4531–4534, **1985.**

Prusiner, S. B.: Some speculations about prions, amyloid and Alzheimer's disease. *N. Engl. J. Med.*, **310:**661–663, **1984.**

Rogers, J., and Bloom, F. E.: Neurotransmitter metabolism and function in the aging central nervous system. In Finch, C. E., and Schneider, E. L. (eds.): *Handbook of the Biology of Aging*, Van Nostrand Reinhold, New York, **1985.**

Samorajski, T., and Persson, K.: Neurochemistry of ageing. In Pathy, M. S. J. (ed.): *Principles and Practice of Geriatric Medicine*, John Wiley & Sons, New York, **1985.**

Scheibel, A. B., and Tomiyasu, U.: Dendritic sprouting in Alzheimer presenile dementia, *Exp. Neurol.*, **60:**1–8, **1978.**

Scheibel, M. E.; Lindsay, R. D.; Tomiyasu, U.; and Scheibel, A. B.: Progressive dendritic changes in aging human cortex, *Exp. Neurol.*, **47:**392–403, **1975.**

Sladek, J. R., and Gash, D. M. (eds.): *Neural Transplants: Development and Function*, Plenum Press, New York, **1984.**

Tanzi, R. E.; Gusella, J. F.; Watkins, P. C.; Bruns, G. A. P.; St. George-Hyslop *et al.*: Amyloid β protein gene: cDNA, mRNA distribution, and genetic linkage near the Alzheimer locus, *Science*, **235:**880–884, **1987.**

Terry, R. D.: The fine structure of neurofibrillary tangles in Alzheimer's disease, *J. Neuropathol. Exp. Neurol.*, **22:**269–292, **1963.**

Terry, R. D.: Brain disease in aging especially in senile dementia. In Terry, R. D.; Bolis, C. L.; and Toffano, G. (eds.): *Neural Aging and Its Implications in Human Neurological Pathology*, Aging, Vol. 18, Raven Press, New York, **1982.**

Timiras, P. S.; Cole, G.; Croteau, M.; Hudson, D. B.; Miller, C.; and Segall, P. E.: Changes in brain serotonin with aging and modification through precursor availability. In Agnoli, A.; Crepaldi, G.; Spano, P. F.; and Trabucci, M. (eds.): *Aging Brain and Ergot Alkaloids*, Aging, Vol. 20, Raven Press, New York, **1983.**

Timiras, P. S.; Hudson, D. B.; and Miller, C.: Developing and aging brain serotonergic systems. In Giacobini, E.; Filogamo, G.; Giacobini, G.; and Vernadakis, A. (eds.): *The Aging Brain: Cellular and Molecular Mechanisms of Aging in the Nervous System*, Aging, Vol. 20, Raven Press, New York, **1982.**

Timiras, P. S.; Hudson, D. B.; and Oklund, S.: Changes in central nervous system free amino acids with development and aging, *Prog. Brain Res.*, **40:**267–275, **1973.**

Timiras, P. S.; Hudson, D. B.; and Segall, P. E.: Lifetime brain serotonin: Regional effects of age and precursor availability, *Neurobiol. Aging*, **5:**235–242, **1984.**

Vernadakis, A.: The aging brain. In Geokas, M. C. (ed.): *Symposium on the Aging Process*, Clinics in Geriatric Medicine, Vol. 1, W. B. Saunders, Philadelphia, **1985.**

Whitehouse, P.; Price, D.; Struble, R.; Clark, A.; Coyle, L.; and Delong, M.: Alzheimer's disease and senile dementia: Loss of neurons in the basal forebrain, *Science*, **215:**1237–1239, **1982.**

Will, B. E.; Schmitt, P.; and Dalrymple-Alford, J. D. (eds.): *Brain Plasticity, Learning and Memory*, Plenum Press, New York, **1985.**

Wilcox, H. H.: Structural changes in the nervous system related to the process of aging. In Birren, J. E.; Inus, H. A.; and Windle, W. F. (eds.): *The Process of Aging in the Nervous System*, Charles C Thomas, Springfield, IL, **1959.**

CHAPTER

10 AGING OF THE NERVOUS SYSTEM

Functional Changes

The functional integrity of the nervous system is well maintained in most elderly persons despite the morphologic and biochemical changes described in the previous chapter. This ability to conserve neurologic and intellectual competence into old age bears witness to the redundancy present in the system and possibly foretells successful compensation.

We must recognize, however, that in a large proportion of the elderly, especially the very old, the boundaries between health and disease become less precise as the incidence of neurologic and mental impairment increases. Thus, CNS disorders are the most common causes of disability in the aged, producing nearly half the disability in individuals beyond the age of 65 and causing more than 90 percent of the cases of total dependency. Impaired memory, intellect, strength, sensation, balance, and coordination are some of the most frequent disabilities of old age.

One characteristic of the aging nervous system that emerged from the discussion in the previous chapter is the variable vulnerability or resistance of discrete structures or biochemical pathways to the aging process. Similarly, functions are differentially affected. In this chapter we have selected examples from three major functional areas of the nervous system: for motor function, gait and balance; for cognitive function, memory; and for electrical activity, sleep. Disruption of these functions can lead to mental deficits, as occurs in the so-called dementias characterized by global loss of cognitive function associated with neurologic deficits and vascular disturbances. The prevalence of dementia is increasing rapidly. Currently the fourth leading cause of death in the 75-to-84-year age group, dementia has been called "the disease of the century"; it has been predicted that it will be "the first killer of the 21st century." Therefore, a brief discussion of this cataclysmic disorder is included.

MOTOR CHANGES: GAIT AND BALANCE

In recent years with increase in the number of elderly and the lengthening of the average lifespan, altered motor function, involving pyramidal and extrapyramidal systems, has become more frequent. These alterations in motor function extend from borderline, barely perceptible and disabling, to overt manifestations of motor dysfunction with severe disability. Disorders of motility and gait in the aged are second only to impaired mental function as the most frequent accompaniments of the aging process.

Control of Posture and Movement. Skilled movements are regulated by nerve fibers that originate in the motor cortex and form the "pyramids" in the medulla, hence the term *pyramidal tracts*. Gross movements and posture are regulated by CNS areas (e.g., basal ganglia) other than those connected with the pyramidal tracts, hence, by exclusion, the term *extrapyramidal system*. Coordination, adjustment, and smoothing of movements are regulated by the *cerebellum,* which receives impulses from several sensory receptors. Impulses from all these brain structures ultimately determine the pattern and rate of discharge of the *spinal motor neurons* and neurons in motor nuclei of *cranial nerves,* thereby controlling somatic motor activity.

With aging, skilled motor movements are slowed, and gross movements, particularly those related to maintenance of posture and gait, are altered. These alterations affect the speed of movement, which may be accelerated (as in hyperkinesias, tremors, tics) or slowed (as in hypokynesias, akinesia), or the contraction of specific muscles, resulting in abnormal movements (as in myoclonus, chorea, ballism, athetosis) or in abnormal posture (as in dystonias). Both alterations of movement and posture lead to imbalance and this to a higher incidence of falls, one of the most frequent and life-threatening accidents of old age.

With advancing age, the normal adult gait changes to a hesitant, broad-based, small-stepped gait with many of the characteristics of early parkinsonism (Chapter 9), often including stooped posture, diminished arm swinging, and turns performed *en bloc*. Rarely do individuals over the age of 75 to 80 walk without the stigmata of age (Klawans and Tanner, 1984). Indeed, it is the ability to walk without serious limitations or falling that distinguishes a normal aged gait from dysfunction. Alterations of locomotion are due to CNS impairment since the peripheral changes seen in normal aging—minor decreases in nerve conduction velocity, decrease in muscle mass, increased muscle tone (rigidity)—are insufficient to account for the disability.

Despite their frequency, relatively little is known of the mechanisms responsible for the changes with aging in neurologic and psychologic regulation of gait and balance. Yet, much can be learned about the overall physiologic competence of the aging individual by observing gait and balance; indeed, disturbances of gait and repeated falls, in the very old, particularly, are signs of serious ill health.

Measurements of gait characteristics, such as speed and length of stride, present no technical difficulty and can provide useful information on the degree of competence or damage of the central and peripheral nervous systems. Several pyramidal and extrapyramidal structures, including visual, vestibular, and proprioceptive sensors, impart finely graded instructions to the muscles of the neck, trunk, and limbs for maintenance of normal posture, balance, and gait. Alteration in any of these functions will reflect impairment and failure of integration of one or more of the CNS structures involved. Further, disturbances of the psychologic and mental status as well as the conditions of the skeleton and joints and orthopedic disorders may also be revealed by the degree of competence or impairment of gait and balance (Isaacs, 1985).

Normal walking is with head erect (without spinal curvature), arms swinging reciprocally (without grabbing at furniture), regular stepping (without stagger or stumbling movements), and feet clearing the ground at each step. Several of these characteristics are altered with aging: velocity and step length are decreased, step-length variability and symmetry and double support ratio (indicative of impaired stability) are increased, while step frequency is unaltered. Such changes may reveal other aspects of aging, for example, sex differences, with females always performing less well than males on all gait parameters, impaired vision or illumination, and cognitive loss with demented patients showing significant decrements in all gait parameters. Gait changes may be useful in providing clinical insight, for example; gait asymmetry gives a clue to hemiplegia or arthritis; alterations of shoulder movements in walking may be a clue to parkinsonism; increase in stride width relates to cerebellar disease and arthritis; trunk flexion suggests unstable balance due to alterations in visual, vestibular, and proprioceptive controls (Barbeau, 1973).

As for gait, balance can be studied clinically by simple measurements such as observation of sway, sweep, and stagger when rising from a chair, standing, walking, or turning. In elderly subjects, obstacles to proper balance include the fear of falling and pain or limitation of joint movement. Disturbances in balance are reflected in the gait pattern. The main adaptation to a balance disorder is the shortening of step length accompanied by slowing of gait and increase in double support ratio. This pattern is particularly noticeable in people who have fallen repeatedly, and, indeed, it is called "postfall syndrome" or "3F syndrome" (fear of further falling). The immediate consequence of alterations in balance is an increased frequency of falls (Overstall, 1985).

Falls are one of the commonest problems of old age, occurring most often indoors in the immediate environment of the house. Trips and accidents account for 45 percent of falls, but the prevalence of this type of fall decreases with aging, probably as a reflection of the reduced mobility of the very old. Other falls may occur without any external cause and may be due to alterations in peripheral (ocular, vestibular, and proprioceptive) and central (cerebellar and cortical) coordination (Drachman, 1979).

There is considserable overall reserve in the locomotor system, and loss of one of the sources of control of postural information or maintenance may be of little consequence. However, in elderly individuals impairment at several functional levels may combine to deplete this reserve. It is not difficult to understand why a fall is the consequence of the simultaneous loss of a number of factors, both neurologic (e.g., extrapyramidal damage) and extraneurologic (drugs, cardiovascular, psychologic). As our methods for the measurement of gait and balance become more sophisticated and quantitative, close examination of these two functions becomes increasingly more important in providing a comprehensive picture of the physiologic or pathologic condition of the old individual. At the same time, improvements of these two functions, although not vital for survival, will considerably increase the well-being and overall health of the elderly.

MEMORY AND AGING

Adaptation to life events occurs over the lifetime. Environmental adjustments modify the nervous system, and as a result, animals can learn and remember. This ability, which can be viewed as an expression of neural plasticity, is altered with aging. Indeed, impairment of memory of varying severity, from benign forgetfulness to memory loss, seems to be a frequent, even regular, manifestation of old age.

THE MECHANISMS OF MEMORY ACQUISITION, RETENTION, AND RECALL are little understood and still controversial. The original idea that information storage is widely and equally distributed throughout large brain regions has been displaced by the view that it is localized in specific areas of the brain. These concepts should not be exclusive; rather memory can be viewed as localized, with discrete brain areas involved in specific aspects of short-term memory, and as widespread, with many areas articulating to form (long-term) memory. Among the prime areas involved are the cerebellum, the limbic system (amygdala and hippocampus), the thalamus, and the cerebral cortex (Thompson, 1986; Squire, 1986). While neurotransmission is undoubtedly involved in memory and learning processes, the identification of which neurotransmitter or which combination of neurotransmitters is responsible for learning and memory continues to elude us. The view of localized discrete brain areas evokes the concept of cell groups producing specific neurotransmitters involved in the memory process. In a model using radioactive tracers (^{14}C-labeled 2-deoxyglucose), increased metabolic activity occurred in response to the presentation of familiar (visual) cues; the distribution of the metabolic changes is compatible with the view of memory localization to specific brain areas, but the large number of neurons involved suggests that most "plastic" (i.e., metabolically responsive) cells participate in multiple memories (John *et al.*, 1986). Indeed, memory is a complex process, difficult to interpret. It must involve the ability to sense an object (visually, audibly, tactily, by smell, etc.) or event, or to formulate a thought, retain this information, and recall it at will. Thus, memory refers to the retention of acquired information regarding specific events, thoughts, and places.

The engram, that is the collection of neural changes representing memory, has been identified differently by various investigators; similarly, different types of memory have been categorized distinguishing between short-term and long-term memory. In *sensory memory,* an image is recorded very briefly, less than a second; the information may pass on to *short-term memory,* which endures for several minutes, then to an *intermediate memory* or labile storage, which lasts minutes to hours, and finally, to *long-term memory,* which needs several hours to days to develop but which lasts a lifetime.

With aging, impairment of memory is sporadic, not specifically related to how long information was retained or to the type of cognitive skills required. Aged normal subjects do not perform as well as young normals on many tasks with a significant memory component. Memory loss in the elderly appears to be restricted to memory for recent events, leaving immediate and remote memory essentially intact. The demented patient does have progressive, severe, memory impairment. Memory loss for recent events is the first severe problem encountered. This is followed by language dysfunction, and at this point, memory function is difficult to assess. It has been hypothesized that deficits in dementia occur in an order that is approximately the reverse of childhood developmental stages. As functional stages merge and overlap at certain points of human development, the broader lines between the various stages of dementia are subtle rather than abrupt. Clearly, severely affected patients have lost the ability to learn and to form new memories.

Of the many models purported to explain memory, one proposes three distinct temporal phases. A first phase, representing short-term memory, may result from ionic changes at the membrane such as increased potassium conductance and increased calcium flux. The second, intermediate phase depends on the activity of membrane-bound enzymes involved in synaptic function such as Na^+K^+-ATPase, and the third phase, or long-term memory, is dependent on new protein synthesis.

Several neurotransmitters have also been implicated in memory processes where they would modulate and facilitate information acquisition and retention. First to be considered were the catecholamines, serotonin, and, particularly, acetylcholine, in the hippocampus. A "cholinergic hypothesis" states that acetylcholine, a major transmitter in the hippocampus, the entorhinal area, and the nucleus of Meynert (all associated with memory), has a key role in the mechanism of memory. Indeed, in Alzheimer's dementia, where memory loss is one of the signs of disease, many neurons are lost. However, neither increase in precursor nor decrease in activity of synthesizing (choline acetytransferase) or metabolizing (acetylcholinesterase) enzymes has normalized impaired memory due to old age, disease, drugs, or experimental lesions. These failures to resolve the impairment have dampened, but not destroyed, interest in acetylcholine. Early intervention in the disease with an acetylcholinesterase inhibitor and careful monitoring of blood levels thereof have shown some promising signs of slight improvement in Alzheimer's dementia (Summers *et al.*, 1986; Davis and Mohs, 1986). Other agents continue to be studied, for example, the use of acetylcholine agonists (see Chapter 9) which bind to postsynaptic receptors.

As with the successful transplantation of fetal dopaminergic neurons into the neostriatum of aged rats with impaired motor coordination (Chapter 9), fetal septal tissue (rich in cholinergic neurons) has been transplanted to the hippocampus, where it remains viable, secretes acetylcholine, and has improved learning in these aged rats (Arendash *et al.*, 1985; Geddes *et al.*, 1985). Such success as has been attained with transplanted neural tissue is certainly encouraging and stimulates the extension of these studies to primates. If future studies provide favorable results, neural transplants to treat SDAT would appear to be a viable option.

Currently, several neuropeptides are being considered in memory processes, the most-studied candidates are vasopressin and cholecystokinin. Vasopressin, a hypothalamic hormone stored in the posterior pituitary, is claimed to facilitate both memory consolidation and retrieval. This action could be mediated through release of catecholamines—a presynaptic action—or through interference with the postsynaptic receptors. Cholecystokinin, an intestinal peptide found also in the brain, seems to possess memory-retaining properties in experimental animals and may act in synergy with catecholamines. While some memory improvement has been reported after administration of these neuropeptides in animals, including humans, the efficacy of neuropeptides in preventing or reducing memory loss in the elderly is controversial.

CHANGES OF SLEEP AND WAKEFULNESS

Alterations of several cyclic functions with aging have been ascribed to changes in neurotransmitter signals. In endocrine function, the cessation of menstrual cycles at menopause (see Chapter 13) exemplifies such an alteration. A prime example of a neural cyclic function is the sleep/wakefulness cycle, which also undergoes characteristic changes with aging. A precise delineation of sleeping changes intrinsic to normal aging is still lacking. However, the incidence of sleep-related abnormalities, designated as pathologic in the young, become increasingly prevalent in old age (Feinberg, 1976). Indeed, it may be suggested that a high percentage of the elderly could benefit from the diagnosis and treatment of sleeping/waking disorders and, vice versa, understanding of the aging changes may help to clarify the pathogenesis of sleep disorders in the young.

As we all know, sleep is a regular and, usually, necessary phenomenon of our daily lives. Yet, its mechanisms and purpose still elude us. Several interpretations of sleep function and characteristics have been suggested, but none has been proven. To quote only the most current:

- sleep is a quiescent period during which the body recovers from the strains of the waking hours, and/or
- sleep represents a descent to a lower level of consciousness characterized by dreaming, and/or
- sleep depends on a specific stage—the rapid-eye-movement or REM sleep—and a selected sleep-wakefulness rhythmicity (as a type of biologic clock) to ensure homeostasis.

Other well-recognized characteristics of sleep include: (1) clear relationship of sleep to brain electrical activity, the so-called electroencephalogram or EEG, and association with whole-body visceral manifestations, such as changes in heart rate, respiration, basal metabolic rate, endocrine function, and so forth; (2) sleep patterns change with age, that is, during growth and development as well as aging; (3) sleep patterns may be modified by the administration of psychotropic drugs and by neuropsychiatric disorders; (4) there are two kinds of sleep: REM sleep, with an EEG resembling the alert, awake state, and a four-phase non-REM, slow-wave (SW) sleep.

EEG Changes with Aging. The EEG represents the background electrical activity of the brain, with a particular rhythm represented by characteristic wave patterns with different frequencies: alpha, 8 to 12 waves/sec; beta, 18 to 30/sec; theta, 4 to 7/sec; delta, less than 4 waves/sec. The amplitude is highest in the alpha waves. The alpha rhythm, eyes closed and mind at rest, slows with normal aging throughout the brain as well as focally (temporal region). The beta activity increases in aged persons (Muller and Schwartz, 1978; Obrist, 1963). With respect to evoked potential, the data suggest latency is prolonged after stimulation through a variety of sensory modalities, perhaps due to decreased conduction velocity (Dorfman and Bosley, 1979) or a change in the sense organ itself (see Chapter 11). These spontaneous and evoked potential alterations are aggravated in SDAT (Shaw and Cant, 1980; Katz and Horowitz, 1982; Syndulko *et al.*, 1982; Coben *et al.*, 1983a,b).

When a person falls asleep, he/she goes from stage 0, quiet wakefulness, to stage 1 (the first of four stages of slow-wave sleep) characterized by low-voltage, mixed-frequency EEG; stage 2, which follows, is characterized by the appearance of the so-called "sleep spindles"; in stages 3 and 4 electrical activity is characterized by a relative predominance (stage 3: 20 to 50 percent; stage 4: >50 percent) of high-amplitude, slow-frequency activity. These last two stages represent the period of deepest sleep and, possibly, of physiologic recuperation. Muscular electrical activity is low and ocular activity is generally quiescent.

By contrast, REM sleep is characterized by an active brain wave pattern similar to the EEG of the waking brain. Rapid, binocularly synchronous eye movements occur (hence the name). Tonic muscular activity is absent and spinal reflexes cannot be elicited.

In the normal adult, the total amount of sleep per day is approximately 7 hours, of which 23 percent is spent in REM sleep and 57 percent in stage 2 sleep. Of the other stages, stage 1 accounts for 7 percent and stages 3 and 4 for about 13 percent (Figure 10–1). Generally, the episodes of REM sleep occur at about 90-minute intervals. They lengthen as the night progresses and they are the stage wherein dreaming occurs.

With aging, sleep patterns undergo significant changes leading to deterioration of circadian organization (Figure 10–1). While the total amount of sleeping time changes little, sleep is interrupted and is distributed more widely over the 24-hour period in short naps (Kales *et al.*, 1967; Miles and Dement, 1980; Prinz *et al.*, 1982; Dement *et al.*, 1985). Likewise, while there is little change in REM sleep time, there are significant changes in the distribution of the other stages, that is:

- lengthening of the period of quiet wakefulness: it takes longer to fall asleep and the number of wakenings per night increases;
- almost complete disappearance of stage 3 and disappearance of stage 4 so that there is little deep sleep time. This may explain

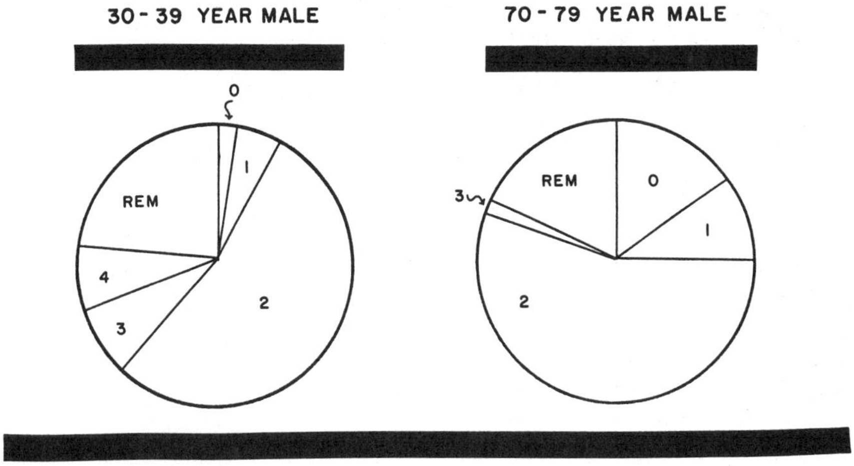

Figure 10–1. *Relative distribution of sleep stages in adult (30–39 years) and aged (70–79 years) male individuals.*

Stage 0 of quiet wakefulness is followed by four (1 through 4) stages of slow-wave (SW) sleep with periods of rapid-eye-movement (REM) sleep. In the aged, the major changes involve lengthening of the period of quiet wakefulness, preceding the onset of sleep, and the almost complete disappearance of SW 3 and 4 stages of deep sleep.

why older individuals complain subjectively of little sleep despite an overall near normal sleeping time, and why they are much more easily aroused than the young. In addition, although the statistics vary widely, there seems to be a progressive reduction of sleep during the night, and about 40 percent of the elderly suffer from insomnia so defined.

Respiratory, Cardiovascular, and Motor Changes During Sleep in the Elderly. Periods of apnea (cessation of respiration) or hypoapnea (slowing of respiration) increase with aging from an average of five respiratory disturbances/night at 24 years of age to 50 disturbances/night at 74 years. These respiratory disturbances are terminated by an arousal and may account for a great deal of the fragmentation of sleep in the elderly. Since in young and adult individuals five to eight apneas per hour of sleep are considered as the upper limit of normal, a number of elderly who are judged to be normal by other criteria would fall, according to their respiratory pattern during sleep, in the category of subjects with sleep apnea syndrome. Another aspect of impairment of respiration, in this case of upper airway function, is the increased prevalence of snoring with aging. It seems that 60 percent of males and 45 percent of females in the sixties are habitual snorers (Lugaresi *et al.*, 1975, 1978, 1980). The significance of respiratory dysfunction associated with sleep in otherwise normal elderly is not understood but has been related to impairments of neural and chemical regulation of respiration (see also Chapter 19).

Cardiac arrhythmias and pulmonary hypertension are common during the apneic periods; apnea, arrhythmia, and hypertension appear to be most frequent during REM sleep and have been associated with an increased release of norepinephrine from sympathetic stimulation (Vitiello *et al.*, 1982). Periodic movements (sleep-related leg movements) occur in one-third of elderly during large parts of the night and are associated with a brief arousal. The origin of these movements is little known, but they seem to be related to loss of coordination between motor excitation and inhibition, they occur during large parts of the night, and are associated with a brief arousal (Coleman *et al.*, 1982).

The genesis of the sleep pattern seems to involve the reticular system. This system, formed of a network of interconnecting neurons distributed in the core midbrain, controls alertness. Alertness, in turn, modulates sensory, motor, and visceral inputs as well as consciousness. Changes in sleep with aging may, perhaps, be related to alterations in the reticular formation and the level of alertness as manifested in EEG and neurotransmitter changes. Serotonin, in particular, has been implicated in the generation of sleep. Insomnia, common in the elderly, might be related to several factors superimposed on the aging process itself. Anxiety, depression, and stress, which always affect sleep, are prevalent among the elderly and may account for some of the sleep disturbances.

THE RETICULAR ACTIVATING AND THE LIMBIC SYSTEMS

Aging changes in the reticular activating system become manifest as changes not only in sleep but also in alertness and behavior. Thus, a decrease in sensory input to the higher centers results from failure of the reticular formation to properly receive, integrate, and relay the signals to the sensory cortex as well as from decrements in peripheral sensory perception, as described in Chapter 11. Impairment of sensory input would likewise impair motor responses and behavior. Such sensory-motor alterations can be detected in EEG recordings and physiologic responses.

Another brain system, the limbic system, which regulates many types of behavior, is also affected by aging. For example, we have already underlined the relationship between the hippocampus and the amygdala, limbic structures, and memory. Memory declines with aging, particularly in some aging-associated diseases such as dementia. Another, more complex, example is the change in mood and personality with aging. These changes involve not only the limbic system, but also other modalities strongly operative in the elderly population, who are profoundly affected by diminished socioeconomic status and often exposed to isolation due to abandonment by the family and to bereavement upon loss of a spouse.

Because depression and insomnia in some people, and anxiety, restlessness, and aggressiveness in others, always complicate the clinical disorders of the elderly, a variety of drugs are administered either to stimulate or to tranquilize. Drugs such as phenothiazines, barbiturates, dibenzazepines, monoamine oxidase inhibitors, and so forth are a part of the medicinal armamentarium for old people. None of these drugs is without side effects, and the metabolism of these drugs—as of most drugs—is impaired in the elderly (Chapter 24).

SENILE DEMENTIAS

Dementia (from the Latin de-mens, without mind) is defined as a global deterioration of intellectual and cognitive functions characterized by a defect of the five major mental functions (orientation, memory, intellect, judgment, and affect) but with persistence of a clear consciousness. Dementia (also referred to in the past as "organic brain syndrome") does occur at all ages and is caused by a variety of factors. It may be reversible or irreversible and progressive. Reversible dementia is generally due to known causes and, once these are removed (e.g., drugs) or cured (e.g., infections), the dementia disappears. A handy mnemonic to list the main causes of reversible dementia is presented in Table 10–1. In the elderly, "senile" dementia may be secondary to any of the factors listed in Table 10–1, or may be primary, due to unknown causes. According to etiopathogenesis and clinical manifestations, it has been categorized into several types, the distribution of which is illustrated in Figure 10–2: senile dementia of the Alzheimer type (SDAT) accounts for 50 to 60 percent of all senile dementia cases; multiple infarct dementia accounts for 20 to 30 percent; reversible dementias, for 10 to 20 percent; depression or pseudodementia for 1 to 5 percent; the remainder is represented by miscellaneous disorders such as Parkinson's and Pick's diseases. The relative proportion of the dementias varies somewhat with the population, the age of the patient, and the particular time of

Table 10–1. REVERSIBLE CAUSES OF DEMENTIA

D	*D*rugs
E	*E*motional disorders
M	*M*etabolic or endocrine disorders
E	*E*ye and ear dysfunctions
N	*N*utritional deficiencies
T	*T*umor and trauma
I	*I*nfections
A	*A*rteriosclerotic complications, i.e., myocardial infarction, stroke, or heart failure

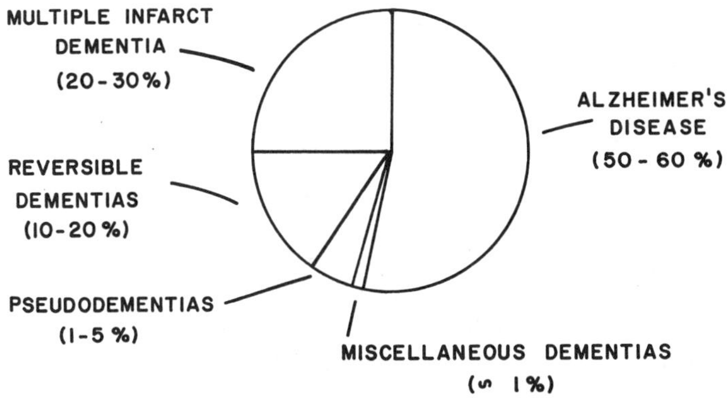

Figure 10–2. *Percentage of major forms of dementias in the elderly.*

the study, but overall, SDAT remains the most frequent.

Differences between normal and pathologic aging of the brain may be essentially quantitative. In the normal brain, neurofibrillary tangles and neuritic plaques are few (Chapter 9), whereas they are numerous and widely distributed in SDAT, where their accumulation represents a definite diagnostic feature of the disease. Whether normal aging is simply an early stage of pathology without obvious clinical expression and whether aging-associated diseases are merely "accelerated aging" or distinctive disease processes remain to be evaluated. Another prevalent view is that normal and pathologic aging are distinct entities and that the aged cell may represent a favorable environment in which some pathologic changes can be superimposed.

Undoubtedly, the larger proportion of the elderly remain lucid and mentally competent until death. That dementia is not an inevitable consequence of aging is evident from the current statistics: severe dementia can be found in only 4 to 5 percent of the population over 65 years and mild to moderate forms in 10 percent. However, the incidence of severe dementia increases with age from 0.01 percent per year at age 65, to 3.5 percent per year beyond 85. Likewise the prevalence also increases from less than 1 percent at age 65 to 70 to greater than 15 percent at age 85 and over. Indeed, age is the single most important risk factor for dementia in the older population (Mortimer and Hutton, 1985), even though some studies seem to indicate a slight decline in SDAT after age 90 (Hagnell *et al.,* 1981). It is predicted that, with the decrease in mortality in these age groups from other causes, the prevalence of dementia will double within 60 years. Currently, two-thirds of the patients in nursing homes have dementia; therefore, two-thirds of the 21 billion dollars spent in nursing home care in the United States (1985) are expended on patients with dementia. Thus, the problem of caring for demented patients is a serious one, which is likely to become worse as the segment of the population apt to be affected continues to grow.

A Capsule View of the Clinical Picture. Of all possible complaints from a patient or the family, none evokes (or should evoke) as much concern and anxiety than that of a change in mental function. ("I'm lost, lost somewhere in the corridors of my mind," an Alzheimer's victim explained to his devoted wife, in one of his more lucid moments.) Part of the tragedy of this terrible dementia is that it takes a developed personality with family, friends, intelligence, and dignity, and slowly destroys it. It is a disease that kills the mind years before it takes the body.

Alzheimer's disease begins as simple forgetfulness, which can be found in roughly 80 percent of the normal healthy elderly (Reisberg, 1983). For most, this is the extent of the problem, but in roughly 10 percent of those over 65 there is progression to a confusional phase of mild to moderate dementia. Many, perhaps most, of these cognitively impaired and confused elderly people appear to decline further to the point where they can no longer care for themselves and are frankly demented. By the time dementia has developed, the life expectancy is about 2.5 additional years and the whole clinical course of the disease averages about 8 years. With increasing numbers of elderly receiving better medical care, and significant inroads into deaths from the leading causes of cancer and heart disease, the numbers of SDAT patients are growing steadily in the United States and Western Europe. Each year several hundred thousand more Americans develop the disease and at least a hundred thousand die with it; we now have 1.5 to 2 million patients. SDAT is considered today the fourth leading cause of death in the 75 to 84 age group, an estimate considered quite conservative by many (Mortimer and Hutton, 1985).

PATHOLOGY OF SDAT

In 1907, Alois Alzheimer, a German neurologist, described the case of a 51-year-old woman with a 5-year history of progressive dementia that led to her death. At autopsy, he found many neurofibrillary tangles and neuritic plaques in her cerebral cortex and hippocampus. Today, the diagnosis of SDAT remains essentially a clinicopathologic one, requiring dementia in life and the two pathologic lesions of tangles and plaques at autopsy. Clinically, it remains a diagnosis of exclusion, that is, once all other possible causes of mental confusion and dementia have been examined and excluded.

Differential Diagnosis of SDAT. Confusional states in the elderly may indicate several conditions, which must be differentiated from dementia. Some of the most common are listed in Table 10–2 and include: *delirium,* an acute or subacute alteration of mental status characterized by clouding of consciousness, fluctuation of symptoms, and improvement of mental function after the underlying medical condition has been treated (reversible dementia); *depression* (or pseudodementia), a specific psychiatric entity that can precede or be associated with dementia, which can be differentially diagnosed and treated; *benign senescent forgetfulness,* which is not progressive and not of sufficient severity to interfere with everyday functions; *paranoid states and psychoses,* again with specifically diagnostic psychiatric correlates; and *amnesic syndrome,* characterized by short-term memory losses without delirium or dementia.

Once dementia has been diagnosed, SDAT must be differentiated from several other forms, the most frequent, in the elderly, being *multiinfarct dementia.* This condition results from recurrent cortical or subcortical strokes; the infarcts can sometimes be detected with an x-ray, CT scan (computerized tomography) or other imaging and

Table 10–2. TYPES OF COGNITIVE IMPAIRMENT IN THE ELDERLY

Delirium
Dementia
Depression (pseudodementia)
Benign senescent forgetfulness
Paranoid states and psychoses
Amnestic syndromes

Table 10–3. CHARACTERISTICS OF MULTIINFARCT DEMENTIA

History of abrupt onset of stepwise deterioration
History of transient ischemic attack or stroke
Presence of hypertension or arrythmia
Presence of any neurologic focal symptoms or signs

metabolism-measuring devices (nuclear magnetic resonance and positron emission tomography), which have been suggested as diagnostic tools for SDAT (Friedland *et al.,* 1984). If the infarcts are too small to be visualized, a clinical diagnosis can be made by the presence of the following elements (Table 10–3): a history of abrupt onset or stepwise deterioration related to the transient ischemic attacks and strokes; the presence of other symptoms of cardiovascular pathology, such as hypertension and arrhythmias; the presence of focal neurologic signs or symptoms, related to the focal nature of the cardiovascular damage. Unfortunately, as in SDAT, once the diagnosis has been made, therapeutic measures to cure or improve the dementia are not currently available. However, prevention of stroke through control of hypertension and cardiac arrhythmias continues to provide a means to reduce the incidence and progression of this disease (Chapter 17).

The relatively young age of the patient first described by Alzheimer indicates that Alzheimer's dementia does also occur at younger ages (40 to 50 years) than those so far discussed. In general, the "adult" or "presenile" form of Alzheimer's dementia presents the same symptoms and pathology as the "senile" form, but these are generally more severe and progress more rapidly. Major signs of SDAT include:

1. Decreased gross brain weight, as occurs in normal aging, but more severe and associated with flattening of gyri and widening of sulci and cerebral ventricles (see Chapter 9).
2. Loss of neurons, particularly in such areas as the nucleus basalis of Meynert (cholinergic neurons) and the locus cer-

uleus (adrenergic neurons) and the hippocampus (associated with memory).

3. Accumulation of lipofuscin in the remaining neurons and severe denudation (i.e., stripping) of dendrites (see Chapter 9).
4. Accumulation of neurofibrillary tangles, neuritic plaques, and perivascular amyloid, the most characteristic pathologic sign of SDAT, generally distributed throughout the brain, but highly concentrated in the same regions as in 2.
5. Increased levels of aluminum, especially in cells with tangles.

Despite active research the origin and nature of the characteristic lesions, tangles, plaques, and perivascular amyloid, remain controversial. One reason is the technical difficulty of solubilizing the proteinaceous material. With better purification and the use of antibodies to neurofilament and microtubule proteins, it appears that the same or similar proteins are present in all three lesions. Whether these proteins are unique to the lesion, such as the Alz-50 protein (Wolozin *et al.,* 1986), or are alterations of normal constituents, such as the microtubule-associated, low-molecular-weight, "tau" protein, remains to be determined (Kosik *et al.,* 1986). Equally uncertain at present is whether the lesions originate in the neurons and then spread to the extracellular and perivascular spaces, or whether they are bloodborne and carried to the brain through an altered blood-brain barrier (Wisniewski and Kozlowski, 1982).

Etiology of SDAT. One-third of patients with Alzheimer's dementia have a positive family history, with some instances of autosomal dominant inheritance. Epidemiologic studies would exclude the influence of toxic environmental exposure, animal contacts, smoking, drinking, dietary habits, or prior viral infections, as well as any change in the frequency of neoplasms. However, they have found an increased frequency of history of head trauma, an association with Down's syndrome and, a less convincing association with thyroid disease. Down's syndrome, characterized by a well-defined chromosomal abnormality and associated with mental impairment, shows an increased frequency of a positive family history with Alzheimer's. Virtually all Down's patients who live long enough to reach 35 to 40 years develop Alzheimer's dementia with the classic clinical and pathologic findings.

Table 10–4. PROPOSED ETIOLOGIES OF SDAT

Autoimmunity
Aluminum toxity
Prions—slow virus theory
Free radical damage

The etiology of Alzheimer's dementia remains unknown despite several proposed theories (Table 10–4). An autoimmune theory is supported by the increased incidence of head trauma in affected patients. According to this theory, an autoimmune process, possibly stimulated by a virus or damage to the blood-brain barrier, would induce deposition of immunoglobulinlike material leading to amyloid production; or alternatively, free radical damage of intracellular neurofilaments and microtubules would lead to the production of abnormal proteins (Chapter 1). Another theory involves the action of metals such as aluminum, which accumulates in the brain of Alzheimer's patients; however, it is more likely that this metal is just sequestered in the diseased cells rather than being a causative agent.

Still another theory suggests that the dementia is caused by a slow virus or slow virus particles called prions. However, epidemiologic evidence that the disease might be transmissible is lacking. The prions would either participate in or induce the formation of the plaque amyloid, would induce the formation of the paired helical filaments, or be responsible for the loss of cholinergic neurons in certain brain areas.

AIDS-Related Dementia. A pattern of neurologic symptoms occurs in individuals affected by acquired immune deficiency syndrome (AIDS). The exact incidence is unknown, but it is claimed that 60 percent of AIDS patients will develop dementia. Early stages of the disease are characterized by forgetfulness, failure to concentrate, confusion, and slow mentation, rapidly followed by progressive loss of cognition. Simultaneously motor problems appear, such as leg weakness, unsteady gait, poor coordination, and trouble with handwriting. Neuropathology includes brain atrophy, ventricular enlargement, demyelination, and multinucleated giant cells. The virus has been cultured from CSF and brain tissue (Barnes, 1986).

Management of SDAT. While there is presently no cure for SDAT, various treatments have been proposed to prevent or slow down its progression or to alleviate associated symptoms. The basic medical workup for dementia consists of a complete history and physical examination and a formal mental status examination, in severe cases, with the help of family or friends. Laboratory tests should include, besides the usual blood tests, an electrocardiogram and chest x-ray. The value of a head CT scan, NMR, and PET or cerebrospinal fluid analysis remains controversial, and probably each case should be judged individually. CT scan has been recommended in cases where reversible dementia is suspected, and PET appears to provide some useful information.

Once reversible causes of dementia have been excluded, the medical therapeutic modalities for intervening are disappointing at best. A wide range of drugs have been or are being tried, but none appears to be clinically useful. These include vasodilators, such as hydergine, cholinomimetic agents as well as choline, lecithin, vasopressin, procaine hydrochloride (Gerovital), desferoxamine (a chelating agent), antiviral agents such as interferon, calcium channel blockers and endorphin blockers.

However, the lack of specific medical therapy for Alzheimer's dementia should not discourage the physician from helping the patient and his/her family. The basic goals of management are:

- to maintain the patient's safety while allowing as much independence and dignity as possible;
- to optimize the patient's function by treating underlying medical conditions and avoiding the use of drugs with side effects on the nervous system;
- to avoid catastrophic reactions or exacerbations by preventing stressful situations;
- to identify and manage complications that arise, such as agitation, depression, and incontinence;
- to provide medical and social information to the patient's family in addition to any needed counseling.

Dementia is a condition that requires the attention not only of the physician, but also of the other branches of the health care system in order to be effectively managed.

SDAT AND THE CELLULAR STRESS RESPONSE

The greater susceptibility of the aging brain to MPTP (discussed in Chapter 9) prompts consideration of SDAT as a consequence of nonspecific cellular stress. Indeed, the etiology of Alzheimer lesions has been related to a variety of superficially different types of damage or chronic stress, such as persistent infection, metal poisoning, or genetic abnormalities. The most salient phenomenon of cellular stress (e.g., heat shock) (Fleming *et al.*, 1986; Ananthan *et al.*, 1986) overlaps with those of SDAT, as illustrated by reduced transcription and protein synthesis, nuclear alterations, and cytoskeletal disruption (Lim *et al.*, 1984; Cole and Timiras, 1987). It is to be recalled that whole-body stress also serves as a model of experimental aging (see Chapters 3 and 12).

References

Ananthan, J.; Goldberg, A. L.; and Voellmy, R.: Abnormal proteins serve as eukaryotic stress signals and trigger the activation of heat shock genes. *Science,* **232:**522–524, **1986.**

Arendash, G. W.; Strong, P. N.; and Mouton, P. R.: Intracerebral transplantation of cholinergic neurons in a new animal model for Alzheimer's disease. In Hutton, J. T., and Kenny, H. D. (eds.): *Senile Dementia of the Alzheimer's Type,* Alan R. Liss, New York, **1985.**

Barbeau, A.: Aging and the extrapyramidal system. *J. Am. Geriatr. Soc.,* **21:**145–149, **1973.**

Barnes, D. M.: AIDS-related brain damage unexplained. *Science,* **232:**1091–1093, **1986.**

Coben, L. A.; Danziger, W. L.; and Berg, L.: Frequency analysis of the resting awake EEG in mild senile dementia of Alzheimer type. *Electroenceph. Clinical Neurophysiol.,* **55:**372–380, **1983a.**

Coben, L. A.; Danziger, W. L.; and Huges, C. P.: Visual evoked potentials in mild senile dementia of the Alzheimer type. *Electroenceph. Clin. Neurophysiol.,* **55:**121–130, **1983b.**

Cole, G. M., and Timiras, P. S.: Aging-related pathology in human neuroblastoma and teratocarcinoma cell lines. In Vernadakis, A. (ed.): *Model Systems of Development and Aging of the Nervous System,* M. Nijhoff, Boston, **1987.**

Coleman, R. M.; Roffwarg, H. P.; Kennedy, S. J.; Guilleminault, C.; *et al.*: Sleep-wake disorders based on a polysomnographic diagnosis, a national cooperative study. *JAMA,* **247:**997–1003, **1982.**

Davis, K. L., and Mohs, R. C.: Cholinergic drugs in Alzheimer's disease. *N. Engl. J. Med.,* **315:**1286–1287, **1986.**

Dement, W.; Richardson, G.; Prinz, P.; Carskadon, M.; Kripke, D.; and Czeisler, C.: Changes of sleep and wakefulness with age. In Finch, C. E., and Schneider, E. L. (eds.): *Handbook of the Biology of Aging,* 2nd ed., Van Nostrand Reinhold, New York, **1985.**

Dorfman, L. J., and Bosley, T. M.: Age-related changes in peripheral and central nerve conduction in man. *Neurology,* **29:**38–44, **1979.**

Drachman, D. A.: Dizziness and vertigo. In Beeson, P.; McDermott, W.; and Wyngaarden, J. (eds.): *Textbook of Medicine,* 15th ed., W. B. Saunders, Philadelphia, **1979.**

Feinberg, I.: Functional implications of changes in sleep physiology with age. In Gershon, S., and Terry, R. D. (eds.): *Neurobiology of Aging,* Aging Series, Vol. 3, Raven Press, New York, **1976.**

Fleming, J. E.; Guattroce, E.; Latter, G.; Miquel, J.; Marcusson, R.; Zucherkandl, E.; and Bensch, K. G.: Age-dependent changes in protein in *Drosophila melanogaster. Science,* **231:**1157–1159, **1986.**

Friedland, R. P.; Budinger, T. F.; Brant-Zawadski, M.; and Jagust, W. J.: The diagnosis of Alzheimer-type dementia. A preliminary comparison of positron emission tomography and proton magnetic resonance. *JAMA,* **252:**2750–2752, **1984.**

Geddes, J. W.; Monaghan, D. T.; Cotman, C. W.; Lott, I. T.; Kim, R. C.; and Chui, H. C.: Plasticity of hippocampal circuitry in Alzheimer's disease. *Science,* **230:**1179–1181, **1985.**

Hagnell, O.; Lanke, J.; Rorsman, B.; and Ojesjo, L.: Does the incidence of age-psychosis decrease? A prospective, longitudinal study of a complete population investigated during the 25-year period 1947–1972: The Lundby Study. *Neuropsychobiology,* **7:**201–211, **1981.**

Isaacs, B.: Gait and balance. In Pathy, M. S. J. (ed.): *Principles and Practice of Geriatric Medicine,* John Wiley & Sons, Chichester, UK, **1985.**

John, E. R.; Tang, Y.; Brill, A. B.; Young, R.; and Ono,

K.: Double-labeled metabolic maps of memory. *Science,* **233:**1167–1175, **1986.**

Kales, A.; Wilson, T.; Kales, J. D.; Jacobson, A.; Paulson, M. J.; Kollar, E.; and Walter, R. D.: Measurements of all-night sleep in normal elderly persons: Effect of aging. *J. Am. Geriatr. Soc.,* **15:**405–414, **1967.**

Katz, R. I., and Horowitz, G. R.: Electroencephalogram in the septagenerian: Studies in a normal geriatric population. *J. Am. Geriatr. Soc.,* **30:**273–275, **1982.**

Klawans, H. L., and Tanner, C. M.: Movement disorders in the elderly. In Albert, M. (ed.): *Clinical Neurology of Aging,* Oxford University Press, Oxford, **1984.**

Kosik, K. S.; Joachim, C. L.; and Selkoe, D. J.: Microtubule-associated protein, tau, is a major antigenic component of paired helical filaments in Alzheimer's disease. *Proc. Natl. Acad. Sci. USA,* **83:**4044–4048, **1986.**

Lewin, R.: Age factors loom in Parkinson's disease research. *Science,* **234:**1200–1201, **1986.**

Lim, L.; Hall, C.; Leung, T.; and Whatley, S.: The relationship of the rat brain 68 kDa microtubule-associated protein with synaptosomal plasma membranes and with the Drosophila 70kDa heat-shock protein. *Biochem. J.,* **224:**677–680, **1984.**

Lugaresi, E.; Coccagna, G.; Farneti, P.; Mantovani, M.; and Cirignotta, F.: Snoring. *Electroenceph. Clin. Neurophysiol.,* **39:**59–64, **1975.**

Lugaresi, E.; Coccagna, G.; and Cirignotta, F.: Snoring and its clinical implications. In Guillenimault, C., and Dement, W. (eds.): *Sleep Anea Syndromes,* Alan R. Liss, New York, **1978.**

Lugaresi, E.; Cirignotta, F.; Coccagna, G.; and Piana, C.: Some epidemiological data on snoring and cardiocirculatory disturbances. *Sleep,* **3:**221–224, **1980.**

Miles, L. E., and Dement, W. C.: Sleep and aging. *Sleep,* **3:**119–220, **1980.**

Mortimer, J. A., and Hutton, J. T.: Epidemiology and etiology of Alzheimer's disease. In Hutton, J. T., and Kenny, H. O. (eds.): *Senile Dementia of the Alzheimer's Type,* Alan R. Liss, New York, **1985.**

Muller, H. F., and Schwartz, G.: Electroencephalograms and autopsy findings in geropsychiatry. *J. Gerontol.,* **33:**504–513, **1978.**

Obrist, W. D.: Problems of aging. In Remond, A. (ed.): *Handbook of Electroencephalography and Clinical Neurophysiology,* Elsevier, Amsterdam, **1963.**

Overstall, P. W.: Falls. In Pathy, M. S. J. (ed.): *Principles and Practice of Geriatric Medicine,* John Wiley & Sons, Chichester, UK, **1985.**

Prinz, P. N.; Peskind, E. R.; Vitaliano, P. P.; Raskind, M. A.; Eisdorfer, C.; Zemcuznikov, N.; and Gerber, C. J.: Changes in the sleep and waking EEG of nondemented and demented elderly subjects. *J. Am. Geriatr. Soc.,* **30:**86–93, **1982.**

Reisberg, B.: An overview of current concepts of Alzheimer's disease, senile dementia, and age-associated cognitive decline. In Reisberg, B. (ed.): *Alzheimer's Disease: The Standard Reference,* Free Press, New York, **1983.**

Roberts, M. A.; McGeorge, A. P.; and Caird, F. I.: Electroencephalography and computerized tomography in vascular and non-vascular dementia in old age. *J. Neurol. Neurosurg. Psychiatry,* **41:**903–906, **1978.**

Shaw, N. A., and Cant, B. R.: Age-dependent changes in the latency of the pattern visual evoked potential. *Electroenceph. Clin. Neurophysiol.,* **48:**237–241, **1980.**

Squire, L. R.: Mechanisms of memory. *Science,* **232:**1612–1619, **1986.**

Summers, W. K.; Majovski, L. V.; Marsh, G. M.; Tachiki, K.; and Kling, A.: Oral tetrahydroaminacridine in long-term treatment of senile dementia, Alzheimer type. *N. Engl. J. Med.,* **315:**1241–1245, **1986.**

Syndulko, K.; Hansch, E. C.; Cohen, S. N.; Pearce, J. W.; Goldberg, Z.; Montan, B.; Tourtellotte, W. W.; and Potvin, A. R.: Long-latency event-related potential in normal aging and dementia. *Adv. Neurol.,* **32:**279, **1982.**

Thompson, R. F.: The neurobiology of learning and memory. *Science,* **233:**941–947, **1986.**

Vitiello, M. V.; Giblin, E. C.; Schoene, R. B.; Halter, J. B.; and Prinz, P. N.: Obstructive apnea, sympathetic activity, respiration and sleep, a case report. *Neurobiol. Aging,* **3:**263–266, **1982.**

Wisniewski, H. M., and Kozlowski, P. B.: Evidence for blood brain barrier changes in senile dementia of the Alzheimer type (SDAT). *Ann. NY Acad. Sci.,* **396:**119–130, **1982.**

Wolozin, B. L.; Pruchnicki, A.; Dickson, D. W.; and Davies, P.: A neuronal antigen in the brains of Alzheimer patients. *Science,* **232:**648–650, **1986.**

CHAPTER

11 AGING OF THE NERVOUS SYSTEM: SENSORY CHANGES

Esmail Meisami

INTRODUCTION

Sensory impairments such as diminished vision and hearing occur so commonly with aging that they often tend to characterize the aged and the aging process. Some of these impairments are due to intrinsic aging process occurring in the sense organs and their associated nervous systems. Others are caused by environmental effects and still others represent manifestations of aging diseases.

The study of aging process in the sensory systems of humans and other mammals, in addition to its worth and applicability to geriatrics, also provides some of the most interesting and challenging cases of gerontological investigation as the elements comprising the various senses portray the entire spectrum of cellular, tissue, organ, and system aging. Thus, while the peripheral receptor cells of the ear's cochlea and the eye's retina are permanently established at birth with no turnover and regeneration in later life, those of the olfactory and cutaneous senses are endowed with these properties. Functional decrement with aging, however, occurs in all of these systems. The aging changes in the eye's lens provide another interesting model system for the study of aging process as they begin so early in life and lend themselves to a wide variety of investigations ranging from molecular biology to physiological optics.

This chapter describes normal aging changes in the various sensory structures and functions. The account is limited to the changes in humans and to the senses of vision, hearing, taste, smell, and certain aspects of somatic sensation such as touch, vibration, and complex somesthesia. The sensations of pain and temperature are not included mainly owing to lack of space and also because less is known about the physiological and structural aspects of these senses in the elderly; appropriate references are provided for the interested reader, however.

In addition to normal aging changes, certain aspects of the sensory disorders and diseases associated with aging are also discussed. Nearly three-fourths of the elderly suffer from significant impairments in their sensory functions. In particular, impaired vision and hearing reduce the capacity for social communication, one of people's cardinal needs and functions, and may result in social isolation and deprivation. Reduced capacities in somatic sensation may interfere with professional activities requiring fine touch and manipulative sensations. Impairments in taste and smell may interfere with appetite, food selection, good nutrition, and the feelings of pleasure and well-being. The reduced sensory abilities may lead to depression; in those already suffering from depression, it may hinder the progress of recovery. Because sensory losses in the old age are so common and their consequences so widespread, understanding of the impact of these deficits is now essential for those interested in geriatrics and/or management of the elderly.

VISION

The eye is the sensory organ for vision. It serves both optical and nervous functions. The neural functions are carried out by the retina while the cornea, lens, pupil, and the aqueous and vitreous humors of the eye's chambers carry out the optical functions. Both neural and optical compartments undergo aging changes, although those of the optical compartment are more pronounced and better known; in fact some of these changes like those in the lens start very early in life. The changes in the optical compartment are probably the primary causes of the serious decline in the visual capacities of the elderly (Graham, 1985; Kuwabara, 1979; Sekuler *et al.*, 1982; Weale, 1963; Wale, 1982). We will review the structural changes in the eye's optical components and attempt to correlate these to the known functional impairments. Then an overview of the changes in visual functions will be presented.

OPTICAL COMPONENTS

Cornea. The *cornea,* which is responsible for most of the refraction of the light rays, becomes thicker and less curved with aging. The loss of curvature is due mainly to an increase in the horizontal diameter. These changes alter the refractive properties of the cornea, making the eye more susceptible to *astigmatism,* a condition characterized by defective curvature and diffusion of light rays. Frequently, in individuals over 60, a gray ring, *arcus senilis,* forms around the cornea's outer edges. This ring would interfere with passage of light rays, especially when the pupil is dilated. However, because normally the pupil is partially constricted in the elderly, the effects of arcus senilis are not detrimental to visual function (Graham, 1985; Kuwabara, 1979; Weale, 1982).

Anterior Chamber. The size and volume of the eye's *anterior chamber* decrease with age mainly due to the thickening of the lens. This growth occasionally exerts pressure on the *canal of Schlem,* an outflow channel at the junction between the iris and cornea, causing a reduction in flow of the *aqueous humor* and an increase in intraocular pressure. Obstruction of this channel leads to markedly increased intraocular pressure and the serious eye disease, glaucoma (Graham, 1985).

Iris. The *iris* is a muscular ring forming the *pupil* of the eye. In the elderly, the iris appears paler in the middle, mainly due to loss of pigmentation. The pigment is associated with a particular type of smooth muscle whose aging changes are discussed later in connection with *miosis* in the elderly (Weale, 1982). With aging, there is also a mild but constant increase in the density of collagen fibers in the iris stroma and noncellular perivascular zone (Kuwabara, 1979).

Vitreous Humor. The *vitreous humor,* a mass of gelatinous substance filling the eye's *posterior chamber,* gives the eye globe its shape and support. It loses some water during old age and shows aging changes in the fibrous skeleton which provides its support. There are also some changes in the color and an increase in the number of inclusion bodies, the so-called *floaters* (Kuwabara, 1979; Marsh, 1980).

Miosis. One of the characteristic ocular impairments in the elderly is a persistent reduction in the pupil size (diameter), the so called *senile miosis* (Weale, 1982). Senile miosis is particularly notable in the fully dark-adapted eye; the reduction in diameter occurs gradually with aging, decreasing from a mean of 8 mm in the twenties to 6 mm in the sixties and 5 mm in the nineties (Figure 11–1).

It is believed that senile miosis results from a relatively higher rate of aging atrophy in the *radial dilator* muscles, which dilate the pupil, compared to the *sphincter constrictor* muscles, which constrict it. As a result, the sphincter is constantly dominant in the aged, causing persistent constriction (Weale, 1982). Compared to youth, the reduced pupil aperture of the elderly results in a one-third reduction in the amount of light entering the eye.

The Lens: Development and Aging. The increase in the opacity (optical density) and the hardness of the *lens* with age are two of the best known changes in the eye's optical properties. In the process of image formation the lens performs two functions, *refraction* and *accommodation*. For refraction, the lens requires an appropriate crystalline structure and transparency, while for accommodation it needs to be elastic, amenable to changes in its curvature. The aging changes in the lens interfere with both these functions.

A knowledge of the lens's structure and development is essential for understanding

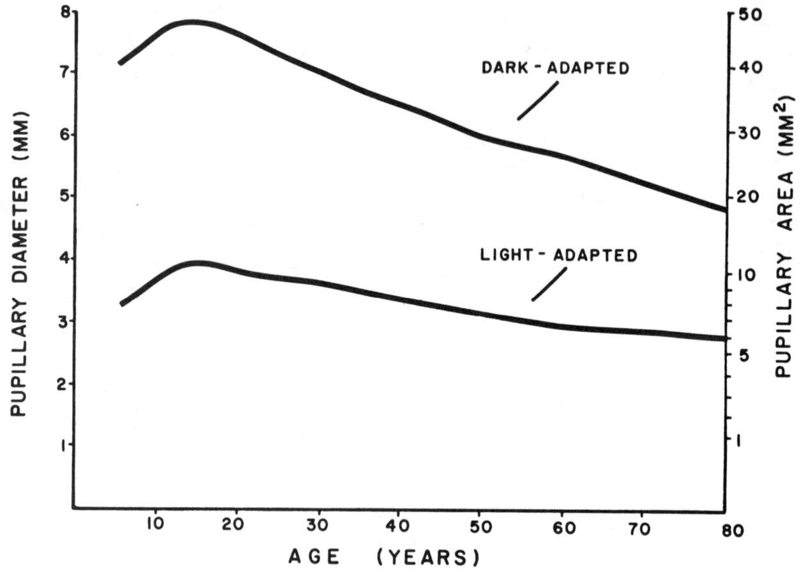

Figure 11–1. *Changes with age in pupillary diameter and area, measured in light-adapted and dark-adapted individuals; note more pronounced effects in dark-adapted eyes.* (Adapted from Weale, 1982; original data from Verriest, 1971.)

its aging. The biconvex lens is formed prenatally, during the embryonic period. It is initially fairly spherical and has a basically fibrous and acellular structure. During postnatal development and throughout maturity the lens continues to grow by addition of new layers of protein fibers laid down by the capsular epithelial cells located in front of the lens. This results in a horizontal growth in the lens, so that between 20 and 80 years, the lens' anterior-posterior diameter increases by about 50 percent (Marsh, 1980).

Increased Opacity. Since the fiber layers in the lens interior are not regenerated during postnatal growth, they tend to cross-over, becoming more dense and less elastic with age; they also become increasingly more yellow (Dark *et al.,* 1969; Marsh, 1980; Weale, 1982). With the passage of years, these changes make the lens gradually less transparent and less refractive. The increased opacity of the human lens with aging has been determined by measuring its optical density at different ages. The results indicate a threefold increase in optical density (at 460 nm, blue) between 20 to 60 years (Weale, 1982). This results in increased light scattering, particularly in the blue and yellow range but much less so in the red range. In addition to impairing refraction these changes may also affect color perception. When the lens opacity becomes very extensive, a pathological condition known as *cataract* is produced whereby the lens becomes cloudy (Graham, 1985).

Decline in Accommodation and Presbyopia. Lens elasticity is extremely important for visual *accommodation.* During accommodation the lens becomes more convex in order to focus the image of the near objects on the retina. This is accomplished by the *ciliary muscle,* one of the most intensively used body muscles. Due to the particular arrangement of the ciliary muscle and the lens *suspensory ligaments* and the lens itself, whenever the ciliary muscles contract, the ligaments relax, causing the lens to relax; in the resting state, the lens has higher curvature; this increases the refractive power, decreases the focal point, and assists in sharp focusing.

The reduced elasticity of the capsule and lens during aging makes the lens less resilient to accommodate for near vision. Indeed the *point of near vision,* i.e., the minimum

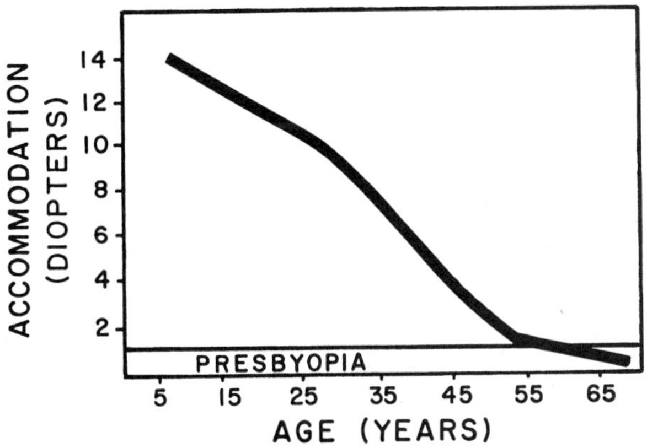

Figure 11–2. *Changes in visual accommodation in humans with age; note decline occurs throughout life resulting in presbyopia in the early fifties.* (Adapted from various similar sources, e.g., Duane, 1931.)

distance between the object and the eye for formation of a clear image, increases ten times during human life, from 9 cm at the age of 10 years to 10 cm at 20 years, 20 cm at 45 and 84 cm at 60 years.

The loss of accommodation with aging can also be determined by studying the changes in the eye's *refractive power,* measured in diopters (reciprocal of the principal focal distance of the lens in meters). Thus, the newborn's lens, being more spherical, shows the highest refractive power (about 60 diopters). As shown in Figure 11–2, accommodation power of the human lens decreases to about 14 diopters at the age of 10, 5 at 40 years, reaching a minimum of 1 in the sixth decade (Duane, 1931). At this age the lens becomes hard and nonresilient, unable to accommodate for near-vision tasks. This condition, known as *presbyopia* (Figure 11–2), is of major clinical significance as practically everyone over 55 years old needs corrective convex lenses or eyeglasses for reading and other near-vision tasks.

Other Factors Influencing Reduced Accommodation. Although the increased hardness of the lens capsule and interior, caused by the intrinsic aging process of the lens proteins, is the principal cause of accommodation loss, environmental effects such as heat and temperature may also enhance this process. People residing in warmer climates show earlier presbyopia (Weale, 1982). It is also quite likely that in addition to the hardening of the lens, aging changes in the suspensory ligaments, the ciliary muscles, their parasympathetic nerve supply, and the associated synapses contribute to the decline in accommodation with aging. Latency of accommodation reflex decreases during aging but in general less is known about the neural aging aspects of accommodation.

Aging Changes in the Retina. The human *retina* shows considerable age-related structural changes, particularly in its *peripheral zones,* although the *macula* is not spared. The aged retinal periphery is thinner (10 to 30 microns), containing lesser number of *rods* and other nerve cell types. The aging loss of rods appears to be a very slow process, beginning in the third and fourth decades, and may be related to accumulated damage due to physiological exposure to light (Kuwabara, 1979). With aging, the rods outer segments shorten and disengage from pigment epithelium microvilli, resulting in lesser amount of *membranous discs* and *rhodopsin.* Cones survive better and become more conspicuous in the aged retinas. Nerve cell loss, particularly evident for the population of *bipolar, amacrine,* and *horizontal cells,* is in the range of 30 percent. *Muller cells* (a type of glia cell in the retina) take over the space left by the lost cells and form cysts, which are common in the aged retina (Kuwabara, 1979; Graham, 1985). The degeneration of macula in advanced ages is discussed below under diseases of eyes in the aged.

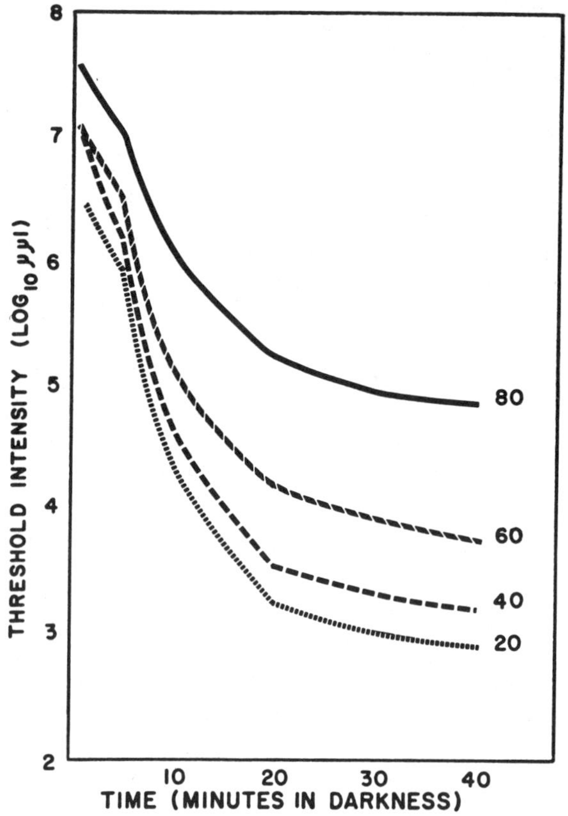

Figure 11–3. *Decline in light sensitivity with age; data show changes in visual threshold after dark adaptation in different age groups (20, 40, 60, 80 years).* (Adapted and redrawn in part from a figure in Marsh, 1980, based on original data of McFarland, 1960.)

VISUAL FUNCTIONS

Sensitivity and Visual Threshold. As discussed previously, with age, the pupillary aperture decreases, resulting in less light input. The decline in the number of photoreceptor cells (rods) and other aging changes in the retina result in reduced availability and regeneration capacity of photoreceptor pigment (rhodopsin), leading to reduced light utilization in the aged eye. As a result, the *visual threshold,* i.e., the minimum amount of light necessary to see an object, increases with age. This is tested by measuring the change in visual threshold as a function of time spent in darkness (*dark adaptation*). It is known that the threshold for light detection decreases with increased duration of dark adaptation, because rhodopsin regeneration is enhanced in the dark. With advancing age this regeneration is presumably deficient, resulting in higher light thresholds (i.e., lower sensitivity).

As illustrated in Figure 11–3, the enhanced light sensitivity after dark adaptation is markedly reduced with aging (McFarland *et al.*, 1960); in fact the visual thresholds in the completely dark-adapted eyes of the aged group (80 years) is 100 times higher than that of the young group (20 years). As evident from the data, however, the pattern of change in sensitivity during dark adaptation is basically similar in the different age groups. This indicates that the retinal function is quantitatively impaired, not qualitatively. Some believe that the decline in threshold is due to reduced oxygenation of retina and the rods in the aged (Marsh, 1980).

Critical Flicker Frequency. The rate at which consecutive visual stimuli can be presented and still be perceived as separate is called the *critical flicker frequency* (CFF). Determination of CFF in the different age groups provides one way by which changes in visual function with age can be measured. These tests reveal a decline in CFF with aging from a value of 40

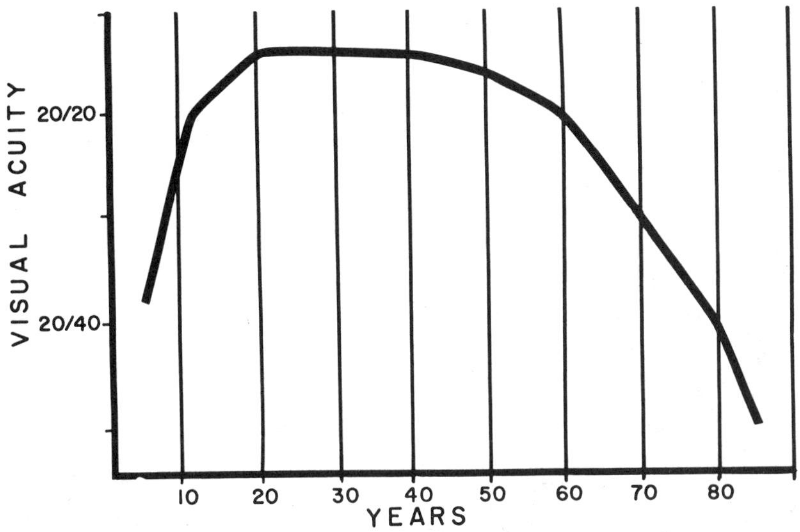

Figure 11–4. *Changes in visual acuity measured in Snellen index with age; note that decline begins after 60 and visual acuity is seriously impaired after 80.* (From Pitts, 1982.)

Hz (cycles/sec) during the fifth decade, to about 30 Hz in the eighth decade (McFarland *et al.*, 1958). The persistent miosis in the elderly must contribute to this decline since the decline is less marked with fully dilated pupils.

Visual Acuity. *Visual acuity* reflects the ability to detect details and contours of objects; it is defined as the minimum separable distance between objects and is basically a measure of the visual system's *spatial* discrimination ability. Several studies (see Figure 11–4) have shown a decline in visual acuity, particularly during and after the eighth decade (Friedenwald, 1930; Pitts, 1982), when it becomes detrimental to vision. The decline in visual acuity with age may be the result of alterations in both optical and neural factors. Thus, (1) the altered refraction of the light rays by the cornea and the lens, (2) the decline in accommodation, (3) the decreased light input due to constricted pupils (senile miosis), (4) any decline in the density and number and function of visual receptor cells, particularly in the fovea, and finally (5) central neural visual changes, may all contribute to the decline of visual acuity with age. It is important to note that elimination of glare and improved illumination can help enhance visual acuity substantially in the aged population.

Color Perception. Beginning with the fourth decade of life, color perception shows a progressive decline with age. Women are relatively less affected than men. During the fourth and fifth decades, the deficiency in color perception is mostly in the short wavelength range, i.e., yellow to blue. This is explained by the changes in the lens, as it becomes more yellowish with age. In the later decades, i.e., after the sixties, a deficiency in the green range also becomes manifest, probably due to retinal or more central factors, as it is evident even after removal of the lens (Marsh, 1980).

Changes in Central Visual Pathways. With advancing age, considerable changes in the *optic nerve* (Dolman *et al.*, 1982) and *visual cortex* (Brody and Vijayashankar, 1977) have been reported. Changes in the visual cortex have included thinning and cell loss. Earlier electrophysiological investigations had indicated marked flattening of the *evoked potential* responses to light flashes in the different parts of the cortex (Schenkenberg, 1970). Another study has found that the amplitude of some of the components of visual evoked potentials are

Table 11–1. SUMMARY OF THE USUAL AGING CHANGES IN THE HUMAN EYE

Structural Changes

Cornea: increased thickness; decreased curvature; some loss of transparency; pigment/lipid accumulation (*arcus senilis*); good epithelial regeneration

Anterior chamber: decreased volume and flow of aqueous humor

Iris: decreased dilator muscle cell number, pigment and activity; mild increase in density of collagen fibers in stroma

Lens: increased size and anterior-posterior thickness; decreased curvature; increased pigment accumulation (yellowishness) and opacity (optical density); decreased epithelial cell number; decreased new fiber formation; increased collagen fiber cross-over; increased hardness in capsule and body

Vitreous body: increased inclusion bodies; decreased water content; lesser support to globe and retina

Ciliary body and muscles: decreased number of smooth muscles (radial and circular); increased hyaline substance and fiber in ciliary process; decreased ciliary pigment epithelial cells

Retina: decreased thickness in periphery; defects in rod outer segments; loss of rods and associated nerve cells; but lesser cone loss; expansion of Muller cells; increased cyst formation; formation of Drusen filled lesions and degeneration of macular region in diseased condition

Pigment epithelium: loss of melanin granules; increased lipofuscin granules

Functional Changes

Corneal and lens functions: decreased accommodation power (*presbyopia*); increased accommodation reflex latency; increased near point of vision; increased lenticular light scattering; decreased refraction; decreased lens elasticity

Retinal function: decreased critical flicker frequency; decreased light sensitivity (increased light thresholds before and after dark-adaptation); reduced color vision initially in yellow to blue and later in the green range

General optical functions: increased pupillary constriction (*senile miosis*); reduced visual acuity

Major Pathologies

Lens: *cataract*; retina: *senile macular degeneration, glaucoma*

markedly reduced while the latency of response is increased (Allison *et al.,* 1984). The latter changes are significantly more marked in elderly men than women. For a summary of normal and pathological aging changes in the human eye see Table 11–1.

AGING AND EYE DISEASES

Various degrees of vision loss and blindness, commonly caused by senile cataract, betic retinopathy, represent the extreme consequence of age-related ocular pathologies. Diabetic retinopathy will be discussed in Chapter 16. In the United States, for patients in the age range 75 to 85 years the prevalence of cataracts is 46 percent, macular degeneration 28 percent and glaucoma 7.2 percent (Kine *et al.,* 1978). Screening for these disorders includes testing visual acuity, ophthalmoscopic examination and checking intraocular pressure (Graham, 1985).

Cataracts. In some individuals the accumulated normal aging changes in pigment and fiber composition in the lens assume pronounced and pathological dimensions, leading to a condition known as *cataract*. In these cases of senile cataracts the lens interior becomes cloudy and opaque. Light refraction is greatly reduced and light scattering markedly increased, resulting in loss of visual acuity. This reduces pattern vision and leads to functional blindness; only a degree of light perception may remain. Cataracts may occur in the lens periphery (cortical cataract) or center (nuclear cataract). Cortical cataract is particularly detrimental to visual acuity while nuclear cataract interferes more with color perception. A mild cataract can be managed with periodic examination and eyeglasses. When the reduction in visual acuity interferes with the patient's daily activities, however, cataract surgery may be necessary (Graham, 1985).

In the United States about 400,000 cataract operations are performed every year, resulting in improved vision in 97 percent of the cases. All cataract operations involve removal of the opacified lens via a corneal incision followed by fine suturing (Salz, 1981). In most cases the operation is done under local anesthesia and sedation. The postoperative patient requires a means for optical correction due to loss of the lens. Several options are available: (1) *Eyeglasses*; these are thick and heavy, increasing object size by 25 percent; they induce optical distortions and interfere with peripheral vision. Although they provide good central vision, eyeglasses cannot be used after surgery, if the other eye is normal. (2) *Contact lenses*; hard or soft extended-wear contact lenses have been used. They are more difficult to use and adjust to, and eyeglasses are still required for reading. However, they do correct central and peripheral vision, increase image size by only 6 percent, and can be used after surgery on one or both eyes. (3) *Intraocular lens*; this is surgically placed inside the iris at the time of cataract surgery. It requires the use of bifocal eyeglasses and does have a higher incidence of surgical and postsurgical complications. However, it increases image size by only 1 percent, corrects central and peripheral vision, and can be used on one or both eyes. (4) *Refractive keratoplasty,* which is still an experimental procedure, whereby the cornea is cut and reshaped.

Glaucoma. Another treatable eye disease is *glaucoma*, which is characterized by the following triad: first the intraocular pressure increases; this leads to progressive excavation of the optic disc, the site where the optic nerve leaves the eye, and cupping of the disc. The latter event causes ischemic damage to the optic nerve fibers, leading to blindness.

Open-angle glaucoma is the commonest type and is also characterized by an insidious and slow onset, initially asymptomatic and then gradually leading to blindness. *Closed-angle* glaucoma is rare and is characterized by an acute attack of severe eye pain and marked loss in vision due to a rapid increase in intraocular pressure compressing the entire retina.

Whereas cataracts are usually treated surgically, glaucoma is often treated medically with eyedrops. Miotics (substances that constrict the pupil) such as pilocarpine are most commonly used. Beta-blockers, which block specific sympathetic innervation, such as Timolol, are also used but caution is warranted since systemic side effects such as heart failure have been shown to occur. Sometimes systemic medications are used such as carbonic anhydrase inhibitors, or surgery may be necessary in the case of an acute-angle attack.

Senile Macular Degeneration. An important cause of visual impairment in the elderly, often leading to legal blindness within 5 years after onset, is *senile macular degeneration* (Lewis, 1979). The macula is an area of retina 6 mm in diameter located just posterior to the lens on the optic axis of the eye. Through its high density of cones and involvement in day and color vision, the macula and in particular its centeral zone, the fovea, provide the structural basis for high visual acuity. Hence macular degeneration, more than any other eye disease, affects visual acuity and central vision dramatically. This disease occurs generally in both eyes and more often (50 percent) in women; it is believed to be a hereditary disorder, not caused by simple aging of the retinal nerve cells, but largely related to manifestation of inherited pathologies in the nonneural retinal elements such as the pigment epithelium (Sarks, 1976). The patients also show an increased incidence of *hyperopia* (farsightedness). The disease may result from disturbances in the walls of subretinal capillaries or in the thickness of subretinal membrane or the retinal pigment epithelium itself (Graham, 1985).

Senile macular degeneration is accompanied by any of the following pathologic changes depending on the stage and extent of the disease (Graham, 1985; Lewis, 1979; Sarks, 1976): (1) white excrescences in the subretinal membrane, called *Drusen* (nodules); these are hyaline deposits ranging in size from punctate lesions to dome-shaped structures 0.5 mm in diameter and are often observed during the early stages of disease; the Drusen occur mostly around the macula but can be found dispersed throughout the fundus; (2) atrophy of *retinal pigment epithelium*; (3) *serous detachment* of retinal pigment epithelium; (4) subretinal *neovascularization*, and (5) *disciform scars* that result from the retinal pigment epithelium detachment.

Unfortunately, treatment of macular degeneration is not nearly as successful as cataract and glaucoma. The only realistic goal of treatment is to prevent subretinal detachment and hemorrhage, disorders that lead to an acute loss of vision. To accomplish this, the sites of subretinal neovascular formation are located using fluorescin angiography. This is followed by laser photocoagulation. This procedure is limited to certain cases and is still considered risky (Graham, 1985).

HEARING

Changes in auditory functions with age provide some of the classic and important case-studies in gerontology and the physiology of aging. The incidence of hearing problems increases from about 10 (per 100,000) during the third decade of life to more than 100 in the sixth, and 1000 in the eighth decade (Weiss, 1963). Hearing disorders afflict a very large segment of the elderly population. Indeed, more than one third of the people over 65 suffer from hearing impairments. Inasmuch as hearing disorders interfere with the perception of speech, both one's own and that of others, they may produce behavioral and social disabilities; deafness, in the extreme, may lead to depression and social isolation (Mauer and Rupp, 1979).

As in the visual system, the age-related problems of the auditory system may stem from structural and functional disorders of both the peripheral auditory components and the central neural aspects. Here, too, more is known about the aging of the ear than about that of the central auditory system.

Age-Related Hearing Loss (Presbycusis). Loss of hearing associated with aging is called *presbycusis*. Numerous studies have reported loss of hearing with age, particularly for sounds in the high frequency range, i.e., more than 1 KHz. (Weiss, 1964; Marsh, 1980; Schuknecht, 1974). Presbycusis occurs in both ears but not necessar-

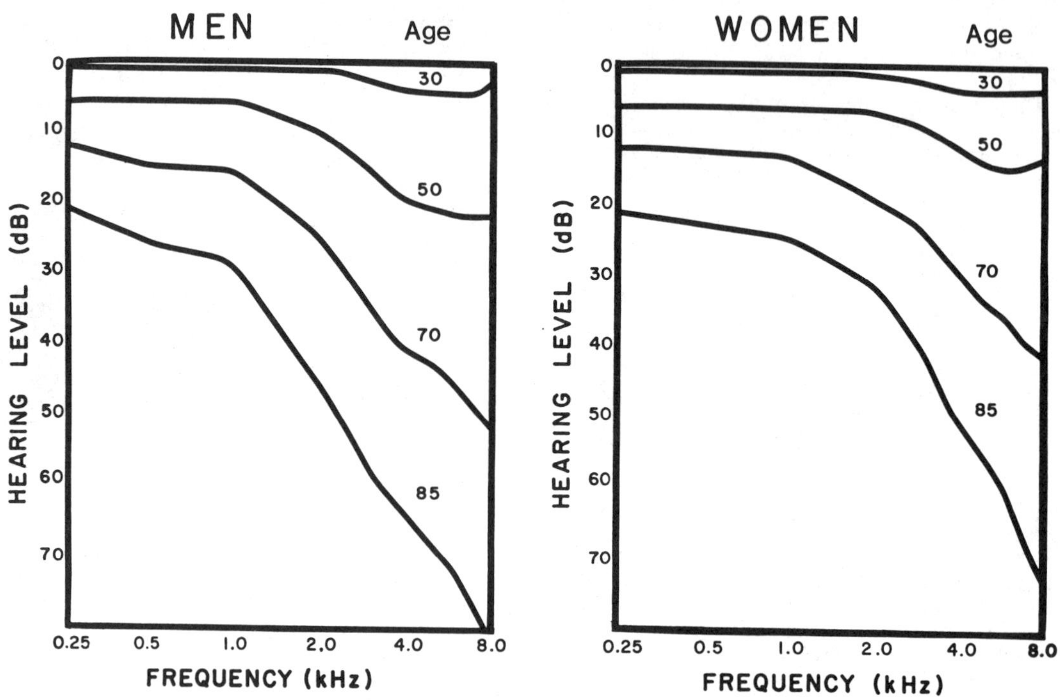

Figure 11–5. *Amount of hearing loss (in decibels) for different pure tones in various age groups of men and women.*

Note the greater loss at higher frequencies and later ages; also, there is a more pronounced hearing loss in men. (Adapted and redrawn in part from a figure in Marsh, 1980 based on original data of Spoor, 1967.)

ily at the same time. In fact the elderly often have a "better ear." To assess auditory loss with age, pure tone audiograms of subjects in different age groups are determined. That is, the threshold in decibels (unit of sound intensity) for hearing sounds of increasing frequency is determined; the results are presented as relative loss of decibels (dB) at different frequencies.

These studies indicate that in the low frequency range (125 to 1000 Hz), young subjects have no hearing deficits while old subjects show deficits of about 10 to 15 dB. In the high frequency range, hearing loss for the young group is very mild, while in the old group it becomes progressively worse with increase in sound frequency (Marsh, 1980; Mills, 1985). A typical amount of hearing loss is 30 dB for 2 KHz, increasing by about 10 dB for each additional KHz (Weiss, 1964); in octogenarian men living in urban areas, the hearing loss may be as much as 80 dB. Another way of determining the hearing loss is by measuring the maximum frequency of sound capable of being heard. This frequency is 20 KHz for children (10 years) decreasing to only 4 KHz for the elderly (80 years); the decline is steady, at the rate of about 2.3 KHz per decade (Weiss, 1964).

Typical pure tone audiometric curves for normal men and women at different age groups is shown in Figure 11–5, which is based on a study by Spoor (1967). In this study the hearing loss was found to be higher in men than women; the sex difference, which begins after the age of 35 years, may possibly reflect the effects of higher exposure of men to work-related noise. The result of the latter study and another (Rosen, 1962), showing that the elderly from noise-free rural areas show lesser hearing loss compared to those in the urban environment, suggest that exposure to environmental noise contributes importantly to the causation of presbycusis. Another cause of presbycusis may be due to vascular (atherosclerosis) and similar disorders related to elevated blood lipids (hyperlipoproteinemia). Thus according to

Spencer (1973), incidence of hearing loss and inner ear diseases is very high in patients with elevated cholesterol levels.

Presbycusis Related to Ear Structure. The major structures of the ear include: (1) the external ear (pinna, external auditory canal, and tympanic membrane); (2) the middle ear (the ossicular chain); (3) the inner ear (cochlea and the organ of Corti). The *organ of Corti* contains the *hair cells,* which are the auditory receptors and the mechanoelectrical transducing organs. The cell bodies of the primary auditory neurons are in the cochlea's *spiral ganglia,* and the axons comprising the auditory nerve enter the medulla to synapse with central auditory neurons. Auditory pathways in the brain include the *medullary* and *midbrain* centers for signal transmission and auditory reflexes, the *inferior colliculi,* and the *auditory cortex* in the temporal lobe of the cerebral cortex. The selective nature of presbycusis indicates that it is probably not associated with aging changes in the outer or middle ear (tympanic membrane and ossicles), but is more likely due to changes in the inner ear (cochlea) or the central auditory system (Schuknecht, 1974).

Types of Presbycusis. Presbycusis may occur due to damage to different parts of the auditory systems. Based on the source of damage, the following types are recognized (Schuknecht, 1974; Maur and Rupp, 1979; Mills, 1985): sensory, neural, strial and cochlear conductive. The pure tone audiogram in these types are often different and may provide clues about the cause and source of the problem (Figure 11–6). The standard type of presbycusis with hearing loss at high Hz is associated often with *neural* or *sensory presbycusis* (Figure 11–6A). Sensory type involves the organ of Corti and deficits in mechanisms involved in transduction of high frequency sounds, while neural type is due to selective degeneration or loss of corresponding primary auditory neurons in the spiral ganglia. Individual cases may present symptoms of both neural and sensory types. In fact, detailed examination of whole human cochleas of the aged (Figure 11–7) suffering from sensory/neural presbycusis reveals loss of outer and inner hair cells of the organ of Corti (Johansson and Hawkins, 1972). The loss is diffuse or patchy and mainly limited to the first quadrant of the cochlea's lower basal turn and is often accompanied with nerve degeneration in the corresponding spiral ganglia (see Johnsson and Hawkins, 1979, for review). This part of the cochlea is specialized for detection of high frequency sounds.

In the *cochlear conductive* type of presbycusis, the audiogram indicates that a loss occurs at all frequencies but the magnitude of the loss increases linearly with increasing frequency (Figure 11–6B). This type of presbycusis is believed to be due to mechanical damage to the basilar membrane of the cochlea. In the *strial* type of presbycusis the audiogram shows a flat curve (Figure 11–6C), indicating equal loss in audibility at all frequencies. This type is believed to be associated with atrophic changes in the vascular supply to the cochlea (Schuknecht, 1974; Johnsson and Hawkins, 1979).

Sound Localization. Tests of sound localization indicate a decline in this ability with aging, beginning in the fourth decade (Marsh, 1980). It is known that localization of low frequency sounds depends on *temporal* discrimination (i.e., time of sound arrival) between the two ears, while in the high frequency range, localization depends on discrimination of sound *intensity* between the two ears. Aging changes occur in both ears, though the rate of aging may be different in the two ears (Schuknecht, 1974). Thus deficits in localization of sound will be apparent for all frequencies but may be more marked for sounds of higher frequency as the perception of these are particularly impaired in old age (see above).

Presbycusis and Speech Perception. The marked hearing deficits in the high frequency range have important bearing on impaired speech perception in the elderly (Jerger and Hays, 1977). Thus *vowels,* generated by low frequency sounds, are heard better than the *consonants,* which are produced by high frequency sounds. Since consonants make speech intelligible while vowels make it more audible, a common

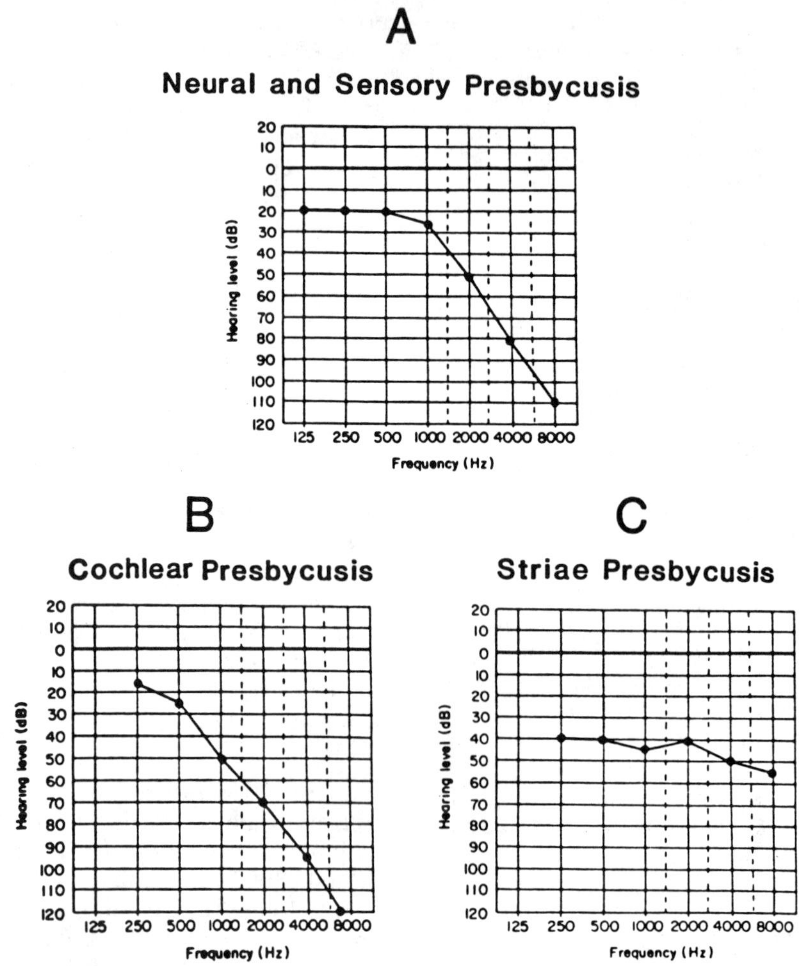

Figure 11–6. *Typical pure tone audiograms of aged individuals suffering from different types of presbycusis.*

A. Neural and sensory: note hearing loss mainly for high Hz; *B.* Cochlear type: note hearing loss is present for all frequencies but increases steadily with higher Hz; *C.* Striae type: note moderate and equal hearing loss for all frequencies.

complaint of the elderly is that they can not understand spoken words although they can hear them (Marsh, 1980). Fortunately lip reading, which is associated more with the expression of consonants, can greatly help this deficiency.

Other Speech Comprehension Problems. As indicated in the data of Figure 11–8, if speech is presented to the aged subjects too fast or with reverberations (i.e., echoing or booming), its comprehension declines markedly (Bergman *et al.*, 1976). The greatest decline in comprehension is observed if speech is presented with repeated interruptions, such as 8 times per second, as is the case with many modern telephone systems (Marsh, 1980). This presents an unfortunate situation for the elderly.

The ability to mask sounds, important for speech comprehension in a crowd of talking people, is considerably diminished in the elderly. Indeed, tests of hearing loss for pure tones provide usually conservative estimates of hearing deficits, as the tests are usually performed under quiet laboratory conditions, eliminating the need for masking. One example of loss of masking ability

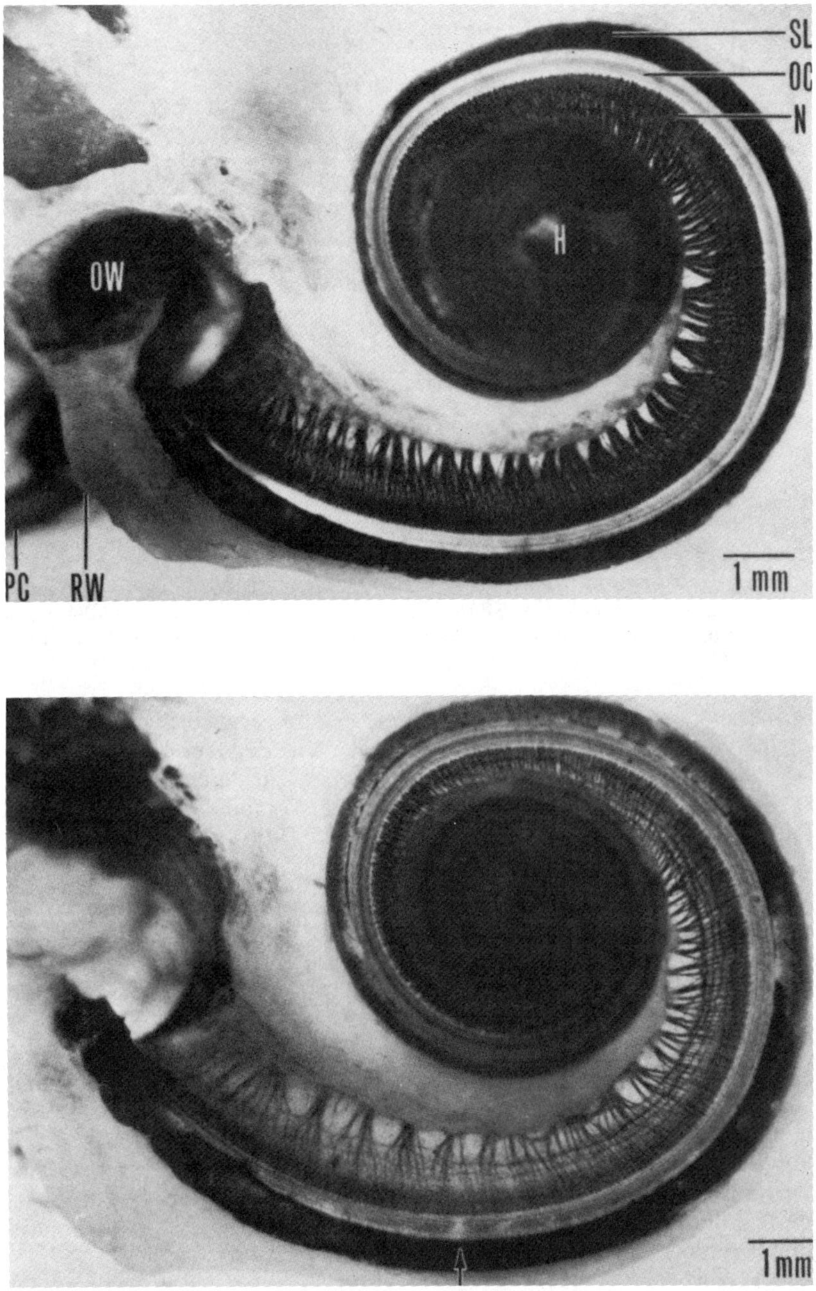

Figure 11–7. *Comparison of human cochlea of an elderly female (92 years,* bottom*) with a young adult female (25 years,* top*).*

Note diffuse degeneration of nerve cells as indicated by the sparseness of myelinated nerve fibers in the lower half of the basal turn; arrow points to a patchy degeneration of organ of Corti. (OW, oval window; RW, round window; PC, posterior canal and ampulla; SL, spiral ligaments; OC, organ of Corti seen as a dark band on the translucent basilar membrane; N, network of myelinated fibers and intralaminar spiral nerve fibers; H, helicotrema.). (Reproduced from Johnsson and Hawkins, 1972.)

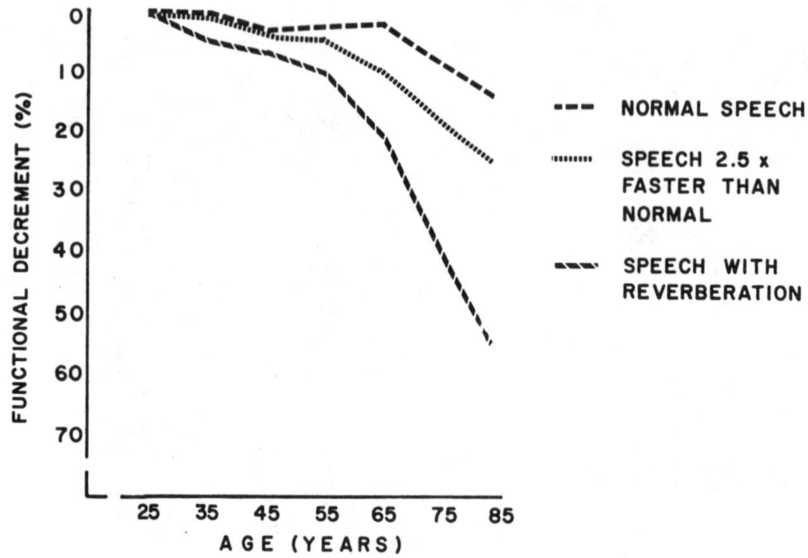

Figure 11–8. *Deficits in hearing speech at different ages; note the normal aging deficits are accentuated when speech is presented faster or with reverberations.* (Adapted and redrawn from a drawing in Marsh, 1980, based on original data of Bergman *et al.*, 1967.)

with age is the increase, with advancing age, in reporting the incidence of ringing in the ear, even though this problem is manifested at all ages. Perhaps the elderly cannot mask these unusual sounds, while the young can (Marsh, 1980).

Aging Changes in Auditory Centers. The frequently encountered degenerative aging changes in the neurons of spiral ganglia was discussed above (Schuknett, 1974; Johnsson and Hawkins, 1979). Aging changes in the central auditory structures were reviewed by Feldman and Vaughn (1979). Among the central auditory structures of the human brain no significant cell loss in the cochlear nuclei of medullary centers were found, although nuclear volume was significantly diminished after the age of 50, indicating loss of neuropil (dendrites, etc.). Neurons of cochlear nuclei show evidence of increased pigmentation (lipofuscin) with aging. Superior olivary nuclei also show shrunken neurons with pale and pyknotic nuclei; lipofuscin is absent, however. There is slight neuronal loss and some shrinkage in the midbrain and thalamic auditory centers (inferior colliculi and medial geniculate body).

In contrast to the lower centers, the human auditory cortex shows very marked and clear degenerative aging changes, consisting of a general thinning of the cortex and disrupted organization of the vertical columns; this is caused by heavy neuronal loss and degeneration. In his well-known study of the aging human cortex, Brody (1955) found the highest degree of cell loss to occur in the superior temporal gyrus, the anatomical locus of the auditory cortex; the loss, amounting to about 50 percent between the ages of 20 to 90, occurred across the cortical thickness. Golgi studies of pyramidal neurons of the auditory cortex by Scheibel *et al.* (1975) revealed marked degenerative changes in the basal dendrites of layers III and V neurons in old subjects (eighth to tenth decades).

Allison *et al.* (1984) have described significant changes in the auditory evoked potentials in the elderly, including increases in the latency and decreases in the amplitude of the response. The changes are more marked in males than in females and occur generally after age 60. Undoubtedly these degenerative changes contribute to the observed disorders of hearing and speech comprehension in the elderly, although an exact cause and effect relationship is still not established. For a summary of the nor-

Table 11–2. SUMMARY OF THE USUAL AGING CHANGES IN THE HUMAN EAR

Structural Changes

Hair cells degeneration:
- basal cochlea: frequent, especially in first quadrant; diffuse and patchy; main cause of *sensory presbycusis*
- apical cochlea: infrequent

Nerve cell degeneration:
- observed in spiral ganglia often with basal cochlear hair cell loss but not with apical cases (involved in *neural presbycusis*)
- is accompanied by loss of myelinated auditory nerve fibers

Atrophic changes:
- generally occur in nonneural components (vascular and connective tissue) of cochlea and lead to *strial* or *conductive* types of *presbycusis*
- in striae vascularis; frequent in the middle and apical turns of cochlea
- in spiral ligaments; accompanied with devascularization
- in inner and outer spiral vessels
- in Reissner's membrane, due to vacuolization
- in basilar membrane leading to mechanical damage

Central neural changes:
- little neuronal loss in lower auditory centers
- heavy loss in cortical auditory centers
- dendritic degeneration of cortical pyramidal neurons
- increased latency and decreased amplitude of auditory evoked potentials; effects more marked in elderly males than females

Functional Changes

Pure tone hearing:
- loss of hearing in the high frequency range (*presbycusis*): loss progressively worsens with age; effects more pronounced in males; noise exposure enhances loss
- decline in maximum sound frequency capable of being heard, from 20 KHz at 10 years to 4 KHz at 80 years

Speech perception:
- diminished ability to hear consonants; speech is heard but is unintelligible
- diminished ability to perceive reverberated and interrupted speech

Sound localization:
- diminished ability to localize sound sources, particularly high frequency ones

mal aging changes in the human ear see Table 11–2.

OLFACTION

The value of the sense of smell in life is underestimated by many except those who study it. Olfaction may be much more important for the elderly than is commonly appreciated, as is evidenced by the consequences of its loss. Anand (1964) found that a high proportion of the elderly die of accidents involving household gas poisoning, indicating that they are unable to smell gas leakage and be warned. Stevens and Cain (1986) have confirmed this and shown that the elderly have thresholds 10 times higher than the young for mercaptan substances added to natural gas for warning. Even when the elderly are able to smell gas, their perception of the stimulus intensity is generally poor, compared to the young groups. Similarly the sense of smell plays a great role in appetite regulation and food selection; its loss in the elderly may be one of the causes of poor appetite and irregular eating habits that result in deficient nutrition and weight loss. Indeed the perception of many flavors is thought to be dependent on the associated food odors (Murphy, 1987; Stevens and Cain, 1984). Additionally other aspects of the good life and a feeling of well-being depend in part on awareness of the aromas of flowers and perfumes and the avoidance of the putrid smells of rotten and infectious matter. Unfortunately olfactory deficiency or loss (hyposmia and anosmia), which is now believed to be widespread in the elderly, is bound to hinder these assets.

FUNCTIONAL CHANGES

Traditionally two types of approaches have been employed to study the functional aging of human olfaction. One approach measures changes in olfactory sensitivity by determining the threshold for various odors in subjects at different ages. In the second approach, designed to measure olfactory recognition and discrimination, the changes in the ability to identify different odors in a mixture are determined in different age groups.

Olfactory Sensitivity. In general, since the earliest study by Toulouse at the turn of the century (see McCartney, 1968 for references to this and other early works), several studies have indicated a decline in olfactory sensitivity with age as measured by increase in odor thresholds (minimum perceptible). For camphor odor, Toulouse found a threshold of a few parts in 100,000 in the young; in the old group, threshold

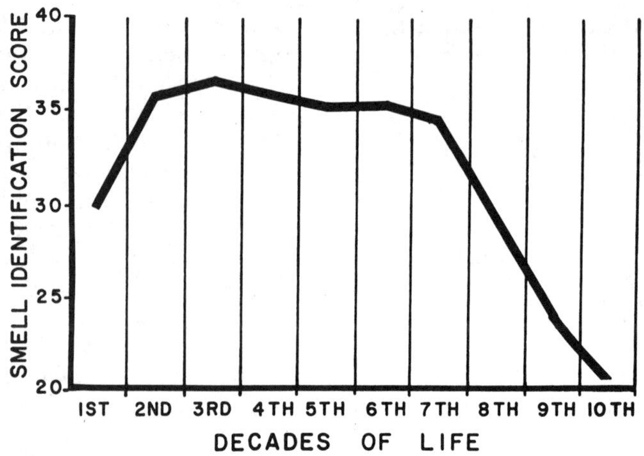

Figure 11–9. *The effect of aging on smell identification performance of humans at different ages.*

Testing is based on the UPSIT test, in which subjects are asked to identify 40 odorants using name cues provided in a forced-choice system. Maximum score is 40. Note marked decline in smell identification ability after the seventh decade. (Redrawn from data of Doty *et al.*, 1984.)

was about 10,000 times higher, women showing higher sensitivity in both age groups. Although the magnitude of this loss appears to be unusually high, the presence of hyposmia in the elderly is now an accepted fact.

More recent and controlled studies like those of Venstrom and Amoore (1968) and Strauss (1970) employing different methods have confirmed the decline in odor sensitivity with aging, although the decline is not as marked as indicated in the early works. In Venstrom and Amoore's study, thresholds in the different ages were compared to that of a middle age group (early forties), finding better sensitivity in the younger group and lower sensitivity in the older group; mean sensitivity showed a steady decline throughout the adult life from the early twenties to the late seventies. Stevens and Cain (1987) found higher absolute thresholds in the elderly compared to the young group. The increase varied depending on the odorant (ninefold for limoline, threefold for benzaldehyde and twofold for isoamylbutyrate).

Odor Identification Ability. Olfactory discrimination may be measured by the ability to identify the constituent odors of a mixture or identify by name or by visual association a host of odors presented to a subject. The effect of aging on these olfactory capacities have been determined in several studies. In one study Anand (1964) presented to subjects in different age groups a mixture containing odors of coffee, peppermint, coal tar, and almond oil. He found that with increasing age the ability to identify the constituent odors diminished. Thus, whereas nearly 70 percent of the subjects in the 20 to 40 years age group were able to detect all four odors, in the 40 to 60 age group, only 50 percent could do the same, and in the subjects in their sixties, 10 percent and those in their seventies, a mere 3 percent identified all four odors.

In a comprehensive study of changes in odor identification throughout the lifespan by Doty *et al.* (1984), 2,000 subjects in different age groups were tested for their smell identification ability according to the University of Pennsylvania Smell Identification Test (UPSIT). The results shown in Figure 11–9 indicated that the ability to identify the odors of different substances improves from childhood to adolescence, reaches a peak by the late teens and begins to decline in the sixth decade. The decline during the seventh and eighth decades is quite drastic; in the latter group nearly 60 percent show impairment in olfactory function and 25 percent are actually anosmic, in terms of identifying smells. In those over 80, 80 percent show impairments and 50 percent are anosmic. A major finding of these and previous similar studies is that women outperform men in olfactory abilities across all age groups, although they too show a similar pattern of aging decline.

NEURAL BASES OF OLFACTORY DECLINE

Olfactory Structures. The physiological and anatomical bases of the decline in olfactory abilities are not well understood, although cell loss seems to play a major part. Peripherally, the sense of smell is served by the bipolar olfactory receptor neurons located in the olfactory mucosa, a sheet of neuroepithelium covering the walls of superior nasal cavities. Dendrites of the olfactory neurons are ciliated. The cilia that protrude into the nasal cavity contain the presumed receptor sites for odor and are the chemoelectrical transducing elements. The axons of receptor cells enter the olfactory bulb after passage through the cribriform plate pores to synapse, in the olfactory glomeruli, with the dendrites of the mitral cells, the bulb's principal relay neurons. The axons of the mitral cells move through the olfactory tract into the brain to end in the cortical olfactory areas. The internal granule cells and the periglomerular cells of the olfactory bulb are small inhibitory neurons involved in integrative activity in the bulb.

As evident from this account, the cilia of the olfactory neurons are directly exposed to the environment of the nasal cavity. Therefore, the olfactory receptor neurons, more than any neurons of the nervous system, are subjected to environmental hazards, e.g., smoking and other airborne pollutants. It should be noted, however, that olfactory receptor neurons are unique in that they regenerate throughout life (Graziadei and Monti-Graziadei, 1978) in contrast to the other neurons of the nervous system. This ability is well proven for rodents, may be present in monkeys, but is not clearly proven in man.

Aging Changes. The human olfactory mucosa begins to show aging rather early in life. Thus while the mucosa in the fetus has a very healthy appearance, in the adult it contains patches of respiratory epithelium; even the olfactory epithelium shows a diminished number of receptor neurons and of other cellular elements like the basal and supporting cells (Nakashima *et al.*, 1984). With aging, this degeneration becomes so marked that in some aged humans there is complete loss of the olfactory sensory neurons (Naessen, 1971). Presumably the neuronal replacement process occurring in lower mammals does not occur in humans, or if it does, it is not successful in maintaining the olfactory mucosa of the adult and elderly in a healthy state.

Loss of neurons has been also demonstrated in the higher nerve centers associated with smell. Thus Smith (1942) showed that in the human olfactory bulbs a gradual atrophy of olfactory *glomeruli* occurs with age, at a rate of about 10 percent per decade so that in very old subjects fewer than 20 percent of the glomeruli remain. In a comprehensive study, Bhatnagar *et al.* (1987) have demonstrated a substantial loss of *mitral cells* in the human olfactory bulb. Thus, while total mitral cell number at age 25 is about 50,000, this is reduced to 30,000 at 60 years and 15,000 by the age of 90. Although the loss in mitral cells amounts to about 5000 per decade, most of the decline occurs after the sixth decade. These atrophic changes in the olfactory bulb are likely to be secondary to transneuronal effects caused by gradual loss of olfactory receptor neurons, as suggested by Liss and Gomez (1958) and Naessen (1971), although factors intrinsic to the bulb and brain cannot be ruled out. As the extremely high sensitivity of the olfactory system in odor detection is in part ascribed to the great number of the olfactory receptor neurons and to the high convergence ratio of these on the mitral cells, then a loss in these neuronal components may underlie the gradual decline in olfactory sensitivity. The causes of decline in odor identification ability may be more complex and relate to factors in the higher central nervous system as well.

Olfaction and Alzheimer's Disease. Recent research has linked the olfactory system with Alzheimer's disease, the major disease of the aging brain (see Serby, 1986 for review). Thus it has been argued that (1) Alzheimer's patients show particularly marked olfactory deficits, and (2) brain lesions (plaques and tangles) are found abundantly in the primary and secondary olfactory brain areas whereas they are absent from the primary sensory areas of other sensory systems. One speculation emerging is that agents causing Alzheimer's disease may enter the brain through the olfactory pathways and that the aging atrophy of the olfactory system may facilitate this transmission.

TASTE

Taste is served by special taste buds located in the taste papillae of the tongue and other parts of the oral cavity. Taste buds contain the taste cells, which are in synaptic contact with the gustatory sensory neurons; the latter transmit taste signals to the lower and higher brain gustatory sensory neurons. Four primary taste qualities—sour, sweet, salty, and bitter—are known for which specialized receptor sites within the taste cells are presumed to exist. The tongue is believed to be regionally specialized so that sweet sensation is detected in the tip, bitter in the back, salty and sour in the sides.

Aging Studies. Earlier studies indicated considerable loss of gustatory perception in the elderly, the loss being very marked for the salty taste and especially in men. Bitter tastes were affected less with aging than sweet and sour (see Marsh, 1980). Later studies, however, suggest that, compared to olfaction, taste is relatively spared by aging (Stevens *et al.,* 1984) and when affected, gustatory abilities decline less markedly with age. There is also less male-female differences, in contrast to olfactory aging.

Taste Sensitivity. Hughs (1969) and Murphy (1979) have summarized the studies on the effects of age on taste sensitivity. Although the findings of the different investigators are not as consistent as in olfaction studies, many report declines in sensitivity. Murphy measured absolute thresholds for various taste modalities in subjects ranging in age from 6 to 73 years, and found taste sensitivity to vary as a function of age and tastant, with no sex difference. Loss in sensitivity was steady and gradual, being in the order of 1 log unit, from a mean of about one part per 10,000 in the young adults to 1 per 1000 in the elderly group. The sensitivity decline is less marked for some substances (e.g., HCl) and marked for others (e.g., tartaric acid). Sucrose and NaCl showed similar decline patterns.

Quantitative measurement of taste threshold may be carried out in a different way by determining the amount of bitter-sour sensation produced by the passage of a mild galvanic current over the tongue surface (Hughs, 1969), the minimum current causing sensation being proportional to the taste threshold. This threshold current is found to increase linearly with age from a value of about 10 μamp during the third decade to 60 μamp in the elderly (Fig. 11–10).

Taste and Flavor Identification. When suprathreshold amounts of tastants are used, however, the aging decline in sensitivity is less noticeable. Nevertheless, a study by Schiffman (1977) concluded that the elderly's performance in recognition of various foods and complex flavors presented in real life situations is considerably diminished. Furthermore, while the elderly seems to rate the food qualities mainly on hedonic dimensions, the young group uses both the hedonic and tactile dimensions to describe their ratings.

Neural Basis of Gustatory Decline. Causes of the increase in taste threshold with aging may be related to the peripheral and/or central components of the gustatory system. Among the aging changes the best known is the decline in the number of taste buds and papillae (see Bradley, 1979 for review). Thus the number of fungiform papillae on the tongue tip shows a steady decline (50 percent) throughout the adult life, from about 60 in the young to about 30 in the sixth decade. In another study the number of taste buds on the circumvallate papillae (located on the back of the tongue) was found to decrease by more than 50 percent, but only after 50 years. Taste buds in the foliate papillae (on the lateral regions) show little aging decline. According to reports cited by Marsh (1980) the major loss of taste buds occurs earlier in women (40 to

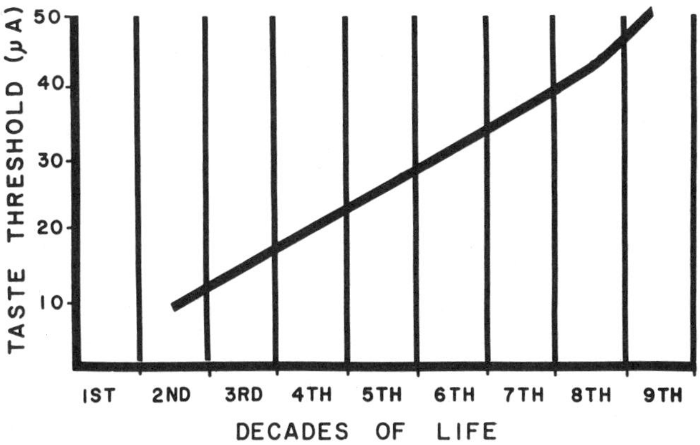

Figure 11–10. *Changes in taste threshold with age.*

Note steady increase in threshold with age, indicating gradual loss of sensitivity. Here taste thresholds are measured by determining minimum current (in microamperes) necessary to perceive a "taste" sensation. (Redrawn from data of Hughs, 1969.)

45 years) compared to men (50 to 60), suggesting involvement of gonadal hormones. Nevertheless, Mistretta (1984), who has reviewed the recent studies on taste buds and aging in humans and monkeys (who do not show any decline in taste bud number), considers the aging loss of taste buds to be less noteworthy than was formerly believed.

It is often assumed that the changes in the number of taste buds are one of the underlying causes of decline in sensitivity. However, this reduction may not affect the behavioral capacities related to taste, which are normally evoked with suprathreshold amounts of tastants (Bradley, 1979). In addition, aging changes in the tongue tissue (surface texture) and salivary secretion may play a part. Indeed the mouth in the elderly is drier due to decreased volume of salivary secretion and increased mucin content (Murphy, 1979). Activity of the salivary enzyme amylase, needed for the sensation of sweetness, is reduced in old age and may contribute to the functional results (Marsh, 1980). Little is known about the aging changes in the cerebral centers for the gustatory system. Nevertheless these changes must be occurring, since perception of complex flavors relating to foods and recognition of food qualities is considerably diminished in old age (Shiffmann, 1977) and it is reasonable to ascribe these effects to aging changes in the higher nervous centers.

SOMATIC SENSATIONS

Somatic sensory systems comprise a large group of sensations (touch, pressure, vibration, proprioception, heat and cold, pain) whose receptors are located in the skin, tendons, joints and viscera. A detailed account of aging changes in all these systems is clearly beyond this chapter's scope; hence only certain selected senses will be discussed.

FUNCTIONAL CHANGES

Touch. In humans, tactile sensitivity shows a wide variation in different parts, being very high in the palmar surface of fingertips, lips, and tongue tip while relatively low in the back, volar surfaces of hands and feet. Most studies have shown a decrease in tactile sensitivity with aging as measured by increased thresholds to touch stimuli. The aging effects may be illustrated by a recent study by Bruce (1980) who compared tactile thresholds on the different surfaces of the little finger in two groups of healthy elderly and young subjects and found the following significant elevations in thresholds with aging: 2.2 times on the palmar surface, 2.2 times on the lateral surface and 2.6 times on the dorsal surface.

Although tactile studies are more readily associated with areas such as hands, the eye's cornea has been a favorite test case, as the contribution of aging changes in the connective tissue to threshold determinations is less critical in the cornea than in the skin; in fact the skin shows great aging changes, including wide individual variation. Also corneal tactile receptors are simple and uniform nerve nets. Boberg-Ans (1956) found that in subjects 10 to 90 years corneal threshold to touch increases by threefold during the life span, the aging change being slow between 10 to 40 years and faster thereafter. Similar patterns of aging loss were found by Millodot with different absolute threshold values (see Kenshalo, 1979 for details).

Vibrotactile Sensation. A number of studies have reported a decline in sensitivity to vibrotactile stimulation. According to Cosh (1953), in the great toe pad, the threshold to vibratory stimulation at 100 Hz frequency shows about threefold increase between childhood (5 years) and extreme old age (90 years). This decline in sensitivity is significantly less marked for the index finger pad. Indeed, most of the clinical investigations in this area have indicated that the decline in vibratory sensitivity is more conspicuous for the lower extremities than in the upper ones (Kenshalo, 1979). The reason for this differential loss may lie in the higher loss of sensory nerve fibers from the lower spinal nerves (see also below).

It appears that the loss of sensitivity to vibratory stimuli may be valid only for the high frequency stimulation and not, as previously believed, for all frequencies. In a comprehensive study Verrillo (1980) also finds that vibrotactile sensitivity, measured at the thenar eminence of the right hand, progressively decreases with age. The decrease is negligible for low frequency stimuli (25 to 40 Hz) and very pronounced for high frequency ones (160 to 250 Hz). In Verrillo's study, the magnitude of the increase in vibrotactile threshold was found to be 3.00 dB per decade for 80 Hz stimulation; in the 160 to 250 range, the increase was 1, 1.5, 2.25, 3.5, and 6 dB in the second to sixth decades of life respectively.

Complex Somesthetic Abilities. Complex tactile abilities have also been tested in relation to aging. In the two-point discrimination test, which measures somatic spatial discrimination ability, the minimum separable distance between two-point stimuli (limen) presented simultaneously on the skin and still perceived as two points, is determined for the various body parts. Lowest limens are found for fingertips and lips (1 to 2 mm) and largest for the back of trunk and neck (30 to 70 mm). As evident by the data in Table 11–3, during aging the two-point limen increases in all body parts, although not to the same extent. The largest change occurs in the great toe pad (15 times) and the smallest in the palms (1.2 times).

Another complex tactoperceptual ability markedly affected by aging is stereognosis (shape recognition by touch). Thus, the elderly score consistently poorly in using blindfold manipulation to identify the objects (Kenshalo, 1979; Marsh, 1980). Similarly, objects placed on the tongue are identified with less precision by the aged group. A third interesting ability involves the ability to recognize body parts. When blindfolded subjects are touched simultaneously on the cheek and hand and asked to identify the parts contacted, they often reply, "the face." Upon successive testing, this "face-dominant" response diminishes in young adults but not in the elderly and young children (Bender *et al.*, 1952). Also brain-damaged patients retain face-dominant responses. The decline in stereognosis and perception of body parts is clearly connected to central neural changes related to the aging process.

Pain and Thermal Sensitivity. The study of the effect of aging on these sensory modalities are complicated by the fact that the responses of the subjects involve not just purely sensory elements, but also affective and cognitive factors such as tolerance, emotions, and habituation. There is also the problem of the descending central inhibitory systems of pain—the influence of which on the perception of pain in the el-

Table 11–3. COMPARISON OF SOME PARAMETERS OF SOMATIC SENSATION BETWEEN YOUNG AND ELDERLY HUMANS

PARAMETER	YOUNG*	ELDERLY*	CHANGE*
Two-point limen (mm)†			
hand palm	6	8	1.24x
thumb pad	2	4	1.7x
volar ring finger	2	4	2x
dorsal middle finger	3	7	2.5x
little finger pad	2	6	3x
thumb-index web space	6	18	3x
great toe pad	2	30	15x
Vibrotactile thresholds‡			
index finger pad	13	18	1.2x
great toe pad	16	34	2.1x
Tactile thresholds			
cornea (mg/sq mm)¶	12	30	2.5x
little finger (g)§			
lateral surface	0.16	0.36	1.9x
dorsal surface	0.19	0.50	2.6x
palmar surface	0.07	0.19	2.7x

*Young group, 20 to 30 years; elderly group, 60 to 80 years; the change is expressed as the elderly/young ratio of means.
†Two-point limen data are from Bolton, *et al.* (1966) and Gellis and Pool (1977), as quoted in Kensahalo (1977); means are rounded off to nearest mm.
‡Means in decibels (re: 1 micron displacement) from Cosh (1953) measured at 100 Hz vibration frequency, as quoted in Kenshalo (1979); according to Verrillo (1980) sensitivity loss is much greater at higher frequency, 160/250 Hz (19 dB in the thenar eminence between second to seventh decade).
¶From Boberg-Ans (1956) as quoted in Kensahalo, 1977.
§From Bruce (1980).

derly is not known. These problems may explain the contradictory reports in the literature as to the direction of change in sensitivity to pain and temperature with aging. Introduction of new methods to eliminate other biases has indicated decreased sensitivity to pain in the elderly. Sensitivity to temperature appears to show little change. The issues relating to perception of pain and temperature in the elderly are, however, far from resolved, and they are discussed in detail by Kenshalo (1979) and Marsh (1980) (see Chapter 26).

AGING LOSS OF CUTANEOUS MECHANORECEPTORS

The Meissner end organs and the Pacinian corpuscles are believed to mediate the sensations of fine touch and pressure/vibration respectively. The Meissner end organs are found mainly in the glabrous skin of the hand and feet; they show differential distribution even within the hand's palmar surface; their density is high in the fingertips (particularly in the index finger) and low in the thenar eminence. The high density of Meissner end organs in fingertips is believed to be responsible for the great tactile sensitivity of these areas. Pacinian corpuscles are found not only in the deeper layers of the palmar and solar skin but also around the joints and tendons.

Many studies, dating back to Meissner's own works (see Kenshalo, 1979; and Witkin, 1979 for reviews) have indicated a continuous decrease in the density of Meissner corpuscles with aging. According to Bolton *et al.* (1966) the density of Meissner corpuscles in the little finger declines nearly three times, from about 25/mm^2 during the second to third decades to about 8/mm^2 in the eighth decade; this is confirmed in a study by Bruce (1980), who notes similar declines in the lateral and dorsal surfaces of the finger and in both men and women. In the great toe pad where the density is 10/mm^2 in early adulthood, a comparable decline with aging occurs. Loss of similar magnitudes in the index finger have been reported by others (Cauna, 1965). Such declines are not limited to humans and have been observed in other primates as well. In the pigtail macaque monkey, between the ages of 5 to 20 years, a reduction of more than 50 percent in Meissner corpuscle density is observed in the thumb, index finger, and great toe (Witkin, 1979).

Aging changes in the Meissner corpuscles are not limited to a decline in number. They also show qualitative changes with aging (Cauna, 1965; Kenshalo, 1979). In the newborn infant the corpuscles are nearly spherical, growing in size and becoming elongated with age. In the young adult, each receptor organ, being cylindrical in shape, is attached to the epidermis superficially and to the elastic elements of the dermis basally. In old age the receptors appear more loosely anchored and become dissociated from the epidermis.

Loss of Pacinian corpuscles with age has also been demonstrated. During infancy the Pacinian corpuscle is small and oval, containing few concentric lamellae; with aging, addition of new lamellae increases the size and rigidity of the corpuscle and distorts its shape. There is also a gradual decrease in the number of Pacinian corpuscles with aging in the glabrous (hairless) skin (Cauna, 1965).

The causes of aging changes in the tactile receptors is not well understood. Clearly these receptors are able to regenerate throughout life, as evidenced by the return of tactile sensibility following repair of skin damage. On the other hand the regenerative capacity of many of these receptors depends on the integrity of their innervation. Therefore the age-related loss in number may reflect changes in fiber branching or fiber number. Physiologic declines in fiber activity or axoplasmic transport of trophic substances may also be involved. Declines in the number of sensory fibers innervating the periphery may also occur with old age. A decrease of up to 30 percent in the number of myelinated fibers in the sensory nerve and in the spinal sensory roots have been observed in old age (Gardner, 1940). In extreme cases these declines may underlie the observed senile peripheral neuropathies.

Although morphological aging changes in the Meissner and Pacinian corpuscles clearly influence their physiologic properties, it is generally believed that, at least with regard to simple tactile abilities, such as sensitivity, the loss in receptor number can best explain the observed functional deficits in the aged, particularly at the peripheral level. Specifically, a reduction in tactile receptor number, by decreasing receptor recruitment, can cause increased tactile thresholds; also decline in receptive field overlap may explain the decreased capacity for spatial discrimination as revealed by the two-point discrimination test. Qualitative aging changes in the morphology of the tactile receptors may be involved in causation of the more complex functional changes.

CENTRAL NEURAL CHANGES

As mentioned previously, loss of sensory fibers and neurons in peripheral nerves and spinal sensory roots have been reported, particularly for the lower extremities (Gardner, 1940). Thinning of the cortex and cell loss in the somatic sensory area are also observed, although not to the same extent as in the auditory cortex (Brody, 1977). Nevertheless, electrophysiological studies indicate that somatic sensory evoked potentials show diminished amplitude and increased latency in the elderly (after 60 years), suggesting significant structural and functional changes, such as fiber loss, reduced myelination, and decreased conduction velocity, as well as synaptic changes in the peripheral and central sensory pathways and sensory cortex (Allison *et al.*, 1984). Here, as in visual and auditory systems, the changes are more marked in males than females.

Bibliography

Allison, T.; Hume, A. L.; Wood, C. C.; and Goff, W. R.: Developmental and aging changes in somatosensory, auditory and visual evoked potentials. *Electroenceph. Clin. Neurophysiol.*, **58:**14–24, **1984.**

Anand, M. P.: Accidents at home. In Anderson, W. F., and Isaacs, B. (eds.): *Conference on Medical and Surgical Aspects of Aging. [Current Achievements in Geriatrics]*, Cassell, London, **1964,** pp. 239–245.

Bender, M. B.; Fink, M.; and Green, M.: Patterns in perception on simultaneous tests of the face and hand. *Arch. Neurol. Psychiat.*, **66:**355–362, **1952.**

Bolton, C. F.; Winkelman, R. K.; and Dyke, P. J.: A quantitative study of Meissner's corpuscles in man. *Neurology*, **16:**1–9, **1966.**

Bergman, M.; Blumensfeld, V. G.; Cascardo, D.; Dash, B.; Levitt, H.; and Margulies, M. K.: Age related decrement in hearing for speech: Sampling and longitudinal studies. *J. Gerontol.*, **31:**533–538, **976.**

Bhatnagar, K. P.; Kennedy, R. C.; Baron, G.; and Greenberg, R. A.: Number of mitral cells and the bulb volume in the aging human olfactory bulb: A quantitative morphological study. *Anat. Rec.,* **218**:73–87, **1987.**

Boberg-Ans, J.: On the corneal sensitivity. *Acta Ophthalmol.,* **34**:149–162, **1956.**

Bradley, R. M.: Effects of aging on the sense of taste: Anatomical considerations. In Han and Coons (eds.), *op. cit.,* pp. 3–8, **1979.**

Bradley, R. M.: The effect of aging on the olfactory sense. In Han and Coons (eds.), *op. cit.,* pp. 34–42, **1979.**

Brody, H.: Organization of the cerebral cortex. III. A study of aging in the human cerebral cortex. *J. Comp. Neurol.,* **102**:511–556, **1955.**

Brody, H., and Vijayashankar, N.: Anatomical changes in the nervous system. In Finch, C., E., and Hayflick, L. (eds.): *Handbook of the Biology of Aging,* Van Nostrand, New York, **1977,** pp. 241–261.

Bruce, M. F.: The relation of tactile thresholds to histology in the fingers of the elderly. *J. Neurol. Neurosurg. and Psychiat.,* **43**:730–734, **1980.**

Cauna, N.: The effects of aging on the receptor organs of the human dermis. In Montagna, W. (ed.): *Advances in Biology of Skin—Aging,* Vol. VI, Pergamon Press, New York, **1965.**

Dark, A. J.; Streeten, B. W.; and Jones, D.: Accumulation of fibrillar protein in the aging human lens capsule. *Arch. Ophthal.,* **82**:815–821, **1969.**

Dolman, C. L.; Mccormick, A. O.; and Drance, S. M.: Aging of the optic nerve. *Arch. Ophthalmol.,* **98**:2052–2058, **1980.**

Doty, R. L.; Shaman, P.; Applebaum, S. L.; Giberson, R.; Sikorski, L.; and Rosenberg, L.: Smell identification ability changes with age. *Science,* **226**:1441–1443, **1984.**

Duane, A.: Accommodation. *Arch. Ophthalmol.,* **5**:1–14, **1931.**

Feldman, M. L., and Vaughn, D. W.: Changes in the auditory pathway with age. In Han and Coons (eds.), *op. cit.,* pp. 143–162, **1979.**

Friedenwald, J. S.: Permeability of the lens capsule, with special reference to etiology of senile cataract. *Arch. Ophthalmol.,* **3**:182–193, **1930.**

Gardner, E. D.: Decrease in human neurons with age. *Anat. Rec.,* **77**:529–536, **1940.**

Graham, P.: The eye. In Pathy, M. S. J. (ed.): *Principles and Practice of Geriatric Medicine,* Wiley, London, **1985,** pp. 833–844.

Graziadei, P. P. C., and Monti-Graziadei, G. A.: Continuous nerve cell renewal in the olfactory system. In Jacobson, M. (ed.): *Handbook of Sensory Physiology,* Vol. IX, *Development of Sensory Systems,* Springer-Verlag, Berlin, **1978,** pp. 55–83.

Han, S. S., and Coons, D. H. (eds.): *Special Senses in Aging,* Institute of Gerontology, University of Michigan, Ann Arbor, **1979.**

Hughs, G.: Changes in taste sensitivity with advancing age. *Gerontol. Clin.,* **11**:224–230, **1969.**

Jerger, J., and Hays, D.: Diagnostic speech audiometry. *Arch. Otolaryngol.,* **103**:216–222, **1977.**

Johnsson, L., and Hawkins, J. E., Jr.: Sensory and neural degeneration with aging, as seen in microdissections of the human inner ear. *Ann. Otol.,* **81**:1–15, **1972.**

Johnsson, L., and Hawkins, J. E., Jr.: Age related degeneration of the inner ear. In Han and Coons (eds.), *op. cit.,* pp. 119–136, **1979.**

Kenshalo, D. R., Sr.: Aging effects on cutaneous and kinesthetic sensibilities. In Han and Coons (eds.), *op. cit.,* pp. 189–218, **1979.**

Kuwabara, T.: Age related changes of the eye. In Han and Coons (eds.), *op. cit.,* pp. 46–78, **1979.**

Lewis, R. A.: Macular degeneration in the aged. In Han and Coons (eds.), *op. cit.,* pp. 93–100, **1979.**

Liss, L., and Gomez, F.: The nature of senile changes of the human olfactory bulb and tract. *Arch. Otolaryngol.,* **67**:157–171, **1958.**

Marsh, G. Perceptual changes with aging. In Busse, E. W., and Blazer, D. G. (eds.): *Handbook of Geriatric Psychiatry,* Van Nostrand, New York, **1980.**

Mauer, J. F., and Rupp, R. R.: *Hearing and Aging: Tactics for Intervention,* Grune and Stratton, New York, **1979.**

McCartney, W.: *Olfaction and Odours,* Springer, Berlin, **1968,** pp. 176–182.

McFarland, R. A.; Warren, A. B.; and Karris, C.: Alterations in critical flicker frequency as a function of age and light-dark ratio. *J. Expt. Psychol.,* **56**:529–535, **1958.**

McFarland, R. A.; Domey, R. G.; Warren, A. B.; and Ward, D. C.: Dark adaptation as a function of age. I. A statistical analysis. *J. Gerontol.,* **15**:149–154, **1960.**

Mills, R.: The auditory system. In: Pathy, M. S. J. (ed.) *Principles and Practice of Geriatric Medicine,* Wiley, London, **1985,** pp. 841–853.

Mistretta, C. M.: Aging effects on anatomy and neurophysiology of taste and smell. *Gerodontology,* **3**:131–136, **1984.**

Murphy, C.: The effect of age on taste sensitivity. In Han and Coons (eds.), *op. cit.,* pp. 21–32, **1979.**

Murphy, C.: Olfactory psychophysics. In Finger, T. E., and Silver, W. L. (eds.): *Neurobiology of Taste and Smell,* Wiley, New York, **1987,** pp. 251–274.

Naessen, R.: An enquiry on the morphological characteristics and possible changes with age in the olfactory region of man. *Acta Otolaryngol.,* **71**:49–62, **1971.**

Nakashima, T.; Kimmelman, P.; and Snow, J. B.: Structure of human fetal and adult olfactory neuroepithelium. *Arch. Otolaryngol,* **10**:641–646, **1984.**

Ordy, J. M., and Brizzee, K. (eds.): *Sensory Systems and Communication in the Elderly,* Raven Press, New York, **1979.**

Pitts, D. G. The effects of aging on selected visual function: Dark adaptation, visual acuity, steriopsis, and brightness contrast. In Sekuler, R.; Kline, D.; and Dismukes, K. (eds.): *Aging and human visual function,* Liss, New York, **1982,** pp. 131–159.

Rosen, S. *et al.*: Presbycusis study of a relatively noise-free population in the Sudan. *Ann. Otol.,* **71**:727–743, **1962.**

Sarks, S. H.: Aging and degeneration in the macular region. A clinicopathological study. *Brit. J. Ophthalmol.,* **60**:324–341, **1976.**

Scheibel, M.; Lindsay, R. D.; Tomiyasu, V.; and Scheibel, A. B.: Progressive dendritic changes in aging human cortex. *Exp. Neurol.,* **47**:392–403, **1975.**

Schuknett, H. F.: *Pathology of the Inner Ear,* Harvard University Press, Cambridge, Mass., **1974,** pp. 388–403; *ibid.* Further observations on the pathology of presbycusis, *Arch. Otolaryngol.,* **80**:369–382, **1964.**

Sekuler, R.; Kline, D.; and Dismuskes, K. (eds.): *Aging and Human Visual Functions,* Liss, New York, **1982.**

Serby, M.: Olfaction and Alzheimer's disease. *Prog. Neuro-Psychopharmacol. & Biol. Psychiat.,* **10**:579–586, **1986.**

Shiffman, S. S.: Food recognition by the elderly. *J. Gerontol.,* **32**:586–592, **1977.**

Smith, C. G.: Age incidence of atrophy of olfactory nerves in man. A contribution to the study of the process of aging. *J. Comp. Neurol.,* **77**:589–596, **1942.**

Spencer, J. T., Jr.: Hyperlipoproteinemia in the etiology of inner ear disease. *Laryngoscope,* **83**:639–678, **1973.**

Spoor, A.: Presbycusis values in relation to noise induced hearing loss. *Inter. Audiol.,* **6**:48–57, **1967.**

Stevens, J. C.; Bartoshuk, L. M.; and Cain, W. S.: Chemical senses and aging: taste versus smell. *Chemical Sens.,* **9**:167–179, **1984.**

Stevens, J. C., and Cain, W. S.: Aging impairs the ability to perceive gas odor. *Chem. Senses,* **11679, 1986.**

Stevens, J. C., and Cain, W. S.: Old age deficits in the sense of smell as gauged by thresholds, magnitude matching and odor identification. *Psychology and Aging,* **2**:36–42, **1987.**

Strauss, E. L.: A study on olfactory acuity. *Ann. Otol.,* **79**:1–10, **1970.**

Venstrom, D., and Amoore, J. E.: Olfactory thresholds in relation to age, sex or smoking. *J. Food Sci.,* **33**:264–265, **1968.**

Verriest, G.: L'influence de l'age sur les fonctions visuelles de l'homme. *Bull. Acad. R. Med. Belg.,* **11**:527–577, **1971.**

Verrillo, R. T.: Age related changes in the sensitivity to vibration. *J. Gerontol.,* **35**:185–193, **1980.**

vibration. *J. Gerontol.,* **35**:185–193, **1980.**

Weale, R. A.: *The Aging Eye,* H. K. Lewis, London, **1963.**

Weale, R. A.: *Focus on Vision,* Harvard University Press, Cambridge, Mass., **1982,** Chap. 3.

Weiss, A. D.: Auditory perception in relation to age. In Birren, J. *et al.* (eds.): *Human Aging,* U.S. Government Printing Office, Washington, D. C., **1963,** pp. 111–140.

Witkin, J.: Peripheral tactile innervation. In Bowden, D. M. (ed.): *Aging in Nonhuman Primates,* Van Nostrand, New York, **1979,** pp. 158–170.

CHAPTER

12 AGING OF ADRENALS AND PITUITARY

Neuroendocrinology of Homeostasis and Stress

Together with the nervous system, the endocrine system coordinates homeostatic responses to environmental signals for the protection of the individual organism and regulates reproductive functions for the perpetuation of the species. With aging, the main expressions of declining functional competence are cessation of reproduction and diminishing capacity to adapt to external demands, especially those involving stress conditions (see Chapters 1 to 3). The aging-related decline in physiologic competence has been ascribed to endocrine deficiency because of the wide range of action of hormones, many necessary for reproduction and survival, and because of the possibility of restorating "vitality" and "well-being" through hormonal replacement therapy.

Endocrine glands are organs that produce and secrete hormones. Reciprocally hormones are molecules synthesized and secreted by specialized (endocrine) cells and released into the blood. They exert biochemical effects on target cells at a distance from their site of origin. This view has expanded, however, and we are now aware of cells or groups of cells that do not form discrete organs but are interspersed with other cells and also produce and secrete hormones. Examples of classic endocrines include the pituitary, adrenals, thyroid and parathyroids, testes, and ovaries. Example of the more diffuse hormone-producing cells are those of the pancreas and intestinal mucosa. Some of the neurotransmitters, described previously (Chapter 9), are also considered hormones. Local-acting substances that either directly stimulate neighboring cells, such as prostaglandins, or promote growth, such as the various growth factors, are also considered hormones and, therefore, part of the endocrine system. The wide distribution of hormone-secreting cells, peripheral nerves, and neural ganglia and the multiciplicity and diversity of secretory products underline the critical role of endocrine and neural coordination of body functions.

Among the endocrine glands, the adrenals regulate certain aspects of metabolism, behavior, and nervous function and, as such, play a key role in homeostasis. The pituitary secretes several hormones and peptides that stimulate peripheral targets, either other endocrine glands or specific tissues and organs; its location in close vicinity to the hypothalamus, with which it articulates through a vascular net (the portal system) and through direct neuronal connections, gives the pituitary the unique function of intermediary between nervous and endocrine systems. Like all endocrine glands, the adrenals and pituitary do not act in isolation, but are dependent both on neuroendocrine signals, usually relayed through or initiated in the hypothalamus, and on the functional status of the target cells. Thus, aging of these and, in fact, of all endocrines depends on aging changes within the gland as well as various age-related factors: aging changes of other endocrines and of the nervous system, of metabolism and body composition, of cellular and molecular responses; the complications of disease, medications, drugs; and the influence of diet and exercise (Table 12–1). Also important are socioeconomic and emotional conditions and methods of assessment (see Chapter 2). In this, as in the subsequent chapters on endocrine aging, we shall consider (1) changes of the endocrine glands themselves, here adrenals and pituitary, and (2) their neuroendocrine and metabolic interrelations, here their role in homeostatic adjustments and adaptation to stress.

Endocrine and neural involvement in aging has led to the formulation of neuroendocrine theories of aging (see Chapter 4). These theories propose that aging is not due to intrinsic deterioration of cells or molecules, but rather to a programmed regulation by "pacemaker cells," possibly situated in the brain and acting through neural and endocrine signals. These signals would orchestrate the passage from one stage of the lifespan to the other, thereby timing the

Table 12–1. FACTORS CONTRIBUTING TO ENDOCRINE AGING

1. Endogenous Factors
   Endocrine
   Neural
   Body composition
   Target cells and molecules
   Disease
2. Exogenous Factors
   Disease
   Medications
   Drugs, including smoking and alcohol
   Diet
   Exercise
   Social factors

entire life cycle, including development, growth, maturation, and aging. While these theories remain for the most part speculative and their general applicability remains difficult in view of the large range and diversity of senescent phenomena among multicellular organisms, they are amenable to experimental manipulation and therefore provide a useful tool to investigate aging processes. Some of the clinical observations and experimental evidence in support of the involvement of neural and endocrine factors in aging are presented in this and in the subsequent chapters on aging of endocrines.

ASSESSMENT OF ENDOCRINOLOGIC FUNCTION

Evaluation of endocrine function in humans often relies on measurements of blood levels under basal (resting or steady state) and stress conditions. However, such an evaluation is not only incomplete but may, in fact, lead to erroneous conclusions. An adequate endocrine evaluation must include several levels of endocrine action as well as interendocrine and neuroendocrine relations, hormone receptor interaction at the target cell, and molecular events inside the cell. A prototypic endocrine system, illustrated in Figure 12–1, shows hierarchical levels of endocrine regulation and provides a framework for investigating endocrine changes with aging. Although aging changes may occur at several levels of the CNS-endocrine axis, none of these changes may, by itself, be sufficient to alter homeostatic competence, but a cascade of minor alterations may result in a desynchronization of the appropriate signal at the target cell or molecule and lead to alterations in hormonal actions.

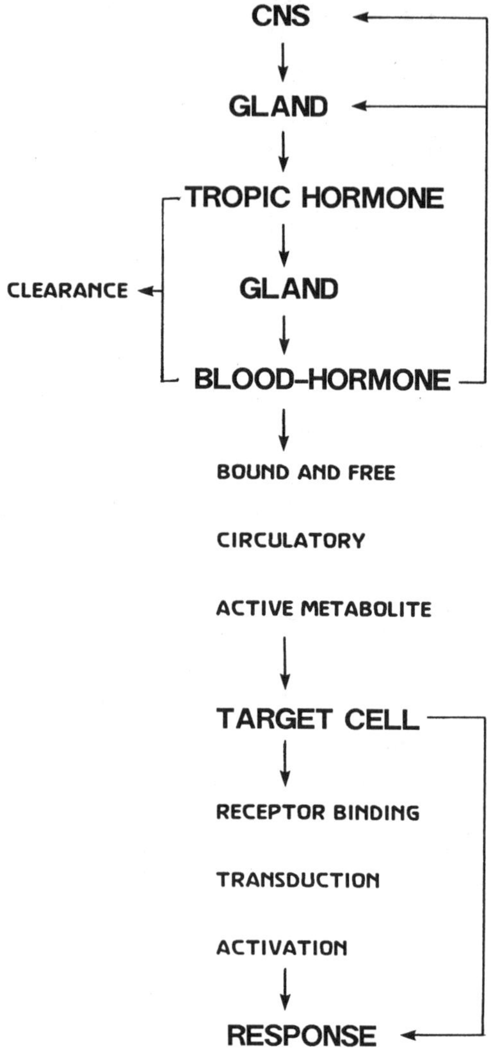

Figure 12–1. *Diagrammatic representation of a typical sequence of hormone action and regulation.*

This more "global" approach to the study of endocrine aging cannot be easily undertaken in humans with current biomedical knowledge. Experimental animals and cultured tissues or cells serve as *in vivo* and *in vitro* models for human studies.

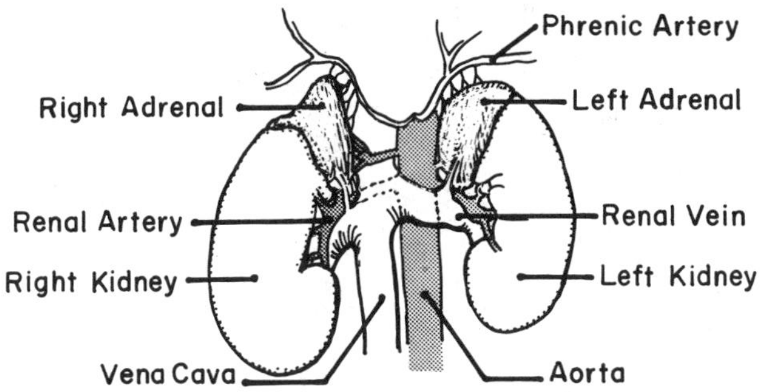

Figure 12–2. *Diagram of the kidney and adrenals. (Drawing by S. Oklund.)*

SOME GENERIC ENDOCRINE CHANGES WITH AGING

Following the diagram in Figure 12–1, changes with aging may occur at all levels of the endocrine system. At the endocrine gland level, weight loss, with atrophy, vascular changes, and fibrosis occur in most cases with or without the accompaniment of adenomas. Basal hormone levels (free, biologically active hormones or hormones bound to plasma proteins) in humans and animals are generally not influenced by age, although some hormones decrease significantly. Regulation of hormone release depends on nervous and environmental stimuli as well as positive and negative feedback from circulating hormones.

Some hormones act exclusively on one target; other hormones act on many cell types by various mechanisms. Thus, the same hormone may have different actions on different tissues. With aging, one of the many actions or one of the many targets may be selectively affected while other actions and targets are preserved.

Secretory and clearance rates often decrease, although it is not clear whether the primary defect involves hormone secretion or hormone clearance, but the question is to what extent the capacity to maintain stable levels of plasma hormones is preserved. The study of the generation of active metabolites may reveal how the rate of hormone production is altered with advancing age.

The specificity of hormones depends on the particular receptors located on target cells, whereas the cellular response is determined by the genetic programming of the particular cell. With aging, receptor binding and intracellular responses vary greatly depending on the hormone and target cell.

Several reviews on the aging of endocrines have been published in the last few years and the reader is referred to these for a detailed discussion (Gregerman and Bierman, 1974; Everitt and Burgess, 1976; Andres and Tobin, 1977; Dilman, 1981; Adelman and Roth, 1982; Frolkis, 1982; Cole *et al.*, 1982; Green, 1985; Minaker *et al.*, 1985; Timiras, 1985). In this and in the following four chapters, we shall succinctly summarize the salient actions of each endocrine gland in the adult and then outline the major changes during aging, with emphasis on neuroendocrine regulation and metabolic interactions.

THE ADRENAL CORTEX

The adrenals are paired glands that lie above the kidneys (Figure 12–2). They have an inner *medulla* and an outer *cortex* (Figure 12–3). The medulla can be considered a sympathetic ganglion: it secretes catecholamines, epinephrine, and norepinephrine. The cortex secretes several hormones, aldosterone—necessary to sustain life—and cortisol—involved in important metabolic functions.

Major Adrenocortical Hormones and Their Actions. Hormones of the adrenal cortex are steroids; they can be distinguished as: glucocorticoids, such as cortisol; and sex hormones, such as dehydroepiandrosterone (DHEA) secreted by the cells of the zona fasciculata and zona reticularis; mineralocorticoids, such as aldosterone, secreted by the cells of the zona glomerulosa; and corticosterone secreted by all three cortical layers (Figure 12–3).

The metabolic actions of *glucocorticoids* are to

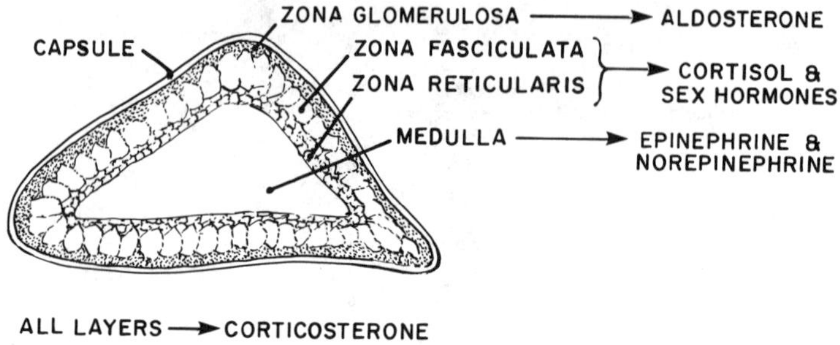

Figure 12–3. *Diagram of a section of the adrenals illustrating the various zones and hormones. (Drawing by S. Oklund.)*

increase amino acid uptake and gluconeogenesis in liver but to decrease amino acid uptake and protein synthesis in muscle. They inhibit somatic growth due to a general catabolic (decreased protein synthesis) action and suppression of pituitary growth hormone secretion; they possess an antiinsulin effect with consequent exacerbation of diabetes; they mobilize serum lipids and cholesterol.

Glucocorticoids have antiinflammatory activity, when administered in supraphysiologic doses. They inhibit inflammatory and allergic reactions, including immune responses. These immunosuppressive actions, utilized for the prevention of transplant rejections and the symptomatic treatment of allergies, have been explained by several mechanisms (e.g., inhibition of leukocyte migration from blood to tissues, decreased number of circulating lymphocytes, and reduced antibody production).

Glucocorticoids also have effects on the nervous system, primarily excitatory, evidenced by the presence of hormone receptors on neurons and glia, induction of neurotransmitter enzymes, EEG changes, and increased convulsibility.

Through their negative feedback on hypothalamus and pituitary, they inhibit the secretion of adrenocorticotropic hormone (ACTH) from the pituitary and corticotropin-releasing hormone (CRH) from the hypothalamus—the higher the levels of the circulating hormones, the lower the secretion of ACTH and CRH; the lower their levels, the greater the ACTH and CRH release.

Other actions of glucocorticoids include: retention of sodium by renal tubules (but much less efficacious than aldosterone), reabsorption of bone and altered calcium metabolism, promotion of appetite and increased stomach acid and pepsin secretion, maintenance of work capacity.

Aldosterone, the major mineralocorticoid, is indispensable for survival. It increases sodium reabsorption from the renal tubular fluid, saliva, and gastric juice. In the kidney, aldosterone acts on the epithelium of the distal tubule and collecting duct where it facilitates the exchange of sodium for potassium and hydrogen ions. It may also increase potassium and decrease sodium in muscle and brain cells.

Secondary actions include: maintenance of blood pressure (as a consequence of sodium-water retention and increased blood volume); moderate potassium diuresis; and increased urine acidity (sodium taken up is exchanged for potassium and hydrogen ions that are excreted).

Sex hormones (primarily androgens, but also some estrogens) have minor masculinizing effects and anabolic actions (i.e., promote protein synthesis).

CHANGES UNDER BASAL CONDITIONS

With aging, the adrenal cortex decreases in weight in men and women and several animals and shows the frequent occurrence of nodules (i.e., multifocal adenomas or localized hyperplastic changes perhaps reactive to a reduced blood supply). The adrenocortical cells, typical secretory cells, rich in mitochondria and endoplasmic reticulum, with droplets indicating steroid hormones storage, undergo numerous changes. The most important are accumulation of lipofuscin granules (see Chapter 5) and the thickening of the connective support tissue shown by the thick capsule and the perivascular fibrous infiltrations.

Despite these anatomic and histologic changes, basal plasma glucocorticoid levels do not differ significantly from maturity to old age in humans and other animal species (cows, goats, dogs, monkeys) (Riegle and Nellor, 1967; Riegle *et al.,* 1968; Bowman and Wolf, 1969; Jensen and Blichert-Toft, 1971; Breznock and McQueen, 1970). In contrast to glucocorticoids, aldosterone values are almost undetectable past age 65 (Flood *et al.,* 1967), and DHEA, with values at age 60 and older approximately one-third of those at age 30 (Migeon *et al.,* 1957), declines with aging.

Hormonal secretion rate appears to be

reduced for all steroids (Samuels, 1957; Romanoff *et al.*, 1961; Serio *et al.*, 1969). In the case of glucocorticoids with plasma levels normal, the lower secretory rate is compensated by decreased clearance, that is, reduced excretion and metabolism. The reduced urinary excretion rate, however, disappears when the urinary values are adjusted to creatinine excretion, which is also decreased with aging (see Chapter 20). Compensation, therefore relies primarily on a decreased rate of removal of cortisol from the circulation, well demonstrated in individuals aged 60 and older (West *et al.*, 1961). This decline has been ascribed to a number of factors: decreased blood flow to the liver (a metabolizing organ), or decreased liver size associated with aging, or decreased activity of liver enzymes involved in cortisol metabolism (Singer and Burns, 1978), or decreased cortisol binding to liver cytosol (Latham and Finch, 1976). It is apparent that, at least for cortisol, metabolic compensatory mechanisms remain intact during aging, with the body adapting either to the decline in rate of removal of the hormone by decreasing production rates of this compound or, vice versa, reducing the rate of removal to maintain normal circulating hormonal levels. The latter explanation may be the most appropriate when considering the declining secretory rate and levels of aldosterone (Hegstad *et al.*, 1983) and DHEA (Orentreich *et al.*, 1984). In the case of these hormones, however, metabolic compensatory adjustments fail to occur.

DHEA Replacement Therapy. The marked reduction in DHEA secretion and levels with aging has led to the speculation that reduction of this major androgen may be responsible for some of the aging decrements. Historically, it may be recalled that one of the first associations between endocrines and aging, as well as one of the primary secretory actions attributed to an organ (the testis), were drawn by the French physiologist Brown-Sequard who extolled the antiaging properties of testicular secretions (androgens) (Timiras, 1983). Testicular transplants and administration of androgens as rejuvenating measures have been attempted repeatedly to delay or reverse aging, but with little success. On this same basis, replacement therapy with DHEA has been suggested and its effects explored in animals. Indeed, long-term DHEA administration in mice has reduced the incidence of mammary cancer, increased survival, and delayed onset of immune dysfunction. The simultaneous reduction in body weight and food intake suggests that the hormone may act in a manner similar to caloric restriction, which also retards tumor development and immunologic senescence (see Chapter 25). Use of this hormone in humans as an antiaging agent is, until now, not warranted without adequate proof of its direct efficacy.

CHANGES UNDER DYNAMIC CONDITIONS

The response of adrenocortical hormones to stimulation has been studied extensively because of its relation to adaptative capability (which is decreased) and survival (which is endangered) in the elderly.

Regulation of Adrenocortical Secretion. As illustrated diagrammatically in Figure 12–4, the adrenal cortex has a hierarchy of regulation, from the hypothalamus, to the pituitary and then to the adrenal. With aging and under conditions of stress, a disruption of this complex regulatory system at one or more levels may result in failure of homeostasis and adaptation.

Corticotropin-releasing hormone (*CRH*), a polypeptide, is released from the median eminence of the hypothalamus; it is transported, via the portal system, a special capillary system carrying, directly, secretory products from hypothalamus, to the anterior pituitary where it stimulates synthesis and release of the adrenocorticotropic hormone (ACTH).

ACTH, a protein, stimulates the adrenal cortex to synthesize and release the glucocorticoids and sex hormones from the two inner zones of the cortex. Thus, after ablation of the pituitary, these two zones atrophy and the levels of the corresponding hormones decrease. Conversely, in tumors of the pituitary in which ACTH levels are increased (as may occur in Cushing's disease), the two adrenocortical zones hypertrophy and the hormonal levels are increased. CRH, ACTH, and glucocorticoid secretions are interregulated by feedbacks operating at each level, with low levels of adrenocortical hormones acting to increase CRH secretion and CRH stimulating ACTH release, which, in turn, stimulates adrenal cortex secretion.

Aldosterone secretion is stimulated only to a minor degree by ACTH and, therefore, removal of the pituitary does not produce atrophy of the outer adrenal layer. Aldosterone secretion is regulated in part by the circulating levels of sodium and potassium: that is, low sodium levels and high potassium levels stimulate secretion. Most important in the control of aldosterone secretion is the *renin-angiotensin system*: that is, the secretion of the enzyme renin from the juxtaglomerular cells of the kidney and its action to transform the circulating hepatic protein, angiotensinogen, into the decapeptide angiotensin I. This, in turn, is

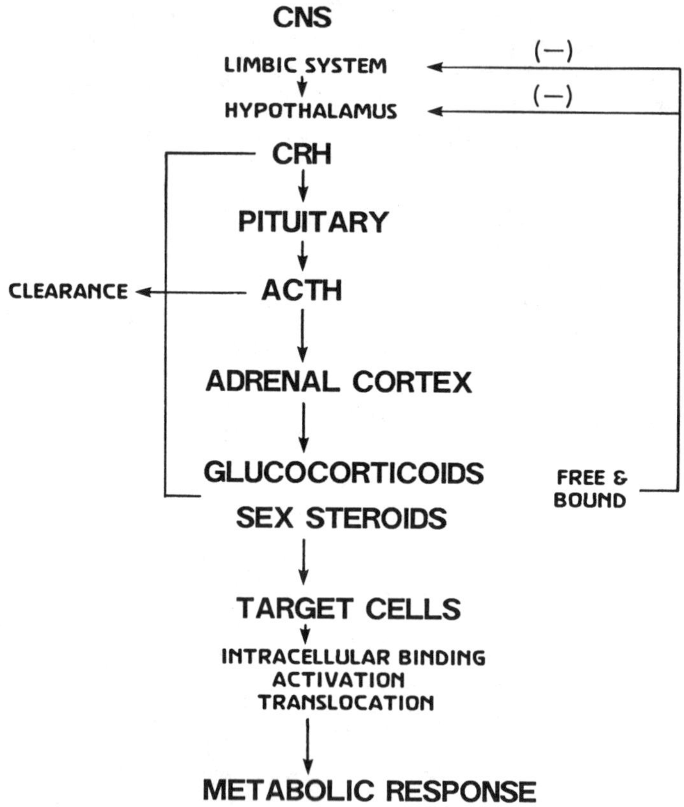

Figure 12–4. *Diagrammatic representation of the hypothalamo-pituitary-adreno-cortical axis.*

transformed into the octapeptide angiotensin II, which, then, stimulates the release of aldosterone.

Excess glucocorticoids, as in Cushing's disease, lead to abnormalities of intermediary metabolism; excess aldosterone, as in Conn's disease, leads to hypertension and electrolyte disturbances; adrenocortical insufficiency, involving both gluco- and mineralocorticoids, as in Addison's disease, leads to hypotension, shock, and death.

A number of animal species have been examined for glucocorticoid response to ACTH administration or to endogenous ACTH increase by a variety of stressful stimuli at young, adult, and old ages. Several animals have responded with a lesser increase in glucocorticoid levels in old age, but others did not show any change with aging (Severson, 1981).

In humans, all the surveys of old individuals seem to agree that the increase in plasma cortisol in response to ACTH is preserved (Blichert-Toft, 1975). However, the response of DHEA to ACTH appears significantly reduced with aging (Vermeulen *et al.,* 1982). Similarly, the aging-related reduction in aldosterone remains lower even under conditions of sodium restriction, which otherwise stimulate aldosterone secretion in young and adult individuals (Flood *et al.,* 1967).

ACTH is secreted in irregular bursts throughout the 24-hour day, with the bursts being more frequent in the early morning and least frequent in the evening. This circadian (diurnal) rhythm of ACTH secretion is associated with a corresponding circadian rhythm in cortisol secretion, and both are preserved during aging in humans (Colucci *et al.,* 1975). However, sustained nighttime cortisol levels (i.e., blunting of the nocturnal drop in cortisol levels compared with daytime levels) have also been reported (Murray *et al.,* 1981) and have been ascribed (1) to reduced renal clearance of the hormone, (2) to reduced muscle mass and generally reduced basal metabolism (thereby reducing need of the organism for cortisol), and (3) to alterations in sleep patterns and insomnia (Friedman *et al.*, 1969). Other tests (e.g., metyrapone-induced decreases in plasma cortisol) indicate that the feedback mechanism for ACTH control as well as the stimulatory action of ACTH on adrenocortical secretion are maintained in old age and allow cortisol production to be adjusted to challenging stimuli. Secretion and levels of aldosterone also undergo in young adults circadian rhythmicity, which is not significantly altered with aging, although it may be somewhat dampened in women after 70 and in older males (Halberg, 1982; Cugini *et al.*, 1983).

In vitro experiments show that isolated adrenal cortical cells from old (24 months of age) rats are less responsive than those of young (3 months of age) rats to a synthetic subunit of ACTH and to cAMP; the marked reduction in corticosterone production in adrenal tissue from old rats suggests intracellular changes involving either impaired steroidogenesis or receptor function (Malamed and Carsia, 1983) perhaps secondary to increased free radical production and membrane alterations (see Chapter 7).

CHANGES IN ADRENAL STEROID RECEPTORS

Adrenal steroids exert their cellular and molecular actions through their binding to intracellular receptors, and the degree of cellular responsiveness is directly proportional to the number of specific receptor molecules. Hormone-mediated responses are controlled partly by the binding of the hormone to specific intracellular receptors and, then, by translocation of the hormone-receptor complex to nuclear acceptor sites (Roth, 1981; Kalimi, 1984) (Figure 12–5). All molecular events subsequent to receptor binding are subject to alteration with age although the nature and magnitude of these age-related changes are variable depending on the hormone, the target cell, and the animal species. In general, the concentration of corticosteroid receptors decreases either in early adulthood or during senescence (Roth, 1981; Kalimi, 1984; Sharma and Timiras, 1986a,b). For example, in the rat brain, glucocorticoid receptors are detectable on day 17 of gestation; they increase gradually after birth and reach adult levels by 15 days of age. These levels are significantly reduced in aged (24-month-old) rats as compared to adults (Kitraki *et al.*, 1984; Roth, 1974). However, in mice, regional differences in brain glucocorticoid receptors were present, but age-related changes were absent (Nelson *et al.*, 1976). In the rat hippocampus, the primary glucocorticoid-concentrating region of the brain (Pfaff *et al.*, 1976), receptors decrease with aging owing to decreased concentration of cytosolic corticosterone receptors without change in receptor affinity or capacity for nuclear translocation (Sapolsky *et al.*, 1985). Some of the physicochemical properties (e.g., activation, transformation) of the receptors seem to be more susceptible to aging than receptor number. Such age-related changes have been reported for glucocorticoid receptors in liver (Kalimi, 1984), skeletal muscle (Sharma and Timiras, 1986b), and cerebral hemisphere (Sharma and Timiras, 1987). Age-related changes in corticosteroid receptors, by altering the responsiveness of target cells and molecules to hormones, may contribute to the decline in the effectiveness of the adrenal cortex to respond to stress.

Aldosterone receptors in target tissues, such as renal cells, have been demonstrated *in vivo* and *in vitro* (Moguilewsky and Raynaud, 1980; Lan *et al.*, 1981; Watlington *et al.*, 1982; Lombes *et al.*, 1984), but little is known of eventual changes with aging. Observations in rats indicate an increase in the number of receptors in renal cells with aging, perhaps as an attempt (i.e., upregulation) to compensate for the low levels of circulating aldosterone (Frolkis *et al.*, 1985).

THE ADRENAL MEDULLA

The adrenal medulla is part of the sympathetic division of the autonomic nervous system and, as such, functions in unison with the other sympathetic structures. It is also interrelated anatomically by a rich vascular network to the cortex and functionally by interactions of glucocorticoids with some of the metabolic actions of medullary hormones (e.g., mobilization of free fatty acids in emergency situations) and

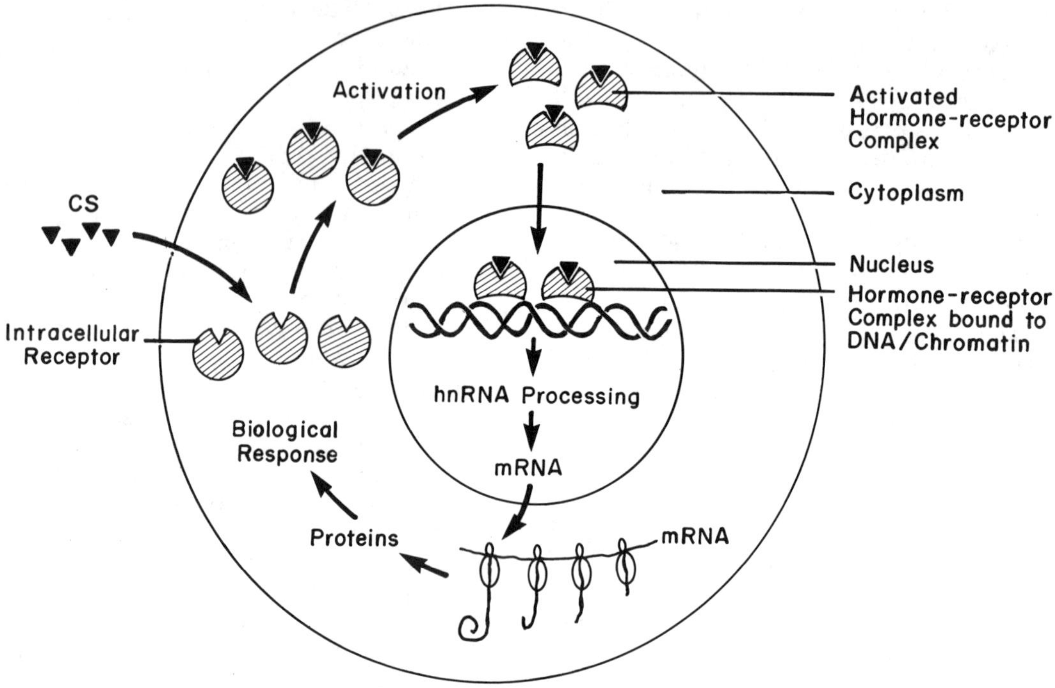

Figure 12–5. *Schematic diagram of corticosteroid (CS) action in a target cell.*

CS molecules diffuse across the plasma membrane and bind to specific receptor proteins in the cytoplasm. The resulting hormone-receptor complexes are activated and translocate to the nucleus where they bind to DNA/chromatin. This stimulates the synthesis of heterogenous RNA (hnRNA) which is processed into mature messenger-RNA (mRNA). The mRNA is transported into the cytoplasm where it is translated into protein which causes as biological response.

by the induction of some of the enzymes for catecholamine synthesis (e.g., the enzyme phenylethanolamine-*N*-methyltransferase, PNMT, which catalizes the formation of epinephrine from norepinephrine). The sympathetic system, including the adrenal medulla, is not essential for life. However, one of the functional characteristics of the system is that, under emergency conditions of stress as in rage and fright, it can discharge as a unit, when sympathetically innervated structures are affected simultaneously over the entire body. The heart rate is accelerated, the blood pressure rises, red blood cell are poured into the circulation from the spleen (in certain species), the concentration of blood glucose rises, the bronchioles and pupils dilate, and, on the whole, the organism is prepared for "fight or flight." The contribution of the adrenal medulla to "the emergency function of the sympathoadrenal system" varies with the animal species and the type of stress (Cannon, 1929). It also seems to vary with the age of the animal, reaching optimal efficiency in adulthood and showing some selective decline in old age.

Structure and Function. The medullary cells, also known as chromaffin cells because of their particular staining affinity, are considered as neurons that have lost their axons and become secretory cells. Major secretory products are the catecholamines, *norepinephrine,* which also is produced and released by neurons in the CNS and by sympathetic neurons, *epinephrine,* formed in the medulla by the methylation of norepinephrine, and some *dopamine,* also a CNS neurotransmitter. Opioid peptides are also secreted (most of the circulating enkephalin comes from the medulla) although they do not pass the blood-brain barrier and their action is presently unknown.

Circulating norepinephrine and epinephrine mimic the effects of sympathetic discharge, stimulate the nervous system, and exert metabolic effects that include glycogenolysis in liver and skeletal muscle, mobilization of free fatty acids, and stimulation of metabolic rate. They act through the binding to two classes of receptors—receptors that induce vasoconstriction in most organs and receptors that (1) mediate the metabolic effects and stimulate rate and force of cardiac contraction and (2) dilate blood vessels in muscle and liver. Their secretion is under neural control and is also influenced by other hormones, primarily glucocorticoids and thyroid hormones (see Chapter 15).

The reports of plasma levels and urinary excretion of catecholamines in humans and laboratory animals under basal conditions disagree. According to some, levels remain unchanged with aging, or they may show a reduction in absolute and averaged circadian amplitude. According to yet others, they may increase, the increase being greater (in humans) after standing and isometric exercise. The reported plasma and urinary elevation after a variety of stimuli has been interpreted as a compensatory reaction to the apparently increasing refractoriness of target tissues to catecholamines with aging. However, the apparent increase in norepinephrine plasma levels does not occur with all stimuli and, in addition, the return to baseline levels is prolonged in the elderly. Also the two catecholamines often show differential responses: although plasma norepinephrine is elevated in elderly subjects during a mental stress test, plasma epinephrine is not; this suggests either a reduction of PNMT or hyperactivity of the sympathetic system in general rather than of the adrenal medulla (Barnes *et al.*, 1982).

An unresolved issue is whether the elderly release more norepinephrine or whether the peripheral clearance of the hormone is reduced. Here again, the observations disagree, with some indicating no changes in clearance (Rubin *et al.*, 1982) whereas others report a decrease (Esler *et al.*, 1981).

If we accept the view that overall sympathoadrenal activity is increased in human aging, then we should provide an explanation for such an increase. One proposed explanation is an increased refractoriness (or, vice versa, a decreased sensitivity) of target tissues to catecholamines owing to alterations in transport and/or binding. Clinical and experimental observations show that the responsiveness of several tissues is diminished in some cases, although in many instances there is no decrease and in others an increase has been reported. Examples of decreased responsiveness may be found in the diminished efficiency of hemodynamic and cardiovascular responses to changes in posture (tilting, standing) and to exercise, as well as the slower dark adaption of pupillary size. An opposite effect is manifested in those organs and tissues regulating blood pressure, which progressively increases with aging leading to hypertension (Chapter 17). The ability of dopamine to stimulate adenylate cyclase in the corpus striatum decreases progressively with age (Puri and Volicer, 1977), as does dopamine binding in rats, mice, and rabbits (Finch, 1978; Roth, 1979; Makman *et al.*, 1980), but remains unchanged in adipocytes (Cooper and Gregerman, 1976) or is increased in hepatocytes (Kalish *et al.*, 1977). Even the suggested decreased receptor density as an explanation of target refractoriness is not clear-cut. A decrease in adrenergic receptor number with aging has been reported in some organs and cells (e.g., cerebellum, adipocytes) and in receptor affinity in others (e.g., lung), but in many cases, changes were not observed. This lack of uniformity in pattern has been ascribed to the differential responsiveness of tissues to catecholamines. Sensitivity to catecholamines may also be influenced by other hormones, such as glucocorticoids and thyroid hormones known to affect catecholamine metabolism and receptors themselves undergoing age-related changes. Other factors, such as alterations in structure and function of membranes and intracellular molecules, may also be operative in changing cell responsiveness to adrenal medullary hormones.

THE PITUITARY GLAND

The pituitary gland (also called hypophysis) regulates several peripheral endocrines (adrenal cortex, thyroid, gonads) and target tissues (through the secretion of growth hormone and prolactin), has close functional ties with the hypothalamus and other CNS centers, and produces a number of peptides with hormone-precursor and behavioral activities. Relatively few studies have explored systematically the changes with aging in these important functions; the current observations reveal that the major pituitary functions show with aging: (1) great variability among individuals of the same species and among different species; (2) differential alteration with aging, with some secretions being greatly affected whereas others remain practically unaltered; (3) the possibility of modifying age-related changes and influencing the lifespan by ablation of the gland in rats; and (4) in view of the selective rather than global nature of these changes and their importance for survival, the formulation of a number of neuroendocrine theories of aging based on the hypothesis that disorganization or desynchronization of hypothalamo-pituitary signals may cause, or at least be closely involved in, aging processes.

Structure and Major Hormones. The pituitary gland is comprised of three, more or less, separate endocrine glands that produce a relatively large number of hormonally active substances (Figure 12–6). These include six well-characterized hormones secreted from the anterior lobe of the gland: ACTH, discussed above, the two gonadotropins, thyroid-stimulating hormone, growth hormone, and prolactin. In addition, the anterior lobe secretes lipotropin and proopiomelanocortin, precursors of ACTH, opioid peptides, and melanocyte-stimulating hormone (MSH).

The intermediate lobe, practically indistinguishable from the anterior lobe in humans, contains MSH, lipotropin, opioid peptides, and the large precursor proopiomelanocortin. The posterior lobe secretes two peptides, vasopressin or antidiuretic hormone (ADH) and oxytocin.

The hormones tropic to a peripheral endocrine are discussed in the chapter on the gland; thus, ACTH and the adrenal cortex are discussed in this chapter. Of the other hormones, growth hormone, prolactin, ADH, and oxytocin will be discussed below, briefly.

STRUCTURAL CHANGES

The changes with aging are relatively few in the anterior lobe and include those general cellular changes (e.g, accumulation of lipofuscin) characteristic of aging cells (Chapter 5) and those particular to neural and secretory cells (e.g., changes in dendritic and synaptic morphology, in neurotransmitters) (Chapter 9). The number of the specific cells that secrete the different hormones is not markedly altered except for the gonadotropes (i.e., gonadotropin-secreting cells), which show changes similar to those observed after castration in experimental animals (Chapter 13). Tumor incidence, illustrated primarily by prolactinomas, increases with aging in rats and mice, more so in females than in males.

Histochemical studies of the posterior pituitary in old rats reported a decrease in neurosecretory material. Some contend the decrease is more marked in oxytocin- than ADH-secreting cells, but others the reverse. This decrease was not found in humans and other animals (e.g., cattle). Despite these contradictions, as age increases, reduced amounts of neurohypohyseal hormones are stored in the pituitary, which remains viable although in a depressed state. This conclusion is justified by quantitative ultrastructural analysis of old rodent pituitary showing increased autophagic activity, increased perivascular space, decline in cell volume, decreased size and number of neurosecretory granules, and reduction in endoplasmic reticulum activity (Choy, 1983).

GROWTH HORMONE

Aging may be associated, in very general terms, with decreased protein synthesis, lean body mass and bone formation, as well as increased adiposity—hence the potential involvement of GH because of its anabolic (i.e., promoting protein synthesis) and metabolic actions. Nevertheless, in humans and other species, the number of somatotropes (i.e., pituitary cells secreting GH), pituitary content of GH, basal plasma levels of the hormone, and its clearance remain essentially unchanged into old age. Some studies, however, have reported a decrease in GH basal levels in rats (Sonntag *et al.*, 1980, 1982) and in humans (Schramm *et al.*, 1981). Obesity is known to suppress circulating GH levels in young individuals (Rabinowitz, 1970), and the increased obesity often present in the elderly may contribute to the decreased GH levels (Rudman *et al.*, 1981), although not all reports agree (Elahi *et al.*, 1982).

Similarly, contradictory results have been reported for GH levels after a variety of stimuli: in rats, GH elevation after stim-

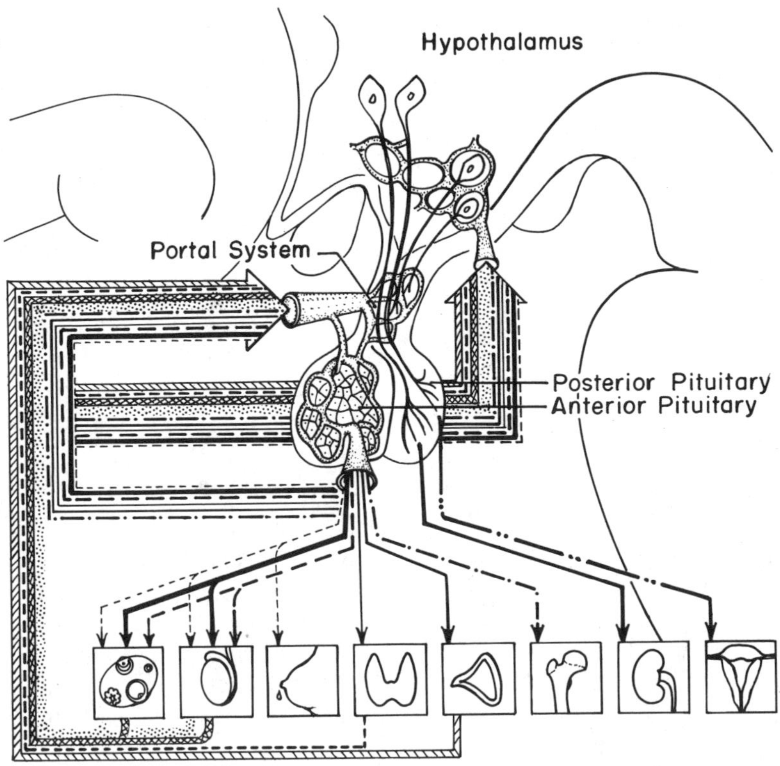

Figure 12–6. *Schematic representation of the hypothalamus, pituitary, and peripheral target sites, drawn to show the multiplicity of tropic hormones, targets, and feedbacks.*

Hypothalamic hormones are carried to the anterior pituitary through the portal system and to the posterior pituitary via axoplasmic flow in nerve fibers.

From the anterior pituitary, a number of tropic hormones are secreted. The tropic organs and their hormones are, from left to right: ovary: prolactin, PL (------), luteinizing hormone, LH (▬▬), follicle-stimulating hormone, FSH (– – –); testes: primarily interstitial-cell-stimulating hormone, ISCH (similar to LH), and to a lesser extent PL and FSH; mammary gland: PL; thyroid gland: thyroid stimulating hormone, TSH (———); adrenal cortex; adrenocortico-tropic hormone, ACTH (▬▬▬); long bones; growth hormone, GH (—•—•).

From the posterior pituitary, continuing from left to right: kidney: antidiuretic hormone or vasopressin, ADH (▬▬▬), smooth muscle, uterus: oxytocin (▬••▬).

The hormones secreted by the peripheral endocrines [sex (▒▒▒) and adrenocortical (▧▧▧) steroids and thyroid hormones (-----)] feedback to stimulate or inhibit secretion from the anterior pituitary or hypothalamus. Likewise, tropic hormones from the pituitary can feedback and regulate hormone secretion by the hypothalamus. In this manner short and long feedback loops are established.

ulation is less marked in old than in young animals (Sonntag *et al.*, 1983), whereas in humans, it may be decreased (Schramm *et al.*, 1981) or remain unaltered (Halbreich *et al.*, 1980).

GH secretion in humans undergoes a nocturnal peak during the first 4 hours of sleep, coinciding with stages 3 and 4 of slow-wave sleep; these are the stages most affected in aging (Chapter 10). Studies in older humans have shown a decrease in sleep-related GH secretion (Prinz *et al.*, 1983), although the relation of GH changes to sleep remains as controversial as that with obesity.

Although there is no complete agreement, the most common hypothesis is that at least some of the effects of GH are not due to a direct action of the hormone on target tissues and cells. GH would instead stimulate the liver and perhaps other tissues to produce several polypeptides, the so-called somatomedins. These possess growth-promoting activity such as insulin-like growth factors I and II, nerve growth factor, epidermal growth factor, fibroblast growth factor, thymosin, and other less-known factors. With aging, a decline in somatomedins has been reported in old rats (Florini *et al.*, 1981) and in humans (Rudman *et al.*, 1981; Sara *et al.*, 1982), as well as a decreased responsiveness of somatomedins to GH administration (Rudman *et al.*, 1981).

Hypothalamic Growth Hormone-Releasing Hormone (GRH) and Growth Hormone-Inhibiting Hormone (Somatostatin or GIH). From the foregoing discussion it emerges that during aging GH release declines, particularly during the night. Whether this decrease is due to a decline in the releasing hormone, GRH, or to an increase in the inhibiting hormone, somatostatin, is not known. Although the major function of GH is to promote growth of whole body as well as several organs during childhood and adolescence, GH, GRH, and somatostatin continue to be secreted throughout life, GH to exert metabolic effects and GRH and somatostatin to regulate GH secretion.

GH secretion depends not only on hypothalamic control (through GRH and somatostatin), but also on several metabolic factors, such as hypoglycemia and fasting, increase in some amino acids (e.g., arginine), in plasma, and on stressful stimuli. It is also influenced by neurotransmitter release, e.g., stimulation by increased norepinephrine and dopamine discharged from brain catecholaminergic neurons. Whether the aging-induced decline in these neurotransmitters that occurs during aging (Chapter 9) accounts for the decrease in GH due to a reduction in GRH release is unsettled, and more research is needed to identify factors regulating GRH, including aging (Frohman and Jansson, 1986).

A number of studies have investigated whether and how somatostatin synthesis and release may be influenced by aging. Somatostatin is a peptide secreted by hypothalamic cells but also present in several brain areas, the gastrointestinal tract, and the pancreas. Its levels in plasma are negligible and its actions are exerted locally in the vicinity of the secretory cells; as such, GIH is representative of that large group of substances produced by diffuse (paracrine) cells in several locations. Its main function is to inhibit GH release from the anterior pituitary. It also inhibits TSH release.

Hypothalamic content of somatostatin decreases with age in rats, and inhibition of its release (by administration of antibodies to somatostatin) causes a greater rise in GH in old than young rats (Sonntag *et al.*, 1980, 1981, 1982). This latter observation suggests a heightened sensitivity of the pituitary GH-secreting cells to the inhibitory action of somatostatin. The hormone content in several brain areas is not altered with aging in normal elderly subjects. However, in individuals affected by senile dementia of the Alzheimer type, brain somatostatin levels are severely depressed in association (but not necessarily in parallel) with the cholinergic deficits (as measured by choline acetyltransferase activity) (Davies *et al.*, 1980; Davies and Terry, 1981). The functional significance of this decrease is not understood. Behaviorally, somatostatin administration to aged monkeys had little ability to reverse their deficits on a memory task (Bartus *et al.*, 1982).

In contrast to the hypothalamic decrease, in the pancreas somatostatin levels are significantly higher in old than in young rats. This increase has been held responsible for, or at least considered as contributing to, the impairment of glucose-stimulated release of insulin and is reversible with antisomatostatin antibodies (Chaudhuri *et al.*, 1983).

PROLACTIN

This hormone, a protein structurally very similar to growth hormone, is present in small amounts in human pituitary except during pregnancy and lactation, when the levels increase and cause milk secretion from the breast. Its role in males is unknown. Among the pituitary hormones, it undergoes the most pronounced changes with aging. Both pituitary content and circulating blood levels are significantly increased in both aged men and women as well as in rodents. This increase has been related to a reduction with aging of the prolactin-inhibiting hormone (PIH), which has been identified as the neurotransmitter dopamine, secreted by the hypothalamic dopaminergic neurons into the portal pituitary vessels. Dopamine content is decreased in several brain areas with aging (Chapter 9); in the hypothalamus this decrease is associated with a reduced capacity to send inhibitory signals to the pituitary to block prolactin synthesis and release. However, some studies in aged subjects (past 80 years) reported (with immunocytochemical techniques) numerous and well-developed prolactin-containing cells in the pituitary but low blood levels in women and high levels in men (Vekemans and Robyn, 1975); the decline in prolactin levels in elderly women has been attributed to the lack of estrogens after menopause, as estrogen stimulates prolactin release (Kovacs *et al.*, 1977).

Plasma prolactin rises during sleep, the

rise starting at the onset of sleep and persisting throughout the sleep period. The differences in day-night levels are somewhat dampened with aging (Halberg, 1982). The changes in rhythmicity of prolactin, as well as those of growth hormone, together with those demonstrated for adrenal and thyroid hormones and the clear-cut changes in ovarian function, may all underlie the progressive failure of chronobiologic regulations with aging.

The high prolactin levels in the elderly may, in some instances, be related to the high incidence with aging of pituitary tumors secreting prolactin. In a study of pituitary tumor incidence, 13 percent were prolactinomas (Kovacs *et al.*, 1980). This high incidence of prolactin-secreting tumor has also been reported in rodents.

Pro-opiomelanocortin (POMC). Corticotropes (adrenocortical hormone-secreting cells) in the anterior pituitary and cells of the intermediate lobe synthesize a large precursor protein that is cleaved to form a family of hormones, primarily ACTH, several forms of lipotropin, MSH, and the opioid endorphin. POMC is also synthesized in the hypothalamus, other CNS structures, the lungs, gastrointestinal tract, and placenta. Of the hormones derived from the large molecule, more is known about ACTH and its relation to adrenocortical function in adult and old individuals than any of the other substances. Of the others, little information is available on their function during development and adulthood and almost nothing during aging. Some controversial evidence suggests decreased endorphin levels with aging in selected brain areas, e.g., the hypothalamus (Barden *et al.*, 1981), but the significance of this decrease is uncertain despite a possible stimulatory action of endorphin on corticosterone secretion in adult rats (Guillemin, 1978). POMC cleavage depends on a family of enzymes (e.g., proteases) currently under active investigation (Marx, 1987). With aging, enzyme activity may be altered, with resulting abnormal hormonal products.

VASOPRESSIN (ADH) AND OXYTOCIN

These nonpeptides are secreted by neurons of the supraoptic and paraventricular nuclei of the hypothalamus and transported along the axons to the posterior lobe of the pituitary, where they are stored before being released into the circulation. Within each hypothalamic nucleus, some neurons produce oxytocin and others ADH. These hormones are synthesized as part of a larger precursor molecule and are associated to neurophysins, which also represent part of the larger molecule. The principal action of ADH is retention of water by the kidney (Chapter 20) and that of oxytocin is stimulation of contraction of the myoepithelial cells of the mammary gland (for milk ejection) and the smooth muscle of the uterus (especially during parturition).

In association with the morphologic alterations described above, normal, aged rats often suffer from functional impairments such as mild diabetes insipidus (resulting from ADH deficiency and failure of water retention by the renal collecting ducts). In addition, the redistribution of water between intracellular and extracellular sites, characteristic of old age, has been ascribed to a decline in ADH levels in humans and rats (Sladek *et al.*, 1981) (Chapter 20). Osmoreceptors are specific cells in the hypothalamus sensitive to changes in osmotic pressure; they are stimulated by increased osmotic pressure as well as decreased extracellular volume of body fluids. With aging, the sensitivity of this hypothalamic "osmostat" appears to be increased. The osmostat set-point would be the same in old and in young people, but more ADH would be secreted for a given stimulus (Chapter 20) (Helderman, 1982; Frolkis *et al.*, 1982). ADH is also a potent vasoconstrictor *in vitro* (hence its alternate name of vasopressin), and when injected in large doses, it elevates blood pressure. However, the amount of endogenous ADH in the circulation of normal individuals does not normally affect blood pressure, and the eventual role of the hormone in the genesis of the hypertension of the elderly remains to be established (Chapter 17).

There have been claims that pituitary peptides act on the CNS to improve memory. ADH administered to old monkeys significantly improves memory performance in some animals, but in no case is the improvement great enough to match that of young animals (Bartus *et al.*, 1982). Clinical tests of vasopressin therapy for dementia of the elderly have been equally equivocal, and the utility of vasopressin therapy remains an open question (Chapter 10).

The pineal gland is considered here briefly because some of its characteristics—rhythmicity and relation to the environment—may have particular import for the regulation of the life cycles, including aging. The production of its main hormone, melatonin, derived from the neurotransmitter serotonin, is cyclic and is synchronized by the light-dark cycle of the environment. Its best-known actions are on reproductive function, which it antagonizes (i.e., possesses antigonadal action). It may also have secondary actions as a synchronizer that entrains physiology to the appropriate seasons of the year (Reiter, 1986). The significance of its 24-hour cycles with its nighttime peak is not understood.

In aged humans, the pineal gland undergoes calcification with loss of pinealocytes, the hormone-secreting cells, but no correlation could be drawn between the degree of calcification and the activity of the major melatonin-synthesizing enzymes (Wurtman *et al.*, 1964; Otani *et al.*, 1968). In general, overall melatonin levels and rhythm do not change until well into old age (85 years and older), when they diminish.

The nighttime melatonin peak, however, undergoes considerable change with age: it is low at birth and increases progressively to reach high values before puberty, at which time it decreases; the night peak remains stable during adulthood and then progressively decreases in old age (Reiter, 1986). Because of the known inhibitory actions of melatonin on reproduction, it has been proposed that the prepuberal decline in nighttime melatonin peak may permit sexual development to take place at puberty (Goldman, 1983; Vaughan, 1983; Ebadi, 1984).

The causes of the changes in melatonin nighttime peak with aging remain unexplained, but it may be hypothesized that they may be part of the general decline in CNS competence and that they may be related to the failure of maintaining the necessary functional rhythm for adaptation to the environment, hence some of the therapeutic applications of pineal gland manipulation. For example, photostimulation has been used with some profit in the treatment of winter depression, in resetting the biologic clock of night shift workers, and in relieving the effects of jet travel (jet lag) across time zones. Alterations in melatonin rhythm may desynchronize adaptation to photoperiodicity and possibly other environmental cues necessary for physiologic adjustments.

CHANGING ADAPTIVE RESPONSES

What are the causes of the decreased ability to respond to stress in old age? One among many hypotheses focuses on the hypothalamo-pituitary-adrenal axis as a key regulator of homeostasis and adaptation (Chapter 4); however, other organs, such as the lungs, kidneys, liver, and gut, are also involved. Maintenance of homeostasis involves a complex series of integrative functions in which almost all body organs and systems participate, although in varying degrees. Thus, homeostatic competence provides a "panoramic view" of overall physiologic performance and explains the current interest among physiologists to identify the control mechanisms involved in this integrated activity.

Under resting (basal) conditions few changes occur in hypothalamo-pituitary-adrenal function with increasing age. Similarly, fasting blood sugar levels remain constant throughout the lifespan, and the blood acidity and bicarbonate content are closely regulated, even into advanced age. In contrast, the rate at which the body is able to readjust and return to normal resting values after the experimental alteration of blood sugar, bicarbonate, or a stress situation stimulating adrenal response, is much slower in old subjects than young. As functional performance declines with increasing age and as pathologic events accumulate and become more severe, the capacity of the organism to synchronize defensive and homeostatic mechanisms is concomitantly impaired. Thus, the failure of the elderly to adapt to internal and external environmental changes reflects more the inability to purposefully coordinate several functions involved in supporting homeostasis than the failure of any single function (although the failure of one may provide a trigger) (Timiras, 1985; Finch and Landfield, 1985).

One of the major problems in the field of gerontology is to relate the functional changes occurring with age to the increasing probability of death. In animals, a particular reflex action or rapid neuromuscular response may be essential to their search for food and shelter, and consequently, a functional failure of this kind could be clearly designated as a mortality risk. On the other hand, death in animals occurs over a narrow age range even when they are maintained under constant optimal laboratory conditions without sudden or excessive demands being imposed on the body. Admittedly, we are largely ignorant of the actual cause of death in normal old age, although failure of homeostatic mechanisms appears to be the most probable candidate. In other words, death would come as a re-

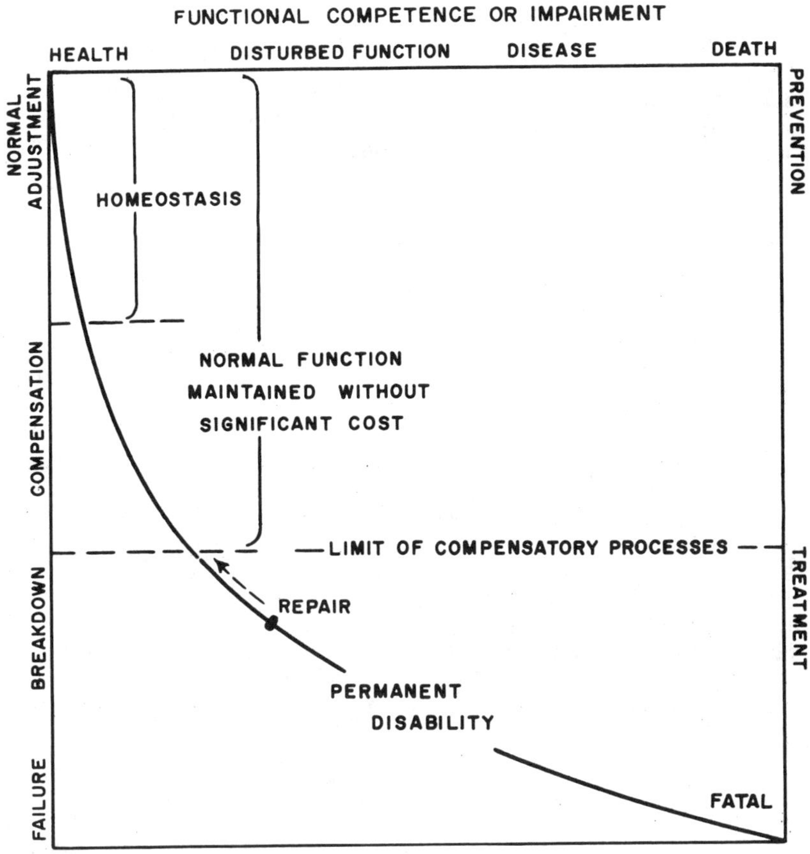

Figure 12–7. *Progressive stages of homeostasis from adjustment (health) to failure (death).*

In the healthy adult, homeostatic processes ensure adequate adjustment in response to stress and even for a period beyond this stage, compensatory processes are capable of maintaining overall function without serious disability. When stress is exerted beyond the compensatory capacities of the organism, disability ensues in rapidly increasing increments to severe illness, permanent disability, and death. When this model is viewed in terms of homeostatic responses to stress imposed on the aged, and to aging itself, a period when the body can be regarded as at the point of "limit of compensatory processes," it is evident that even minor stresses are not tolerable and the individual moves rapidly into stages of breakdown and failure.

sult of an internal fluctuation—a disruption of the constancy of the internal environment—that could not be contained through homeostatic regulation. We know, for example, that a small shift in metabolism, easily counteracted in youth, threatens survival in the elderly (Figure 12–7).

Evidence of decreased resistance to environmental changes accompanying the aging process is plentiful, and the increased risk of death following stress in the elderly is acknowledged. Older people are less resistant than younger subjects to excessively cold or warm temperatures owing to the progressive deterioration of thermoregulatory mechanisms. Equally diminished is the capacity to adapt to hypoxia, traumatic injury, exercise, and physical work, all types of stress that require complex physiologic adjustments. For example, the ability to carry out physical work involves competence of numerous functions, such as oxygen uptake by the lungs and/or tissues, pulmonary ventilation, diffusing capacity of lungs, cardiac work, pulse rate, and production and elimination of blood lactate

(Chapter 25). Alteration in any of these factors or their interrelation will result in a marked decrease in work capacity and a significant increase in the time for recovery from exercise. Emotional stress in the old may also trigger or aggravate a series of physical ailments that, superimposed on an already debilitated state, would lead to disease and death.

Some of the aging changes of the adrenal cortex and medulla described here and those in the nervous system described in Chapters 9 to 11 may be responsible for the decline in adaptive capability. Stressful stimuli activate both the hypothalamo-pituitary-adrenocortical and sympathoadrenal systems, which coordinate physiologic reactions to maintain homeostasis. This coordination is through a series of neuroendocrine signals that involve various hormones and brain centers. Aging disrupts the synchrony of these signals: the capacity to restore the original homeostasis is altered, and the hypothalamus is unable to undergo the major remodeling of its circuitry necessary for adaptation (Meites, 1981).

THE NEUROENDOCRINOLOGY OF STRESS AND AGING

The role of the hypothalamo-pituitary-adrenal system in adaptive responses was first emphasized by Cannon (1929) for the adrenal medulla and by Selye (1950) for the adrenal cortex. This role has been both supported and criticized by many investigators and continues to be controversial. We shall briefly summarize here some aspects of the adrenal cortex' participation as originally formulated by Selye in his "General Adaptation Syndrome" and more current data presented in an extensive review of the "Glucocorticoid Cascade Hypothesis" by Sapolsky and associates (1986a).

"The General Adaptation Syndrome and Aging." Four fundamental observations are at the basis of Selye's theories:

- first, the now classic observation that the adrenal cortex is indispensable for life—the mineralocorticoids, of which aldosterone is the most physiologically active representative, being of primary importance;
- second, that the adrenalectomized (or hypophysectomized) animal can survive indefinitely provided it receives additional salt in its diet (to compensate for the excessive loss of sodium resulting from the failure of renal reabsorption of sodium in the absence of aldosterone) and provided it is maintained under optimal environmental conditions;
- third, that the capacity to survive various types of stress is severely impaired in an adrenalectomized (or hypophysectomized) animal compared to its intact counterpart; and
- fourth, that maintenance doses of adrenocortical hormones to adrenalectomized (or hypophysectomized) animals, although sufficient to maintain life under nonstress conditions, are incapable of supporting adaptive reactions when stress is present—a finding that underlines the necessity for activation of the pituitary-adrenocortical system above normal levels in order for adaptation to occur.

Selye further demonstrated that all harmful agents that act on the body, generally or locally, exert dual actions, i.e., specific and nonspecific. Specific actions are different for each agent; e.g., ether induces anesthesia, *Salmonella typhosa* causes typhoid fever. Nonspecific actions are represented by stereotypical reactions, that is, reactions that are always the same, regardless of the causative agent: both cold and trauma, for example, will cause increased adrenocortical secretion, thymicolymphatic involution, and eosinopenia. In other words, when the organism is challenged by an adverse event, chemical, physical, biologic, or psychologic in nature, it responds both by mobilizing specific physiologic defenses to counterbalance the damaging effects of the stress and by stimulating the adrenal cortex to secrete larger amounts of its hormones; it is on the efficiency of these two sets of responses that the successful adaptation or failure of the organism to the challenging stress will depend. In this respect, it has been recognized since Selye's early experiments in this area, that not all responses to stress can be traced directly to the increased circulating levels of adrenocortical hormones, for some responses of still unknown etiopathology are found to occur also in adrenalectomized animals.

The general adaptation syndrome is characterized by three phases: an initial phase in which defense mechanisms are acutely challenged (alarm reaction), a period of enhanced adaptive capacity (stage of resistance), and the loss of the capacity to adapt (stage of exhaustion) (Selye, 1950). At this stage, there is no reason to believe that life expectancy is shortened, but surprisingly, after a variable period of time (generally inversely proportional to the severity of the stressor) the animal begins to lose weight and in a short time it dies, again manifesting all the signs of the alarm reaction. This general response pattern assumes that some form of energy, finite in amount, is necessary for the performance of adaptive work and can be exhausted under the influence of stress (Figure 12–8).

These considerations have given rise to an analogy between the loss of adaptive capacity in the adrenalectomized animal and its decline in the

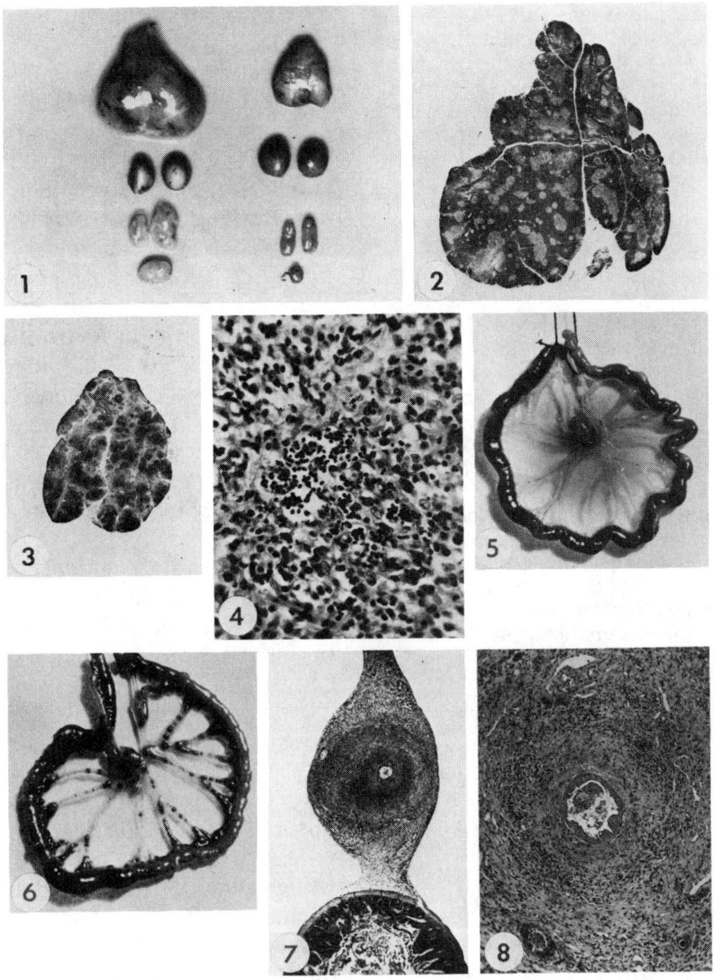

Figure 12–8. *Some physiologic and pathologic responses to stress in selected organs.*

The experimental animal chosen is the rat. (1,left) Naked eye view of adrenal and lymphatic organs of normal rat; (right) same organs during alarm reaction. Three iliac lymph nodes (bottom) and thymus (top) are significantly decreased in size in the stressed animal, whereas adrenals are enlarged and hyperhemic. (2) Low magnification of cross-section of the thymus of a normal rat and (3) of a stressed rat. Note the inversion of the thymus pattern (light-dark areas) due to depletion of the cortex of thymocytes and migration of thymocyte debris into the medulla in the stressed animal. (4) Higher magnification of an area of the thymus during the alarm reaction, dark patches representing nuclear debris from the degenerate thymocytes. Before, direct chemical measurement of adrenocortical hormones in the blood was possible, the involution of the thymus and lymph nodes was taken as an index of adrenocortical activity. (5 to 8) Hormonally induced vascular lesions approximating those occurring in diseases of adaptation. (5) Normal mesenteric vessels. Macroscopic view of a normal intestinal loop of a rat. Note thin and regular mesenteric vessels. (6) Abnormal mesenteric vessels. Macroscopic view from an animal chronically treated with desoxycorticosterone acetate. Note numerous beadlike periarteritis nodosa (resembling atherosclerosis) nodules along the mesenteric vessels. (7 and 8) Low and high magnification of periarteritis nodosa nodules in the mesenteric vessels. Note the thick layer of hyalinized fibrin lining vascular lumen, and the partial necrosis of the arterial wall (from Selye, 1950).

old individual (Selye and Prioreschi, 1960). In this view, old age is regarded as the accumulated result of the stresses and strains that the organism has supported during its lifespan; in other words, old age would correspond to the stage in which the adaptive energy available to the organism from early development has been exhausted. Thus, not only is the resistance of the elderly generally low, but when adaptive energy is employed for resistance against one stressor, resistance to other types of stressors is diminished. This concept could explain, for example, how a certain trauma, physical or psychologic, especially in the elderly, might significantly decrease the resistance of the organism to further stress and lead to death. Indeed, the progressive loss and ultimate exhaustion of adaptive energy may explain the exponential increase in death risk.

It is a common observation that people living in impoverished areas, with insufficient food, poor hygienic conditions, and so on, have a shorter lifespan and that they not only look older but are physiologically older than people of the same age whose standard of living is high. Among the latter group, it has been commonly observed that individuals in positions of heavy responsibility or in very taxing occupations are the most likely to succumb to cardiovascular accidents at an early age, a finding that also has been related to alterations in the mechanisms of adaptation. Accounts of individuals held for relatively long periods of time in concentration camps under extremely unfavorable conditions have also shown that even though they might have survived, they have suffered marked functional impairment. According to Selye's stress theory of aging outlined here, the continuing problem in aging studies of distinguishing between the alterations produced by age and those produced by previous diseases is not an issue. If every stressful episode represents a fundamental component of the aging process and leaves an indelible scar, no distinction needs to be made between these two groups of phenomena: the organism pays for surviving the stress by becoming a little older. Within this theoretic framework, it is assumed that the newborn is endowed with a finite quantity of adaptive energy, and thus, his lifespan is governed by the amount he has inherited and the rate at which he spends it. In this sense, the stresses to which he is exposed throughout life and that draw on his adaptive energy are of paramount concern to health and longevity.

Early investigators established a theoretical framework for a relationship between stress and aging, postulated a finite "adaptive energy" progressively depleted by the stresses of life, and suggested that the "rate of living" could be a pacemaker of aging. Several experimental approaches have supported these concepts and have demonstrated that some biomarkers of aging can mimic or be accelerated by stress (Chapter 3). However, only recently have advances in neuroendocrinologic knowledge and techniques established more solid cellular and molecular bases for these views. For example, at the cellular level, heat shock proteins have been implicated as contributing to the degenerative changes leading to the pathology of dementias (Chapter 10); at the molecular level, loss of glucocorticoid receptors in selected brain neurons may release the hypothalamo-pituitary-adrenocortical system from the inhibitory action of limbic structures with consequent failure to adapt. Another consequence of such failure is the occurrence of diseases prevalent in senescence, such as dementia (SDAT) and depression (Sapolsky *et al.*, 1986b).

Stress-elevated glucocorticoids induce predominantly catabolic reactions (e.g., increased gluconeogenesis from proteins) to provide readily available energy in response to acute emergency conditions. These responses impose a cost on the organism, as already suggested by Selye in the "alarm reaction." They may result in diabetes, hypertension, myopathy, immunosuppression, infertility, loss of weight, or inhibition of growth in children. Thus, while glucocorticoid action (like thyroid hormones, see Chapter 15) may have temporary value for survival, it is important that these actions be terminated rapidly lest they cause damage. Repeated exposure to stress would continuously stimulate adrenocortical secretion, and the ensuing elevated hormone levels might induce, contribute to, or aggravate existing physiologic impairment or disease, the so-called diseases of adaptation suggested by Selye.

Upon exposure to stress, aged rats are as capable as young of initiating an appropriate increase in secretion and levels of corticosterone (the main glucocorticoid in the rat). Corticosterone levels progressively increase with age even under basal conditions. However, after stress the old animals find it more difficult than the young to terminate the stress-induced rise in corticosterone (Figure 12–9) (Sapolsky *et al.*, 1983a). Also altered in the aged rats is the ability to adapt to mild sustained stress. The prolongation of poststress corticoster-

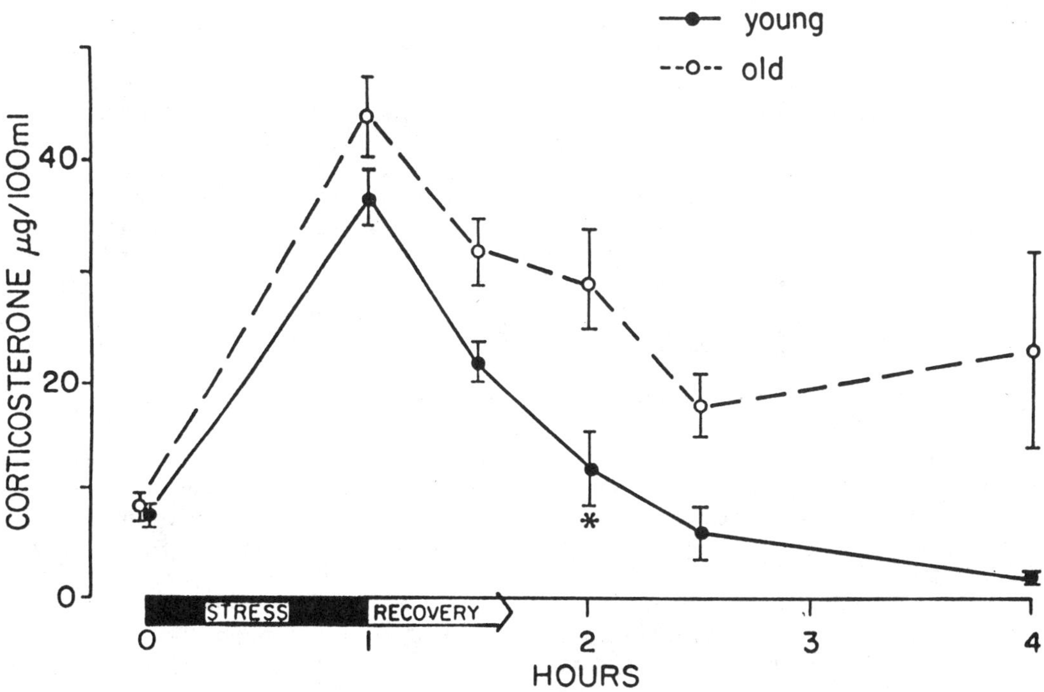

Figure 12–9. *Corticosterone titers in young (3–5 months) and aged (24–28 months) Fischer 344 rats during 1 hour of immobilization stress, followed by 4 hours of post-stress recover.*

*Indicates time when titers are no longer significantly elevated above baseline (determined by two-tailed paired to test). In the case of young subjects, this was after 1 hour of the recovery period; for aged subjects, such recovery did not occur within the monitored time-period. (From Sapolsky, *et al., Endocr. Rev.,* 7:284–301, 1986a.)

one elevation has been ascribed to: (1) structural (e.g., loss of neurons) and functional (e.g., increased excitability) changes in the brain; (2) consequent increase in CRH (?), ACTH, and some of the opioid peptides (e.g., β-endorphin); (3) decreased sensitivity of the adrenal cortex to ACTH (perhaps as a compensatory response to limit the effects of increased ACTH); and (4) dampened sensitivity of the pituitary to CRH, probably associated with (but not proven) higher CRH levels.

That brain sensitivity to corticosterone (and possibly other hormones) is progressively lost with aging is not unique to the hypothalamo-pituitary-adrenal axis. Similar sensitivity changes to hormonal negative feedbacks in hypothalamic and other CNS areas have been described for other pituitary hormones (Chapter 13). The causes for the decreased glucocorticoid sensitivity are in part the loss of neuronal hormone receptors and in part the shift in the brain cell populations with a decrease in neuronal number and an increase in glial cells (Chapter 9) (Sapolsky *et al.,* 1986a). Glucocorticoid receptors in the hippocampus, an area rich in these receptors, fall with aging to 50 percent below adult values, whereas affinity of binding and translocation are unaltered. With aging, the glial population increases (see Chapter 9). Glial cells do not have glucocorticoid receptors; therefore, the progressive loss of neurons with aging and the increase in glial cells may explain the loss of glucocorticoid receptors limited to the neuronal population (Sapolsky *et al.,* 1983b).

Glucocorticoid receptors are lost with aging not only in the hippocampus but also in the amygdala, both limbic structures regulating hypothalamic functions including CRH secretion. If these limbic structures have an inhibitory action on the hypothalamus and CRH secretion, and indirectly also on the adrenal cortex (Keller-Wood and Dallman, 1984), then their loss with aging may reduce inhibition and cause hypersecretion. Increased ACTH and glucocorticoid secretion after lesioning of the hippocampus supports this consent of decreased inhibition (Wilson *et al.*, 1980).

The loss of brain glucocorticoid receptors with aging may be due to a number of insults that damage hippocampal neurons. Among these damaging insults, a first suspect is corticosterone itself. It is significant that the effects of stress on the adrenocortical axis demonstrate that endogenous substances, such as hormones, can induce a number of brain alterations, including neuronal loss and changes in excitability, electrolytes, and metabolism (Timiras *et al.*, 1954; Woodbury *et al.*, 1957; Landfield *et al.*, 1978, 1981). Thus, cumulative exposure to basal concentrations of corticosterone leads to a progressive loss of hippocampal neurons, and stress, with its resultant increase in corticosterone, accelerates this loss. Indeed, hormones have not only metabolic and behavioral actions in the adult, but also organizing functions (i.e., inducing differentiation) during development, and damaging actions (or potentiating the damaging effects of toxic substances and injury) in senescence.

Is the central role of the adrenal cortex in stress-induced responses demonstrated in rodents also applicable to other animal species? Which and how many of these adrenocortical actions extend to humans? A list of these actions, previously discussed, includes: (1) increased secretion and levels of hypothalamic CRH (probable), pituitary ACTH, and adrenal glucocorticoids upon exposure to stress at all ages, including senescence; (2) continuing glucocorticoid excess in old rats (i.e., delayed termination of stress-induced hormonal hypersecretion) after the end of stress; (3) degenerative changes caused by prolonged glucocorticoid excess in discrete brain areas (e.g., limbic structures) that normally inhibit the hypothalamo-pituitary-adrencocortical axis; (4) adrenocortical hypersecretion due to decreased inhibition; and (5) further damage of brain neurons by hormonal hypersecretion: this damage aggravates reduced inhibition and increases adrenocortical secretion, thereby creating a "cascade" of cumulatively altered neuroendocrine signals and responses (Figure 12–10).

Of the foregoing actions, at least the first

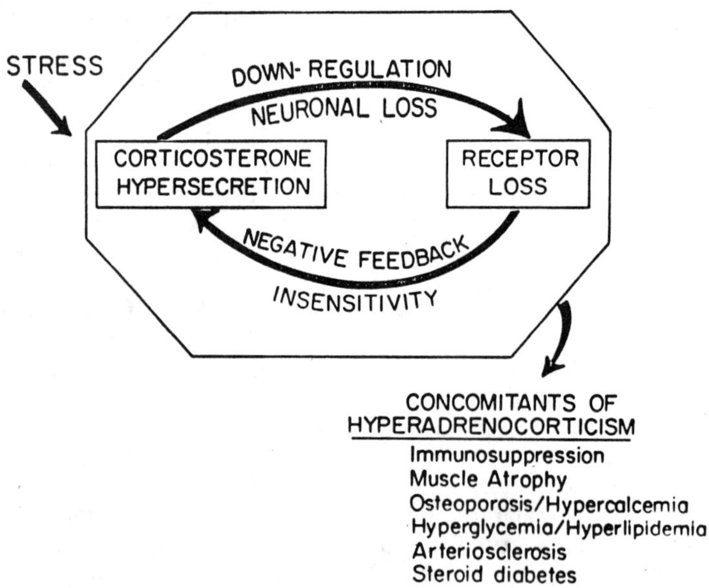

Figure 12–10. *Schematic representation of glucocorticoid cascade hypothesis. © The Endocrine Society.*

two are not operative in humans, in whom basal glucocorticoid levels and responses to ACTH and stress remain normal well into old age. In primates, glucocorticoid excess damages hippocampal neurons and this damage leads to adrenocortical hypersecretion (Gerlach *et al.*, 1976; Krieger, 1982). In humans, while absent in normal aging, some of the features of the adrenocortical "cascade" may be coupled with some pathologic states, such as in patients with SDAT (where hippocampal damage may be associated with adrenocortical hypersecretion) and in depression (an affective disorder frequent in the elderly and associated with several hormonal dysfunctions).

Factors contributing to the decline of ability of the elderly to maintain homeostasis, in addition to the adrenal cortex, include: other endocrines (Chapters 13 to 16), the sympathoadrenal system (implicated in adaptive responses), and, perhaps, the parasympathetic system as well (its stress connections have until now received little attention), the much stronger control in humans by cerebral cortical high centers over the limbic and other structures regulating visceral functions than in lower mammals, and the aging changes in the cellular and molecular properties of the target cells not only in brain but also in other tissues and organs. With aging and repeated exposure to stress throughout the lifespan, alterations may occur at any or several levels that disrupt appropriate articulation and timing of the necessary signals and thereby prevent optimal adjustments to internal and external demands with consequent failure to adapt and death.

References

Adelman, R. C., and Roth, G. S. (eds.): *Testing the Theories of Aging*, CRC Press, Boca Raton, FL, **1982.**

Andres, R., and Tobin, J. D.: Endocrine systems. In Finch, C., and Hayflick, L. (eds.): *Handbook of the Biology of Aging*, Van Nostrand Reinhold, New York, **1977.**

Barden, N.; Dupont, A.; Labrie, F.; Merand, Y.; Rouleu, D.; Vaudry, H.; and Boissier, J. R.: Age-dependent changes in the beta-endorphin content of discrete rat brain nuclei. *Brain Res.*, **208:**209–212, **1981.**

Barnes, R. F.; Raskind, M.; Gumbrecht, G.; and Halter, J. B.: The effects of age on the plasma catecholamine response to mental stress in man. *J. Clin. Endocrinol. Metab.*, **54:**64–69, **1982.**

Bartus, R. T.; Dean, R. L.; and Beer, B.: Neuropeptide effects on memory in aged monkeys. *Neurobiol. Aging*, **3:**61–68, **1982.**

Blichert-Toft, M.: Secretion of corticotrophin and somatotrophin by the senescent adenohypophysis in man. *Acta Endocrinol.*, **78 (Suppl. 195):1–157, 1975.**

Bowman, R. E., and Wolf, R. C.: Plasma 17-hydroxycorticosteroid response to ACTH in M. mulatta: Dose, age, weight, and sex. *Proc. Soc. Exp. Biol. Med.*, **130:**61–64, **1969.**

Breznock, E. M., and McQueen, R. D.: Adrenocortical function during aging in the dog. *Am. J. Vet. Res.*, **31:**1269–1273, **1970.**

Cannon, W. G.: Organization for physiological homeostasis. *Physiol. Rev.*, **9:**399–431, **1929.**

Chang, W., and Roth, G. S.: Changes in the mechanisms of steroid action during aging. *J. Steroid Biochem.*, **11**889–892, **1979.**

Chaudhuri, M.; Sartin, J. L.; and Adelman, R. C.: A role for somatostatin in the impaired insulin secretory response to glucose by islets from aging rats. *J. Gerontol.*, **38:**431–435, **1983.**

Choy, V. J.: Structure and function of the aged hypothalamoneurohypophysial system. In Walker, R. F., and Cooper, R. L. (eds.): *Experimental and Clinical Interventions in Aging*, Marcel Dekker, New York, **1983.**

Cole, G. M.; Segall, P. E.; and Timiras, P. S.: Hormones during aging. In Vernadakis, A., and Timiras, P. S. (eds.): *Hormones in Development and Aging*, S. P. Medical and Scientific Books, New York, **1982.**

Colucci, C. F.; D'Alessandro, B.; Bellastella, A.; and Montalbetti, N.: Circadian rhythm of plasma cortisol in the aged (Cosinor method). *Gerontol. Clin.*, **17:**89–95, **1975.**

Cooper, B., and Gregerman, R. I.: Hormone-sensitive fat cell adenylate cyclase in the rat. Influences of growth, cell size and ageing. *J. Clin. Invest.*, **57:**161–168, **1976.**

Cugini, P.; Scavo, D.; Centanni, M.; Halberg, F.; Haus, E.; Lakatua, D.; Schramm, A.; Pusch, H. J.; Franke, H.; and Kawasaky, R.: Circadian as well as circannual rhythms of circulating aldosterone have decreased amplitude in aging women. *J. Endocrinol. Invest.*, **6:**17–20, **1983.**

Davies, P.; Katzman, R.; and Terry, R. D.: Reduced somatostatin-like immunoreactivity in cerebral cortex from cases of Alzheimer's disease and Alzheimer's senile dementia. *Nature*, **288:**279–280, **1980.**

Davies, P., and Terry, R. D.: Cortical somatostatin-like immunoreactivity in cases of Alzheimer's disease and senile dementia of the Alzheimer's type. *Neurobiol. Aging*, **2:**9–14, **1981.**

Dilman, V. M.: *The Law of Deviation of Homeostasis and Diseases of Aging*, John Wright, Boston, **1981.**

Ebadi, M.: Regulation of the synthesis of melatonin and its significance to neuroendocrinology. In Reiter, R. J. (ed.): *The Pineal Gland*, Raven Press, New York, **1984.**

Elahi, D.; Muller, D. C.; Tzankoff, S. P.; Andres, R.; and Tobin, J. D.: Effect of age and obesity on fasting levels of glucose, insulin, glucagon, and growth hormone in man. *J. Gerontol.*, **37:**385–391, **1982.**

Esler, M.; Skews, H.; Leonard, P.; Jackman, G.; Bobik, A.; and Korner, P.: Age-dependence of noradrenaline kinetics in normal subjects. *Clin. Sci.*, **60:**217–219, **1981.**

Everitt, A. V., and Burgess, J. A. (eds.): *Hypothalamus Pituitary and Aging*, Charles C Thomas, Springfield, IL, **1976.**

Finch, C. E.: Age-related changes in brain catecholamines: A synopsis of findings in C57BL/6J mice and the rodent models. In Finch, C. E.; Potter, D. E.; and Henny, A. D. (eds.): *Advances in Experimental Medicine and Biology*, Plenum Press, New York, **1978.**

Finch, C. E., and Landfield, P. W.: Neuroendocrine and

autonomic functions in aging mammals. In Finch, C. E., and Schneider, E. L. (eds.): *Handbook of the Biology of Aging*, 2nd ed., Van Nostrand Reinhold, New York, **1985.**

Flood, C.; Gherondache, C.; Pincus, G.; Tait, J. F.; Tait, S. A. S.; and Willoughby, S.: The metabolism and secretion of aldosterone in elderly subjects. *J. Clin. Invest.*, **46:**960–966, **1967.**

Florini, J. R.; Harned, J. A.; Richman, R. A.; and Weiss, J. P.: Effects of rat age on serum levels of growth hormone and somatomedins. *Mech. Ageing Dev.*, **15:**165–176, **1981.**

Friedman, M.; Green, M. F.; and Sharland, D. E.: Assessment of hypothalamic-pituitary-adrenal function in the geriatric age group. *J. Gerontol.*, **24:**292–297, **1969.**

Frohman, L. A., and Jansson, J. O.: Growth hormone releasing hormone. *Endocr. Rev.*, **7:**223–253, **1986.**

Frolkis, V. V.: *Aging and Life-Prolonging Processes*, Springer-Verlag, New York, **1982.**

Frolkis, V. V.; Verkhratsky, N. S.; and Magdich, L. V.: Regulation of aldosterone secretion in old rats. *Gerontology*, **31:**84–94, **1985.**

Gerlach, J.; McEwen, B. S.; Pfaff, D.; *et al.*: Cells in regions of Rhesus monkey brain and pituitary retain radioactive estradiol, corticosterone and cortisol differentially. *Brain. Res.*, **103:**603, **1976.**

Goldman, B. D.: The physiology of melatonin in mammals. *Pineal Res. Rev.*, **1:**145–182, **1983.**

Green, M. F.: The endocrine system. In Pathy, M. S. J. (ed.): *Principles and Practice of Geriatric Medicine*, John Wiley & Sons, Chichester, UK, **1985.**

Gregerman, R. I., and Bierman, E. L.: Aging and hormones. In Williams, R. H. (ed.): *Textbook of Endocrinology*, W. B. Saunders, Philadelphia, **1974.**

Guillemin, R.: Peptides in the brain: The new endocrinology of the neuron. *Science*, **202:**390–402, **1978.**

Halberg, F.: Biological rhythms, hormones, and aging. In Vernadakis, A., and Timiras, P. S. (eds.): *Hormones in Development and Aging*, S. P. Medical & Scientific Books, New York, **1982.**

Halbreich, U.; Asnis, G. M.; Halpern, F.; Tabrizi, M. A.; and Sachar, E. J.: Diurnal growth hormone responses to dextroamphetamine in normal young men and post-menopausal women. *Psychoneuroendocrinology*, **5:**339–344, **1980.**

Hegstad, R.; Brown, R. D.; Jiang, N. S.; Kao, P.; Weinshilbou, R. M.; Strong, C.; and Wisgerhof, M.: Aging and aldosterone. *Am. J. Med.*, **74:**442–447, **1983.**

Helderman, J. H.: The impact of normal aging on the hypothalamic-neurohypophysealrenal axis. In Korenman, G. (ed.): *Endocrine Aspects of Aging*, Elsevier Biomedical, New York, **1982.**

Jensen, H. K., and Blichert-Toft, M.: Serum corticotrophin, plasma cortisol, and urinary excretion of 17-ketogenic steroids in the elderly (age group 66–94 years). *Acta Endocrinol. (Copenhagen)*, **66:**25–34, **1971.**

Kalimi, M.: Glucocorticoid receptors: From development to aging. A review. *Mech. Ageing Dev.*, **24:**129–138, **1984.**

Kalish, M. I.; Katz, M. S.; Pineyro, M. A.; and Gregerman, R. I.: Epinephrine- and glucagon-sensitive adenylate cyclases of rat liver during aging: Evidence for membrane instability associated with increased enzymatic activity. *Biochim. Biophys. Acta.*, **483:**452–466, **1977.**

Keller-Wood, M., and Dallman, M.: Corticosteroid inhibition of ACTH secretion. *Endocr. Rev.*, **51:**1–24, **1984.**

Kitraki, E.; Alexis, M. N.; and Stylianopoulo, F.: Glucocorticoid receptors in developing rat brain and liver. *J. Steroid Biochem.*, **20:**263–269, **1984.**

Kovacs, K.; Ryan, N.; Horvath, E.; Penz, G.; and Ezrin, C.: Prolactin cells of the human pituitary gland in old age. *J. Gerontol.*, *32*:534–540, 1977.

Kovacs, K.; Ryan, N.; Horvath, E.; Singer, W.; and Ezrin, C.: Pituitary adenomas in old age. *J. Gerontol.*, **35:**16–22, **1980.**

Krieger, D. T. (ed.): *Cushing's Syndrome*, Springer-Verlag, Berlin, **1982.**

Lan, N. C.; Natulich, D. T.; Morris, J. A.; and Baxter, J. D.: Mineralocorticoid receptor-like aldosterone binding protein in cell culture. *Endocrinology*, **109:**1963–1981, **1981.**

Landfield, P.; Waymire, J.; and Lynch, G.: Hippocampal aging and adrenocorticoids: A quantitative correlation. *Science*, **202:**1098, **1978.**

Landfield, P.; Braun, T.; Pitler, J.; Lindsay, J.; and Lynch, G.: Hippocampal aging in rats: A morphometric study of multiple variables in semithin sections. *Neurobiol. Aging*, **2:**265, **1981.**

Latham, K. R., and Finch, C. E.: Hepatic glucocorticoid binders in mature and senescent C57B1/6J male mice. *Endocrinology*, **98:**1480–1489, **1976.**

Lombes, M.; Claire, M.; Pinto, M.; Michaud, A.; and Rafestin-Oblin, M. E.: Aldosterone binding in the human colon carcinoma cell line HT29: Correlation with cell differentiation. *J. Steroid Biochem.*, **20:**329–333, **1984.**

Makman, M. H.; Ahn, H. S.; Thal, L. J.; Sharpless, N. S.; Dvorkin, B.; Horowitz, S. G.; and Rosenfeld, M.: Evidence for selective loss of brain dopamine and histamine-stimulated adenylate cyclase activities in rabbits with aging. *Brain Res.*, **192:**177–184, **1980.**

Malamed, S., and Carsia, R. V.: Aging of the rat adrenocortical cell: response to ACTH and cyclic AMP *in vitro*. *J. Gerontol.*, **38:**130–136, **1983.**

Marx, J. L.: A new wave of enzymes for cleaving prohormones. *Science*, **235:**285–286, **1987.**

Meites, J.: Changes in hypothalamic regulation of pituitary function in aging rats. In Enna, S. J.; Samorajski, T.; and Beer, B. (eds.): *Brain Neurotransmitters and Receptors in Aging and Age-Related Disorders*, Raven Press, New York, **1981.**

Migeon, C.; Keller, A.; Lawrence, B.; and Shepard, T.: Dehydroepiandrosterone and androsterone levels in human plasma. Effect of age and sex; day to day and diurnal variation. *J. Clin. Endocrinol. Metab.*, **17:**1051–1061, **1957.**

Minaker, K. L.; Meneilly, G. S.; and Rowe, J. W.: Endocrine systems. In Finch, C. E., and Schneider, E. L. (eds.): *Handbook of the Biology of Aging*, Van Nostrand Reinhold, New York, **1985.**

Moguilewsky, M., and Raynaud, J. P.: Evidence for a specific mineralocorticoid receptor in rat pituitary and brain. *J. Steroid Biochem.*, **12:**309–314, **1980.**

Murray, D.; Wood, P. J.; Moriarty, J.; and Clayton, B. E.: Adrenocortical function in old age. *J. Clin. Exp. Gerontol.*, **3:**255–268, **1981.**

Nelson, J. F.; Holinka, C. F.; Latham, K. R.; Allen, J. K.; and Finch, C. E.: Corticosterone binding in cytosols from brain regions of mature and senescent male C57BL/GJ mice. *Brain Res.*, **115:**345–351, **1976.**

Orentreich, N.; Brind, J. L.; Rizer, R. L.; and Vogelman, J. H.: Age changes and sex differences in serum dehydroepiandrosterone sulfate concentrations throughout adulthood. *J. Clin. Endocrinol. Metab.*, **59:**551–555, **1984.**

Otani, T.; Gyorkey, F.; and Farrel, G.: Enzymes of the human pineal. *J. Clin. Endocrinol. Metab.*, **28:**349–354, **1968.**

Pfaff, D. W.; Gerlach, J. L.; McEwen, B. S.; Ferin, M.; Carmel, P.; and Zimmerman, E. A.: Autoradiographic localization of hormone concentrating cells in the brain of the female Rhesus monkey. *J. Comp. Neurol.*, **170:**279–294, **1976.**

Pincus, G.; Romanoff, L. P.; and Carlo, J.: The excretion or urinary steroids by men and women of various ages. *J. Gerontol.*, **9:**113–132, **1954.**

Prinz, P. N.; Weitzman, E. D.; Cunningham, G. R.; and

Karacan, I.: Plasma growth hormone during sleep in young and aged men. *J. Gerontol.*, **38**:519–534, **1983.**

Puri, S. K., and Volicer, L.: Effects of aging on cyclic AMP levels and adenylate cyclase and phosphodiesterase activities in the rat corpus striatum. *Mech. Ageing Dev.*, **6**:53–58, **1977.**

Rabinowitz, P.: Some endocrine and metabolic aspects of obesity. *Annu. Rev. Med.*, **21**241–258, **1970.**

Reiter, R. J.: The pineal gland: An important link to the environment. *News in Physiological Sciences*, **1**:202–205, **1986.**

Riegle, G. D.; Przekop, F.; and Nellor, J. E.: Changes in adrenocortical responsiveness in ACTH infusion in aging goats. *J. Gerontol.*, **23**:187–190, **1968.**

Riegle, G. D.; Przekop, F.; and Nellor, J. E.: Changes in adrenocortical responsiveness to ACTH infusion in aging goats. *J. Gerontol.*, **23**:187–190, **1968.**

Romanoff, L. P.; Morris, C. W.; Welch, P.; Rodriguez, R. M.; and Pincus, G.: The metabolism of cortisol 4-C^{14} in young and elderly men 1. Secretion rate of cortisol and daily excretion of tetrahydrocortisol, allotetrahydrocortisol, tetrahydrocortisone, and cortalone (20 alpha and 20 beta). *J. Clin. Endocrinol. Metab.*, **21**:1413–1435, **1961.**

Roth, G. S.: Age-related changes in specific glucocorticoid binding by steroid responsive tissues of rats. *Endocrinology*, **94**:82–90, **1974.**

Roth, G. S.: Hormone action during aging: Alterations and mechanisms. *Mech. Ageing Dev.*, **9**:497–514, **1979.**

Roth, G. S.: Changes in hormone receptors during adulthood and senescence. In Florini, J. R. (ed.): *Handbook of Biochemistry in Aging*, CRC Press, Boca Raton, FL, **1981.**

Rubin, P. C.; Scott, P.; McLean, K.; and Reid, J. L.: Noradrenaline release and clearance in relation to age and blood pressure in man. *Eur. J. Clin. Invest.*, **12**:121–125, **1982.**

Rudman, D.; Kutner, M. H.; Rogers, C. M.; Lubin, M. F.; Fleming, G. A.; and Bain, R. P.: Impaired growth hormone secretion in the adult population: Relation to age and adiposity. *J. Clin. Invest.*, **67**:1361–1369, **1981.**

Samuels, L. T.: Factors affecting the metabolism and distribution of cortisol as measured by levels of 17-hydroxycorticosteroids in blood. *Cancer*, **10**:746–751, **1957.**

Sapolsky, R. M.; Krey, L. C.; and McEwen, B. S.: The adrenocortical stress-response in the aged male rat: Impairment of recovery from stress. *Exp. Geront.*, **18**:55–64, **1983a.**

Sapolsky, R. M.; Krey, L. C.; and McEwen, B. S.: Corticosterone receptors decline in a site-specific manner in the aged rat brain. *Brain Res.*, **289**:235, **1983b.**

Sapolsky, R. M.; Krey, L. C.; and McEwen, B. S.: Prolonged glucocorticoid exposure reduces hippocampal neuron number: Implications for aging. *J. Neurosci.*, **5**:1222–1227, **1985.**

Sapolsky, R. M.; Krey, L. C.; and McEwen, B. S.: The neuroendocrinology of stress and aging: The glucocorticoid cascade hypothesis. *Endocr. Rev.*, **7**:284–301, **1986a.**

Sapolsky, R. M.; Krey, L. C.; and McEwen, B. S.: The adrenocortical axis in the aged rat: Impaired sensitivity to both fast and delayed feedback inhibition. *Neurobiol. Aging*, **7**:331–335, **1986b.**

Sara, V. R.; Hall, K.; Enzell, K.; Gardner, A.; Morawski, R.; and Wetterberg, L.: Somatomedins in aging and dementia disorders of the Alzheimer type. *Neurobiol. Aging*, **3**:117–120, **1982.**

Schramm, V. A.; Pusch, H. J.; Franke, H.; and Haubitz, I.: Hormonal adaptability in the elderly. *Fortschr. Med.*, **27**:1255–1260, **1981.**

Selye, H.: *Stress—The Physiology and Pathology of Exposure to Stress*, Acta Inc., Montreal, **1950.**

Selye, H., and Prioreschi, P.: Stress theory of aging. In Shock, N. W. (ed.): *Aging . . . Some Social and Biological Aspects*, American Association for the Advancement of Science, Washington, DC, **1960.**

Serio, M.; Piolanti, P.; Cappelli, G.; DeMagistris, L.; Ricchi, F.; Anzalone, M.; and Gusti, F.: The miscible pool and turnover rate of cortisol with aging and variations in relation to time of day. *Exp. Gerontol.*, **4**:95–101, **1969.**

Severson, J. A.: The adrenal gland. In Masoro, E. J. (ed.): *Handbook of the Physiology of Aging*, CRC Press, Boca Raton, FL, **1981.**

Sharma, R., and Timiras, P. S.: Changes in glucocorticoid receptors in different regions of brain of immature and mature male rats. *Biochem. Int.*, **13**:609–614, **1986a.**

Sharma, R., and Timiras, P. S.: Regulatory changes in glucocorticoid receptors in the skeletal muscle of immature and mature male rats. *Mech. Ageing Dev.*, **37**:249–256, **1987.**

Sharma, R., and Timiras, P. S.: Activation of glucocorticoid receptors in the cerebral hemispheres of weanling and adult male rats. INS-ASN 1987 Joint Meeting of Neurochemistry, La Guaira, Venezuela, June **1987.**

Singer, S. S., and Bruns, L.: Enzymatic sulfation of steroids. VII. Hepatic cortisol sulfation and glucocorticoid sulfotransferases in old and young female rats. *Exp. Gerontol.*, **13**:425–429, **1978.**

Sladek, C. D.; McNeill, T. H.; Gregg, C. M.; Blair, M. L.; and Baggs, R. B.: Vasopressin and renin response to dehydration in aged rats. *Neurobiol. Aging*, **2**:293–302, **1981.**

Sonntag, W. E.; Forman, L. J.; Miki, N.; Steger, R. W.; Ramos, T.; Arimura, A.; and Meites, J.: Effect of CNS active drugs and somatostatin antiserum on growth hormone release in young and old male rats. *Neuroendocrinology*, **33**:73–78, **1981.**

Sonntag, W. E.; Forman, L. J.; Miki, N.; Trapp, J. M.; Gottschall, P. E.; and Meites, J.: L-Dopa restores amplitude of growth hormone pulses in old male rats to that observed in young male rats. *Neuroendocrinology*, **34**:163–168, **1982.**

Sonntag, W. E.; Hylka, W.; and Meites, J.: Impaired ability of old male rats to secrete GH *in vivo* but not *in vitro* in response to hpGRF 1-44. *Endocrinology*, **113**:*2305–2307*, **1983.**

Sonntag, W. E.; Steger, R. W.; Forman, L. J.; and Meites, J.: Decreased pulsatile release of growth hormone in old rats. *Endocrinology*, **107**:1875–1879, **1980.**

Timiras, P. S.: Neuroendocrinology of aging: Retrospective, current, and prospective views. In Meites, J. (ed.): *Neuroendocrinology of Aging*, Plenum Press, New York, **1983.**

Timiras, P. S.: Physiology of ageing: Aspects of neuroendocrine regulation. In Pathy, M. S. J. (ed.): *Principles and Practice of Geriatric Medicine*, John Wiley & Sons, Chichester, UK, **1985.**

Timiras, P. S.; Woodbury, D. M.; and Goodman, L. S.: Effect of adrenalectomy, hydrocortisone acetate and desoxycorticosterone acetate on brain excitability and electrolyte distribution in mice. *J. Pharmacol. Exp. Ther.*, **112**:80–93, **1954.**

Timiras, P. S.; Woodbury, D. M.; and Baker, D. H.: Effect of hydrocortisone acetate, desoxycorticosterone acetate, insulin, glucagon and dextrose, alone or in combination on experimental, convulsions and carbohydrate metabolism. *Arch. Int. Pharmacodyn. Ther.*, **105**:450–467, **1956.**

Vaughan, G. M.: Melatonin in humans. *Pineal Res. Rev.*, **2**:142–202, **1983.**

Vekemans, M., and Robyn, C.: Influence of age on serum prolactin levels in women and men. *Br. Med. J.*, **4**:738–739, **1975.**

Vermeulen, J. P.; Deslypere, J. P.; Shelfhout, W.; Verdonck, L.; and Rubens, R.: Adrenocortical function in old age: Response to acute adrenocorticotropin stimulation. *J. Clin. Endocrinol. Metab.,* **54:**187–191, **1982.**

Watlington, C. O.; Perkins, F. M.; Munson, P. J.; and Handler, J. S.: Aldosterone and corticosterone binding and effects on Na^+ transport in cultured kidney cells. *Am. J. Physiol.,* **242:**F610–F619, **1982.**

West, C. D.; Brown, H.; Simons, E. L.; Carter, D. B.; Kumagai, L. F.; and Engelbert, E. L.: Adrenocortical function and cortisol metabolism in old age. *J. Clin. Endocrinol. Metab.,* **21:**1197–1207, **1961.**

Wilson, M.; Greer, M.; and Roberts, L.: Hippocampal inhibition of pituitary-adrenocortical function in female rats. *Brain Res.,* **197:**433, **1980.**

Woodbury, D. M.; Timiras, P. S.; and Vernadakis, A. Influence of adrenocortical steroids on brain function and metabolism. In Hoagland, H. (ed.): *Hormones, Brain Function and Behavior,* Academic Press, New York, **1957.**

Wurtman, R. J.; Axelrod, J.; and Barchas, J. D.: Age and enzyme activity in the human pineal. *J. Clin. Endocrinol. Metab.,* **24:**299–301, **1964.**

CHAPTER

13 AGING OF THE FEMALE REPRODUCTIVE SYSTEM

The Menopause

Anne M. Holehan and Brian J. Merry

DEFINITIONS

The "menopause" is the permanent cessation of menstruation which is preceded, in the majority of women, by a period of approximately 12 months of perimenopause when cycles are irregular. Spontaneous menopause follows the loss of ovarian follicular function, but the term menopause also refers to the cessation of menstruation due to surgical procedures. As normal ovarian function may persist for some time after simple hysterectomy, the World Health Organization (WHO) (1981) suggested that the term "surgical menopause" be applied only to the procedure of bilateral ovariectomy with or without hysterectomy. The WHO recommended the following definitions (Figure 13–1):

Menopause—the permanent cessation of menstruation resulting from a loss of ovarian follicular activity.

Perimenopause of Climacteric—the period immediately prior to and at least 1 year after the menopause, characterized by physiologic and clinical features of ovarian involution.

Postmenopause—the period of life remaining after the menopause.

Premenopause—an ambiguous term used variously to describe the 1 to 2 years previous to the menopause or the whole reproductive period prior to the menopause. The WHO recommended that users define the term precisely and it is used in this chapter in the latter sense.

Evolutionary Considerations. The menopause appears restricted to the human female although, if they survive long enough in captivity, *Macaca mulatta, M. nemestrina,* and possibly *Papio* spp. undergo hormonal and other physiologic changes similar to those seen in menopausal *Homo sapiens*. However, the Pongidae (evolutionarily our closest living relatives) do not exhibit a menopause (Graham, 1981; Hogden *et al.*, 1977; Lapin *et al.*, 1979).

The origin of the menopause is a source of controversy. In the wild state the reduction or cessation of reproduction precedes senescence, and the postreproductive period is theoretically irrelevant to natural selection. Consequently, selection against genes that have a potentially deleterious effect later in life will be very weak. The lifespan of a species depends on a balance between positive selection pressures, which favor long life, and negative factors, which cause a decline in reproductive function in later life. The evolutionary value of an individual will rest on its ability to produce the maximum number of surviving offspring; therefore, selective pressures favor survival of young reproductively active individuals (Chapter 1). The menopause evolved because women survived to an age where natural selection no longer favored the maintenance of reproductive capacity (Charlesworth, 1980). The menopause may be a pleiotropic effect of a gene or gene cluster that has selection value earlier in life.

The contrasting argument suggests that the menopause is advantageous to the individual female; as early hominids increased population growth, the greater number of children required more parental care and protection (Mayer, 1982). In the hunter-gatherer hominids this would have required the presence of nonreproductive group members. Selection in older females favored cessation of reproduction and these postreproductive women became the "surrogate" mothers. Alternatively, the costs of the menopause i.e. increased mortality and morbidity of women and their offspring in the period of declining reproduction, would far outweigh any benefits that might accrue from "grandmotherly" behavior: "the menopause is an artefact of human civilization which emerged when our growing mastery of the environment increased our survivorship" (Gosden, 1985).

FUNCTIONAL CHARACTERISTICS OF MENOPAUSE

Age at Natural Menopause

Determining the age at menopause is subject to analytic inaccuracies. Serious sam-

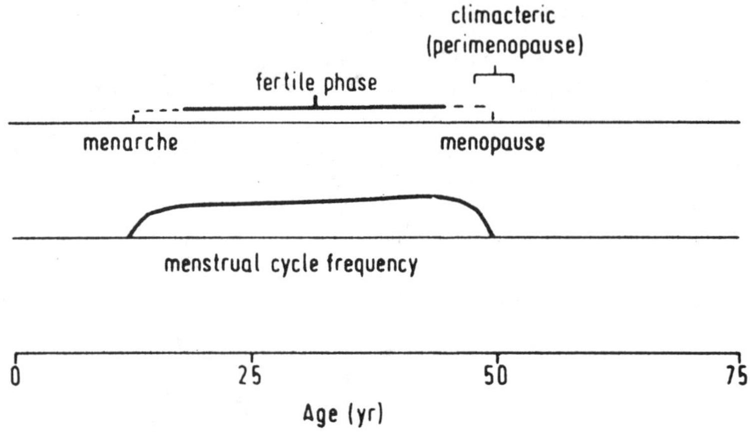

Figure 13–1. *Schematic diagram illustrating definitions and timing of events in the reproductive lifespan of women.* (Reprinted with permission from Gosden, R.G.: *Biology of the Menopause: The Causes and Consequences of Ovarian Ageing,* Academic Press Inc. (London) Ld., London, 1985.)

pling errors may occur in a population study, and two populations may not be comparable on the basis of age and birth cohort. Random sampling is essential. Hospital patients are already self-selected on the basis of illness and may introduce bias into the data. Retrospective sampling (asking women to recall the date of their last menstrual period) can be biased by memory error, understating the age at menopause, recalling age at last birthday in menopause year rather than actual date of last menstrual flow (which can lead to an underestimation of up to six months) and the tendency to round up age to the nearest five years resulting in an artificially high incidence of menopause at age 40, 45 and 50 (McKinley *et al.,* 1972).

Methods to Detect Menopausal Age. Two recent methods, although still associated with the risk of bias by including more women who have an early menopause, have avoided the problems associated with retrospective studies. The first is a cross-sectional design where age and menopausal status of women are determined at the time of interview and the second, a longitudinal cohort design in which groups of women are followed over time until they reach natural menopause.

The frequency distribution of age at menopause is asymmetric as there is a wider scatter of women at a lower menopausal age (i.e., negatively skewed data); therefore, use of the mean age at menopause leads to an underestimate of the age. It is statistically more accurate to use the median age, i.e., the age at which 50 percent of the population has reached menopause. A probit or logit transformation of the percentage of postmenopausal women at each age makes the distribution more symmetric (Table 13–1). In Caucasian women the median age of menopause is between 49 and 51.

FACTORS INFLUENCING THE AGE AT MENOPAUSE

Race. The median age at menopause in Caucasian women is remarkably similar, but less is known about other racial groups. The median age at menopause for Caucasian and Negro women in the USA and South Africa differs by less than one year (Table 13–1). However, the Punjabis in India, the Melanesian women of New Guinea, and the Indians in Mexico (age at the menopause = 40) all have lower median ages at the menopause (Chavez and Martinez, 1982). These discrepancies may occur because of poor nutrition, health, or socioeconomic situation.

Nutrition. In the Melanesian population of New Guinea, median age at the menopause (43.6 years) is lower in women suffering protracted malnutrition with mean height of only 144.5 cm and mean weight 40.22 kg. The nonmalnourished group had a median age at menopause of 47.3 years, a mean height of 153.8 cm, and a mean weight of 51.14 kg (Scragg, 1973). Thinner women, particularly with small stature, tend to have an earlier menopause (Van

Table 13–1. ESTIMATES OF THE AGE AT MENOPAUSE FROM SELECTED STUDIES

COUNTRY AND YEAR OF STUDY	RACE	MEAN OR MEDIAN AGE AT MENOPAUSE (YEARS)		STUDY DESIGN
Scotland 1970	Caucasian	50.1	Median	Cross-sectional
England 1965	Caucasian	50.78	Median	Cross-sectional
		47.49	Mean	
England 1951–1961	Caucasian	49.82	Median	Cross-sectional
U.S.A. 1934–1974	Caucasian	49.8	Median	Cohort
		49.5	Mean	
U.S.A. 1966	Caucasian	50.02	Median	Cross-sectional
	Negro	49.31	Median	
	Both races	49.8	Median	
Germany 1972	Caucasian	49.06	Mean	Retrospective
Finland 1961	Caucasian	49.8	Mean	Retrospective
Switzerland 1961	Caucasian	49.8	Mean	Retrospective
Israel 1963	Caucasian	49.5	Mean	Retrospective
Netherlands 1969	Caucasian	51.4	Median	Cross-sectional
New Zealand 1967	Caucasian	50.7	Median	Cross-sectional
South Africa 1971	Caucasian	50.4	Median	Cross-sectional
	Negro	49.7	Median	
South Africa 1960	Negro	48.1	Median	Retrospective
		47.7	Mean	
South Africa 1960	Caucasian	48.7	Mean	Retrospective
Punjab 1966	Asian	44.0	Median	Cohort and cross-sectional
New Guinea 1973	Melanesian	47.3 (nonmalnourished)	Median	Cross-sectional
		43.6 (malnourished)	Median	

Reprinted from Gray, R.H.: The menopause—Epidemiological and demographic considerations. In Beard, R.J. (ed.): *The Menopause*, MTP Press Ltd., Lancaster, England, 1976. With the permission of MTP Press Ltd.

Keep *et al.*, 1979), and in well-nourished women, age at menopause is associated with percentage of body fat in early adulthood (Sherman *et al.*, 1981).

Marital Status and Age at Parity. Single and/or employed women may reach the menopause at a slightly earlier age, an effect that cannot be accounted by parity (i.e., bearing of children) or age at first pregnancy (Brand and Lehert, 1978). The age at menopause may also be slightly lower in nulliparous (not having borne children) women (Benjamin, 1960; Hauser *et al.*, 1963). The relationship between parity and age at menopause is unclear: some studies report no relationship (Jaszmann *et al.*, 1969b; Masters and Johnson, 1966) while others demonstrate a positive correlation between higher parity and later menopause in women of upper but not lower socioeconomic status.

Use of Oral Contraceptives. Little is known on this subject. Oral contraception could mask the transition from menstruation to menopause. A slightly higher median age at menopause follows use of oral contraceptives (Van Keep *et al.*, 1979).

Smoking. Smoking tobacco is associated with an earlier menopause (Lindquist and Bengtsson, 1979; Van Keep *et al.*, 1979) (Kaufman *et al.*, 1980). Naturally postmenopausal women aged 60 to 69 from the USA, Canada and Israel who had never smoked had a mean age at menopause of 49.4 years, whereas, in those who smoked one to 14 cigarettes per day from before the age of 35, the age was 48.0 years and fell to 47.6 when cigarette consumption was 15 or more per day. The tar constituents and tobacco smoke reduce the oxygen carrying capacity of hemoglobin, have adverse effects on ovarian blood vessel walls, may affect neuroendocrine status and steroid metabolism and one component, benzo(a)pyrene, destroys mouse oocytes and affects follicular reserve (Mattison and Thorgeirsson, 1978).

THE ENDOCRINOLOGY OF MENOPAUSE AND POSTMENOPAUSE PERIODS

The Female Reproductive Tract. The major components of the female reproductive tract are the two ovaries, the two oviducts (or Fallopian tubes), the uterus, the cervix, and the vagina. The ovaries, located in the pelvic cavity, are small (in humans, walnut-sized), oval structures containing the germinal cells, the ova, and the endocrine cells which secrete the two major hormones, estrogen(s) and progesterone. Estrogens are secreted from granulosa and thecal cells lining the follicles and by cells of the corpus luteum; these latter cells are formed at the site of the ruptured follicle at ovulation and produce both estrogens and progesterone. Thecal cells also secrete weak androgens. The ovaries lie on either side of the uterus and are covered by the fimbriae, the fringed ends of the oviducts, the tubes that lead to the uterus and in which fertilization occurs. The uterus serves as a gestation sac for the developing embryo and fetus and the vagina as the receptive organ during intercourse and the birth canal at parturition. The ovary is the primary sex organ or gonad and the other structures are secondary sex organs, which also include the breast or mammary gland and the external genitalia (vulva). Dependent on the ovarian hormones are the secondary sex characteristics, which include hair distribution, voice pitch, adipose tissue distribution, stature, muscle development, and so forth.

Major Hormones Regulating Sexual and Reproductive Function. These hormones are operative at four different levels which are all affected by aging:

- in the brain and, particularly, the hypothalamus, the gonadotropin-releasing hormone, GnRH, is a polypeptide secreted into the portal blood vessels which carry it to the anterior pituitary where it stimulates the synthesis and release of the two gonadotropins, follicle-stimulating hormone, FSH, and luteinizing hormone, LH. The midbrain, the limbic system specifically outputs from the amygdala) sustain ovulation and an increase in LH secretion;
- in the anterior pituitary, the two glycoproteins FSH and LH are synthesized and released in response to stimulation by the GnRH and are also stimulated or inhibited by the positive and negative feedbacks from the plasma ovarian hormones;
- in the ovary, the major hormones are steroids, estrogens (in humans, the most potent estrogen is 17-β estradiol followed in decreasing order of potency by estrone and estriol) progesterone and androgens (e.g. testosterone, in very small amounts). Androgens, especially weak androgens, i.e., dehydroepiandrosterone (DHA) are synthesized by the ovary; this is especially true in the postmenopausal ovary. During pregnancy, the ovary also secretes the polypeptide relaxin.
- in the periphery, ovarian steroid hormones are bound to plasma proteins, metabolized in the liver, and excreted in the urine. At the target cells, estrogens and progesterone follow the same mechanism of action as the other steroid hormones (from the adrenal cortex) and bind to the nuclear receptors and stimulate the RNA and protein synthesis responsible for the many actions of these hormones.

Reproductive Cyclicity. In the female, but not in the male, the reproductive function shows cyclic changes viewed as periodic preparations for fertilization and pregnancy and is associated with underlying cyclic endocrine and behavioral changes. The reproductive cycle of varying length in lower animals is called the estrous cycle; in primates the reproductive cycle is called the menstrual cycle with ovulation at midcycle. The major function of the menstrual cycle is *ovulation*, but another feature is menstruation.

Endocrine cyclicity involves all hormones active in reproductive function. In brief: (1) at the beginning of the menstrual cycle (the first day of menstruation) several follicles begin to grow but only one is dominant and continues to grow and will ovulate. The others degenerate, forming atretic follicles. Levels of ovarian hormones FSH and LH are low, but FSH levels are rising due to the low levels of sex hormones and therefore the reduced negative feedback of these hormones on the hypothalamo-pituitary axis; (2) with the maturation of the follicle in the ovary under the influence of FSH stimulation, estrogen levels increase and, through a positive feedback, stimulate the release of LH, which triggers ovulation, at about the 14th postmenstrual day; (3) at ovulation, the ovum is released into the oviduct to be fertilized. The site of the ruptured follicle is transformed into the corpus luteum, which secretes abundant amounts of both estrogens and progesterone, and finally (4) in case of pregnancy the corpus luteum continues to secrete estrogens and progesterone necessary for survival and implantation of the new organism; in the absence of fertilization, the corpus luteum recedes and is replaced by scar tissue (corpus albicans). Estrogens and progesterone levels fall and the hypertrophic and hyperhemic uterine mucosa is shed and menstruation occurs.

The transfer from regular menstrual cycles to amenorrhea (i.e. cessation of menstruation) is preceded by a period of menstrual cycle irregularity characterized by a decline in length of the follicular phase in the two decades prior to the menopause (Vollman, 1977) and an increase in anovulatory cycles (3 to 7 percent of cycles at 26 to 40 years and 12 to 15 percent at 41 to 50 years;) (Doring, 1969). In normal regularly cycling menstruating women over 45 years of age, cycle length is significantly shorter than in younger women and estradiol levels are lower (50 to 120 ng/l as opposed to 150 ng/l). FSH levels are increased particularly in the follicular phase of the cycle

(Sherman *et al.,* 1976) but LH remains unchanged when compared to younger women. When menstrual irregularities occur, a variety of hormonal patterns are recorded, including phases of rising and falling estradiol concentrations with or without elevations in progesterone, elevated levels of FSH alone, or FSH and LH. These data suggest that ovarian follicles are maturing in an irregular fashion and ovulation is no longer occurring in each cycle.

Prior to menopause, estrogen is mainly produced by aromatization of weak androgens to estradiol in the granulosa cells of the ovarian follicle with smaller amounts from extraglandular aromatization of plasma androstenedione. In postmenopausal women, estrogen production is almost exclusively due to peripheral aromatization of circulating adrenal androstenedione (Judd *et al.,* 1982). The ratio of androstenedione to estrone is inversely related to the androstenedione level, which falls after the menopause. The degree of conversion is also a function of excess body fat (Marshall *et al.,* 1978; Siiteri and MacDonald, 1973). The androstenedione is aromatized to estrone in stromal tissue of fat, bone, muscle, hair, and brain. Little, if any, ovarian or adrenal secretion of estrogen occurs in postmenopausal women (Edman, 1983a). During the first 6 months after the menopause, significant amounts of estrogen may be secreted intermittently from the ovary, probably from residual follicles (Sherman *et al.,* 1979), but subsequently, plasma estradiol levels fall to low stable values for the remainder of life. The production rates of estradiol and estrone fall at different rates so that the mean blood production rate (BPR) of estradiol in postmenopausal women is 0.006 mg/24 hr which is less than 1 percent of the level in menstruating midcycle females. The BPR of estrone only falls by approximately 50 percent to 0.04 mg/24 hr and estrone is, therefore, the most abundant estrogen of the postmenopausal period (Roberts *et al.,* 1980). Estrone can be produced by peripheral conversion of androstenedione via estradiol and testosterone. This pathway is, however, much less active than the direct conversion of androstenedione to estrone, as levels of testosterone are lower than those of androstenedione. Despite low levels, testosterone becomes the principal steroid hormone secreted by the ovarian stroma. As the estrogen levels fall, testosterone action becomes unopposed and may be responsible for hair growth on the chin and upper lip of many elderly women (Edman, 1983a).

With the onset of menopause, serum levels of FSH and LH rise so that, one year after the menopause, FSH is 10 to 15 times higher than in young women and LH is about three times higher (Chakravarti *et al.,* 1976; Wide *et al.,* 1973). The maximum levels of LH are found 2 to 3 years after the menopause and remain constant thereafter (Scaglon *et al.,* 1976) or show a steady downward trend after the age of 60 (Chakravarti *et al.,* 1976). The high levels of FSH are presumably due to the loss of negative feedback of estradiol at the hypothalmo-pituitary level. The levels of both FSH and LH show a marked pulsatility, pulsing every 1 to 2 hours in a frequency similar to that seen in young women, although the amplitude of the pulses is much greater. This increased amplitude is believed to be due to increased gonadotropin-releasing hormone (GnRH). The amplitude of the pulses of GnRH is coincident with LH secretion and the increased amplitude is consistent with increased hypothalamic activity after ovarian failure (Yen *et al.,* 1972).

SYMPTOMS OF THE MENOPAUSE

The most common symptoms of the menopause can be subdivided into three groups (Table 13–2). Not all these symptoms are present in women undergoing the menopause and, when present, they are of differing intensities.

Hot Flushes. The most common and well known symptom is the hot flush (flash), usually associated with inappropriate sweating (Thompson *et al.,* 1973). Women in Aberdeen, Scotland, who were approaching the menopause were examined and 48 percent experienced flushes close to the time of the menopause, the peak incidence being the first 2 postmenopausal years (Table 13–3). In a Netherlands study of women aged 42 to 62 years, 17 percent of

Table 13–2. THE SYMPTOMS OF THE MENOPAUSE

AUTONOMIC NERVOUS SYSTEM IMBALANCE	PSYCHOGENIC	FEATURES RELATED TO METABOLIC CHANGES
Hot flushes	Headaches	Senile vaginitis
Perspiration	Insomnia	Atheromatosis and thrombosis
Palpitations	Mood changes	Skin atrophy
Angina pectoris	Irritability	Breast atrophy
	Depression	Osteoporosis
	Frigidity	Degenerative arthropathy
	Apprehension	Hirsutism

Reprinted from Utian, W.H.: Scientific basis for post-menopausal estrogen therapy: The management of specific symptoms and rationale for long-term replacement. In Beard, R.J. (ed.): *The Menopause*, MTP Press Ltd., Lancaster, England, 1976. With the permission of MTP Press Ltd.

Table 13–3. FLUSHING EXPERIENCE OF WOMEN IN ABERDEEN BY MENOPAUSAL GROUP

MENOPAUSAL STATUS	FLUSHING CURRENT	STOPPED	NEVER	NUMBER OF WOMEN
Premenopausal	11	—	87	98
Menopausal	6	1	9	16
Postmenopausal	37	41	29	107
Years since menopause				
<2 years	11	2	1	14
2–3 years	7	2	1	10
3–4 years	4	3	1	8
4–6 years	8	7	11	26
7–9 years	5	11	8	24
10+ years	1	15	7	23
Not stated	1	1		2
Total number of women	54	42	125	221

Reprinted from Thompson, B.; Hart, S.A.; and Durno, D.: Menopausal age and symptomatology in a general practice. *J. Biosocial. Sci.*, *5*:71–82, 1973. With the permission of the Galton Foundation.

women with regular cycles were already experiencing flushes, in women with irregular cycles this figure rose to 40 percent (Jaszmann *et al.*, 1969a). One to 2 years after menopause, the incidence was 65 percent and remained 35 percent even 5 to 10 years after menopause. The frequency of flushes varies from several each day to one to two per week. After a sensation of pressure in the head, a sudden feeling of heat is felt in the face, neck, and chest associated with cutaneous vasodilation and sweating in most regions of the body. Skin conductance rises beginning about 45 seconds after the pressure sensation, is maximal 4 minutes later, and by 18 minutes has declined to baseline. The concomitant rise in skin temperature (Figure 13–2) has a longer duration and is greatest in the fingers and toes (Tataryn *et al.*, 1980). Because of the sweating and peripheral vasodilation heat loss is increased with a fall of approximately 0.2°C in core body temperature. The flush is accompanied by an increase of 20 percent of heart rate over resting values and a three- to fourfold increase in blood flow to the hand in the first 2 to 3 minutes (Ginsburg *et al.*, 1981; Sturdee *et al.*, 1978).

The flushing is not a direct or specific effect of estrogen withdrawal. Flushes have been experienced by boys and girls with hypothalamic damage in the early stages of puberty before exposure to adult estrogen levels (Witt and Blethen, 1983) and by hypogonadal men following luteinizing hormone-releasing hormone (LHRH) agonist treatment (Ginsburg and O'Reilly, 1983). Although estrogen treatment can alleviate

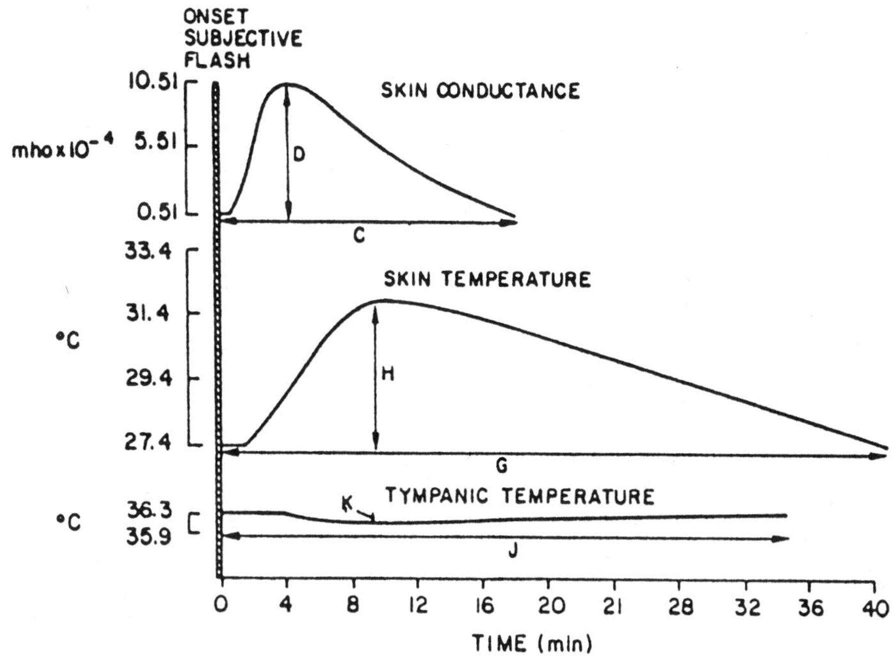

Figure 13–2. *Characteristics of the changes in skin conductance, skin temperature, and tympanic membrane temperature during a hot flush (n = 25).*

Measurements commenced when the onset of the subjective flush was signalled by the patient. [Reprinted from Tataryn, I.V.; Lomax, P.; Bajorek, J.G.; Chesarek, W.; Meldrum D.R.; and Judd, H.L.: *Maturitas,* 2:101–107, 1980. With the permission of Elsevier Science Publishers B.V. (Biomedical Division), Amsterdam.]

flushing, other compounds (progestogens, placebos, Clonidine, and Nalazone) are also effective (Gosden, 1985; Judd, 1983).

Etiology of Hot Flushes. Sweating and hot flushes occur after hypophysectomy and neither LHRH nor exogeneous gonadotropins trigger flushes in young women. Rather, the rise in pituitary gonadotropins during the menopause would be responsible for the hot flushes (Meldrum *et al.*, 1981). The rise in finger temperature (indicative of flush) is related to a pulsatile release of LH (Meldrum *et al.*, 1980) but not estrogen (Figure 13–3). Using LHRH analogs to inhibit pulsatile release of LH by down-regulation of pituitary LHRH receptors, flushing is induced in premenopausal women by lowering gonadotropins (DeFazio *et al.*, 1983), but flushing is not relieved in menopausal women (Casper and Yen, 1981). Therefore, LH pulses are not responsible for the flushing. The flushing may have a central origin as each pulse of LH corresponds to a pulse of LHRH neurosecretion. This would explain the relationship between vasodilation (under adrenergic control) and sweating (sympathetic cholinergic fibers), which is consistent with increased sympathetic reaction when core body temperature must be lowered. The decrease in core body temperature experienced during the flush is itself consistent with a central disorder as, under normal conditions, the peripheral cooling would be compensated by thermoregulatory adjustments to prevent a decrease in core temperature (Judd and Korenman, 1982).

Hypothalamus and Thermoregulation. The hypothalamic LHRH containing neurons are located adjacent to the central thermoreceptors in the posterior preoptic–anterior hypothalamic areas and inappropriate activity of these central thermoregulatory mechanisms would be responsible for the vasomotor symptoms (Figure 13–4). When the hot flush is initiated, the set point of the thermoregulatory systems falls transiently; this indicates the need for heat dissipation and leads to lower core temperature (Tataryn *et al.*, 1980). How this fall in the set point is regulated by estrogen withdrawal is unknown although some evidence implicates catechol estrogens. These metabolic products of estradiol and estrone are competitive inhibitors of the metabolism of catecholamines by catechol-*o*-methyltransferase (Ball *et al.*, 1972; Lloyd *et al.*, 1978). They displace catecholamines from cellular binding sites in nonneural tissue and inhibit the rate-limiting enzyme of catecholamine synthesis, tyrosine hydroxylase (Lloyd and Weisz, 1978; Schaeffer and Hsueh,

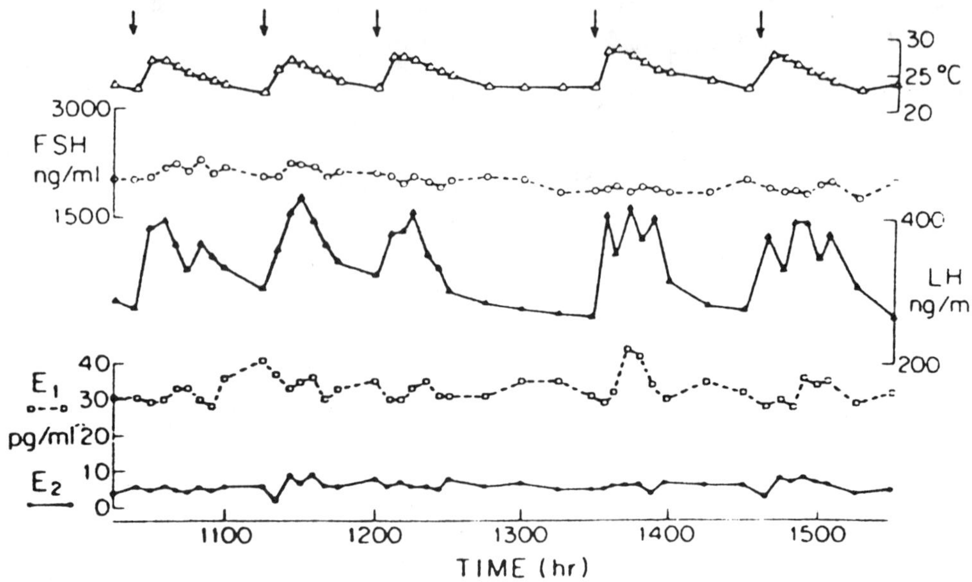

Figure 13–3. *Serial measurements of finger temperature and serum LH, FSH, estrone (E_1), and estradiol (E_2) in an individual subject.*

The onset of the temperature rises are marked by the arrows. (From D.R. Meldrum, I.V. Tataryn, A.M. Frumar, Y. Erlik, K.H. Lu and H.L. Judd, *J. Clin. Endocrinol. Metab.*, 50(4), 685–689, © by The Endocrine Society, 1980.)

1979). The catechol estrogens formed in the hypothalamus might affect menopausal flushing through their actions on synaptic activity.

Psychological Symptoms. Many menopausal women experience anxiety (apprehension, loss of self-image, and fear), nervousness (becoming easily excitable, having mental and physical unrest), irritability (frequent rage or anger and uncontrollable crying fits), and depression (apathy, inability to make decisions, loss of emotional reaction and libido, and psychomotor retardation). The depression appears not to be hormone-dependent (Winokur, 1973). Several studies reported little difference in overall psychologic and psychosomatic symptoms at any age (13 to 64) but certain symptoms (irritability, nervousness, depression, headaches and palpitations) were more common at the menopause than at other ages. The most frequent symptoms reported by menopausal women after flushing were headache, giddiness, obesity, and nervous instability, the latter being experienced by just over 30 percent of the women (Medical Women's Federation, 1933). In a study in the Netherlands, irritability was reported by 28 percent of premenopausal women, 37 percent of menopausal women and 24 percent 2 years later (Jaszmann *et al.*, 1969a,b). The corresponding figures for pre- and postmenopausal women for depression were 20 and 24 percent and for mental imbalance 17 and 23 percent. Fatigue and headache also peaked at menopause, but the frequency of shortness of breath, palpitations, insomnia, and dizziness did not alter.

Sexual behavior has been extensively studied (Kinsey *et al.*, 1953). Sexual interest and activity in men decline continuously from puberty, but the sexual activities of (unmarried) women do not decline until 55 to 60 years. Therefore, the decline in marital coital rates (50 percent of age 20 rates at age 40) is due to declining libido in the male (James, 1974). For every 5 additional years of age of the wife the decline in coitions per month when other variables were controlled was 0.1 but that of the husband was 0.8. Decline in sexual interest in postmenopausal women cannot be explained simply by the decline in husbands' interest (Halls-

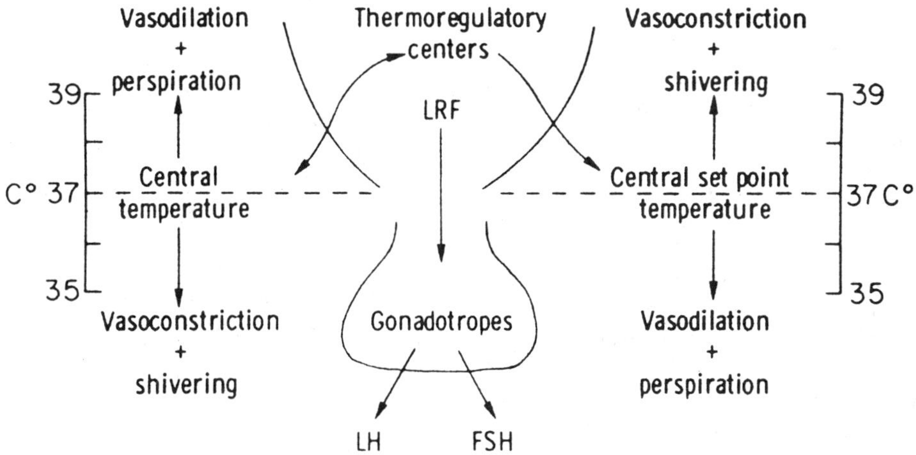

Figure 13–4. *The proposed mechanism of hot flushes is a sudden downward setting of the central set point temperature in the hypothalamic regulatory centers.*

Since central temperature would be higher this would trigger vasodilation and perspiration (hot flush) to dissipate heat. [Reprinted with permission from Judd, H.L.: In Meites, J. (ed.): *Neuroendocrinology of Aging*, Plenum Press, New York, 1983.]

trom, 1973). Rather, postmenopausal women would retain the potential for effective sexual response, particularly when regularly stimulated (Masters and Johnson, 1966). In most of these women, however, the intensity and duration of each phase of the sexual response is reduced. In 3 to 5 percent of women, vaginal dryness and associated dyspareunia (painful intercourse) can lead to a secondary decline in sexual enjoyment and interest (Hallstrom, 1979; Utian, 1972).

EFFECTS OF ESTROGEN DEPRIVATION ON TARGET ORGAN RESPONSE

VULVA

At menopause, pubic hair decreases and the labia majora become very small. The vulvar skin shows atrophy and reduction in the amount of glycogen in the epithelial cells (Voet, 1983). Skin conditions (e.g., lichen sclerosis and hyperplastic dystrophy) are prevalent.

VAGINA

The vaginal epithelium is highly responsive to estrogen and at the menopause when levels decrease, atrophy occurs, leading to shortening of the vagina and loss of elasticity (Lang and Aponte, 1967). Histologically, the vaginal epithelium becomes flattened with a loss of glycogen. The glycogen from vaginal epithelial cells provides energy for the lactobacilli present in the vagina. After the menopause, the population of lactobacilli decreases, reducing the release of lactic acid, with a rise in vaginal pH from 3.5 to 4.5 to above 5.0 (Semmens and Wagner, 1982). The microbial population often includes staphylococci and streptococci, and the postmenopausal vagina is at a greater risk of bacterial infections, which, if treated with antibiotics, may encourage the growths of yeasts responsible for postmenopausal vaginitis (Ross, 1978). The reduction in thickness of the epithelium (from 8 to 10 cell layers to three to four layers) associated with the withdrawal of estrogen results in a vagina that is vulnerable to mechanical injury and bleeds readily (atrophic vaginitis). This condition is aggravated by vaginal dryness and may lead to painful intercourse but is responsive to exogeneous estrogen treatment.

CERVIX

The uterine cervix becomes atrophic with epithelial atrophy and loss of fibromuscular stroma during the menopause

(Singer, 1975). The cervix often becomes flush with the apex of the vagina as it shortens and the cervical os (opening) is visible. The epithelium becomes thinner with a flattened superficial layer and the glandular tissue is much less active, producing little mucus. Cytological examination of the cervix becomes difficult at the menopause due to the predominance of parabasal cells as estrogen is withdrawn (Tweeddale, 1970) and the atrophic vaginitis and accompanying inflammation often exacerbate this problem. A more reliable interpretation of the smears can be obtained after a short course of vaginal or systemic estrogen.

UTERUS

As estrogen levels fall, the uterus gradually reduces in size. The total collagen and elastin content as well as the wet weight of uterine tissue reaches a maximum around age 30 (approximately 120 g wet weight) and remains constant until about age 50. Over the next 15 years the fibrous tissue content and wet weight decline by 30 to 50 percent (Woessner, 1963) and the uterus atrophies to as little as 1 cm in very old women (Lang and Aponte, 1967). The uterine endometrium becomes atrophic with a residual cystic dilation of the glands; these show no cyclic changes of activity and very little sign of secretion as the columnar epithelium becomes flattened to a cuboidal shape. In the perimenopausal period, the estrogen stimulation of the uterus, unopposed by progesterone, can stimulate proliferation of the atrophic endometrial glands that can lead to cystic changes. At this time the stromal and epithelial cells hypertrophy and glandular hyperplasia is seen in some women. This can lead to confusion when endometrial curettings are taken, as the disordered proliferative pattern can be confused with adenocarcinoma (Hendrickson and Kempson, 1980). Active hyperplasia after the menopause is confined almost exclusively to the first 5-year period; in curettage of postmenopausal women with no irregular bleeding, 31.5 percent had simple atrophy, 40.7 percent had inactive cystic glands, and only 1 percent showed actively secreting glands indicative of progesterone stimulation (McBride, 1954).

OVIDUCTS

Postmenopausally the oviducts shorten and their diameter decreases, conditions ameliorated by estrogen. As the epithelium becomes atrophic over a period of years, the stromal layer underneath forms blunted villi and the smooth muscle layer becomes replaced by fibrous tissue (Gaddum-Rosse *et al.*, 1975). After the age of 60, cilia are gradually lost and tubal secretion and peristalsis are decreased or absent (Hafez, 1982).

OVARY

As the ovary ages, it becomes smaller and more fibrotic. The number of primordial and Graafian follicles diminishes markedly, but the follicles persist in small numbers although most of those present are atretic (Chang and Judd, 1981; Talbert, 1978). The stromal tissue becomes fibrotic with a high incidence of hyperplasia, usually attributed to stimulation by the high level of gonadotropins (Rakoff and Nowrooz, 1978). Postmenopausally, the ovarian surface becomes convoluted with deep clefts where the germinal epithelium can be preserved; inclusion cysts, which may become cystoadenomas, form from the surface epithelium when the clefts become covered (Figure 13–5) (Voet, 1983). The postmenopausal medulla has a characteristic accumulation of corpora albicanta (scar tissue), which are composed of fine collagen fibers with very few cells. These may be formed from degenerating corpora lutea or from relatively recent atretic follicles (Mossman and Duke, 1973). The blood vessel walls of the medulla and hilus become sclerotic, there is hyalinization of collagen elements (Thung, 1961) and stromal calcification and/or hemorrhage (Kuppe *et al.*, 1976).

SKIN

The skin contains estrogen receptors and can actively metabolize estrogens which affect the hyaluronic acid and water content of the sex skin and increase its thickness (Marks and Shahrad, 1976). With aging, the dermis and epidermis become thinner, lose water and elasticity, and accumulate in-

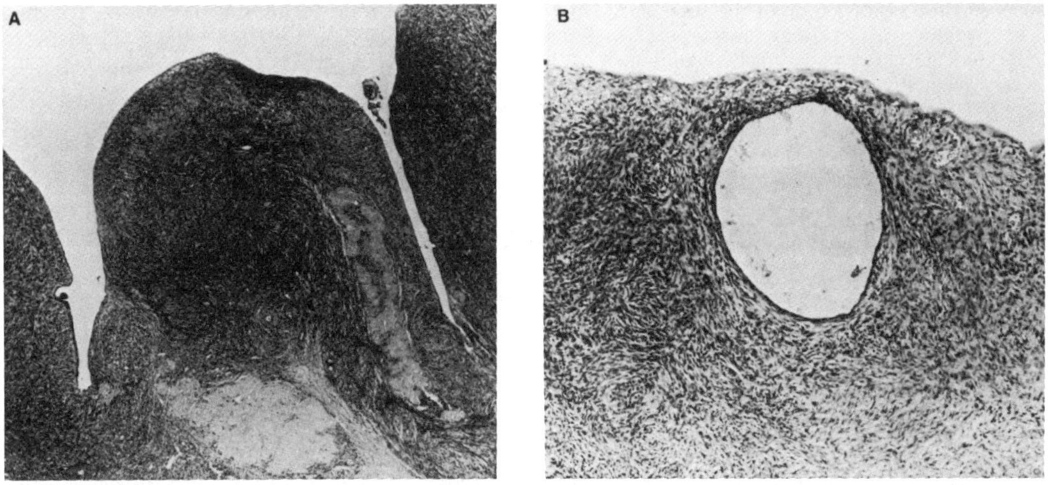

Figure 13–5.

A. Section of postmenopausal ovary showing the deep convolutions that give rise to the cerebriform convolutions characteristic of the postmenopausal ovaries. There are scattered corpora albicanta with preservation of the germinal epithelium in some of the clefts. H + E ×50. *B*. Section of a postmenopausal ovary demonstrating a germinal inclusion cyst. The convolutions shown in A that retain the germinal epithelium can be covered and produce the inclusion cysts from the surface epithelium. H + E ×120. [Reprinted with permission from Voet, R.L.: In Buchsbaum, H.J. (ed.): *The Menopause*, Springer-Verlag, New York, 1983.]

creasing amounts of pigment giving rise to "aging spots" and lose pigmentation (vitiligo), producing pale areas (Chapter 23). The reduced activity of the sebaceous and sweat glands, together with the thinning of the epidermis, makes the skin more sensitive to temperature, humidity, and trauma.

BLADDER AND URETHRA

The atrophy of the urethra parallels that of the vagina as both tissues have a common embryonic origin. Both the urethra and the trigone region of the bladder are rich in estrogen receptors and are responsive to estrogen withdrawal. As the bladder and urethra atrophy, the incidence of cystitis, urinary frequency, dysuria, and noninflammatory urethritis increases (Chapter 20). Problems with incontinence can also be caused by relaxation of the pelvic floor and atrophy of pelvic structures, but this correlates more closely with other factors (parity, obesity, constipation, race) than with withdrawal of estrogen (Edman, 1983a; Smith, 1972).

CARDIOVASCULAR SYSTEM

Both normal and surgical menopause are related to increased incidence of coronary heart disease (CHD), development of atherosclerosis and accompanying alterations in levels of serum lipids and lipid metabolism (Chapters 17 and 18).

The cessation of menstruation is associated with a rise in hemoglobin and serum cholesterol, a moderate increase in low-density lipoproteins (LDL), and a gradual rise in high-density lipoproteins (HDL) possibly associated with the high gonadotropin levels of postmenopausal women (Krauss, 1982) (Chapter 18). The high estrogen levels found in premenopausal women would protect against CHD, thus accounting for the lower incidence than in men of the same age (Chapter 17). Postmenopausally, where estrogen levels have fallen, this protection is withdrawn and the incidence of the disease increases in women.

Increased Incidence of CHD After Menopause. Postmenopausal women aged 45 to 54 years have CHD incidence 2.4 to 3.0 times greater than that of premenopausal women of the same age. However, women with a history of ischemic heart disease had a tendency to early menopause with myocardial infarct before age 48 and were still menstruating at the time of the cardiovascular incident (Bengtsson, 1973). Several studies of surgical menopause have shown that incidence of CHD and angina was more prevalent in ovariectomized women due to loss of estrogen, although the subjects studied were few, other risk variables not accounted for, and, thus, the interpretation of the data was uncertain.

Factors other than estrogen withdrawal may account for the progressive increase in CHD deaths in postmenopausal women. In ovariectomized women, serum cholesterol levels did not increase significantly for at least two years after surgery, no difference could be demonstrated in the level of coronary atherosclerosis when control and castrate women were compared, and the age at onset of myocardial infaction did not correlate with age at menopause (Utian, 1972).

Estrogen therapy increases HDL cholesterol levels in postmenopausal women but also increases LDL and VLDL. Adding a progestogen results in a pattern characteristic of atherosclerosis, i.e. lowered HDL, increased LDL, and increased cholesterol esters, and certain combinations of estrogen/progestogen may greatly increase the risk of cardiovascular disease in the postmenopausal woman (Edman, 1983a). Present evidence does not suggest that estrogen therapy produces the atherosclerotic pattern and it is insufficient to ascribe CHD development to reduction in estrogen. The progressive decrease in male:female deaths from CHD from 8:1 at age 45 to 1:1 at age 85 (Edman, 1983a) may be due, not to a rapid acceleration in the rate of mortality in women after the menopause but to a slowing of the rate in men at this age (Figure 13–6) (Heller and Jacobs, 1978). Around age 50, men appear to begin to lose some factor that had increased their risk of developing CHD, possibly the male sex hormones or an alteration in the estradiol-to-testosterone ratio.

THE SKELETAL SYSTEM

Postmenopausal osteoporosis is manifest approximately 4 to 5 years after the menopause and the frequency increases thereafter. It may produce a variety of symptoms associated with the musculoskeletal system, one of the most common being low back pain. In osteoporosis the total bone mass is reduced while retaining the normal mineral-to-matrix ratio, resulting from a greater amount of bone resorption than formation. This leads to an increased incidence of fractures, particularly in bones which have a high proportion of trabecular bone and/or are weight bearing (spinal column, particularly the lumbar area; proximal femur; pelvis and distal radius). The rate of bone resorption is greater in women than in men. Black women have a higher bone density and lower incidence of osteoporosis than Caucasian women, but bone density is lowest and osteoporosis most prevalent in Asian women. By age 60, the incidence of compression fractures of the lumbar area of the spinal column in white women is 25 percent and distal radius fractures are 10 times more frequent in women than men of the same age. In women, for every 10 years of life after 60, the incidence of proximal femur fractures doubles, and by age 75, 50 percent of all women have compression fractures of the spinal column (Edman, 1983a).

While genetic factors may have some influence on bone density and increased risk of osteoporosis, nutritional and hormonal factors may be more important. Two distinct types of osteoporosis can be identified on the basis of the pattern of loss of cortical and trabecular bone. Type II (senile osteoporosis) is associated with accelerated bone loss and poor absorption of calcium and is seen in women older than 75 years. Type I osteoporosis is associated with estrogen deficiency after menopause (Riggs and Melton, 1983). The rate of bone formation and loss involves a complex relationship between dietary intake of calcium and its absorption, the serum levels of calcium and phosphorus, and the secretion of calcitonin, parathyroid hormone, and 1,25-dihydroxy-vitamin D (Chapter 22). Total body calcium levels are lower in women than in men and decline from middle age at a much faster rate in women. Bone loss is aggravated by inadequate calcium intake due to a poor diet, or an impaired ability of the gut to absorb calcium due to vitamin D deficiency (Gosden, 1985) (Chapter 21). This leads to an increased calcium requirement with increasing age. The levels of plasma estrogen are inversely related to fasting urine levels of calcium hydroxyproline and the degree of metacarpal bone loss. The transferral of calcium from bone to blood may be inhibited by estrogen. This increases parathyroid hormone which acts on the kidney to stimulate 1αhydroxylase activity producing 1,25-dihydroxy-cholecalci-

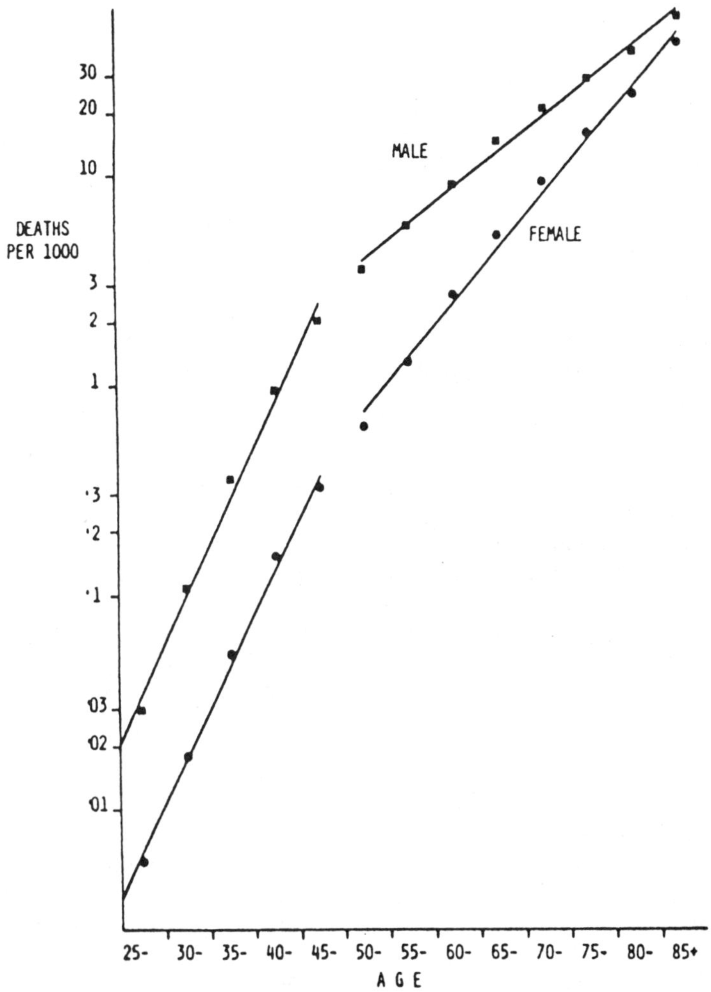

Figure 13–6. *Death rates from ischemic heart disease in men and women according to age (England and Wales, 1970–1974).*

The change occurring at the menopausal age is in men rather than women. (From Heller, R.F., and Jacobs, H.S.: *Br. Med. J.*, 1:472–474, 1978. With the permission of the British Medical Journal.)

ferol, the active metabolite of vitamin D. Estrogen lack would cause a reduction in the synthesis of this active metabolite. Giving estrogen to patients with postmenopausal osteoporosis results in retention of calcium and phosphorus, decreased serum and urinary calcium and phosphorus, urinary hydroxyproline, fasting urinary calcium and bone resorption, and increased serum immunoreactive parathyroid hormone (Pak, 1983). These effects support the concept that estrogen decreases the responsiveness of bone to endogeneous parathyroid hormone (which promotes bone resorption) and that the development of bone disease in postmenopausal females may be due in part to a loss of the protective effect of estrogen. Further evidence is seen in the finding that postmenopausal osteoporosis increases in nonobese women while obese women have a greater bone mass and are less likely to develop symptomatic osteoporosis presumably because of the higher circulating estrogen levels (Pak, 1983).

Not all investigators, however, accept the concept of estrogen withdrawal as a cause of osteoporosis. While circulating estrone levels are decreased in osteoporotic women compared to age-matched controls, plasma estrogen levels do not differ when women with and without osteoporotic fractures are compared (Edman, 1983a). It has been impossible to demonstrate the existence of estrogen receptors in bone, and there is unlikely to be any impaired responsiveness of target tissues to estrogen action. Further evidence indicates that bone loss normally begins during the third decade of life, and although the rate of osteoporosis is greatest during the first 5 years after menopause, it actually declines with increasing age.

On the basis of present evidence it is impossible to establish a simple causal effect between decreased estrogen levels and the development of postmenopausal osteoporosis. It is apparent that estrogen treatment does have some protective effect against bone loss, as does supplementation of the diet with calcium, although the mechanism of action is different (increased absorption of calcium results in decreased parathyroid hormone, and 1,25-dihydroxycholecalciferol). Calcium supplements do not conserve bone as effectively as estrogen (Recker *et al.*, 1977).

THE RISKS AND BENEFITS OF HORMONE REPLACEMENT THERAPY

Hormone replacement therapy, particularly with estrogen, is used to alleviate menopausal symptoms. Not all these symptoms are eliminated or relieved by the therapy, and concern is increasing over the dangers of uninterrupted estrogen therapy in postmenopausal women. Certain specific symptoms of the menopause are related to estrogen withdrawal, i.e., hot flushes, atrophic vaginitis; short-term estrogen therapy has been used to treat these successfully in some women. Both the frequency and duration of the flushes can be reduced and associated insomnia relieved by estrogen, and it is possible to titrate the dose so that the minimum possible is given to ensure relief of symptoms. Ethinyl estradiol (0.02 to 0.05 mg) or conjugated estrogen (0.62 to 1.25 mg) given daily is the usual treatment for these symptoms (Edman, 1983b) but relief has been obtained with dithiocarbamoylhydrazine (a mild tranquilizer), clonidine (an α-adrenergic agonist), and, in some cases, mild sedatives (possibly acting through a placebo effect). Intramuscular injections of 150 mg medroxyprogesterone acetate given monthly reduce flushing by 90 percent (Judd, 1983) but this progestin produces mild depression, fluid retention, and irregular uterine bleeding in approximately 10 percent of women. For the treatment of atrophic vaginitis and urethritis lower doses of estrogen are required to relieve the symptoms and may be administered as vaginal creams.

The beneficial effect of estrogen treatment on hot flushes and night sweats, by improving the sleep pattern, may be responsible in part for the reported action of estrogen in relieving some of the minor psychiatric symptoms of the menopause (i.e. irritability, minor depression, insomnia). Estrogens may directly reduce the latency period required to fall asleep and increase the amount of rapid eye movement sleep (Thomson and Oswald, 1977) and the resulting enhanced ability to sleep will improve mood and enhance concentration.

The protective effect of estrogen on bone resorption is dose-dependent. If therapy is started shortly after the menopause, bone resorption is retarded for up to 8 years, the incidence of fractures is reduced, and the development of bone fragility is prevented. The effects on bone density, however, are reversed, if the therapy is discontinued. Because of the risks attendant on long-term estrogen therapy, it is recommended only for those women most at risk from osteoporosis, i.e., small-framed Caucasian women who smoke or who had a surgical menopause before the age of forty. Increasing the levels of calcium is advisable in postmenopausal women with negative calcium balance. As the requirement for calcium rises with age, a supplement is likely to be beneficial to many postmenopausal women. The rate of vertebral fracture was reduced by 36 percent when 1500 mg/day calcium carbonate was given (Riggs *et al.* 1982), and this figure increased to 50 percent with the addition of vitamin D and 65 percent with sodium fluoride. The best results were obtained with combinations of calcium and estrogen (78 percent reduction in fracture rate) or calcium, estrogen, and sodium fluoride (94 percent reduction). Vitamin D should not be used alone as it induces hypercalcemia and hypercalciuria (Edman, 1983b), thus accelerating mineral bone loss. A daily regime of light exercise can promote deposition of calcium in bone and increase muscle tone. It also has beneficial effects on atherosclerosis by increasing the HDL cholesterol levels (Gosden, 1985).

Dangers of Estrogen Replacement Therapy. Estrogen replacement therapy must not be given to any woman who has breast or genital tract carcinoma, chronic liver disease, neuroophthalmologic vascular disease, undiagnosed vaginal bleeding or who has a history of thromboembolism. Caution should be observed in prescribing this treatment when endometriosis, familial hyperlipidemia, gall bladder disease, fibrocystic breasts or porphyria is diagnosed and when the woman is a heavy cigarette smoker, severely overweight, or has severe varicose veins or preexisting hypertension.

One major problem associated with estrogen therapy is endometrial hyperplasia and the risk of developing endometrial cancer. A dose-dependent effect results in a 16 to 32 percent incidence of cystic glandular and atypical hyperplasia. The relative risk of developing endometrial cancer increases four to eight times with estrogen therapy (Utian, 1980) and hyperplastic changes develop rapidly, sometimes within 6 to 7 months of the start of therapy. However, the development of estrogen-dependent endometrial cancer is a localized process and early diagnosis and treatment result in a 5-year survival rate of 95 percent. The addition of cyclic progestational therapy to the estrogen reduces the risk and incidence of endometrial cancer. Administration of progestins for 10 or more days per month to mimic the characteristic pattern of the normal cycle result in withdrawal bleeding for 3 to 4 days per month in the majority of women. This treatment has a protective effect on the endometrium.

It is unclear whether long-term estrogen or estrogen/progestogen therapy has an adverse effect on the incidence of carcinoma of the breast. The presence of fibrocystic breast disease is a contraindication for estrogen therapy as there is some evidence of breast tumor formation in these women when doses of estrogen (0.62 mg conjugated estrogen) are given that have no effect on healthy breasts (Ross *et al.*, 1980). The evidence that breast tumor formation in women with no fibrocystic breast disease is linked to estrogen therapy is inconclusive. The risk of developing breast cancer increased after long-term therapy but only in women with very high doses of estrogen (Hulka, 1980; Ross *et al.*, 1980).

Short-term, low-dose estrogen therapy does not apparently increase hypertension and thrombosis or alter glucose metabolism (Studd and Thom, 1980), but postmenopausal women using this treatment are more at risk of developing gallstones (Chapter 21), particularly when overweight (Boston Collaborative Drug Surveillance Program, 1974).

Estrogen replacement therapy has a role to play in the management of menopausal symptoms, particularly hot flushes, atrophic vaginitis, and osteoporosis. It is important that the risks associated with this treatment are understood and proper examination of the patient undertaken while therapy is administered. It is recommended that regular checkups should assure no changes in blood pressure, regular breast and pelvic examinations should be undertaken and histological evaluation of the endometrium is necessary, particularly if any unexplained vaginal bleeding has occurred. Doses of estrogen should be kept as low as possible to ensure relief of symptoms and the therapy should be given in a cyclic fashion with the addition of progestin in order to protect the uterus if present (Edman, 1983b; Utian, 1980).

AGE-RELATED LOSS OF FERTILITY

Reproductive Lifespan in Humans

Fertility patterns in modern human populations are subject to the outside influences of contraception and abortion but one group has been studied in which these confounding parameters are eliminated. The Hutterite communities of North America are an Anabaptist sect whose beliefs prohibit extramarital coitus, contraception, and abortion, and whose good diet and standards of medical care produce high fertility rates (Eaton and Mayer, 1953; Laing, 1980). Early marriage is not usual among the Hutterites and the degree of fertility is high among the older age groups (Table 13–4). The average age at birth of the last child is 40.9 years, and the number of births per thousand women falls rapidly once the fourth decade is reached with a rapid increase in the percentage of sterile couples from 33 percent at age 35 to 39 to 100 percent a decade later (Gosden, 1985). These figures are in agreement with other data from earlier populations in which contraception was less common (Henry, 1961) and would indicate that births after the age of 50 are extremely rare although the oldest documented age at birth is 57 years and 129

Table 13–4. AGE-SPECIFIC FERTILITY RATES FOR THE ETHNIC HUTTERITES, 1926–1930, 1936–1940, 1946–1950

	ANNUAL NUMBER OF LIVE BIRTHS PER 1000 WOMEN		
AGE OF MOTHER (YEARS)	1926–1930	1936–1940	1946–1950
15–19	16.9	13.1	12.0
20–24	268.0	259.1	231.0
25–29	417.4	465.6	382.7
30–34	397.1	461.9	391.1
35–39	355.0	430.6	344.6
40–44	238.9	202.9	208.3
45–49	23.5	47.6	42.1
TOTAL	236.5	258.0	226.6

Reprinted from *Human Biology*, vol. 25, No. 3 (1953), by Joseph W. Eaton and Albert J. Mayer by permission of the Wayne State University Press. Copyright (1953) by the Wayne State University Press.

days (Fergusson *et al.*, 1982). In the Hutterite society, fertility is highest at age 25 to 34, whereas highest fertility in a modern society where contraceptive methods are practiced lies between the ages of 20 and 29, with a rapid decline in the older age groups (Table 13–5). Comparison of the birth rate for 1955 and 1985 in Scotland reveals a decline in all age groups except the 15-to-19-year-olds, with the greatest rate of decline seen from age 30 onward. This apparent drop in fertility was confirmed by data from an AID (Artificial Insemination by Donor) program in which the average time to achieve a pregnancy by donor sperm rose from 6 months below age 30 to over a year when the woman was older than 35 (Federation CECOS *et al.*, 1982). In this study any possibility of male infertility or alteration in coital rates was eliminated and only the fertility of the female was studied. The results seem to indicate a drop in human fertility at a relatively early age.

Table 13–5. AGE-SPECIFIC FERTILITY RATES, SCOTLAND, 1955 AND 1985

	ANNUAL NUMBER OF LIVE BIRTHS PER 1000 WOMEN	
AGE OF MOTHER (YEARS)	1955	1985
15–19	23.1	30.9
20–24	149.2	95.1
25–29	161.0	123.1
30–34	103.0	67.9
35–39	56.0	20.7
40–44	15.5	3.4
45–49	72.5	52.6

Reprinted with the permission of the Registrar General of Scotland.

REPRODUCTIVE LIFESPAN IN LABORATORY ANIMALS

In the typical laboratory rat or mouse there is an initial juvenile period of 3 months, followed by a fertile period of approximately 12 months. In these polytocous species (i.e., producing many eggs or young at the same time) the number of ovulations increases at the second or third litter, resulting in a greater litter size (Kennedy and Kennedy, 1972). Subsequently, after a plateau period, the size of the litters declines progressively, the interval between litters increases, delivery of young becomes difficult, and lactation becomes poor in the older mothers (Asdell *et al.*, 1941; Roman and Strong, 1962).

In mice, the genetic constitution of the strain may influence the decline in litter size and the eventual termination of fertility (Jones and Krohn, 1961). Inbreeding represents a definite disadvantage with respect to reproductive capacity, leading to a significant postreproductive portion of the lifespan in hamsters, mice, rats, guinea pigs, rabbits, and gerbils (Talbert, 1977).

Although the ability of Long-Evans rats to reproduce successfully falls sharply and continuously with age, the age at which repeated pregnancies were initiated (2 or 9 months) did not influence the litter size or average pup weight at birth (Miller *et al.*, 1979). This is in marked contrast to the results of other studies, where decreases in average litter size were found in the aged rat (Asdell *et al.*, 1941; Ingram *et al.*, 1958).

The parental age of mice may influence the length of the fertilization plus gestation period, litter size and the stillborn mortality rate (Roman and Strong, 1962). In C57BL/6J mice, age did not alter the fraction of matings in previously parous mice (>80 percent at 3 to 7, and 11 to 12 months), rather the effects of age were smaller than the effects of virgin status (Holinka and Finch, 1981). In another study, the reproductive performance of mothers kept virgin or continuously pseudopregnant for 9 months before mating was not significantly different to that of mothers bred continuously from puberty. It was concluded that in these mice, the decline in litter size with age which was associated with a high level of embryonic loss after implantation, was an effect of chronological aging and not of parity (Finn, 1963), a finding since confirmed in rats (Holehan, 1984; Holehan and Merry, 1985).

Reproductive Lifespan in Domesticated Animals

Few data are available on total reproductive capacity in domestic animals as it is unusual to keep breeding stock once reproductive capacity begins to decline. The most accurate records are those kept for thoroughbred horses, which show a decline in fertility from about 19 years, although some horses have been bred successfully at 27 to 33 years, almost their normal lifespan. Reproduction also declines in cattle and sheep as well as in dogs, with the peak reproductive capacity followed by a plateau and then decline (Anderson, 1965; Talbert, 1977). All these animals are in a protected environment, and it is impossible to draw conclusions from these data about the situation pertaining in wild animals as reproductive senescence is rare, and disease and predators remove animals from the population before reproductive potential is exhausted.

Reproductive Lifespan in Primates

As with domestic animals, data concerning the end of the reproductive lifespan in primates are scarce. Only a few centers maintain primate colonies and the length of life is such that these data are only just becoming available. At the Wisconsin Primate Research Center, pregnancy in rhesus monkeys has been reported to occur as late as 26 years (Dierschke *et al.*, 1983), although in other studies, menopause in this species occurred between the ages of 25 and 30 and the latest age for carrying a pregnancy was 19 (van Wagenen, 1972). Chimpanzees continue to menstruate at the age of 44 (Talbert, 1977), but the fertility at this age is poor (Graham, 1979).

The Basis for Declining Fertility

Various explanations may account for the decline in fertility with advancing age: a reduction in the number of ova shed, an increase in abnormal ova or a wearing out of the accessory organs so that the ova cannot be fertilized or embryos carried to term or disruption of the hormonal control of the ovary or the uterine environment (Asdell *et al.*, 1941; King, 1916) (Jones and Krohn, 1961). Here, again, comparative animal physiology provides useful models for human aging.

Oocyte Depletion. Most mammals begin extrauterine life with a finite stock of oocytes that is not added to in adult life (Franchi *et al.*, 1962). Aging is accompanied by a progressive loss of oocytes at a rate apparently determined by the genetic makeup of the species or strain (Jones and Krohn, 1961). Normal disappearance of oocytes by ovulation after puberty accounts for a small proportion of the total loss, but this is insignificant when compared to the effects of atresia (involution of follicles that failed to mature).

In the human female there is a rapid decline in oocyte number from birth to 25 or 30 years (Block, 1952; 1953), a plateau period until around 38, and then a rapid decline. Very little data are available on women over 45 years old. A qualitative assessment in a group of women past the age of 50 observed only an occasional follicle or corpus luteum indicating that few ova may persist to the sixth decade (Novak, 1970). However, primordial follicles and remnants of old tertiary follicles and corpora lutea were found in ovarian samples from women up to 80 years of age (Costoff and Mahesh, 1975).

Despite this progressive loss of oocytes, reproduction in most rodents, unlike humans, comes to an end long before the ovaries are depleted of oocytes. The ovaries of rats that ceased breeding around 550 days still had 1200 to 1500 oocytes at this age (Mandl and Shelton, 1959) and in mice of different strains between 500 and 1000 oocytes were still present when the last litter was born. The only known exception among the rodents are CBA mice in which total depletion of oocytes occurs soon after reproduction ends.

Unilateral ovariectomy in rodents leads to compensatory hypertrophy of the remaining ovary, which becomes more responsive to gonadotropin and produces approximately double the normal number of ovulations (Biggers *et al.*, 1962a, Jones and Krohn, 1960). The overall number of litters born and the mean litter size were reduced and reproduction ceased earlier than in the intact animals, but the early cessation of breeding was not due to premature exhaustion of the oocytes. Intensive breeding had no effect on the rate at which oocyte number declined, and prevention of ovulation after prolonged steroid-induced infertility in mice did not counteract the decline in fertility. It was concluded that the decline of reproductive capacity in rodents and rabbits does not depend on the diminished number of oocytes available in the aging ovary.

Ovulation does not significantly affect the rate of loss of oocytes since only one ovum is lost by ovulation for every 1000 lost by atresia in the human. In virgin rats and mice which ovulate regularly every 4 to 5 days throughout their reproductive lifespan, the rate of loss of oocytes is no greater than in repeatedly bred females which ovulate less frequently. The greatest influences on the rate of loss of oocytes are the factors that control the rate of atresia. Hypophysectomy decreases the rate of loss of oocytes by reducing the rate of atresia. Another method used to slow the rate of loss of oocytes in mice is restriction of caloric intake (Chapter 25).

Developmental Abnormalities. With advanced age, increased losses prior to implantation and increased intrauterine mortality lead to resorption of fetuses in polytocous species or to spontaneous abortions in humans. Although one in every 200 live births in older women is associated with a chromosomal disorder, about 50 percent of all spontaneous abortions are genetically abnormal. As the spontaneous termination rate of clinically recognizable pregnancies in humans is 10 to 15 percent this would indicate that at least 5 to 10 percent have abnormal chromosome complements mainly reflecting an increasing maternal age (Schneider, 1981).

Chromosomal Abnormalities and Down's Syndrome. Although the incidence of clinically recognizable chromosomal disorders rises with increasing maternal age in humans, the distribution of some of these disorders is J-shaped because of a small, but significant increase among the offspring of teenage mothers. This increase, in the case of Down's syndrome, is thought to arise from environmental effects on the ova or from hereditary causes. Down's syndrome (trisomy of chromosome 21) is the most common age-related disorder in humans, rising from an incidence of 1:2000 to 2500 in women under 30 years to 1:300 between the ages of 35 and 39 and as high as 1:45 after 45 (Roberts, 1967). Edwards' and Patau's syndromes involving chromosomes 18 and 13 respectively, are the two other most common autosomal trisomies showing a dramatic increase with maternal aging (Figure 13–7) (Hook, 1981). Also associated with advanced maternal age are two sex chromosome trisomies, XXY, the Klinefelter syndrome, and XXX, the triple X syndrome. Trisomies arise in the majority of cases at the first meiotic division of oocytes because of maternal chromosome nondisjunction. Paternal nondisjunction is thought to be responsible for the most common chromosome monosomy XO (Turner's syndrome), which is not related to maternal age.

The mechanism(s) involved in the production of genetically abnormal offspring with increased maternal age are little known: they include increased exposure to radiation or chemicals, autoantibodies, infectious agents, genetic predisposition and pre- and postovulatory aging of oocytes. Mothers of Down's syndrome offspring may have been exposed to a greater cumulative dose of radiation than controls and X-irradiation has been shown to affect sex-chromosome nondisjunction in *Drosophila* and to produce decreased chiasmata frequency (visible cross formation seen in homologous chromosomes during prophase, thought to be due to crossing over) in mammalian oocytes. Chronic or acute exposure to specif-

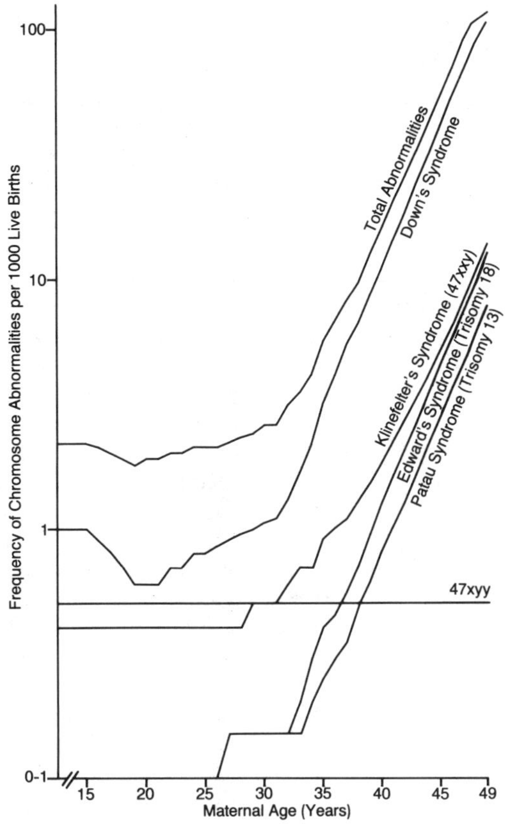

Figure 13–7. *Incidence of autosomal and sex chromosome trisomies in American live births according to maternal age.*

Data presented for autosomal trisomies represents the midpoint of the range at each age. (Adapted from Hook, E.B., *Obstet. Gynecol.*, 58:282–285, 1981. With permission from the American College of Obstetricians and Gynecologists.)

ic chemicals (e.g., methadone, mercury compounds, methotrexate, diethylstilbestrol diphosphate, 6-aminonicotinamide) may lead to the production of abnormal offspring. There are strong correlations between Down's syndrome and thyroid autoantibodies, although these may be involved in postzygotic chromosomal abnormalities rather than maternal age-dependent meiotic nondisjunction. It seems unlikely that infectious agents are involved in the etiology of Down's syndrome or that there is a strong genetic influence (Schneider, 1981).

The study of the relationship between age and frequency of chromosomal abnormalities in mouse oocytes revealed a higher number of alterations at the first meiotic division in aged mice than young adults (Henderson and Edwards, 1968). A gradient in oocyte development was proposed, the oocytes formed earliest in the ovary being the ones to ovulate first. When the total number of oocytes available for ovulation is reduced later in life, the frequency of ovulation of chromosomally abnormal oocytes would be increased. This, however, has not been confirmed in the fetal mouse ovary (Speed and Chandley, 1983). It would be expected, if a gradient existed, that the frequency of abnormal offspring should increase as the age of the mother increases. It has been pointed out, however, that many spontaneously aborted human embryos or fetuses are physically malformed or chromosomally aberrant, or both (Kalter, 1978). Loss of such conceptuses would reduce the frequency of liveborn offspring with congenital malformations and chromosomal abnormalities to a small fraction of what it would be otherwise, and the existence of a gradient of oocyte development is uncertain. The decreased incidence of liveborn malformed offspring with increasing age of mother may be due to a decreased ability of the uterus to support embryos, the abnormal fetuses being resorbed (Parsons, 1963).

Postovulatory Aging. In humans, decreased sexual activity with age and duration of marriage might delay fertilization in older women. Delayed fertilization cannot be the sole factor responsible for Down's syndrome but might be a contributory factor to the maternal-age effect (Schneider, 1981). In rabbits, postovulatory aging was induced by a two-step procedure: first, the females were mated with vasectomized males to induce ovulation, and second, they were mated several hours later with normal males for fertilization. The litter size decreased as the ovulation-to-fertilization interval increased. In guinea pigs, a 20-hour delay between ovulation and insemination induced cytolysis prior to implantation associated with an increase in gross structural abnormalities of the embryo and abortion after implantation (Blandau *et al.*, 1949). In the rat a 9-to-12 hour delay induced 60 percent abnormal ova, and polyspermy increased as the period of delay lengthened. An increase in the number of resorbed fetuses was seen but those coming to term were normal. In hamsters, a 3-to-9 hour delay between ovulation and fertilization increased the number of triploid embryos (Chang and Fernandez-Castro, 1958).

Preovulatory Aging. In both humans and rats preovulatory aging of oocytes is detrimental to development. Since coital activity in the human is not restricted to the period of ovulation, the human ovum is vulnerable to fertilization late in the menstrual cycle, leading to malformation and abortion. Aging of human ova is associated with a high risk of abortion (Guerrero and Rojas, 1975; Hertig *et al.*, 1956). The oocyte undergoes preovulatory aging as a consequence of prolonged menstrual cycles during late reproductive life. An examination of embryos from patients with dated coitus revealed that of those women who ovulated after day 14 of the cycle, over 50 percent exhibited developmental abnormalities. In a study of over 1000 spontaneously aborted fetuses from women with known reproductive histories, 62 percent of these abortions were classified as relating to factors in the ovum. The similarity of the anatomic and chromosomal anomalies found in human spontaneous abortions to those observed in laboratory animals has led to the suggestion that the fertilization of overripe ova (probably intrafollicular overripeness) is a cause of abortion (Mikamo, 1970). The incidence of human trisomies precedes any extension in cycle length; thus, extension is unlikely to be the primary causative factor. However, the endocrine changes prior to and consequent on any alterations in cycle length may have a considerable effect, for ovarian steroids are known to impair segregation of meiotic chromosomes when ova are matured in vitro (McGaughey, 1977). Teenage women with irregular cycle length have an increased incidence of Down's syndrome among their offspring, and hormonal imbalance due to oral contraception has also been implicated (Read, 1982).

Role of Estrogen in Preovulatory Aging. Aged rats with 4 or 5 days of persistent estrus appear to have an increase in developmental abnormalities when compared to younger controls. Extension of the estrous cycle to 6 days markedly increases the number of abnormal and unfertilized one-cell ova, degenerating embryos and conceptuses (Butcher, 1971). Artificial extension of the estrous cycle in the mature rat by injections of pentobarbital is also associated with developmental defects, decreased implantation and fertilization rates, increased polyspermy and a threefold increase in the number of aneuploid fetuses, including trisomies, polyploidy and mosaicism. During the naturally and artificially prolonged period of ovulatory delay the oocytes remain in meiotic arrest. In these rats there is an early rise in the plasma level of estradiol-17β in relation to ovulation. Therefore, a role for estrogen in the alteration of follicularly aged oocytes seems probable. Detrimental effects of delayed ovulation were prevented by binding of the endogenous estrogen with an antiserum (Butcher and Pope, 1979) but were reinstituted by administration of diethylstilbestrol, an estrogenic compound not bound by the antiserum (Tables 13–6 and 13–7). The early rise in estrogen has the consequence that the preovulatory oocyte is contained for a prolonged time in an environment of elevated es-

Table 13–6. EFFECTS OF NEUTRALIZATION OF CIRCULATING ESTROGEN EARLY IN THE ESTROUS CYCLE ON EARLY EMBRYONIC DEVELOPMENT

	% RECOVERED EMBRYOS			
GROUPS[a]	NORMAL BLASTULA	NORMAL MORULA	ABNORMAL	DEGENERATING
Control	89.7 ± 2.5	5.6 ± 2.2	3.1 ± 1.4	1.5 ± 0.8
Nemb[b]	64.5 ± 8.5	13.4 ± 4.2	11.1 ± 3.3	11.1 ± 7.7
ASE[c] + Nemb	83.6 ± 4.2	7.7 ± 2.9	5.9 ± 1.5	2.9 ± 1.4
DES[d] + ASE + Nemb	50.0 ± 6.8	22.5 ± 7.4	20.2 ± 3.5	7.6 ± 2.2

[a]n = 15 pregnant rats/group on day 4 of gestation.
[b]Sodium pentobarbital (Nembutal) delay of ovulation for 48 hours.
[c]ASE = antisera to estradiol on day 1 and 2 of the cycle.
[d]DES = diethylstilbestrol (0.25 μg day 1 and 0.5 μg day 2).
Reprinted from Butcher, R.L., and Pope, R.S.: Role of estrogen during prolonged estrous cycles of the rat on subsequent embryonic death or development. *Biol. Reprod., 21*:491–495, 1979. With the permission of the Society for the Study of Reproduction.

Table 13–7. EFFECTS OF NEUTRALIZATION OF ESTROGEN EARLY IN THE ESTROUS CYCLE ON EMBRYONIC DEVELOPMENT BY MIDGESTATION

			% SURVIVING EMBRYOS			
GROUPS[a]	IMPLANTATION RATE (%)	POSTIMPLANTATION DEATH (%)	NORMAL	ABNORMAL	<3/4 SIZE	<1 to >3/4 SIZE
Control	84.7 ± 1.9	4.7 ± 1.4	91.9 ± 1.5	0.8 ± 0.5	2.7 ± 0.9	4.6 ± 1.5
Nemb[b]	43.4 ± 5.3	21.6 ± 6.2	57.0 ± 5.8	8.9 ± 5.5	22.7 ± 4.7	11.4 ± 3.7
ASE[c] + Nemb	89.1 ± 3.5	7.5 ± 2.4	80.6 ± 4.6	1.3 ± 0.7	6.4 ± 1.7	11.7 ± 3.8
DES[d] + ASE + Nemb	75.0 ± 5.4	18.2 ± 5.0	70.4 ± 5.6	7.4 ± 3.8	11.9 ± 2.7	10.3 ± 2.8

[a]n = 27 to 29 litters/group at day 11 of gestation.
[b,c,d]See Table 13–6 for definitions.
Data from Butcher and Pope (1979) with the permission of the Society for the Study of Reproduction.

trogen, which appears to result in an increased incidence of subsequent abnormal development or death of the embryo; such an endocrine change also has the effect of producing an altered uterine environment and a decreased implantation rate (Butcher and Page, 1981).

AGING OF THE UTERUS

Alterations of the uterus with aging in humans were described earlier in this chapter. In old C56BC/6J mice the reduced number of offspring at term may be ascribed, at least in part, to aging-related changes in uterine structure and function. Indeed, ovulation rate is not altered nor is the number of implantation sites. Progesterone levels are low in early (and then again in late) pregnancy, and the rise in estradiol that precedes parturition is delayed and reduced (Holinka *et al.*, 1979a,b). Most of the hormonal alterations occurring in middle and late pregnancy are associated with increased resorption of fetuses at midgestation. If blastocysts from old mothers are transplanted to the uteri of young, hormonally prepared females, the survival rate ranges from 48 to 50 percent in rabbits, hamsters, and mice. In the reverse procedure, blastocysts from young to old mothers, survival rate is reduced to 1.5 to 14 percent in the same species (Adams, 1970; Blaha, 1964; Talbert and Krohn, 1966). The old uterus in these species is clearly a hostile environment for the fertilized egg. Similarly reduced is the capacity of old hamsters, rats, and mice to respond to hormonal and mechanical stimuli to simulate pregnancy. This unfavorable environment offered by the uterus may be ascribed to characteristic structural changes (Finn and Martin, 1969), decreased responsiveness to hormones (Holinka and Finch, 1977), and alteration in blood flow (Sorger and Soderwall, 1981; Finch and Holinka, 1982).

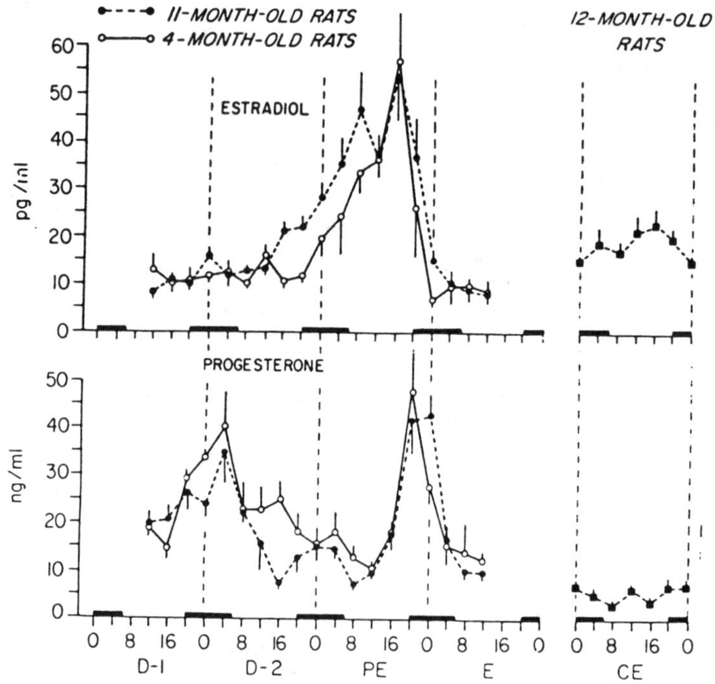

Figure 13–8. *Circulating concentrations of estradiol and progesterone in 4 and 11 month old regularly cycling female rats and in 12-month-old constant-estrous (CE) females.*

D-1 = diestrus day one; D-2 = diestrus day two; PE = proestrus, E = estrus. The solid bars on the abscissa indicate the dark phases of the dark-light photoperiod, and the numbers are hours of the day. From D-2 afternoon until PE noon, estradiol values appear to be higher in old than in young cyclic animals, and estradiol levels in CE are similar to those of old cyclic animals on D-2 evening. By contrast progesterone values in CE rats are persistently low. [Reprinted with permission from Lu, J.K.H.: In Meites, J.: (ed.): Neuroendocrinology of Aging, Plenum Press, New York, 1983.]

REPRODUCTIVE DECLINE IN FEMALE RODENTS

The foregoing discussion underlines the usefulness of laboratory animals, especially rodents, to serve as models for understanding the aging of reproductive function. Keeping in mind the notable difference between animals and humans as well as among animals, the following section focuses on reproductive aging in the female rodent, perhaps the most extensively studied animal in this area.

Reproductive function in rodents follows the estrous cycle with respect to morphology and function of ovary and secondary sex organs, role of hormones in the regulation of estrous cyclicity, fertilization, and pregnancy. Rats, mice, hamsters, and guinea pigs are polyestrous species that, unlike the "reflex ovulators" such as the rabbit, repeat the cycles (lasting 4 to 5 days in the rat) throughout the year without much variation unless interrupted by pregnancy or pseudopregnancy (the latter, as the name indicates, with hormonal signs of pregnancy but without the occurrence of fertilization). In these species, eggs are normally released from the ovary during "heat" or estrus when the sexual interest of the female is aroused. The days of the cycle are numbered from the day(s) of estrus (in the rat: estrus, diestrus, proestrus, and again estrus). A number of interventions—hormonal, nutritional, psychologic—can alter the rhythmicity and duration of reproductive function and interact with the effects of age in directing both onset and cessation of reproduction.

Aging and the Estrous Cycle in Female Rodents. Beginning at approximately 10 to 12 months of age female rats show gradual changes

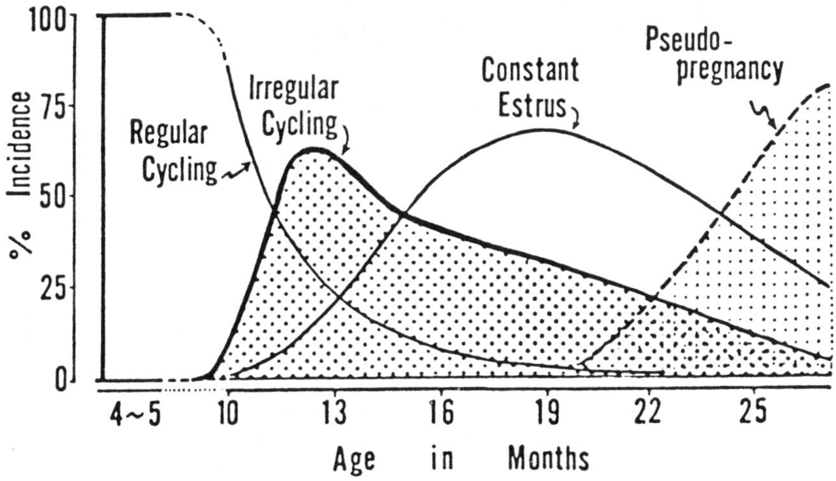

Figure 13–9. *Chronological changes in reproductive pattern in aging female rats (Long-Evans).*

Many females change from regular cycles to irregular cycles at about 10 to 12 months of age. Thereafter aging rats become chronically anovulatory, and display constant-estrus vaginal smears. Older animals exhibit repetitive pseudopregnancies. (From Lu, K.H., Hopper, B.R., Vargo, T.M. and Yen, S.S.C.: *Biol. Reprod.*, 21:193–203, 1979. With the permission of the Society for the Study of Reproduction.)

in the estrous cycle. The cycles become irregular and lengthened, usually characterized by an increase in the number of days of diestrus or estrus. At this age, circulating estradiol levels are high on day 2 of diestrus and on proestrus (Figure 13–8) which is of interest in view of the work on preovulatory aging of oocytes already discussed.

In 8- to 10-month-old rats, the LH surge is delayed (Cooper *et al.*, 1980; van der Schoot, 1976) and its magnitude significantly decreased (Wise, 1982). Serum progesterone is decreased at proestrus in the middle-aged rat (Miller and Riegle, 1979) and FSH levels are elevated and sustained on the day of estrus, probably in association with increased estradiol (Lu, 1983). The progressive cessation of regular estrous cycles may be preceded in middle-aged rats undergoing regular cycles by an enhanced FSH secretion, resulting in advanced follicular growth and increased ovarian estrogen production. Repeated exposure to high estrogen levels may eventually reduce the responsiveness of the hypothalamus to the feedback effect of ovarian steroids: LH surge is delayed and its magnitude is decreased; the timing of the follicular maturation and ovulation in the estrous cycle is altered and the regular cycles gradually become irregular.

This period of irregular cycling is followed by a constant estrus (or persistent vaginal cornification (that is, continuous estrus with only an occasional diestrus) or persistent pseudopregnancy (characterized by long periods of dietrus with occasional estrus and ovulation) and finally an anestrus state (characterized by continuous diestrus) (Figure 13–9). Not all rats follow this pattern; some may continue to cycle regularly until approximately 2 years old, and some may proceed directly from irregular cycles to persistent pseudopregnancy (Clemens and Meites, 1971; Huang and Meites, 1975).

While rats in constant estrus or persistent pseudopregnancy may revert to irregular cycling, reversion of the anestrus state to any other form has not been reported. Anestrus is seen in the oldest rats, seems to represent the final form of reproductive decline and could be pathological (Aschheim, 1983). Its manifestation in mice has been likened to the postmenopausal period in humans (Gosden, 1985).

Steroid Feedback Regulation of the Hypothalamus. In ovariectomized old rats, injection of estradiol or estradiol-progesterone increases LH secretion only in rats that were formerly in persistent pseudopregnancy and not in those showing constant estrus. However, 5 weeks after ovariectomy, the positive feedback effect of estrogen and progesterone on LH secretion was present in constant-estrus females. Chronic estrogen implants abolished the ability of both groups to produce a surge of LH in response to administered ovarian steroids. The constant-estrus syndrome is associated with sustained, but moderate amounts of estrogen in the presence of low progesterone, and in persistent-pseudopregnancy animals, estrogen levels are low and progesterone values high. In constant estrus rats the positive feedback mechanism of steroids on LH is present, but the high estrogen levels may act through a neurotoxic action on the hypothalamus to pre-

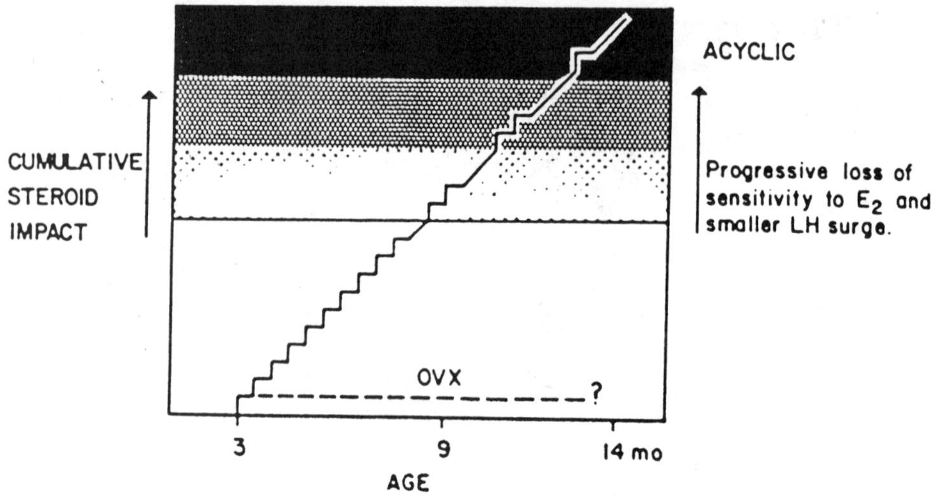

Figure 13–10. *Hypothetical mechanism of ovary-dependent neuroendocrine aging processes in which ovarian steroids have a cumulative impact on unspecified hypothalamic and pituitary loci.*

The steroid impact may be incremental over some or all estrous cycles as depicted by the stair-step ascending line. At some point the cumulative steroid impact causes a loss of neuroendocrine sensitivity to estradiol and a smaller LH surge, shown by the shaded area at the top. The theory postulates that a reduction in the availability of ovarian steroids (e.g., by long-term ovariectomy) would markedly attenuate ovary-dependent neuroendocrine aging. [From C.E. Finch, L.S. Felicio, C.V. Mobbs and J.F. Nelson, *Endocr. Rev.*, 5(4), 467–497, © The Endocrine Society, 1984.]

vent pituitary secretion of LH. This action is perhaps alleviated by the high progesterone levels of persistent pseudopregnancy animals in which the central nervous system mechanisms that regulate the positive feedback of steroids on pituitary secretion of LH are still functioning (Lu *et al.*, 1980; 1981).

In young, cycling female rats chronic elevation of circulating estrogen alters dopamine neurotransmission in the tuberoinfundibular region associated with high prolactin secretion and causes neuronal degeneration accompanied by astrocytic and microglial hyperactivity (histologic indices of hypothalamic aging) in the hypothalamic arcuate nucleus (Brawer *et al.*, 1980; Casanueva *et al.*, 1982). This is accompanied by impairment of the LH surge. In Wistar rats and C57BL/6J mice, astrocytic and microglial activity increased significantly from 6 to 14 and 4 to 13 months respectively. Ovariectomy at 2 months of age markedly retarded the development of gliosis in 14-month-old rats and 13-month-old mice (Schipper *et al.*, 1981). These authors suggested that the changes seen in these old animals were similar to the arcuate lesion found in young estrogen-treated rats (Brawer *et al.*, 1980). This was thought to represent a chemical deafferentation (i.e., separation) of the arcuate nucleus from the medial preoptic area.

In senescent female rodents the age-related functional impairment of reproduction may be due to deterioration of the preoptic arcuate pathway although the disruption may be incomplete as it is possible to reinitiate ovarian cyclicity by stimulation of the hypothalamic-pituitary axis, as discussed below.

In rodents, sex steroids, like glucocorticoids (Chapter 12), may initiate a series of functionally damaging events whereby the hormones induce neuronal and endocrine cell loss in the hypothalamus and pituitary throughout the period of reproductive activity, culminating with cessation of reproduction. These losses, in turn, would lead to alterations of hypothalamopituitary responsiveness to hormonal feedbacks with consequent impairment or cessation of cyclicity and reproduction. Thus, while in humans menopause is essentially due to termination of ovarian function, in rodents failure of the hypothalamopituitary axis may be the prevalent cause. This failure may be prevented or modified by a number of interventions that may delay or accelerate reproductive aging or may reactivate damaged reproductive function.

Reactivation of Regular Estrous Cycles. A variety of agents has been used to reactivate regular cycles in irregularly cycling rodents. They include progesterone, adrenocorticotrophic hormone (ACTH), vitamin E, ether or cold stress, L-Dopa, ergotrile mesylate, iproniazid and epinephrine. In constant-estrus rats regular or irregular cycling is reinitiated by L-Dopa, progesterone, ACTH, ether, stress, and iproniazid, which increase hypothalamic catecholamines (Huang *et al.*, 1976). Old persistent-pesudopregnancy rats respond to ergotrile mesylate (a dopamine agonist) and prostaglandin, which reduce progesterone secretion (Clemens and Bennett, 1977). LH release and ovulation in constant-estrus rats can be induced by electrical stimulation of the anterior hypothalamus or preoptic area or administration of synthetic LHRH (Meites *et al.*, 1978) or by injection of LH (Aschheim, 1979).

Experimental Delay of the Age-Related Changes in Reproductive Function. When rats were ovariectomized at 6 to 12 months and given kidney capsule grafts of young ovaries at 2 years, reproductive cycles were reinstated (Aschheim, 1965). This work has been repeated and extended in C57BL/6J mice (Finch *et al.*, 1980, 1984). In these long-term ovariectomized mice with grafts, normal numbers of corpora lutea and growing follicles were produced and apparently normal ova were shed. The capacity for cyclic LH releases was retained 6 to 12 months beyond the usual age, and the magnitude of the responses was equal to that found in young controls. Histologic changes in the arcuate nucleus thought to be caused by estrogen can be retarded by long-term ovariectomy and ovarian grafting.

A mechanism has been proposed whereby cumulative steroid impact is envisaged to have a detrimental effect on unspecified hypothalamic and pituitary loci (Figure 13–10) during some or all of the estrous cycles, resulting in a loss of neuroendocrine sensitivity to estrogen, a smaller LH surge, and cycle lengthening. After cessation of estrous cyclicity, further exposure to estrogen in constant-estrus rodents causes additional damage to the neuroendocrine system. The lengthening of the estrous cycle can be prevented if animals are ovariectomized at a young age, and some of the additional neuroendocrine impairments in constant estrus animals can be reversed by prolonged ovariectomy. Indeed, aging of the neuroendocrine regulating system may be viewed as suspended, at least temporarily, during the postovariectomy period by lack of steroidal action.

The period of ovarian cyclicity has been extended in rats by addition of L-tyrosine to the diet from 7.5 months of age (Cooper and Walker, 1917). This probably resulted in the achievement of an appropriate catecholamine to serotonin balance within the central nervous system. Dietary restriction of rats from weaning also slows down the rate of reproductive aging and is associated with reduced circulating levels of estradiol (Chapter 25).

References

Adams, C. E.: Aging and reproduction in the female mammal with particular reference to the rabbit. *J. Reprod. Fertil.* (Suppl.), **12**:1–16, **1970**.

Anderson, A. C.: Reproductive ability of female beagles in relation to advancing age. *Exp. Gerontol.*, **1**:189–192, **1965**.

Aschheim, P.: La reactivation de l'ovaire des rattes seniles en oestrus permanent au moyen de'hormones gonadotropes ou de la mise a l'obscurite. *C.R. Acad. Sci.*, **260**:5627–5630, **1965**.

Aschheim, P.: Relation of neuroendocrine system to reproductive decline in female rats. In Meites, J. (ed.): *Neuroendocrinology of Aging*, Plenum Press, New York, **1983**.

Asdell, S. A.; Bogart, R.; and Sperling, G.: The influence of age and rate of breeding upon the ability of the female rat to produce and raise young. *Mem. Cornell Univ. Agric. Exp. Stn.*, **238**:3–26, **1941**.

Ball, P.; Knuppen, R.; Haupt, M.; and Brueur, H.: Interactions between estrogens and catechol amines III. Studies on the methylation of catechol estrogens, catechol amines and other catechols by the catechol-o-methyl-transferase of human liver. *J. Clin. Endocrinol. Metab.*, **34**:736–746, **1972**.

Bengtsson, C.: Ischaemic heart disease in women. *Acta Med. Scand.*, **49** (Suppl. 549):1–128, **1973**.

Benjamin, F.: The age of the menarche and of the menopause in White South African women and certain factors influencing these times. *S. Afr. Med. J.*, **34**:316–320, **1960**.

Biggers, J. S.; Finn, C. A.; and McLaren, A.: Long term reproductive performance of female mice. I. Effect of removing one ovary. *J. Reprod. Fertil.*, **3**:3303–312, **1962**.

Blaha, G. C.: Effect of age of the donor and recipient on the development of transferred golden hamster ova. *Anat. Rec.*, **150**:413–416, **1964**.

Blandau, R.; Kaunitz, H.; and Slanetz, C.: Ovulation, fertilization, and transport to ova in old vitamin E deficient rats. *J. Nutr.*, **38**:97–104, **1949**.

Block, E.: Quantitative morphological investigations of the follicular system in women. Variations at different ages. *Acta Anat.*, **14**:108–123, **1952**.

Block, E.: A quantitative morphological investigation of the follicular system in newborn female infants. *Acta Anat.*, **17**:201–206, **1953**.

Boston Collaborative Drug Surveillance Program: Surgically confirmed gallbladder disease, venous thromboembolism, and breast tumors in relation to postmenopausal estrogen therapy. *New Engl. J. Med.*, **290**:15–19, **1974**.

Brand, P. C., and Lehert, P.: A new way of looking at environmental variables that may affect the age at menopause. *Maturitas*, 121–132, **1978**.

Brawer, J. R.; Schipper, H.; and Naftolin, F.: Ovary-dependent degeneration in the hypothalamic arcuate nucleus. *Endocrinology*, **107**:274–279, **1980**.

Butcher, R. L., and Page, R. D.: Role of the aging ovary in cessation of reproduction. In Schwartz, N. R., and Hunzicker-Dunn, M. (eds.): *Dynamics of Ovarian Function*, Raven Press, New York, **1981**.

Butcher, R. L., and Pope, R. S.: Role of estrogen during prolonged estrous cycles of the rat on subsequent embryonic death or development. *Biol. Reprod.*, **21**:491–495, **1979.**

Casanueva, F.; Cocchi, D.; Locatelli, V.; Flavo, C.; Zambotti, F.; Bestetti, G.; Rossei, G. L.; and Muller, E.: Defective central nervous system dopaminergic function in rats with estrogen-induced pituitary tumors, as assessed by plasma prolactin concentrations. *Endocrinology*, **110**:590–599, **1982.**

Casper, R. F., and Yen, S. S. C.: Menopausal flushes: Effect of pituitary gonatropin desensitization by a potent luteinizing hormone-releasing factor agonist. *J. Clin. Endocrinol. Metab.*, **53**:1056–1058, **1981.**

Chakravarti, S.; Collins, W. P.; Forecast, J. S.; Newton, J. R.; Oram, D. H.; and Studd, J. W. W.: Hormonal profiles after the menopause. *Br. Med. J.*, **2**:784–787, **1976.**

Chang, M. C., and Fernandez-Castro, L.: Effects of delayed fertilization on the development of the pronucleus and the segmentation of hamster ova. *Anat. Rec.*, **132**:307–317, **1958.**

Chang, R. J., and Judd, H. L.: The ovary after menopause. *Clin. Obstet. Gynaecol.*, **24**:181–191, **1981.**

Charlesworth, B.: *Evolution in the Age-Structured Populations,* Cambridge University Press, Cambridge, **1980.**

Chavez, A., and Martinez, C.: *Growing up in a Developing Community,* Institute of Nutrition of Central America and Panama, Mexico, **1982.**

Clemens, J. A., and Bennett, D. R.: Do aging changes in the preoptic area contribute to loss of cyclic endocrine function? *J. Gerontol.*, **32**:19–24, **1977.**

Clemens, J. A., and Meites, J.: Neuroendocrine status of old constant estrous rats. *Neuroendocrinology,* **7**:249–256, **1971.**

Cooper, R. L.; Conn, M.; and Walker, R. F.: Characterization of the LH-surge in middle-aged female rats. *Biol. Reprod.*, **23**:611–615, **1980.**

Cooper, R. L., and Walker, R. F.: Potential therapeutic consequences of age-dependent changes in brain physiology. In von Hahn, H. P. (ed.): *Interdisciplinary Topics in Gerontology,* Vol. 15, S. Karger, Basel, **1979.**

Costoff, A., and Mahesh, V. B.: Primordial follicles with normal oocytes in the ovaries of postmenopausal women. *J. Am. Geriatr. Soc.*, **23**:193–196, **1975.**

DeFazio, J.; Meldrum, D. R.; Laufer, L.; Vale, W.; Rivier, J.; Lu, J. K. H.; and Judd, H. L.: Induction of hot flashes in premenopausal women treated with a long-acting GnRH agonist. *J. Clin. Endocrinol. Metab.*, **56**:445–448, **1983.**

Dierschke, D. J.; Koening, J.; Krueger, G.; and Robinson, J. A.: Reproductive and hormonal patterns in perimenopausal rhesus monkeys. *Program Endocr. Soc.*, Abstr. No. 678, **1983.**

Doring, G. K.: The incidence of anovular cycles in women. *J. Reprod. Fertil. Suppl.*, **6**:77–81, **1969.**

Eaton, J. W., and Mayer, A. J.: The social biology of very high fertility among the Hutterites. The demography of a unique population. *Hum. Biol.*, **25**:206–264, **1953.**

Edman, C. D.: The Climacteric. In Buchsbaum, H. J. (ed.): *The Menopause,* Springer-Verlag, New York, **1983a.**

Edman, C. D.: Estrogen replacement therapy. In Buchsbaum, H. J. (ed.): *The Menopause,* Springer-Verlag, New York, **1983b.**

Federation CECOS; Schwartz, D.; and Mayaux, M. J.: Female fecundity as a function of age. Results of artificial insemination in 2193 nulliparous women with azoospermic husbands. *New Engl. J. Med.*, **306**:404–406, **1982.**

Fergusson, I. L. C.; Taylor, R. W.; and Watson, J. M.: *Records and Curiosities in Obstetrics and Gynaecology,* Bailliere, London, **1982.**

Finch, C. E.; Felicio, L. S.; Flurkey, K.; Gee, D. M.; Mobbs, C.; Nelson, J. F.; and Osterburg, H. H.: Studies on ovarian-hypothalamic-pituitary interactions during reproductive aging in C57BL/6J mice. *Peptides,* **1** (Suppl. 1):163–175, **1980.**

Finch, C. E.; Felicio, L. S.; Mobbs, C.; and Nelson, J. F.: Ovarian and steroidal influences on neuroendocrine aging process in female rodents. *Endocrine Reviews,* **5**:467–497, **1984.**

Finch, C. E., and Holinka, C. F.: Aging and uterine growth during implantation in C57BL/6J mice. *Exp. Gerontol.*, **17**:235–241, **1982.**

Finn, C. A.: Reproductive capacity and litter size in mice: Effect of age and environment. *J. Reprod. Fertil.*, **6**:205–214, **1963.**

Franchi, L. L.; Mandl, A. M.; and Zuckerman, S.: The development of the ovary and the process of oogenesis. In Zuckerman, S. (ed.): *The Ovary,* Vol. 1, Academic Press, New York and London, **1962.**

Fugo, N. W., and Butcher, R. L.: Effects of prolonged estrous cycles on reproduction in aged rats. *Fertil. Steril.*, **22**:98–101, **1971.**

Gaddum-Rosse, P.; Rumery, R. E.; Blandau, R. J.; and Thiersch, J. B.: Studies on the mucosa of postmenopausal oviducts: Surface appearance, ciliary activity, and the effect of estrogen treatment. *Fertil. Steril.*, **26**:951–969, **1975.**

Ginsburg, J.; Sinhoe, J.; and O'Reilly, B.: Cardiovascular responses during the menopausal hot flush. *Br. J. Obstet. Gynaecol.*, **88**:925–930, **1981.**

Gosden, R. G.: *Biology of the Menopause: The Causes and Consequences of Ovarian Aging,* Academic Press, London, **1985.**

Gosden, R. G.; Laing, S. C.; Felicio, L. S.; Nelson, J. F.; and Finch, C. E.: Imminent oocyte exhaustion and reduced follicular recruitment mark the climacteric in aging mice. *Biol. Reprod.*, **28**:255–260, **1983.**

Graham, C. E.: Reproductive function in aged female chimpanzees. *Am. J. Phys. Anthropol.*, **50**:291–300, **1979.**

Graham, C. E.: Menstrual cycle of the great apes. In Gram, E. C. (ed.): *Reproductive Biology of the Great Apes,* Academic Press, New York, **1981.**

Guerrero, R., and Rojas, O. I.: Spontaneous abortion and aging of human ova and spermatozoa, *New Engl. J. Med.*, **293**:573–575, **1975.**

Hafez, E. S. E.: Scanning electron microscopy of female reproductive organs during menopause and related pathologies. In Fiorette, P.; Martini, L.; Melis, G. B.; Yen, S. S. C. (eds.): *The Menopause: Clinical, Endocrinological and Pathophysiological Aspects,* Serono Foundation Symposium No. 39, Academic Press, New York, **1982.**

Hallstrom, T.: *Mental Disorder and Sexuality in the Climacteric,* Scandinavian University Books, Esselte Studium, Stockholm, **1973.**

Hallstrom, T.: Sexuality of women in middle age: The Goteborn study. *J. Biosocial Sci. Suppl.*, **6**:165–175, **1979.**

Hauser, G. A.; Remen, U.; Valaer, M.; Erb, H.; Muller, T.; and Oribi, J.: Menarche and menopause in Israel. *Gynaecologia,* **155**:39–47, **1963.**

Heller, R. J., and Jacobs, H. S.: Coronary heart disease in relation to age, sex and menopause. *Br. Med. J.*, **1**:472–474, **1978.**

Henderson, S. A., and Edwards, R. G.: Chiasma frequency and maternal age in mammals. *Nature (London),* **218**:22–28, **1968.**

Hendrickson, M. R., and Kempson, R. L.: Endometrial epithelial metaplasia: Proliferations frequently misdiagnosed as adenocarcinoma. *Am. J. Surg. Pathol.*, **4**:525–542, **1980.**

Henry, L.: Some data on natural fertility. *Eugen. Q.*, **8**:81–91, **1961.**

Hertig, A. T.; Rock, J.; and Adams, E. C.: A description of 34 human ova within the first 17 days of development. *Am. J. Anat.*, **989**:435–493, **1956.**

Hogden, G. D.; Goodman, A. L.; O'Connor, A.; and Johnson, D. K.: Menopause in rhesus monkeys: Model for study of disorders in the human climacteric. *Am. J. Obstet. Gynecol.*, **127**:581–584, **1977.**

Holehan, A. M.: *The Effect of Aging and Dietary Restriction upon Reproduction in the Female CFY Sprague-Dawley Rat*, Ph.D. Thesis, University of Hull, **1984.**

Holehan, A. M., and Merry, B. J.: Lifetime breeding studies in fully fed and dietary restricted female CFY Sprague-Dawley rats. 1. Effect of age, housing conditions and diet on fecundity. *Mech. Aging Dev.*, **33**:19–28, **1985.**

Holinka, C. F., and Finch, C. E.: Age-related changes in the decidual response of the C57BL/6J mouse uterus. *Biol. Reprod.*, **16**:385–393, **1977.**

Holinka, C. F.; Tseng, Y- C.; and Finch, C. E.: Reproductive aging in C57BL/6J mice: plasma progesterone, viable embryos and resorption frequency throughout pregnancy. *Biol. Reprod.*, **20**:1201–1212, **1979.**

Hulka, B. S.: Effect of exogenous estrogen on postmenopausal women: The epidemiologic evidence. *Obstet. Gynecol. Survey*, **35**:389–399, **1980.**

Huang, H. H., and Meites, J.: Reproductive capacity of aging female rats. *Neuroendocrinology*, **17**:289–295, **1975.**

Huang, H. H.; Marshall, S.; and Meites, J.: Induction of estrous cycles in old noncyclic rats by progesterone, ACTH, ether stress or L-dopa. *Neuroendocrinology*, **20**:21–34, **1976.**

Ingram, D. L.; Mandl, A. M.; and Zuckerman, S.: The influence of age on litter size. *J. Endocrinol.*, **17**:280–285, **1958.**

James, W. H.: Marital coital rates, spouses' ages, family size and social class. *J. Sex. Res.*, **10**:205–218.

Jaszmann, L.; van Lith, N. D.; and Zaat, J. C. A.: The perimenopausal symptoms: The statistical analysis of a survey. *Med. Gynaecol. Sociol.*, **4**:268–277, **1969a.**

Jones, E. C., and Krohn, P. L.: Effect of unilateral ovariectomy on reproductive lifespan of mice. *J. Endocrinol.*, **20**:129–134, **1960.**

Jones, E. C., and Krohn, P. L.: The relationships between age, numbers of oocytes and fertility in virgin and multiparous mice. *J. Endocrinol.*, **21**:469–495, **1961.**

Judd, H. L.: Pathophysiology of menopausal hot flushes. In Meites, J. (ed.): *Neuroendocrinology of Aging*, Plenum Press, New York, **1983.**

Judd, H. L., and Korenman, S. G.: Effects of aging on reproductive function in women. In Korenman, S. G. (ed.): *Endocrine Aspects of Aging*, Elsevier, New York, **1982.**

Judd, H. L.; Shamonki, I. M.; Frumar, A. M.; and Lagasse, L. D.: Origin of serum estradiol in postmenopausal women. *Obstet. Gynecol. (N.Y.)*, **59**:680–686, **1982.**

Kalter, H.: Elimination of fetal mice with sporadic malformations by spontaneous resorption in pregnancies of older females. *J. Reprod. Fertil.*, **53**:407–410, **1978.**

Kaufman, D. W.; Slone, D.; Rosenberg, L.; Miettinen, O. S.; and Shapiro, S.: Cigarette smoking and age at natural menopause. *Am. J. Public Health*, **70**:420–422, **1980.**

Kennedy, T. G., and Kennedy, J. P.: Effects of age and parity on reproduction in young female mice. *Biol. Reprod.*, **16**:286–291, **1972.**

King, M. D.: The relation of age to fertility in the rat. *Anat. Rec.*, **11**:269–287, **1916.**

Kinsey, A. C.; Pomeroy, W. B.; Martin, C. E.; and Gebhard, P. H.: *Sexual Behavior in the Human Female*, W. B. Saunders, Philadelphia, **1953.**

Krauss, R. M.: Regulation of high density lipoprotein levels. *Med. Clin. North Am.*, **66**:403–430, **1982.**

Kuppe, G.; Metzger, H.; and Ludwig, H.: Aging and structural changes in the female reproductive tract. In Hafez, E. S. E. (ed.): *Aging and Reproductive Physiology*, Ann Arbor Science, Michigan, **1976.**

Laing, L. M.: Declining fertility in a religious isolate: The Hutterite population of Alberta, Canada, 1950–1971. *Hum. Biol.*, **52**:288–310, **1980.**

Lang, W. R., and Aponte, G. E.: Gross and microscopic anatomy of the aged female reproductive organs. *Clin. Obstet. Gynecol.*, **10**:454–465, **1967.**

Lapin, B. A.; Krilova, R. I.; Cherkovich, G. M.; and Asanov, G. H.: Observations from Sukhumi. In Bowden, C. (ed.): *Aging in Nonhuman Primates*, Van Nostrand Reinhold, New York, **1979.**

Lindquist, O., and Bengtsson, C.: The effect of smoking on menopausal age. *Maturitas*, **1**:191–199, **1979.**

Lloyd, T., and Weisz, J.: Direct inhibition of tyrosine hydroxylase activity by catechol estrogens. *J. Biol. Chem.*, **253**:4841–4843, **1978.**

Lu, J. K. H.: Changes in ovarian function and gonadotropin and prolactin secretion in aging female rats. In Meites, J. (ed.): *Neuroendocrinology of Aging*, Plenum Press, New York, **1983.**

Lu, J. K. H.; Damassa, D. A.; Gilman, D. P.; Judd, H. L.; and Sawyer, C. H.: Relationship between circulating estrogens and the central mechanism by which ovarian steroids stimulate luteinizing hormone secretion in aged and young female rats. *Endocrinology*, **108**:836–841, **1981.**

Mandl, A. M., and Shelton, M.: A quantitative study of oocytes in young and old nulliparous laboratory rats. *J. Endocrinol.*, **18**:444–450, **1959.**

Marks, R., and Shahrad, P.: Aging and the effects of estrogens on the skin. In Beard, R. J. (ed.): *The Menopause: A Guide to Current Research and Practice*, MTP Press, Lancaster, **1976.**

Marshall, D. H.; Crilly, R.; and Nordin, B. E. C.: The relation between plasma androstenedione and oestrone levels in untreated and corticosteroid-treated post-menopausal women. *Clin. Endocrinol. (Oxford)*, **9**:407–412, **1978.**

Masters, W. H., and Johnson, V. E.: *Human Sexual Response*, Churchill, London, **1966.**

Mattison, D. R., and Thorgeirsson, S. S.: Smoking and industrial pollution, and their effects on menopause and ovarian cancer. *Lancet*, **1**:187–188, **1978.**

Mayer, P. J.: Evolutionary advantage of the menopause. *Hum. Ecol.*, **10**:477–494, **1982.**

McBride, J. M.: The normal postmenopausal endometrium. *J. Obstet. Gynaec. Brit. Empire*, **61**:691–697, **1954.**

McGaughey, R. W.: The culture of pig oocytes in minimal medium, and the influence of progesterone and estradiol-17B on meiotic maturation. *Endocrinology*, **100**:38–45, **1977.**

McKinley, S.; Jefferys, M.; and Thompson, B.: An investigation of the age at menopause. *J. Biosocial Sci.*, **4**:161–173, **1972.**

Medical Women Federation: An investigation of the menopause in 1000 women. *Lancet*, **1**:106–108, **1933.**

Meites, J.; Huang, H- H.; and Simpkins, J. W.: Recent studies on neuroendocrine control of reproductive senescence. In Schneider, E. L. (ed.): *The Aging Reproductive System*, Raven Press, New York, **1978.**

Meldrum, D. R.; Erlik, Y.; Lu, J. K. H.; and Judd, H. L.: Objectively recorded hot flushes in patients with pituitary insufficiency. *J. Clin. Endocrinol. Metabl.*, **52**:684–687, **1981.**

Meldrum, D. R.; Tatryn, I. V.; Frumar, A. M.; Erlik, Y.; Lu, J. K. H.; and Judd, H. L.: Gonadotropins, estrogens and adrenal steroids during the menopausal hot flush. *J. Clin. Endocrinol. Metab.*, **50**:685–698, **1980.**

Mikamo, K.: Anatomic and chromosomal anomalies in spontaneous abortion. *Am. J. Obstet. Gynecol.*, **106**:243–254, **1970.**

Miller, A. E., and Riegle, G. D.: Endocrine factors associated with the initiation of constant estrus in aging female rats. *Fed. Proc.*, **38**:1248, **1979.**

Miller, A. E.; Wood, S. M.; and Riegle, G. D.: The effect of age on reproduction in repeatedly mated female rats. *J. Gerontol.*, **34**:15–20, **1979.**

Mossman, H. W., and Duke, K. L.: *Comparative Morphology of the Mammalian Ovary*, The University of Wisconsin Press, Wisconsin, **1973.**

Novak, E. R.: Ovulation after fifty. *Obstet. Gynecol.*, **36**:903–910, **1970.**

Pak, C. Y. C.: Post menopausal osteoporosis. In Buchsbaum, H. J. (ed.): *The Menopause*, Springer-Verlag, New York, **1983.**

Parsons, P. A.: Congenital abnormalities and competition in man and other mammals at different maternal ages. *Nature (London)*, **198**:316–317, **1963.**

Rakoff, A. E., and Nowrooz, K.: The female climacteric. In Greenblatt, R. B. (ed.): *Geriatric Endocrinology*, Raven Press, New York, **1978.**

Read, S. G.: The distribution of Down's syndrome. *J. Ment. Defic. Res.*, **26**:215–227, **1982.**

Recker, R. R.; Saville, P. D.; and Heaney, R. P.: Effect of estrogens and calcium carbonate on bone loss in postmenopausal women. *Ann. Intern. Med.*, **87**:649–655, **1977.**

Riggs, B. L., and Melton, L. J. III: Evidence for two distinct syndromes of involutional osteoporosis. *Am. J. Med.*, **75**:899–901, **1983.**

Riggs, B. L.; Seeman, E.; and Hodgson, S. F.: Effect of the fluoride/calcium regimen on vertebral fracture occurrence in postmenopausal osteoporosis. *New Engl. J. Med.*, **306**:446–450, **1982.**

Roberts, J. A. F.: *An Introduction to Medical Genetics*, Oxford University Press, London, **1967.**

Roberts, K. D.; Rochefort, J. G.; Blean, G.; and Chapdelaine, A.: Plasma estrone sulfate levels in postmenopausal women. *Steroids*, **35**:179–187, **1980.**

Roman, L., and Strong, L. C.: Age, gestation mortality and litter size in mice. *J. Gerontol.*, **17**:37–39, **1962.**

Ross, C. A. C.: Post-menopausal vaginitis. *J. Med. Microbiol.*, **11**:209–210, **1978.**

Ross, P. K.; Paganini-Hill, A.; and Gerkins, V. R.: A case-control study of menopausal estrogen therapy and breast cancer. *J.A.M.A.*, **243**:1635–1639, **1980.**

Scaglio, H. M.; Medina, M.; Pinto-Ferreira, A. L.; Vazques, C. G.; and Perez-Palacios, G.: Pituitary LH and FSH secretion and responsiveness in women of old age. *Acta Endocrinol. (Kbh)*, **81**:673–679, **1976.**

Schaeffer, J. M., and Hsueh, A. J. W.: 2-hydroxyestradiol interaction with dopamine receptor binding in rat anterior pituitary. *J. Biol. Chem.*, **254**:5606–5608, **1979.**

Schipper, H.; Brawer, J. R.; Nelson, J. F.; Felicio, L. S.; and Finch, C. E.: Role of the gonads in the histologic aging of the hypothalamic arcuate nucleus. *Biol. Reprod.*, **25**:413–419, **1981.**

Schneider, E. L.: Aging and reproductive performance: Models for the study of age-related chromosomal and point mutations. Maternal age and aneuploidy. In Schimke, R. T. (ed.): *Biological Mechanisms in Aging, Conference Proceedings*, NIH Publication No. 81-2194, U. S. Dept. Health and Human Services, June, **1981.**

Scragg, R. F. R.: Menopause and reproductive span in rural Niugini. In *Proceedings of the Annual Symposium of the Papua New Guinea Medical Society*, Port Moresby, **1973.**

Semmens, J. F., and Wagner, G.: Estrogen deprivation and vaginal function in postmenopausal women. *J.A.M.A.*, **248**:445–448, **1982.**

Sherman, B. J.; Wallace, R. B.; and Treloar, A. E.: The menopausal transition: Endocrinological and epidemiological considerations. *J. Biosocial Sci.*, **6** (Suppl.):19–35, **1979.**

Sherman, B. J.; Wallace, R. B.; and Treloar, A. E.: The menopausal transition: Endocrinological and epidemiological considerations. *J. Biosocial Sci., (Suppl.)***6**:19–35, **1979.**

Siiteri, P. K., and MacDonald, P. C.: Role of extraglandular estrogen in human endocrinology. In Greep, R. O., and Astwood, E. B. (eds.): *Handbook of Physiology*, Vol. II, Part 1, Am. Physiol. Soc., Washington, DC, **1973.**

Singer, A.: The uterine cervix from adolescence to the menopause. *Br. J. Obstet. Gynaecol.*, **82**:81–99, **1975.**

Smith, P.: Age changes in the female urethra. *Br. J. Urol.*, **44**:667–676, **1972.**

Sorger, T., and Soderwall, A.: The aging uterus and the role of edema in endometrial function. *Biol. Reprod.*, **24**:1134–1144, **1981.**

Speed, R. M., and Chandley, A. C.: Meiosis in the foetal mouse ovary. II. Oocyte development and age-related aneuploidy. Does a production line exist? *Chromosoma*, **88**:184–189, **1983.**

Studd, J. W. W., and Thom, M. H.: Ovarian failure and aging. In Green, M. (ed.): *Clinics in Endocrinology and Metabolism*, Vol. 10, No. 1, *Endocrinology and Aging*, W. B. Saunders Company Ltd., Eastbourne, **1981.**

Sturdee, D. W.; Wilson, K. A.; Pipili, E.; and Crocker, A. D.: Physiological aspects of menopausal hot flush. *Br. Med. J.*, **2**:79–80, **1978.**

Talbert, G. B.: Aging of the reproductive system. In Finch, C. E.; Hayflick, L. (eds.): *Handbook of the Biology of Aging*, Van Nostrand Reinhold, New York, **1977.**

Talbert, G. B.: Effect of aging of the ovaries and female gametes on reproductive capacity. In Schneider, E. L. (ed.): *The Aging Reproductive System*, Raven Press, New York, **1978.**

Talbert, G. B., and Krohn, P. L.: Effect of maternal age on viability of ova and uterine support of pregnancy in mice. *J. Reprod. Fertil.*, **11**:399–406, **1966.**

Tataryn, I. V.; Lomax, P.; Bajarek, J. G.; Chesarek, W.; Meldrum, D. R.; and Judd, H. L.: Postmenopausal hot flushes: A disorder of thermoregulation. *Maturitas*, **2**:101–107, **1980.**

Thompson, B.; Hart, S. A.; and Durno, D.: Menopausal age and symptomatology in general practice. *J. Biosocial Sci.*, **5**:71–82, **1973.**

Thomson, J., and Oswald, I.: Effect of oestrogen on the sleep, mood and anxiety of menopausal women. *Br. Med. J.*, **2**:1317–1319, **1977.**

Thung, P. J.: Aging changes in the ovary. In Bourne, J. (ed.): *Structural Aspects of Aging*, Hafner, New York, **1961.**

Tweeddale, D. N.: Cytopathology of cervical squamous carcinoma in situ in postmenopausal women. *Acta Cytol*, **14**:363–369, **1970.**

Utian, W. H.: The true clinical features of postmenopause and oophorectomy, and their response to estrogen therapy. *S. Afr. Med. J.*, **46**:732–737, **1972.**

Utian, W. H.: *Menopause in Modern Perspective: A Guide to Clinical Practice*, Appleton-Century-Crofts, New York, **1980.**

Van der Schoot, P.: Changing pro-oestrous surges of luteinizing hormone in aging 5-day cyclic rats. *J. Endocrinol.*, **69**:287–288, **1976.**

Van Keep, P. A.; Brand, P. C.; and Lehert, P.: Factors affecting the age at menopause. *J. Biosocial Sci. Suppl.*, **6**:37–55, **1979.**

Van Wagenen, G.: Vital statistics from a breeding colony: Reproduction and pregnancy outcome in *Macaca mulatta. J. Med. Primatol.,* **1**:3–28, **1972.**

Voet, R. L.: End organ response to estrogen deprivation. In Buchsbaum, H. J. (ed.): *The Menopause,* Springer-Verlag, New York, **1983.**

Vollman, R. F.: The menstrual cycle. In Friedman, E. A. (ed.): *Major Problems in Obstetrics and Gynecology,* Vol. 7, Saunders, Philadelphia, **1977.**

Wide, L.; Nillius, S. J.; Gemsell, C.; and Roos, P.: Radioimmunosorbent assay of follicle-stimulating hormone and luteinizing hormone in serum and urine from men and women. *Acta Endocrinol.* (Copenh.)(Suppl.)**174**:1–58, **1973.**

Winokur, G.: Depression in the menopause. *Am. J. Psychiatry,* **130**:92–93, **1973.**

Wise, P. M.: Alterations in proestrous LH, FSH, and prolactin surges in middle-aged rats. *Proc. Soc. Exp. Biol. Med.,* **169**:348–354, **1982.**

Witt, M. F., and Blethen, S. L.: The endocrine evaluation of three children with vasomotor flushes following hypothalamic surgery. *Clin. Endocrinol. (Oxford),* **18**:551–555, **1983.**

Woessner, J. F.: Age-related changes of the human uterus and its connective tissue framework. *J. Gerontol.,* **18**:220–226, **1963.**

World Health Organisation: Research on the menopause. *W.H.O. Technical Report Series No. 670,* WHO, Geneva, **1981.**

Yen, S. S. C.; Tsai, C. C.; Naftolin, F.; Vandenberg, G.; and Ajabor, L.: Pulsatile patterns of gonatropin release in subjects with and without ovarian function. *J. Clin. Endocrinol. Metab.,* **34**:671–675, **1972.**

CHAPTER
14 AGING OF THE MALE REPRODUCTIVE SYSTEM

Anne M. Holehan and Brian J. Merry

The aging of the testis does not culminate in the cessation of function as in the ovary, but is rather a long, gradual process. It has been argued that testicular function continues indefinitely or, alternatively, that an "andropause" begins at about age 60. The andropause would be associated with some clinical and emotional symptoms and with minimal endocrine alterations, involving a moderate decline in testosterone and a minimal increase in gonadotropins. Thus, the andropause, if it exists, differs endocrinologically from the menopause, but shares, with the menopause, some of the changes involving nonreproductive organs and functions.

The reproductive system in human males includes the primary organ, the two testes, which produce the germ cells, or sperm, as well as the principal male hormones and a number of secondary sex organs—epididymis, vas deferens—which serve for transport of the sperm, and others—seminal vesicles, prostate—for the production of the seminal fluid.

As for the ovary, the hormones involved in testicular function are operative at four different levels but, unlike the ovary, these are generally little affected by aging:

- in the hypothalamus, GnRH (or LHRH), equivalent to the same polypeptide in females, is secreted and carried through the portal blood system to the anterior pituitary where it stimulates the synthesis and release of the two gonadotropins, FSH and LH, also similar to those in females.
- in the anterior pituitary, the synthesis and release of the two gonadotropins FSH and LH (also called ICSH, interstitial cell stimulating hormone) are regulated by hypothalamic LHRH and, through a negative feedback, by circulating levels of testosterone, for LH, and inhibin for FSH.
- in the testis, the major hormones are steroids: testosterone, secreted by the Leydig cells (the major type of interstitial cell) and extremely small amounts of estradiol, probably secreted by both Leydig and Sertoli cells. Another hormone, inhibin, is a protein secreted by the Sertoli cells; its secretion is stimulated by FSH and its levels inhibit FSH release from the pituitary and may also decrease LHRH.
- at the periphery, testosterone, as the ovarian steroids, is transported in the plasma partly (99 percent) bound to a steroid-binding protein (steroid hormone binding globulin, SHBG) and partly (1 percent) transported in the free, biologically active form; it is metabolized in the liver and excreted in the urine.
- at the target cells, testosterone has the same mechanism of action as other steroid hormones such as corticosteroids and ovarian hormones, already described. It freely passes the plasma membrane, forms a cytoplasmic activated steroid–receptor complex, which is carried to the nucleus, where it stimulates protein synthesis to induce the characteristic masculinizing effects and growth-promoting actions of the hormone.

In the prostate and several other tissues that are primary targets for testosterone, testosterone is converted to dehydrotestosterone (DHT) and it is DHT rather than testosterone that is physiologically active. A small amount of testosterone is also converted (by aromatization) to estrogens.

It should be recalled that androgens are also secreted by the adrenal cortex and, in fact, these androgens represent the major portion of the adrenal sex hormones. In general, their androgen activity is 20 percent less than that of testosterone. Changes with aging have been discussed in Chapter 12.

AGE RELATED CHANGES IN TESTIS

HISTOLOGY, SPERM COUNT, AND FERTILITY

Testis weight does not change significantly with age in men over 40. Data from several strains of rat have opposite results: some studies indicate no change in testis weight although an upward trend with age was seen, while others show a decline in absolute testis weight and volume. In C57BL/6J mice, testis weight did not change between 12 and 28 months, unless disease was present (Steger *et al.*, 1981; Steger and Huang, 1983; Talbert, 1977). Spermatogenesis in men continues until old age; sperm is found in the ejaculate of 48 percent of men between the ages of 80 and 90 although the percentage of seminiferous tubules containing sperm drops from 90 percent at 20 to 30 years to 10 percent in men over 80. The number of spermatocytes is reduced in older rats but the spermatogenic cycle is unchanged at 22 months. In the aging human testis, the tunica propria and basement membrane of the seminiferous tubules thicken with a progressive intertubular fibrosis and a thinning of the spermatogenic epithelium, as well as a decrease in capillary numbers. In 22-month-old Wistar rats, limited thickening of the basement membrane and tubular fibrosis occurs.

Alterations in number and volume of Leydig cells (the major producers of testosterone) vary with age and animal species. In humans, the number of these cells declines or is unchanged in old men, but it increases in Sprague-Dawley rats and stallions (Johnson and Neaves, 1981; Kaler and Neaves, 1981). In the rat, the total Leydig cell volume per testis and volume of interstitial tissue are constant with age, but in the stallion, total volume of Leydig cells increases with age and is seasonally dependent. Total Leydig cell volume and number increase by approximately 40 percent in the midbreeding season.

Barring dysfunction in the reproductive system, fertility in males is retained into old age. The oldest reported case of successful paternity was in a 94-year-old man (Seymour *et al.*, 1935), and in male rats as old as 24 months, 50 percent were still capable of siring litters, although the capacity for repeated matings was reduced (Merry and Holehan, 1981).

TESTICULAR STEROIDS

In the Baltimore Longitudinal Study, using healthy, well-educated volunteers, no decrease was noted in serum testosterone and serum estrogens between the ages of 25 and 90 years (Figure 14–1). The free testosterone index (a measure of biologically active serum testosterone) shows no alteration with age, although the binding of testosterone to sex hormone binding globulin (SHBG) is increased. Levels of 5α-dihydrotestosterone (DHT) remain constant (Harman and Tsitouras, 1980). These findings contrast with other studies in which plasma testosterone declined steadily from around age 50 (Harman, 1983). SHBG capacity increased with age, thus, producing a decrease in free plasma testosterone (Stearns *et al.*, 1974). Plasma levels of unconjugated estradiol and estrone are increased in older men because of increased peripheral androgen conversion. DHT levels decrease in testicular vein and peripheral vein blood with age and increase in

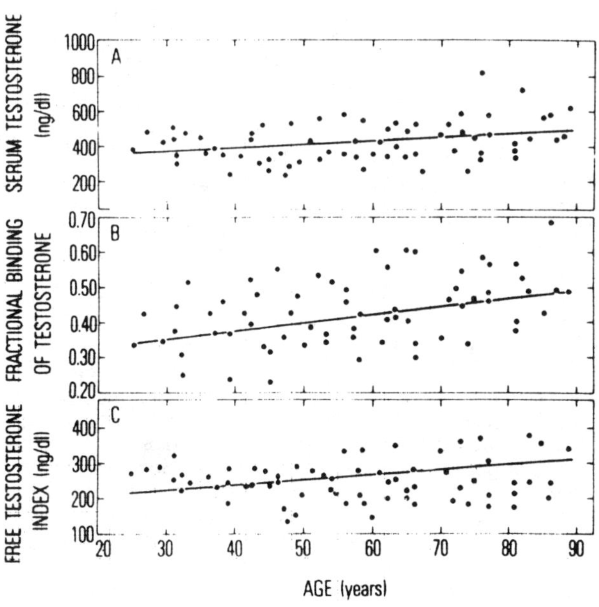

Figure 14–1.

A. Total serum testosterone concentrations in healthy male participants in the Baltimore Longitudinal Study (n = 69, ages = 25–80). *B*. Fractional binding of testosterone to sex-hormone binding globulin in these men. *C*. Free testosterone indices (percent binding × total testosterone concentration). [From S.M. Harman and P.D. Tsitouras, *J. Clin. Endocrinol. Metab.*, 51(1), 35–40, © by The Endocrine Society, 1980.]

serum in men with benign prostatic hyperplasia.

Discrepancies between reports of testosterone production with age are attributed to the inclusion of obese, alcoholic, and/or chronically ill subjects without allowing for medications taken by the subjects. Obesity is associated with a low serum testosterone and reduced SHBG binding capacity. Hepatic metabolism of testosterone is enhanced by barbiturates, benzodiazepines, and alcohol, and hypothyroidism is known to alter A-ring reduction of testosterone, producing more inactive 5β- rather than active 5α-DHT. In old men, the target tissue response to androgens is reduced. Benign prostatic hyperplasia is perhaps due to a disorder of DHT metabolism resulting in accumulation of DHT in the prostate, and possible overstimulation of the gland (Korenman and Stanik, 1984) (Chapter 20).

Comparative Androgen Levels with Aging. Unless the animals were diseased, serum testosterone levels did not decline in old C57BL/6J mice. In the long-lived White-Footed mouse *Peromyscus leucopus,* serum testosterone levels declined steadily after 20 months, although differences between young and old were not statistically significant (Steger *et al.,* 1980). The aging male golden hamster showed a comparable endocrine profile, in that serum testosterone levels had no age-related decrement although there was a greater variance in values at 31 months than at 4 to 24 months (Swanson *et al.,* 1982). In aging male rats, however, testosterone levels declined significantly with age and the diurnal variations found in plasma testosterone levels at 3 to 4 months were not present at 19 to 20 months (Merry and Holehan, 1981; Simpkins *et al.,* 1981; Steger and Huang, 1983). A slight decline in androstenedione and a significant decline in dehydroepiandrosterone with age were noted. 5α-DHT was unchanged, as were levels of estrone and estradiol, unless Leydig cell tumors were present and estradiol values rose. Increased serum pregnenolone and progesterone were present in the old male rat (Saksena and Lau, 1979). In aging male Sprague-Dawley rats, the reduction in testosterone levels may not be as severe as apparently indicated. The blood volume of this strain increases with age and the reduction in serum testosterone levels perhaps resulted from a dilution effect, the steroid release by the old testis being comparable to that of young animals (Kaler and Neaves, 1981). Testosterone reduction with age has been ascribed to decreased secretion, as the ratio of peripheral to testicular venous testosterone was not shown to change with age (Frankel and Mock, 1982).

RESPONSE OF THE TESTIS TO GONADOTROPIN STIMULATION

The ability of Leydig cells to produce testosterone in response to gonadotropin (LH) declines in aging men. Stimulation of these cells by human chorionic gonadotropin (hCG) (a substitute for LH, easily obtainable from the urine of pregnant women), in the dose of 1500 IU for 3 days, elevates testosterone levels significantly less in elderly males than in young men (Vermeulen, 1976). Although the percentage response is unchanged with age, the levels of testosterone, both before and after hCG stimulation, are lower in elderly men. This indicates that the number of responsive Leydig cells in older men is reduced. In recent work, a reduction in levels of testosterone and percentage response to hCG (Harman, 1983) followed a characteristic time course, with age, showing a reduced response to testosterone 15 hours after hCG stimulation in both middle-aged (50 to 69 years) and elderly (70 to 89 years) men; 24 hours later, only in the elderly group, testosterone values remained reduced when compared to young men (25 to 49 years) (Harman and Tsitouras, 1980). Thus, there may be a reduction in the reserve capacity of the Leydig cells with age and/or a reduction in Leydig cell number.

Leydig Cell Changes with Aging. In old rats, Leydig cell number increases possibly in an attempt to compensate for an age-related deficit in Leydig cell function, probably due to a decreased testicular blood flow. Binding of LH, and uptake of hCG by old and young testes did not differ but the old testis was less responsive to a single injection of gonadotropin. The production of testosterone in response to 1, 5, and 20 IU hCG is lower in the old testis when compared to young, although the percentage increase above baseline may be equal at both ages (Riegle and Miller, 1978) (Figure 14–2). If multiple injections of hCG are given for a 3- or 7-day period, the response of young, middle-aged and old rats does not differ significantly although the initial response decreased with age (Harman *et al.,* 1978). Daily injections of hCG in old rats returned to normal metabolic enzyme levels and testicular blood flow but could not restore the circulating levels of testosterone. Leydig cells from old rat testes incubated *in vitro* show a reduced response to hCG stimulation but the *in vitro* secretion of testosterone was unchanged because of the higher Leydig

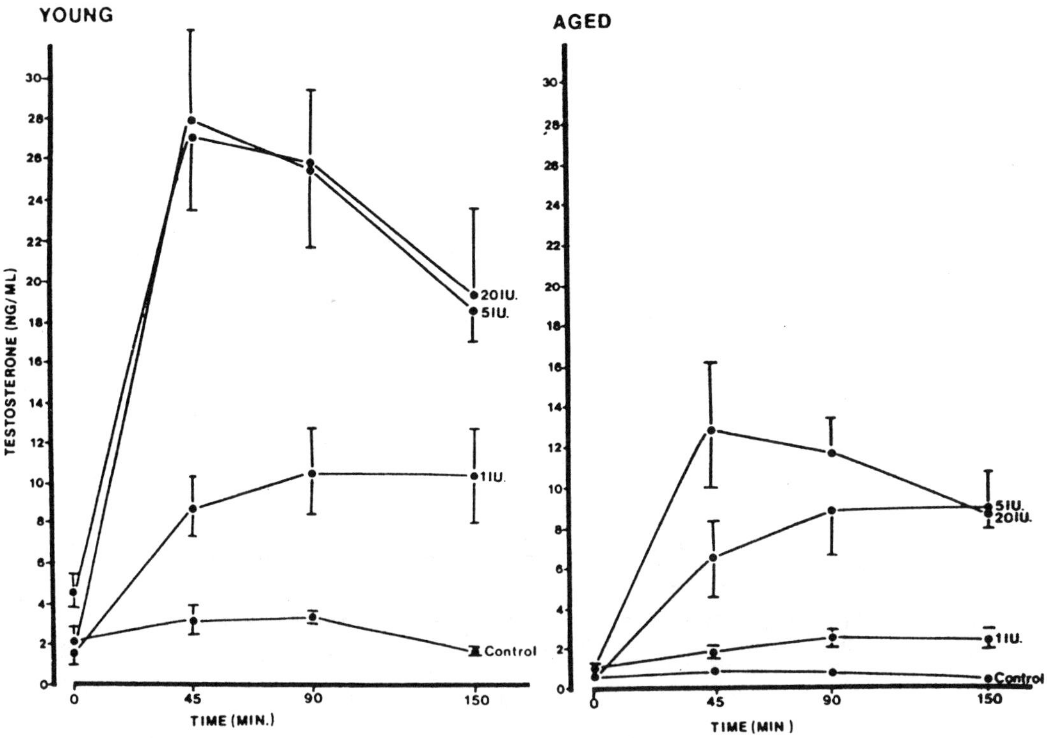

Figure 14–2. *Effect of intravenous injections of 1, 5, and 20 IU hCG on serum testosterone in young (4 month) and aged (22 to 30 months) male Long-Evans rats.*

Testosterone levels are shown as the group mean and SEM from blood samples taken under light ether anesthesia before and at 45, 90, and 150 minutes after hCG injection. [From Riegle, G.D., and Miller, A.E.: In Schneider, E.L. (ed.): *The Aging Reproductive System*, Raven Press, New York, 1978. With the permission of Raven Press.]

cell number in old rats (Steger and Huang, 1983). It seems likely that gonadotropin binding per Leydig cell declines with age despite the absence of alteration in number or affinity of binding sites for hCG, due to the increased number of Leydig cells in the old rat.

Gonadotropins and Steroid Feedback Inhibition

Plasma gonadotropins show variability with age in men. Increased LH but normal FSH levels have been reported or increased FSH but normal LH, or increased both LH and FSH—with the rise in FSH usually greater than that of LH. Both gonadotropins increase, particularly in men over 50, and in some older men (80 to 90). Levels of FSH and LH were equivalent to those seen after castration or in postmenopausal women. Increased gonadotropin secretion is associated with unchanged plasma levels of testosterone (Harman *et al.*, 1982). Thus, a decrease in sex steroid feedback inhibition of the hypothalamo-pituitary axis could result from a decreased Leydig cell function and lead to increased gonadotropin secretion. FSH secretion may be independently regulated by inhibin. As inhibin levels decrease with age, FSH rises, thereby accounting for the greater rise seen in this hormone in some studies (Baker *et al.*, 1976; Harman, 1983).

Release by the pituitary of LH and FSH in response to LHRH in elderly men is lower than would be expected in view of their elevated basal gonadotropin levels (the higher the basal gonadotropin level the greater is the magnitude of response to LHRH) (Harman *et al.*, 1982). A consistent reduction in LH response after blocking hy-

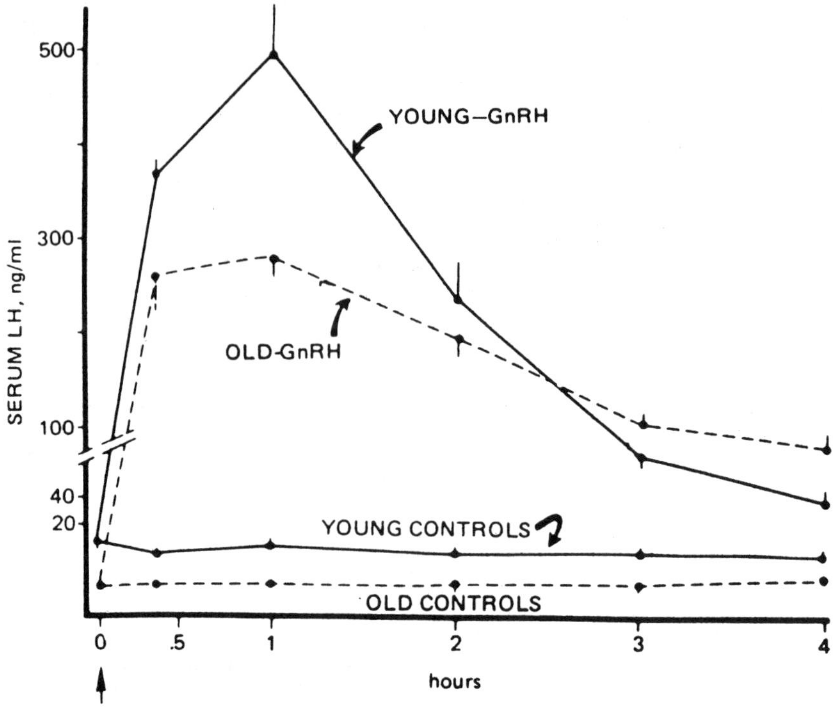

Figure 14–3. *Effects of a single injection (arrow) of GnRH on serum LH in young (4 month) and old (21 months) male Wistar rats.*

Vertical lines indicate SEM. [From Bruni, J.F.; Huang, H.H.; Marshall, S.; and Meites, J.: *Biol. Reprod.*, 17:309–312, 1977. With the permission of the Society for the Study for Reproduction.]

pothalamic estrogen receptors with clomiphene citrate may be the consequence of the freeing of gonadotropin secretion from steroid feedback inhibition in elderly men. As LHRH was not measured in these experiments it was impossible to separate alterations at the hypothalamic and pituitary level (Harman, 1983). Some impairment of the pituitary gonadotropin secretory response in aging men follows and the hypothalamic response may be reduced as well.

Molecular Changes with Aging—LH and FSH. The declining levels of plasma testosterone in old male rats are accompanied by a reduction in plasma levels of FSH and LH and an increase in prolactin (Smith and Conn, 1983). The reduction by 25 percent in the pituitary content of LH in old male rats and the increase in the molecular size of LH (assessed by gel filtration) in the circulation and pituitaries of 20 to 24-month-old male rats (Conn *et al.*, 1980) are possibly due to an alteration in sialic acid content of the LH molecule. The LH in old male rats can be restored to the molecular size of LH in young animals by 12 days of testosterone proprionate injections. This indicates that the decreased testosterone levels in old male rats may affect the LH molecule itself. Following castration, old (23 to 30 months) male rats show a smaller rise in LH and FSH than young animals (3 to 6 months). The high LH levels in old castrated males are significantly reduced by testosterone proprionate injections. This indicates an increase in sensitivity to testosterone negative feedback (Shaar *et al.*, 1975). The relative response of LH and FSH to a single injection of GnRH was equal in old (21 month) and young (4 month) male Wistar rats (Figure 14–3) (Bruni *et al.*, 1977). Multiple injections of GnRH produced significantly smaller increases in LH and FSH in old than in young male rats suggesting that the function of the pituitary changes with age (Figure 14–4).

HYPOTHALAMIC FUNCTION

The lower hypothalamic content of GnRH in 26-month-old compared to 4-month-old male rats suggests a lower re-

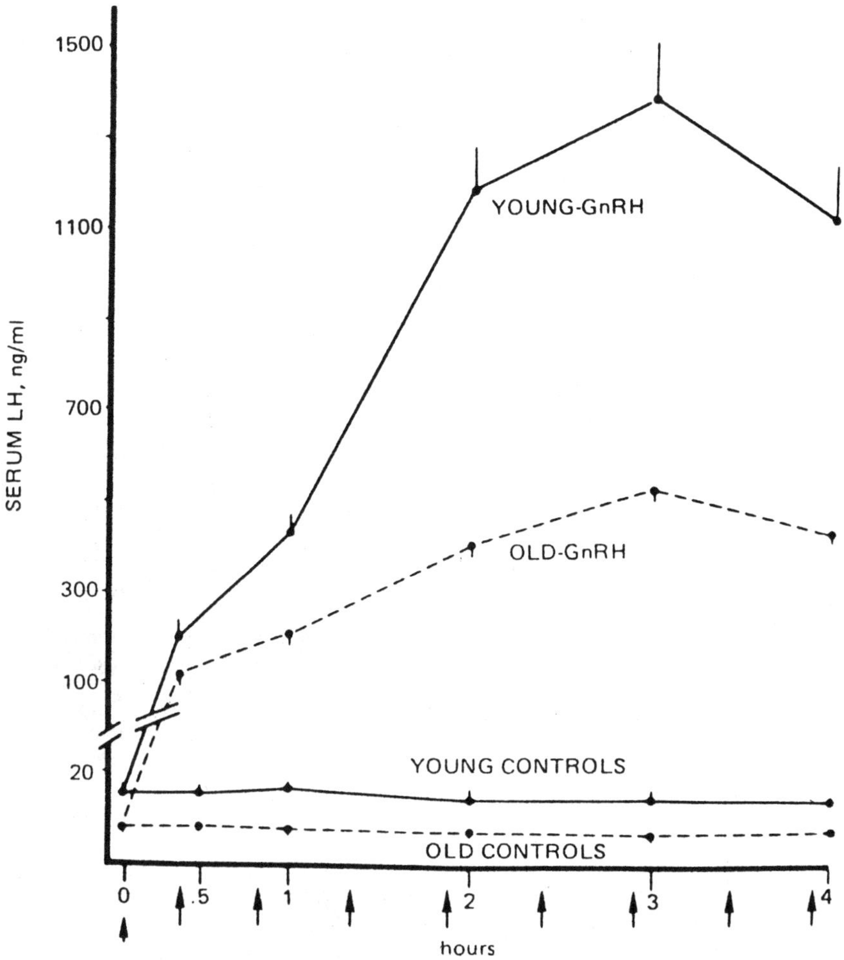

Figure 14–4. *Effects of multiple injections (arrows) of GnRH on serum LH in young (4 month) and old (21 month) male Wistar rats.*

Vertical lines indicate SEM. (From Bruni *et al.*, 1977. With the permission of the Society for the Study of Reproduction.)

lease of GnRH, hence a reduced LH and FSH secretion. Reduced content and turnover rate of dopamine and norepinephrine with increased turnover of serotonin in the hypothalamus of old males is responsible for the decreased LH and FSH and increased prolactin secretion. This neurotransmitter imbalance may also be responsible for the smaller postcastration rise of LH seen in the old rat. Therefore, both the hypothalamus and pituitary of aging male rats show functional defects (Meites *et al.*, 1980; Smith and Conn, 1983).

Accessory Sex Organs

The epididymis grows slowly throughout adult life and shows little evidence of cell renewal. Pigment granules (lipofuscin) are laid down in the epithelial cells of the epididymis, seminal vesicles, and prostate with age. In the human seminal vesicle, fluid volume falls from 5 ml at 21 years to 2.25 ml over the age of 60. Lipofuscin is deposited in the columnar but not basal cells of the epithelium and epithelial cell height decreases. The walls of the seminal vesicles decrease in thickness and the mucosal folds

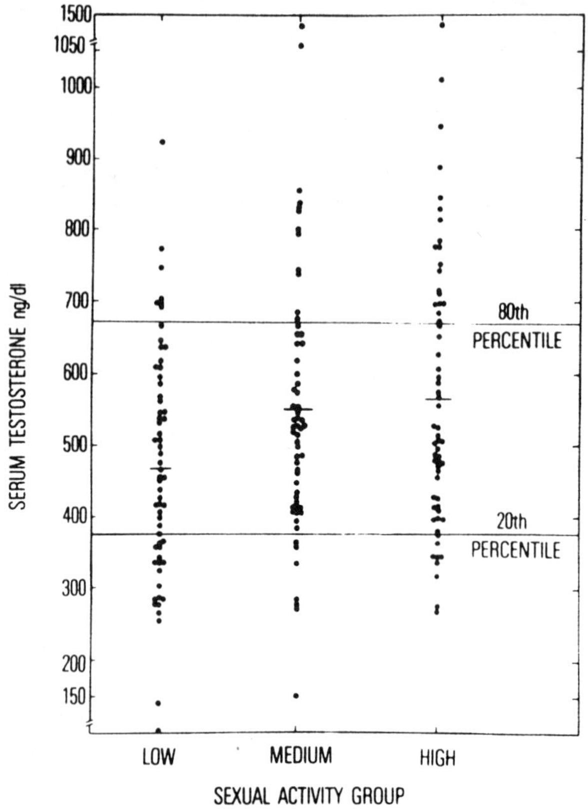

Figure 14–5. *Individvual and mean serum testosterone concentrations in 183 men from the Baltimore Longitudinal Study aged 60 to 79, divided into groups according to sexual activity in the previous year.* (From Tsitouras, P.D.; Martin, C.E.; and Harman, S.M.: *J. Gerontol.*, 37:288–293, 1982. With the permission of The Gerontological Society of America.)

are lost from ages 30 to 40 onward. The weight of the seminal vesicles declines with age in the rat with a gradual decrease in citric acid levels (thought to be an indicator of hormonal stimulation) from 12 to 20 weeks of age. Fructose levels in the seminal vesicles do not change with age, DHT binding remains unchanged, but specific prolactin-binding sites are decreased with age (Steger and Huang, 1983; Talbert, 1977).

Aging changes in the prostate are presented in Chapter 20 and therefore are not discussed here.

SEXUAL FUNCTION

In men, events leading to orgasm decrease with age. The curve of total impotence in men is exponential, with 0.4 percent of men being impotent at age 25, 6.7 percent at age 50, and 55 percent at age 75 (Kinsey *et al.*, 1948). Erotic responsiveness, speed of attaining erection and its duration, the amount of preorgasmic mucus secreted, nocturnal erections and emissions, and the capacity for multiple climax all decline with age (Kinsey *et al.*, 1948).

Testosterone is important for the maintenance of male sex drive and potency in humans. Between 60 to 80 years, men with high testosterone tend to be more sexually active than those with low testosterone (Figure 14–5) (Tsitouras *et al.*, 1982). Muscle mass, smoking, or coronary heart disease does not significantly influence either sexual activity or testosterone levels. Alcohol intake over 4 oz/day reduces sexual activity but not testosterone. Increased percentage of body fat does the reverse. Thus, serum testosterone only slightly coincides with male sexual vigor. Fall in testosterone levels in men did not appear to be correlated with total testosterone and sexual activity, potency, or libido (Davidson *et al.*, 1983); thus, declining androgen levels and reduced sexual potency are separate and only partly related aspects of the aging process.

Declining level of testosterone is only

one of the many factors contributing to the age-related decline in sexual activity. Men with high levels of sexual activity in the first 1 to 2 years of marriage or, generally, between the ages of 20 to 39 are likely to sustain higher levels into their sixties and seventies (Martin, 1981). But age itself appears to be the most important determinant of sexual frequency so far investigated, and further study of this complex area is needed.

Sexual Function in Aged Animals. In middle-aged, sexually experienced rats, the probability of mating is significantly reduced and, when it does occur, the time to intromission and ejaculation is lengthened. Sexual motivation is also decreased in middle-aged (13 to 15-month) rats, as compared to young. In aged rats, erection frequently is reduced, but the number of spontaneous ejaculations is increased (Gray *et al.*, 1981) as is the number of ejaculations required to reach sexual exhaustion (Larsson, 1958; Larsson and Essberg, 1962). In aged male CBF_1 mice, the three component parts of copulation (mounting, intromission, and ejaculation) show independent rates of deterioration with age, (ejaculatory failure in these animals being associated with urogenital pathology) (Huber *et al.*, 1980). The decrease in mounting and intromission behavior observed with age is not due to muscular debilitation, loss of the capacity to arouse or a general reproductive/endocrine lesion, but may be attributable to physiologic changes in the specific neural or neuromuscular tissues responsible for this behavior. In rats, restoring plasma testosterone levels in middle-aged rats to those found in young adults restores the capacity for erection, but sexual motivation and the latency periods for copulatory behavior were not restored to young levels (Gray *et al.*, 1981). Sexual motivation (probability of mating to ejaculation and the rate of mating) decreases in male macaques over the age of 20 years when compared to those about 10 years old. Circulating testosterone levels were not decreased in old rhesus monkeys, but SHBG levels were significantly higher in the older group and showed high negative correlations with ejaculation, intromissions/minute, and contacts/minute (Chambers and Phoenix, 1981). Restoration of testosterone levels in the old males had no effect on sexual behavior. Therefore, at present, it appears that neither an alteration in testosterone levels nor decreased sensitivity to testosterone accounts for the changes shown in sexual behavior in old animals.

References

Baker, H. W. G.; Bremner, W. J.; Burger, H. G.; deKretser, D. M.; Dulmanis, A.; Eddie, L. W.; Hudson, B.; Keogh, E. J.; Lee, V. W. K.; and Rennie, G. C.: Testicular control of follicle stimulating hormone secretion. *Rec. Prog. Horm. Res.*, **32**:429–476, **1976**.

Bruni, J. F.; Huang, H. H.; Marshall, S.; and Meites, J.: Effects of single and multiple injections of synthetic GnRH on serum LH, FSH and testosterone in young and old male rats. *Biol. Reprod.*, **17**:309–312, **1977.**

Chambers, K. C., and Phoenix, C. H.: Diurnal patterns of testosterone, dihydrotestosterone, estradiol and cortisol in serum of rhesus males: Relationship to sexual behavior in aging males. *Horm. Behav.*, **15**:416–426, **1981.**

Conn, P. M.; Cooper, R.; McNamara, C.; Rogers, D. C.; and Schoenhardt, L.: Qualitative change in gonadotropin during normal aging in the male rat. *Endocrinology*, **106**:1549, **1980.**

Davidson, J. M.; Chen, J. J.; Crapo, L.; Gray, G. D.; Greenleaf, W. J.; and Catania, J. A.: Hormonal changes and sexual function in aging men. *J. Clin. Endocrinol. Metab.*, **57**:71–77, **1983.**

Frankel, A. I., and Mock, E. J.: Testis vein testosterone falls in the aging rat: Refutation of the "dilution" hypothesis. *J. Androl.*, **3**:113–116, **1982.**

Gray, G. D.; Smith, E. R.; Dorsa, D. M.; and Davidson, J. M.: Sexual behavior and testosterone in middle-aged male rats. *Endocrinology*, **109**:1597–1605, **1981.**

Harman, S. M.: Reproductive decline in men. In Meites, J. (ed.): *Neuroendocrinology of Aging*, Plenum Press, New York, **1983.**

Harman, S. M.; Danner, R. L.; and Roth, G. S.: Testosterone secretion in the rat in response to chorionic gonadotropin: Alterations with age. *Endocrinology*, **102**:540–544, **1978.**

Harman, S. M., and Tsitouras, P. D.: Reproductive hormones in aging men I. Measurement of sex steroids, basal LH, and Leydig cell response to hCG. *J. Clin. Endocrinol. Metab.*, **51**:35–40, **1980.**

Harman, S. M.; Tsitouras, P. D.; Costa, P. T.; and Blackman, M. R.: Reproductive hormones in aging men II. Basal pituitary gonadotropins and gonadotropin responses to luteinizing hormone releasing hormone. *J. Clin. Endocrinol. Metab.*, **54**:547–551, **1982.**

Huber, M. R. H.; Bronson, F. H.; and Desjardins, C.: Sexual activity of aged male mice: Correlation with level of arousal, physical endurance, pathological status and ejaculatory capacity. *Biol. Reprod.*, **23**:305–316, **1980.**

Johnson, L., and Neaves, W. B.: Age-related changes in the Leydig cell population, seminiferous tubules, and sperm production in stallions. *Biol. Reprod.*, **24**:703–712, **1981.**

Kaler, L. W., Pomeroy, W. B.; and Martin, C. E.: *Sexual Behavior in the Human Male*, W. B. Saunders, Philadelphia, **1948.**

Korenman, S. G., and Stanik, S.: The male reproductive system and aging. In Cristofalo, V. J.; Baker, G. T.; Adelman, R. C.; Roberts, J. (eds.): *Altered Endocrine Status During Aging*, Alan R. Liss, Inc., New York, **1984.**

Larsson, K.: Age differences in the diurnal periodicity of male sexual behavior. *Gerontologia*, **2**:64–72, **1958.**

Larsson, K., and Essberg, L.: Effect of age on the sexual behavior of the male rat. *Gerontologia*, **6**:133–143, **1962.**

Martin, C. E.: Factors affecting sexual functioning in 60–79 year old married males. *Arch. Sex. Behav.*, **10**:399–420, **1981.**

Meites, J.; Steger, R. W.; and Huang, H. H.: Relation of the neuroendocrine system to the reproductive decline in aging rats and human subjects. *Fed. Proc.*, **39**:3168–3171, **1980.**

Merry, B. J., and Holehan, A. M.: Serum profiles of LH, FSH testosterone and 5-DHT from 21 to 1000 days of age in *ad libitum* fed and dietary restricted rats. *Exp. Gerontol.*, **16**:431–444, **1981.**

Riegle, G. D., and Miller, A. E.: Aging effects on the hypothalamic-hypophyseal-gonadal control system in the rat. In Schneider, E. L. (ed.): *The Aging Reproductive System,* Raven Press, New York, **1978.**

Saksena, S. K., and Lau, I. F.: Variations in serum androgens, estrogens, progestins, gonadotropins and prolactin level in male rats from prepubertal to advanced age. *Exp. Aging Res.,* **5**:179–194, **1979.**

Seymour, F. I.; Duffy, C.: and Koerner, A.: A case of authenticated fertility in a man of 94. *J.A.M.A.,* **105**:1423–1425, **1935.**

Shaar, C. J.; Euker, J. S.; Riegle, G. D.; and Meites, J.: Effects of castration and gonadal steroids on serum LH and prolactin in old and young rats. *J. Endocrinol.,* **66**:45–51, **1975.**

Simpkins, J. W.; Kalra, P. S.; and Kalra, S. P.: Alterations in the daily rhythms of testosterone and progesterone in old male rats. *Exp. Aging Res.,* **7**:25–32, **1981.**

Smith, W. A., and Conn, P. M.: Causes and consequences of altered gonadotropin secretion in the aging rat. In Walker, R. F., and Cooper, R. L. (eds.): *Experimental and Clinical Interventions in Aging,* Dekker, New York, **1983.**

Stearns, E. L.; MacDonald, J. A.; Kauffman, B. J.; Lucman, T. S.; Winters, J. S.; and Fairman, C.: Declining testis function with age: Hormonal and clinical correlates. *Am. J. Med.,* **57**:761–766, **1974.**

Steger, R. W.; Huang, H. H.; Hodson, C. A.; Leung, F. C.; Meites, J.; and Sacher, G. A.: Effects of advancing age on hypothalamic-hypophysial-testicular functions in the male white-footed mouse (Peromyscus leucopus). *Biol. Reprod.,* **22**:805–809, **1980.**

Steger, R. W.; Huang, H. H.; and Meites, J.: Reproduction. In Masoro, E. J. (ed.): *CRC Handbook of Physiology in Aging,* CRC Press, Inc., Boca Raton, Florida, **1981.**

Steger, R. W., and Huang, H. H.: The reproductive decline in male rats. In Meites, J. (ed.): *Neuroendocrinology of Aging,* Plenum Press, New York, **1983.**

Swanson, K. J.; Desjardins, C.; and Turek, F. W.: Aging of the reproductive system in the male hamster: Behavioral and endocrine patterns. *Biol. Reprod.,* **26**:791–799, **1982.**

Talbert, G. B.: Aging of the reproductive system. In Finch, C. E., and Hayflick, L. (eds.): *Handbook of the Biology of Aging,* Van Nostrand Reinhold Company, New York, **1977.**

Tsitouras, P. D.; Martin, C. E.; and Harman, S. M.: Relationship of serum testosterone to sexual activity in healthy elderly men. *J. Gerontol.,* **37**:288–293, **1982.**

Vermeulen, A.: Leydig cell function in old age. In Everitt, A. V., and Burgess, J. A. (eds.): *Hypothalamus, Pituitary and Aging,* Charles C Thomas, Springfield, Illinois, **1976.**

CHAPTER

15 AGING OF THE THYROID GLAND AND BASAL METABOLISM

The hormones of the thyroid gland, primarily thyroxine (T_4) and triiodothyronine (T_3), have traditionally sparked the interest of investigators seeking hormonal determinants of aging. Early studies in humans suggested that certain signs of aging resemble those of thyroid insufficiency or hypothyroidism. Individuals affected by hypothyroidism develop a number of signs that could be interpreted as "precocious senility," including a reduced metabolic rate, hyperlipidemia, and accelerated atherosclerosis, early aging of skin and hair, slow reflexes, and slow mental performance. Since these patients improve markedly after hormonal replacement therapy, it has been argued that similar symptoms in normally aging individuals may represent effects secondary to thyroid involution with age. In view of the well-known action of thyroid hormones in controlling development, it seemed logical to suspect that these hormones might also control the rate or site of aging. As early as the turn of this century, experimenters optimistically attempted rejuvenation or prolongation of life through hormone administration. While thyroid hormone administration to some animals (rats) seemed to shorten rather than prolong life (Robertson, 1928), others (fowl) showed an apparent dramatic rejuvenation (Crewe, 1929–1925). Delayed and impaired growth and maturation associated with a significant prolongation of the lifespan were also reported in rats made hypothyroid at an early (first postnatal week) age (Ooka *et al.,* 1983; Ooka and Shinkai, 1986), resembling the effects reported after food restriction (Chapter 25). However, the aging process in euthyroid elderly humans was never significantly slowed or altered by the administration of these hormones nor was the lifespan affected by hypo- or hyperthyroidism.

The capacity to maintain a euthyroid (normal) state continues during aging despite a number of changes in various aspects of thyroid hormone production, secretion, and action. As for all other endocrines, normal thyroid function in the elderly is marginal and easily endangered by repeated challenging demands and stress; the ensuing dysthyroid (abnormal) state may lead to decreased overall physiologic competence, disease, and aging (see reviews by Everitt, 1976; Gregerman and Davis, 1978; Ingbar, 1978; Cole *et al.,* 1982; Green, 1985; Minaker *et al.,* 1985; Timiras, 1985). In the present chapter we shall consider first the aging of the thyroid gland and the hypothalamo-pituitary-thyroid axis and second the possible consequences of this aging on the whole organism and specific functions—basal metabolism, thermoregulation—regulated by thyroid hormones. Included also is aging of the parathyroids, because of their intimate anatomic association with the thyroid gland.

STRUCTURAL AND FUNCTIONAL CHANGES IN HYPOTHALAMO-PITUITARY-THYROID AXIS

During development, the thyroid gland is necessary for whole-body and organ growth and development and maturation of the central nervous system. In adulthood, it has an essentially metabolic function, regulating tissue oxygen consumption and thereby maintaining metabolic rate as well as influencing some aspects of behavior. The thyroid gland is not essential for life, but in its absence, there is poor resistance to cold, mental and physical slowing, and, in children, mental retardation and dwarfism. Reciprocally, in hyperthyroidism, metabolic and behavioral alterations threaten well-being and survival.

Structure and Regulation. The thyroid gland is a bilateral organ that bridges the lower larynx and upper trachea with a narrow isthmus. As

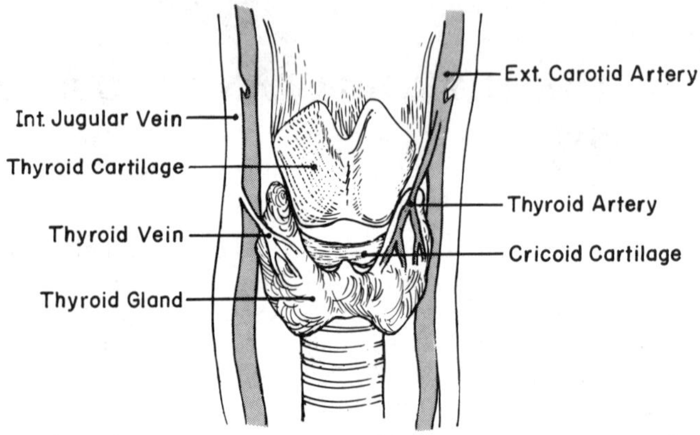

Figure 15–1. *Diagrammatic Representation of the Thyroid Gland.*

The thyroid and cricoid cartilages and the major blood vessels are included. Note that four parathyroid glands are imbedded in the superior and inferior poles of the thyroid gland. C cells secreting calcitonin are dispersed throughout the thyroid gland. (Drawing by S. Oklund)

one of the most vascularized endocrines, it receives blood from the superior thyroid arteries, branches of the external carotid artery, and is drained by corresponding veins into the internal jugular vein (Figure 15–1). In normal individuals, vascularity, size, and microscopic structures vary with the levels of the pituitary tropic hormone, thyroid-stimulating hormone (TSH) or thyrotropin, nutrition, temperature, sex, and age.

The functional units of the thyroid gland are multiple, variable-sized follicles, formed by a single layer of cells, filled with colloid (a proteinaceous material containing thyroglobulin, a glycoprotein necessary for the synthesis of T_3 and T_4) (Figure 15–2). At high magnification the cell surface lining the follicle is rich in microvilli that project into the follicle where they secrete the colloid; hormones are secreted into blood at the opposite cell pole adjoining the rich capillary net (Fujita, 1984).

The control of the thyroid gland in the elderly, as at all other ages, cannot be viewed in isolation but must be considered in the context of (a) regulation at the hypothalamo-pituitary axis, (b) thyroid hormone metabolism, and (c) interrelations with receptors at target cells (Figure 15–3). These connected levels of integration can be briefly outlined as follows:

- At the level of the *hypothalamus,* thyrotropin-releasing hormone (TRH) is a tripeptide secreted into the portal capillaries relaying TRH secretion to the anterior pituitary. In the pituitary, TRH stimulates the synthesis and release of thyroid-stimulating hormone or thyrotropin or TSH. Secretion of TSH is, in turn, inhibited by the negative feedback of thyroid hormones and stimulated or inhibited by stimuli from higher brain centers in response to environmental changes.
- At the *pituitary* level, TSH is a glycoprotein secreted by the basophilic thyrotropes. TSH secretion is regulated by negative feedback of thyroid hormones; i.e., the higher the serum levels of these hormones, the lower TSH release (and vice versa) and stimulation from TRH. In the absence of TSH (e.g., by hypophysectomy in experimental animals) thyroid function is depressed and the thyroid gland atrophies; administration of TSH stimulates the thyroid gland and increases circulating levels of thyroid hormones.
- At the *thyroid* level, thyroid hormone, thyroxine (T_4) triiodothyronine (T_3), and to a much lesser extent, reverse T_3 (rT_3) are synthesized by iodination and condensation of the tyrosine precursor on the thyroglobulin molecule store in the colloid of the thyroid follicle. Thyroglobulin is ingested by endocytosis into the thyroid cell where it is broken down to liberate T_4 and T_3, which are released into the circulation. Cells of the thyroid gland contain TSH receptors. Binding of TSH to its receptors activates the enzyme adenylate cyclase with increase in intracellular cAMP. Most of TSH actions are mediated through this cAMP increase, but some depend on stimulation of cell membrane phospholipids.
- The major product of the thyroid gland is T_4. One-third of circulating T_4 is converted to T_3 in *peripheral tissues.* Both hormones are present in serum either bound to proteins or in the free state. The free hormone is biologically active and interacts with specific receptors localized in the membrane, mitochondria, cytoplasm, and nucleus of responsive cells. T_3 and T_4 are deiodinated and deaminated in the tissues. In the

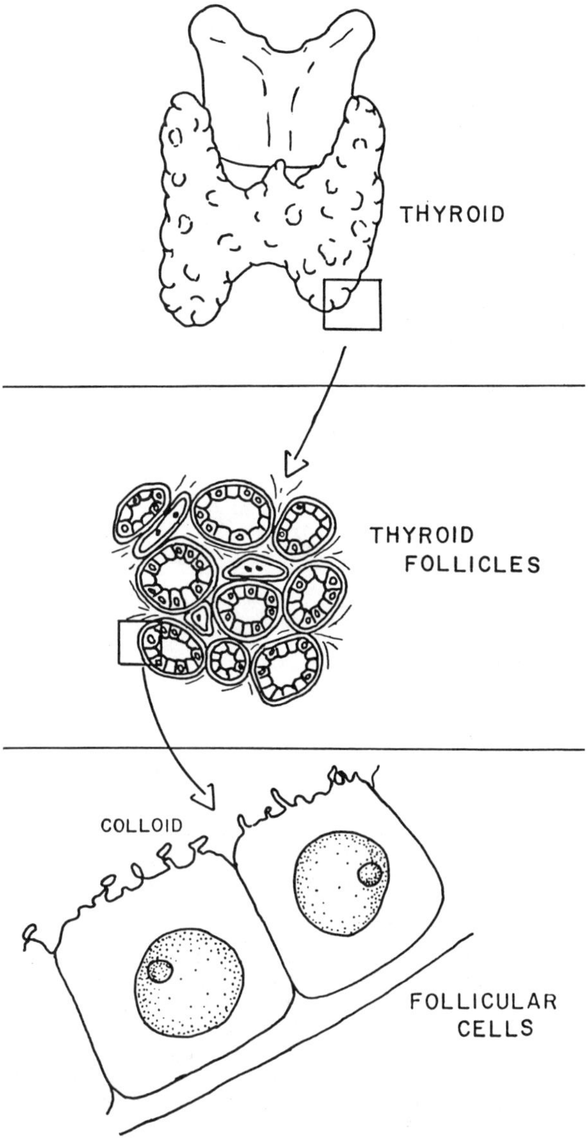

Figure 15–2. *Diagrammatic Representation of the Thyroid (on the top), the Thyroid Follicles (in the middle), and the Follicular Cells (at the bottom): the microvilli from the follicular cells project into the follicular colloid.* (Drawing by S. Oklund)

liver, they are conjugated, pass into the bile and are excreted into the intestine. Conjugated and free hormones are also excreted by the kidney.

Structural Changes in the Thyroid Gland

From maturity to old age, the size of the thyroid gland decreases, although in some cases, the weight of the gland may remain unchanged or even increase (Hegedus *et al.*, 1983). The increase is due most often to the presence of nodules (small lumps or masses of hyperplastic and hypertrophic cells) or to mild endemic goiter (hypothyroidism due to iodine deficiency). The general shape of the gland remains unchanged although microscopic changes are frequent and include: distention of follicles, discoloration of colloid, flattening of the follicular epithelium suggesting reduced secretory activity, decreased number of mitosis, suggesting decreased cell turnover, increased fibrosis of interstitial connective tissue and parenchyma, and vascular changes of atherosclerotic nature suggesting decreased transport between cells, blood, and follicles.

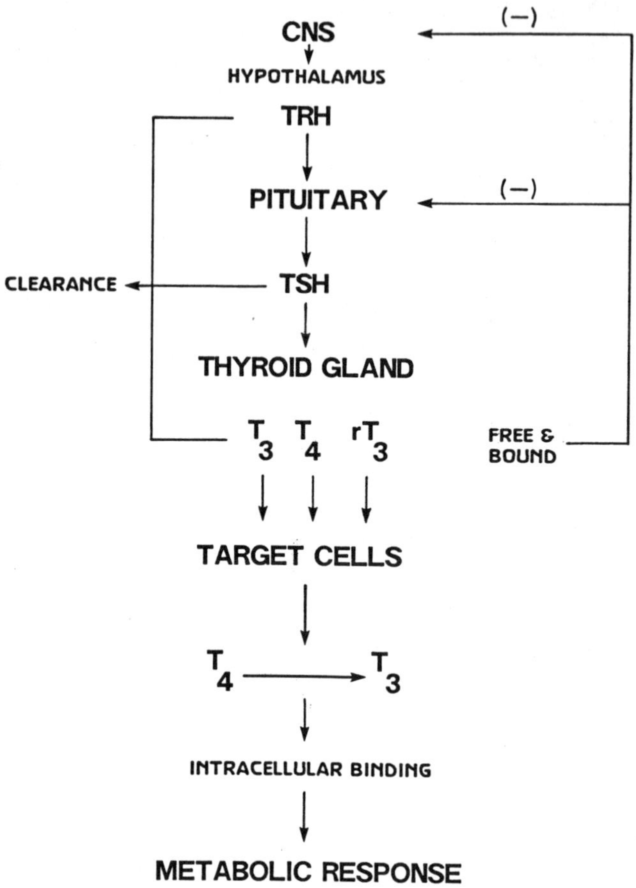

Figure 15–3. *Diagram of the Interrelations of the Hypothalamo-pituitary-thyroid Axis.*

All these changes suggest reduced functional activity. However, in acute illness, thyroid hormonal output may be greatly increased (Gregerman and Solomon, 1967). When thyroid cells are active, as following TSH stimulation, follicles are small, and cells are cuboidal or columnar with signs of active endocytosis, i.e., transport of the colloid into the cell. When the cells are inactive, as in the absence or deficiency of TSH or in some old individuals, follicles are large, more colloid is accumulated in the follicular cavity due to reduction of endocytosis, and the lining cells are flat and display signs of reduced secretory activity.

Nodules, primarily involutional in older individuals, are characterized by localized tissue proliferation with overlapping areas of cell involution or stimulation as occur frequently in the hyperthyroidism of the elderly (Davis and Davis, 1974). The prevalence of micronodules and clinically palpable nodules has been reported both to increase (Studer *et al.*, 1979) and to decrease (Tunbridge *et al.*, 1977) with age. The variability of this finding reflects geographic differences in the prevalence of endemic goiter (overall enlargement of the thyroid) due essentially to iodine deficiency. Endemic goiter is more prevalent in young women than men and may be caused by a relative iodine deficiency associated with poor dietary habits and nutritional deficiencies that may occur at adolescence or the increased nutritional demands created by pregnancy. With aging, the prevalence of goiter tends to decrease while that of multiple nodules increases (Figure 15–4). Multinodular goiter is also associated with increased antithyroid antibodies. The much lower prevalence of goiter and nodules in men does not vary significantly with age.

CHANGES IN THYROID HORMONE SERUM LEVELS

Of the three major hormones from the thyroid gland, T_3 is more active biologically than T_4, and rT_3 is inactive. However, T_4 is the major hormone secreted by the thyroid

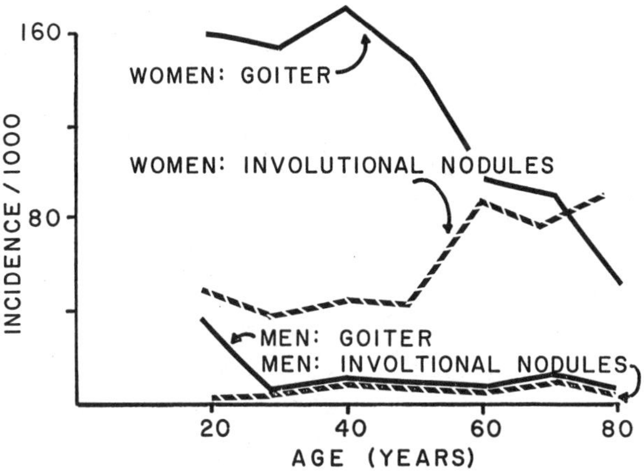

Figure 15–4. *Incidence of Goiter and Involutional Nodules in the Thyroid Gland as a Function of Age in Women and Men.*

gland while T_3 is secreted only in small amounts and derives mainly from the peripheral deiodination of T_4. All thyroid hormones are iodine-containing derivatives of the amino acid tyrosine and are present in blood in the bound-to-plasma proteins and in the free form. T_3 is less tightly bound to plasma proteins than is T_4 and is therefore more readily available for cellular uptake. Intracellularly, T_3 binds to nuclear receptors to a much greater extent than T_4; hence T_3 is more rapidly and biologically active than T_4.

Changes with aging in the levels of these hormones are controversial owing to fluctuations in response to a variety of stimuli and disease (Figure 15–5). Total and free T_4 serum levels may be unchanged, slightly decreased, or increased, depending on age, sex, and general health (Burrows *et al.*, 1975; Chopra *et al.*, 1978; Herrmann *et al.*, 1981). In a study of healthy geriatric euthyroid individuals, serum T_4 levels declined by 15 to 20 percent in some individuals but increased by a similar percentage in others, irrespective of body weight, diagnostic category, drug treatment, or age (ranging from 69 to 95 years). In most studies, however, T_4 levels remain unchanged in advanced age even when thyroid secretion may have decreased, in some cases as much as 50 percent (Gregerman and Solomon, 1967). As for the adrenocortical hormones, a slower metabolism (in the liver and tissues) and excretion (by the kidney) of the hormones compensate for the reduced secretion and the levels remain essentially constant. In elderly individuals, T_4 kinetics show that T_4

	TRH	TSH	T4	T3
Serum Level	↑↓ ↔	↑↑↓ ↔	↑↓ ↔	↔ (↓↓ illness)
T4 and T3 Turnover			↔ ↓↓ (↓ secretion)	↔
T4 and T3 Conversion				↓
$T4_F / T4_B$			↔	
TBG			↑↓ ↔	
Secretion			↓↓ (↑ illness)	
Exogenous TRH		↔ ↓↓	↔ ↓	

(Thyroid ^{131}I Uptake ↔ ↓↓)

Figure 15–5. *Changes with Age in the Levels and Turnover of Hormones of the Hypothalamo-pituitary-thyroid Axis.* ↑ *increase;* ↓ *decrease;* ↔ *no change;* $T4_F$ *– free thyroxine;* $T4_B$ *– thyroxine-bound to thyroxine-binding globulin (TBG).*

metabolism progressively declines with aging. In the ninth decade, T_4 metabolism may be only 50 percent of that found in the adult. As for the hormone, the levels of the T_4-binding proteins (primarily globulin) in serum have been reported unchanged, decreased, or increased. Despite these conflicting reports, the ratio of bound (99.8 percent) to free (0.2 percent) hormone, particularly in the absence of debilitating diseases, remains constant into old age.

Serum T_3 has been reported significantly reduced in some aged individuals (Bermudez *et al.*, 1975; Chopra *et al.*, 1978;

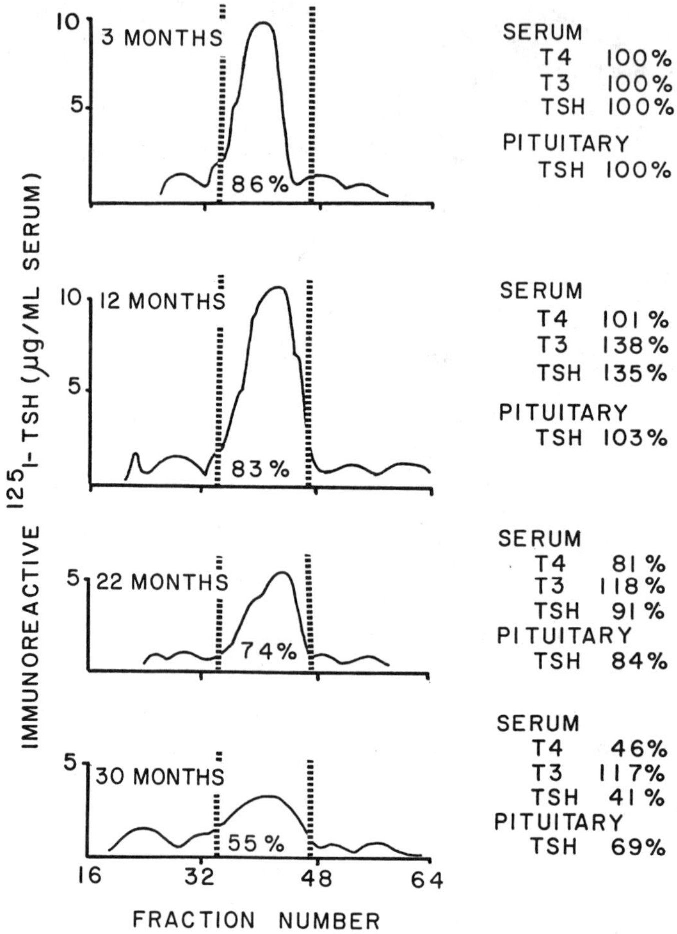

Figure 15–6. *Changes with Age in TSH Immunoreactivity.*

On the left side, changes in the fractionation profiles of TSH at different ages (3, 12, 22, and 30 months) in male Fisher 344 rats. TSH extracted from sera was radioimmune-assayed to obtain the illustrated profiles. The amount of immuno-reactive TSH in each faction was corrected for the original volume of serum and for the recovery from the affinity column so that the four plots are directly comparable. The percentages are relative to the total TSH recovered. On the right side, serum T_4, T_3, and TSH and pituitary TSH values measured at the same corresponding ages, taking 3 months as 100%. (Redrawn from Choy *et al.*, 1982).

Herrmann *et al.*, 1981). However, these reports may have been influenced by the inclusion in the study of subjects who were ill or undernourished. Levels of rT_3 remain essentially unchanged into old age. Any age-related decrease of blood T_3 concentration presumably reflects either (a) impaired T_4 to T_3 conversion in tissues; (b) increased T_3 degradation (metabolism or excretion); (c) decreased T_3 secretion from the thyroid gland due to either failure of stimulation by TSH (see below) or intrinsic, primary alteration of the gland. Based on the current data, it is impossible to distinguish among the foregoing possibilities. However, T_4 to T_3 conversion falls with age, at least in experimental animals (rat) (Ooka, 1979). With respect to laboratory animals, not only are there differences from humans but also intraspecies. For example, in the Sprague-Dawley rat, one of the most used animals for aging research, serum T_4 rather than T_3 is markedly reduced with aging (Figure 15–6) (Choy *et al.*, 1982).

CHANGES IN THE PITUITARY-THYROID AXIS

TSH secretion from the pituitary regulates the function of the thyroid gland and is, in turn, controlled by the hypothalamic-releasing hormone (TRH) and by direct inhibitory feedback of high circulating thyroid hormone levels. In this way, the pituitary-thyroid axis is capable of bringing about the appropriate adjustments to internal and external environmental changes.

When TSH levels are low, the ability of the thyroid gland to secrete thyroid hormones is reduced, and vice versa, when TSH levels are high, the activity of the gland is increased. TSH action on the thyroid gland involves increase in iodide trapping and binding, T_3 and T_4 synthesis, thyroglobulin secretion into colloid, and colloid endocytosis into thyroid cells, as well as increase in blood flow. Prolonged stimulation of the thyroid gland by TSH results in cell hypertrophy with overall enlargement of the gland or goiter.

With aging, TSH circulating levels are usually elevated when T_4 or T_3 circulating levels are lowered. However, in rats, qualitative changes also occur. TSH is a glycoprotein and is present in several forms of different molecular weight and immunoreactivity. In old rats, there is a progressive decrease in the major TSH form, which is also biologically the most active, and an increase in the proportion of high- and low-molecular-weight forms (Figure 15–6) (Klug and Adelman, 1977; Choy *et al.*, 1982). The biologic significance of this age-related increase in TSH polymorphism still remains speculative. Polymorphism is not limited exclusively to TSH but occurs in other glycoproteic hormones of the pituitary, such as the gonadotropins, in which the proportion of polymorphic forms also increases with aging. In rats, not only are TSH levels and TSH polymorphism increased with aging, but the typical circadian cyclicity of the hormone is abolished. The functional significance of TSH rhythmicity is still obscure; however, the loss of specific pulsatile signals may suggest a progressive failure with aging of fine tuning of thyroidal function. Such a failure is supported by the observation that in some species, the low T_3 and T_4 serum levels are associated with normal or reduced (rather than elevated) TSH levels. Inasmuch as the major amounts of pituitary T_3 (effective in the negative feedback inhibition of TSH) may be derived from intrapituitary deiodination of T_4 (Larsen *et al.*, 1979), it is possible that the low thyroid hormone levels are due to decreased systemic deiodination (without affecting the levels of pituitary T_3) or that the thyroid hormone–pituitary feedback is impaired.

The majority of studies describe unchanged or slightly elevated circulating TSH levels without marked changes in circadian periodicity in humans and rats (Klug and Adelman, 1979; Tunbridge *et al.*, 1977; Blichert-Toft *et al.*, 1975). For TSH as well as for hypothalamic TRH, current results are in conflict particularly in relation to sex differences, a decrease in TRH having been reported exclusively in either males or females, depending on the investigator. Other studies show increased TSH responsiveness to TRH in apparently normal elderly subjects in whom T_4 levels are unchanged and basal TSH levels slightly increased (Ohara *et al.*, 1974).

TSH Antibodies and Thyroid Autoimmune Diseases. The frequency of antithyroid antibodies, primarily directed against the cell-surface receptors for TSH on thyroid gland cells, increases with age. This increased incidence may be due to the decline in the self-recognition ability of the immune system (Chapter 8) as well as to the increased TSH polymorphism.

The incidence of two autoimmune diseases of the thyroid—Graves' disease, or toxic diffuse goiter, and Hashimoto's disease, or chronic lymphocytic thyroiditis—increases with age. Graves' toxic goiter is associated with hyperfunction or hyperthyroidism (with low TSH, high T_3 and T_4). Hashimoto's thyroiditis is associated with hypofunction or hypothyroidism (with high TSH, low T_3 and T_4) (Table 15–1). Both are prevalent in women, in whom they reach a peak around 40 years of age.

TSH levels are not detectable in Graves' disease because of continuous stimulation of the thyroid receptors by TSH antibodies and consequent high T_4 and T_3 secretion. TSH levels are either normal or elevated in Hashimoto's disease as a consequence of low T_3 and T_4 levels and TSH blockage by TSH antibodies.

Although the events that trigger the disease are not known, the immune system is strongly implicated. Graves' and Hashimoto's diseases may represent the extremes of a continuum of signs and symptoms resulting from a deranged immune system with hyperthyroidism at one end and hypothyroidism at the other. Antibodies against

Table 15–1. AUTOIMMUNE DISEASES OF THE THYROID

CHARACTERISTICS	GRAVES' DISEASE (TOXIC DIFFUSE GOITER)	HASHIMOTO'S THYROIDITIS (CHRONIC LYMPHOCYTIC THYROIDITIS)
Thyroid status	Hyperthyroid	Hypothyroid
TSH	Generally undetectable	Normal to elevated
T_4, T_3 (serum)	Above normal	Below normal
Antibodies (ABs)	ABs compete with TSH at receptor site Loss of TSH control over thyroid function	Some ABs block TSH action
Autoantibodies against thyroglobulin, T_3, T_4, thyroid microsomal and nuclear components	Generally present	Generally present, destructive of thyroid
Lymphocytic invasion	Limited	Marked
Female : male ratio	As high as 10 : 1	As high as 10 : 1

TSH-receptors or thyroid cell components are present in both disorders, although in different proportions. TSH-receptor antibodies compete with TSH at the receptor site on the thyroid cell. Some of these antibodies stimulate T_3 and T_4 secretion as in Graves', others block access of TSH at the receptor sites and reduce T_3 and T_4 secretion.

TSH-receptor antibodies are not the only antithyroid antibodies present in autoimmune disorders. The most common antibodies, important clinically, are those directed against thyroglobulin, the thyroid cell protein, precursor of T_3 and T_4, antibodies against thyroidal microsomal and nuclear components, and antibodies against T_3 and T_4. All these antibodies lead to thyroid destruction; they are more frequent in Hashimoto's disease.

Another feature of both disorders is invasion of the thyroid tissue by lympathic tissue. This infiltration is more aggressive in Hashimoto's with extensive destruction of the thyroid gland.

THYROID HORMONE RECEPTORS

As it is difficult to reconcile a relatively normal adrenocortical function (at least with respect to glucocorticoid secretion) with a severely decreased capacity to withstand stress with aging, similarly the relative adequacy of the pituitary-thyroid axis into old age seems to belie the apparent symptoms of altered thyroid state of the elderly. One possible explanation is that age-related alterations occur essentially at the peripheral level (Naidoo and Timiras, 1979), primarily within the cell, and involve, to a lesser extent, the hypothalamo-pituitary-thyroid axis. The study, then, of intracellular hormone receptors and their eventual changes with aging and their impact on cell function may prove useful in attempting to elucidate intracellular alterations.

Thyroid hormone receptors, primarily T_3, have been identified in the nucleus, mitochondria, plasma membrane, and cytosol (Eberhardt *et al.*, 1978; Naidoo *et al.*, 1978) (Figure 15–7). The biologic actions of the hormone occur through nuclear binding and stimulation of protein synthesis. The number of receptors appears to be inversely related to hormone levels so that receptors increase in number when the hormone level is low, as in hypothyroidism (up-regulation), and decrease in number when hormone level is high, as in hyperthydoidism (down-regulation). *In vitro* studies of T_3 nuclear binding in rat liver and brain show that receptor number remains unchanged with aging, although low circulating T_4 levels *in vivo* might have forecast an upward regulation. *In vivo* the major source of intracellular T_3 is local conversion from T_4; thus, nuclear receptor binding is dependent on the availability of T_4 and T_3 to the cell and hormone availability is decreased with aging.

After *in vivo* administration of radiolabeled T_4, cytoplasmic free T_4 and T_3 values are lower but bound values are higher in brain (cerebral hemispheres) of old rats. Furthermore, the amount of T_3 derived intracellularly from conversion of T_4 is significantly reduced in the old animals, and nuclear binding of both T_3 and, to a lesser extent, T_4 is also reduced (Margarity *et al.*, 1985). These data indicate a reduction with

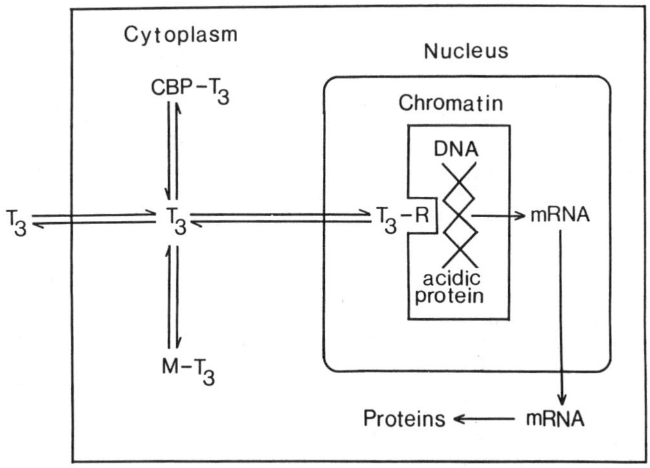

Figure 15–7. *Model for T_3 Interaction with Target Cell: CBP – Cytosol Binding Proteins, M – Mitochondria, R – Nuclear Receptor.*

As T_3 enters the cell, it may be bound to a cytosol-binding protein, in reversible equilibrium with a small pool of free T_3 which can interact reversibly with T_3 receptors in the nucleus and perhaps also with receptors in the mitochondria. (Reproduced from Naidoo *et al.*, 1978).

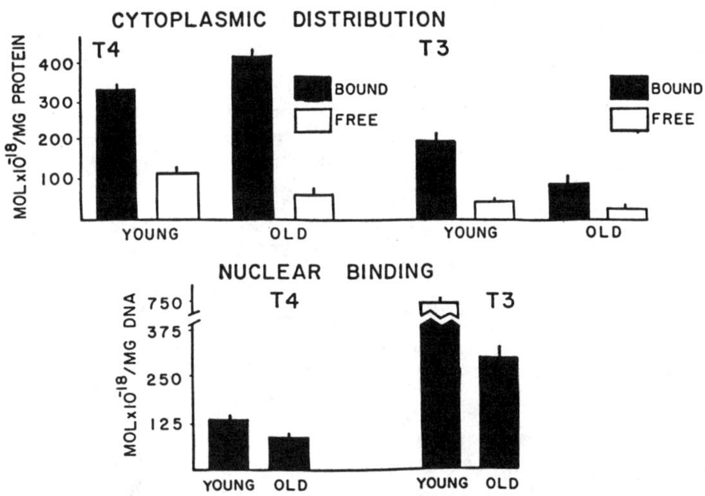

Figure 15–8. *Changes with Age in T_3 and T_4 Cytoplasmic Distribution and Nuclear Binding.*

Bound T_4 increases and free T_4 decreases in the cerebral hemispheres of 24-month old as compared to 2-month old male Long-Evans rats. Lower T_3 levels in older animals suggest depressed T_4 deiodination with aging. The depressed free cytoplasmic T_4 and T_3 levels are also reflected in decreased nuclear binding of these hormones, particularly for T_3. Similar results were also reported in the liver. (Drawn from Margarity *et al.*, 1985).

aging of intracellular production of T_3 (from T_4). At the same time, plasma T_4 levels decrease with aging in Long-Evans rats. These two factors—reduced secretion of T_4 from the thyroid gland and reduced intracellular conversion of T_4 to T_3—would be responsible for a reduced intracellular T_3 binding and consequent reduced T_3 actions (Figure 15–8).

An alternative explanation of the decreased peripheral action of T_3 is the presence of an antithyroid factor of pituitary origin, proposed several years ago but not confirmed (Denckla, 1974). This factor would be secreted in larger amounts with progressive age and its actions would inhibit those of thyroid hormone on the cell. In the absence of verification of this antithyroid factor, the first mechanism, that is, decreased availability of intracellular T_3 for nuclear binding and stimulation of protein synthesis, is the more acceptable.

Table 15–2. THYROID HORMONES REGULATE

Calorigenesis
Metabolism
Brain maturation
Behavior
Growth and development

EFFECTS OF THYROID HORMONES

Of the major actions of thyroid hormones listed in Table 15–2, those directing growth and development cease once adulthood has been reached. In some instances, however, thyroid hormones appear to promote growth of adult tissues, even those that reach maturity early in life, such as the nervous tissue. For example, a facilitatory action of thyroid hormones has been proposed—although it is currently disputed—in the recovery of spinal cord and peripheral nerve injuries in humans and other animals. Catchup whole-body growth and rehabilitation of some behaviors, impaired by thyroid deficiency at an early age, have been described in adult rats after return to the euthyroid state (Meisami, 1984; Tamasy *et al.*, 1986a,b).

Thyroid hormones also modulate such widespread processes as oxygen consumption, regulation of basal metabolic rate, and calorigenesis. Other actions of thyroid hormones that may be relevant to the aging process and affect the lifespan are those involved in (a) intermediary metabolism, particularly cholesterol metabolism, (b) regulation of cardiac output due to stimulatory interaction of thyroid hormones and catecholamines on cardiac rate, (c) decreased peripheral resistance due to increased cutaneous vasodilation, (d) behavioral changes such as rapid mentation, irritability, and restlessness, probably mediated through neurotransmitter effects and not through changes in oxygen consumption, which is unaffected by thyroid hormones in adult and aged brain.

For a better comprehension of some of these actions, the reader is referred to the corresponding chapters (Chapters 9 to 11 for the nervous system and Chapters 17 and 18 for the cardiovascular system). We will consider here metabolic rate, calorigenesis, and cholesterol metabolism.

BASAL METABOLIC RATE

Basal metabolic rate (BMR) is the rate at which oxygen is consumed and carbon dioxide produced under conditions of physical and mental rest and in comfortable ambient temperature (Keys *et al.*, 1973). BMR, significantly influenced by thyroid hormones, decreases consistently with aging, but the magnitude of the fall varies with the study and the criterion of measurement (body weight versus lean body mass). BMR is customarily calculated in terms of oxygen consumption in kilocalories per unit of time and of body surface. With this method, the value for a healthy (euthyroid) male weighing 80 kg and aged 20 to 30 years is 39.5 kcal/m^2 of body surface/hour.

With aging, from adolescence to old age, metabolic rate decreases progressively, in both men and women—in the latter, values are always slightly lower than in men—from 46 kcal in men and 43 kcal in women at 14 to 16 years of age to 35 and 33, respectively, at 70 to 80 years. The cause of this progressive decline in BMR is not definitely known (Masoro, 1985). It may be associated, at least in part, with the age-related declining levels of thyroid hormones, primarily T_3, although this decline is generally slight and does not occur in all aged individuals.

The decreased BMR with aging has also been ascribed to a progressive increase in adipose body mass (less metabolically active) relative to lean body mass (more metabolically active) (Chapter 20). The metabolically active cytoplasmic mass would decrease with aging, as shown by an age-related decline in total body potassium (the major intracellular electrolyte) and urinary excretion of creatine (a product of muscle metabolism). However, these metabolic alterations themselves could also result from the changing thyroid hormone levels.

Is Aging Associated with Alterations in Hormone Metabolism and Tissue Demand Rather Than Inadequate Secretion? As previously discussed in relation to the adrenal, and as will be seen in relation to the pancreas and insulin, the peripheral metabolism of thyroid hormones and tissue demands for these hormones appears to be altered with aging: thus, T_4 and corticosteroid turnover rates decline and insulin resistance appears to develop with age. Because the circulating hormone levels are maintained constant, several authors have concluded that peripheral demand for the metabolic hormones declines with increasing age. The most common explanation offered for this decline in demand is the loss of metabolically active tissue mass with aging, as suggested above. However, this explanation has several flaws: endocrine changes begin early in life, before significant changes in body composition; changes in body composition do not occur in all individuals, and when they occur they may be secondary to the endocrine changes.

If a smaller lean body mass cannot account for the reduction in peripheral hormone metabolism, perhaps an explanation may be found elsewhere, for example in some metabolic alteration in the target tissues, such as an overall decline in protein synthesis with aging. Thus, endocrine changes that occur with aging may ultimately be associated with a decline in overall protein synthesis, which begins with the cessation of growth and continues to fall throughout the duration of the lifespan. Thyroid hormones with their widespread actions on cell metabolism represent an ideal model to illustrate age-related changes in metabolic-endocrine interrelations.

Hypothyroidism as a "Protective" Response in the Elderly. Thyroid hormones, necessary for growth and development when energy requirements are high, may become detrimental when the only energy needed is for homeostasis. A selective impairment of the general anabolic actions of thyroid hormones may occur with cessation of growth and subsequent aging without a concomitant loss of catabolic effects. For example, injections of high doses of T_4 in young animals are tolerated quite well: the animals respond with increased appetite and more rapid growth. The same doses injected to the adult animals result in muscle wasting and weight loss. These and other findings have led to the suggestion that "there is an homeostatic wisdom in the arrangement whereby conversion of T_4 to T_3 is inhibited when catabolism is already overactive" (Chopra *et al.*, 1978). From this perspective, the age-related decline in thyroid hormone metabolism would reflect not so much a reduced demand for tissue utilization as an increased need for protection against the catabolic actions of these hormones (Utiger, 1980). Therefore, the reduced intracellular availability of T_3 for nuclear binding and consequent effects on protein synthesis may represent a compensatory beneficial response to the decreased metabolic needs of the aging individual.

CALORIGENESIS

Thyroid hormones stimulate oxygen consumption in almost all tissues with the exception of adult brain, testes, uterus, lymph nodes, spleen, and anterior pituitary. Increased oxygen consumption leads to increased cellular metabolic rate and this to increased heat production or calorigenesis.

The magnitude of the calorigenic effect of thyroid hormones depends on several factors such as interaction with catecholamines and initial metabolic rate; the higher the levels of catecholamines and the lower the metabolic rate at the time of T_3 administration, the greater the calorigenic effect. The calorigenic effect of thyroid hormones contributes to the maintenance of body temperature together with a number of other metabolic and neural adjustments. With aging, thermoregulation is progressively impaired and this decline may be due in part to alterations in thyroid function.

Thermoregulatory Changes with Aging. Thermoregulation involves a series of adjustments destined to maintain body temperature constant in homeothermic (warm-blooded) animals, including humans. These adjustments maintain a balance between heat production (stimulated by muscular exercise, assimilation of food, and hormones regulating basal metabolism) and heat loss (induced by conduction and radiation through the skin and mucosae, sweat, respiration, urination, and defecation). The balance depends on a group of reflex and hormone responses that are integrated in the hypothalamus and operate to maintain body temperature within a narrow range in spite of wide fluctuations of environmental temperature.

With aging, alterations occur at several levels of thermoregulation: in peripheral temperature sensation (Chapter 11), at hypothalamic autonomic and neuroendocrine centers, and in higher cerebrocortical centers, which control perception and coördinate the multiple inputs that determine the effectiveness of adaptative adjustments. Thus, defects in thermoregulation commonly increase with advancing age (Finch *et al.*, 1969; Wollner and Spalding, 1978). The higher mortality of the elderly during "heat" or "cold waves" is well documented and may be attributed not only to physiologic decrements but often to economic (inadequate diet, poor clothing, housing) and emotional and mental (depression, dementia) impairments.

In rodents, body temperature falls lower and takes longer to return to normal in old rats immersed in cold water than in younger animals (Segall and Timiras, 1975, 1976). Dietary restriction (i.e., tryptophan deficiency), initiated at weaning, continued to 1 year of age and followed by a normal diet, improves thermoregulatory responses. The fall in temperature after cold exposure is less severe and the return to normal more rapid. This persistence of efficient thermoregulation in old animals has been interpreted as a benefit of the delayed aging induced by dietary tryptophan restriction.

Responses to heat are also impaired with aging. For example, the onset of sweating is slower in the elderly (Foster *et al.*, 1976). As a consequence of the impaired thermoregulatory competence, the elderly have also a reduced fever response (Petersdorf, 1980). Fever is the most universal hallmark of disease and depends on a "resetting" of the hypothalamic thermostat in response to a variety of agents such as bacteria responsible for the production of interleukin-1, which acts on lymphocytes (Chapter 8). Interleukin-1 enters the brain where it stimulates the local production of prostaglandins activating the fever response. Fever responses are dampened in old humans and old animals (Finch and Landfield, 1985).

CHOLESTEROL METABOLISM

Serum cholesterol levels rise with aging in both the human and the rat despite a fall in hepatic cholesterol synthesis, indicating a net reduction in overall turnover (Story and Kritchevsky, 1978). A similar situation obtains in hypothyroidism; this effect has prompted several attempts to treat hyperlipedemia with thyroid hormones and their analogs (Burrow, 1978). Several studies suggest that a causal relationship exists between decreased thyroid activity and elevated serum cholesterol. Hruza (1971) found that in young rats thyroidectomy resulted in reduced cholesterol turnover and elevated serum levels while in old rats there was no significant postoperative change. Similar results have been observed in a wide variety of mammalian species (Fleischmann, 1951). The implication is that there is a reduction in thyroid hormone secretion and/or a decrease in the sensitivity of cholesterol metabolism to thyroid hormones (Hruza, 1971). The observation in aging rats of an inverse relation between thyroid response and the increased thyroid secretory rate induced by exercise (Story and Griffith, 1974) suggests that an increase in cholesterol levels may be dependent on reduction of thyroid hormones (Hruza, 1971). In humans, a hyperbolic fall in serum cholesterol occurs with increasing serum T_3 concentrations (Bantle *et al.*, 1980) and a similar inverse correlation is seen between declining serum T_3 and the age-related increase in serum cholesterol levels (Ikejiri *et al.*, 1978). Taken together, these results support the inference that age changes in cholesterol metabolism may be secondary to age changes in the thyroid axis.

The specific defect in cholesterol metabolism that develops in the hypothyroid state would result from a reduction in turnover of the serum low-density lipoproteins, elevated in both hypothyroidism (Walton *et al.*, 1965) and aging (Slack *et al.*, 1977), while metabolism of high-density lipoprotein remains unchanged. The significance of altered lipoprotein metabolism in the development of atherosclerosis suggests that early attempts by investigators to relate declining thyroid function to factors predisposing to atherosclerotic lesions (Wren, 1968) may not be entirely without foundation.

Thyroid Status and Longevity. As noted previously, the lower circulating T_3 in the elderly and T_4 in the aged rat and the reduced conversion of T_4 to T_3 in target tissues may represent a beneficial compensation to the catabolic actions of the hormones, a certain "homeostatic wisdom," reflecting the changing metabolic needs of the organism. This is supported by studies in which rats made hypothyroid neonatally outlived the corresponding controls by about 4 months, for males, and 1 month, for females (Ooka et al., 1983). In these experiments, the mortality of hypothyroid rats was similar to that of controls until 24 months old but markedly lower thereafter. Maximum life duration was 35 months for male hypothyroid and 31 for male controls; it was 37 months for female hypothyroid and 36 months for female controls. The sex difference may be related to the higher T_3 and T_4 levels in males than in females and their greater reduction through neonatal intervention. The life-extending effects of hypothyroidism resemble those found after pituitary ablation (Everitt, 1976). They also resemble effects produced by food restriction, for the body weight of hypothyroid animals is significantly reduced and the inhibition of growth may act as an antiaging factor (Chapter 25).

When the thyroid hormone levels are increased through the administration of exogenous T_4 over many months (12 and 22 months), the average lifespan is significantly shortened in the treated animals (Ooka and Shinkai, 1986). If T_4 treatment is initiated at an already senescent age (26 months), the lifespan is not affected. Thus, the life-shortening effects of excess thyroid hormones are not due to the direct action of the hormones to initiate or promote old age diseases, the direct cause of death, but rather, due to acceleration of the aging process, which may result, in turn, from more rapid timetable of development. Thyroid hormones seem to act as pacemakers capable of controlling not only certain key events during development (the metamorphosis of tadpoles into frogs), but also intervene in initiating the aging processes (Walker and Timiras, 1982).

ABNORMAL THYROID STATES IN THE ELDERLY

The precariousness of the euthyroid state in the elderly is translated in a greater frequency of thyroid disorders with age. This age-related increase is often masked by the atypical manifestations of the disease. Thus, although modalities for treatment of thyroid disease are readily available and straightforward, the subtleties of diagnosis in the elderly often provide a challenge for the clinician. A diagnosis of thyroid disease in the elderly can be delayed or missed entirely because the possibility of thyroid disease is overlooked. In the elderly, signs and symptoms of thyroid disease frequently are minimal or atypical and are commonly assumed to be caused by either the normal aging process or other diseases that are common in the elderly (Gambert, 1985; Hurley, 1983; Klein and Levey, 1984; Heikoff *et al.*, 1984; Green, 1985; Swain *et al.*, 1985).

At all ages, thyroid disease is 3 to 14 times more frequent in women than men. Abnormalities of thyroid function occur more often in older patients who are institutionalized or ill than in the healthier elderly who live in the community. Overall, however, the prevalence of hypothyroidism is said to be between 0.5 and 4.4 percent in the elderly. Likewise, the prevalence of hyperthyroidism has been reported to be between 0.5 and 3 percent (Table 15–3). As already discussed, the prevalence of thyroid nodules increases with age, reaching 5 percent by age 60. Nodules are present in 90 percent of women over the age of 70 and 60 percent of men over the age of 80. This makes it impractical to routinely perform a workup on all elderly patients with thyroid nodules.

Table 15–3. PREVALENCE OF THYROID DISEASES IN ELDERLY

CONDITION	PERCENT OF PERSONS OVER AGE 60
Hypothyroidism	0.5–4.4
Hyperthyroidism	0.5–3
Thyroid Nodule	5–90

HYPERTHYROIDISM

Thyroid hormone excess or hyperthyroidism is caused by either Graves' disease (i.e., diffuse toxic goiter) or nodular toxic goiter. Because the signs and symptoms that occur in older patients are often attributed to another illness, the term "masked hyperthyroidism" has been introduced (Table 15–4). Cardiovascular abnormalities are quite common in older patients with hyperthyroidism. In one study, 79 percent of subjects had an abnormal cardiovascular examination, 67 percent had symptoms of congestive heart failure, 39 percent were in atrial fibrillation, 20 percent had symptoms of angina, and 8 percent presented pulmonary edema. Tachycardia, or fast heartbeat, even in the presence of atrial fibrillation, is less impressive in older than in younger hyperthyroid patients. Typical signs and symptoms such as tremor, nervousness, and muscular weakness may be ignored because they are considered common in the elderly. Weight loss, another common symptom in the elderly, may lead to an evaluation for malignant gastrointestinal lesion. A goiter may or may not be palpable, and the eye findings of Graves' disease may be absent. Since thyroid nodules are common in the elderly, it is difficult to arouse suspicion of significant thyroid disease solely on the basis of their presence.

Apathetic hyperthyroidism is another term used for a thyroid disease in the el-

Table 15–4. COMMON SIGNS AND SYMPTOMS OF HYPERTHYROIDISM IN THE ELDERLY

- Cardiovascular abnormalities
  - Congestive heart failure symptoms
  - Atrial fibrillation
  - Angina
  - Pulmonary edema
- Tremor
- Nervousness
- Weakness
- Weight loss and anorexia (poor appetite)
- Palpable goiter (may not be present)
- Eye findings (may not be present)
- Thyroid nodules (nonspecific)

Table 15–5. CHARACTERISTICS OF APATHETIC HYPERTHYROIDISM

Blunted affect, i.e., withdrawal behavior with apathy and depression
Absence of hyperkinetic motor activity
Slowed mentation
Proximal muscle weakness
Edema of the lower extremity
Droopy eyelids
Cardiovascular abnormalities
Diarrhea

derly, the characteristics of which could potentially be confused with a hypothyroid state (Table 15–5). This condition is characterized by: (1) blunted affect, i.e., withdrawal behavior with apathy and depression, (2) absence of hyperkinetic motor activity, (3) slowed mentation, (4) proximal weakness, (5) diarrhea, (6) edema of the lower extremity, (7) droopy eyelids, (8) cardiovascular abnormalities.

Laboratory diagnosis of hyperthyroidism includes serum T_4 and T_3 determination, and a radionuclide thyroid scan can help differentiate Graves' disease from toxic multinodular goiter.

Treatment of hyperthyroidism includes medical, radiological, and surgical approaches, single or combined. In the medical treatment, the goal is to reduce thyroid hormone production. The most commonly used antithyroid medication is propylthiouracil. The major disadvantage is the recurrence of hyperthyroidism after treatment is stopped.

Administration of radioiodine is usually the preferred treatment in the elderly. The isotope is actively picked up by thyroid gland, particularly in the regions of active proliferation, and the fast-growing and secreting tissue is destroyed. Radioiodine can be administered in conjunction with medical treatment since the effect from radioiodine is gradual and not usually complete until 3 months after treatment. Close follow-up is necessary in view of the possibility of postradioiodine hypothyroidism (Young *et al.*, 1984).

Surgery of the thyroid gland, an uncommon intervention in the elderly, may be necessary for large multinodular glands resistant to radioiodine.

HYPOTHYROIDISM

Thyroid hormone deficiency, or hypothyroidism, is caused by autoimmune thyroiditis or as a consequence of treatment for hyperthyroidism. Just as "masked hyperthyroidism" exists in the elderly, so does "masked hypothyroidism" (Table 15–6).

Table 15–6. FREQUENTLY MISSED COMMON SIGNS AND SYMPTOMS OF HYPOTHYROIDISM IN ELDERLY PATIENTS

Cardiovascular
Dyspnea
Chest pain
Enlarged heart
Bradycardia (slow heartbeat)
Anorexia and constipation
Muscular weakness
Mild anemia
Depression
Cold intolerance
Joint pain

Typical symptoms of hypothyroidism such as fatigue, weakness, dry skin, hair loss, constipation, mental confusion, depression, and cold intolerance may be attributed to old age instead of thyroid disease. In addition, the insidious onset and slow progression of hypothyroidism makes it easier to misdiagnose. Laboratory diagnosis of hypothyroidism is best made with an elevated TSH since T_4 may or may not be decreased in mild cases.

Common signs and symptoms in elderly hypothyroid include the following: (1) Cardiovascular abnormalities such as dyspnea (a sensation of shortness of breath) occur in over one-half of patients; chest pain is present in up to one-quarter; an enlarged heart in most; and bradycardia (or a slow heartbeat). (2) Anorexia (poor appetite) and constipation are common. (3) Muscular weakness is noted by one-half of patients. (4) Mild anemia is present in roughly one-half of patients. (5) Depression is present in up to 60 percent. (6) Joint pain has also been described as a symptom.

Treatment of hypothyroidism is thyroid replacement in the form of L-thyroxine (Rosenbaum and Barzel, 1982). Follow-up TSH levels are the best indicator of adequate replacement. Overreplacement is dangerous in older patients and especially in those with cardiac disease. Safe replacement should be started slowly with low initial doses of 0.025 to 0.05 mg of L-T_4 per day. Maintenance dose in the elderly is generally lower than in younger patients and, once established, usually remains constant (around 0.1 mg/day).

In view of the difficulties in clinically diagnosing thyroid disease in the elderly, the role of laboratory screening becomes very

Table 15–7. CONDITIONS FOR THYROID LABORATORY SCREENING IN ELDERLY PATIENTS

Admission to an acute-care hospital, nursing home, or psychiatric ward
Dementia or altered mental status
Proximal myopathy
Any tachyarrhythmia including atrial fibrillation

important (Walfish and Gryce, 1982). Although arguments have been made that such screening, including a serum TSH, in the healthy ambulatory population of elderly is not worthwhile, certain guidelines can be established (Table 15–7). Thus, patients over 60 years of age should have laboratory screening for thyroid disease under the following conditions: (1) admission to acute-care hospital, nursing home, or psychiatric ward, (2) dementia or altered mental status, and (3) tachyarrhythmia, including atrial fibrillation.

Thyroid disease states, although potentially difficult to diagnose clinically in the elderly, can be detected if the possibility is entertained. The relative ease and success of treatment makes such detection well worthwhile.

THE PARATHYROID

In humans, the four parathyroid glands, embedded in the thyroid gland, secrete the parathyroid hormone (PTH). So-called C cells dispersed throughout the thyroid gland, the parathyroids, and thymus secrete another hormone, calcitonin (CT). Both hormones play a significant role in the maintenance of calcium homeostasis (Chapter 22). They do not appear to be consistently altered with aging.

Major Actions in Parathyroid Hormone and Calcitonin. PTH, a polypeptide, is secreted in response to hypocalcemia; it raises the concentration of plasma calcium by (1) increasing renal calcium reabsorption; (2) mobilizing calcium from bones by stimulating osteoclastic activity (i.e., destruction of bone cells); (3) in the presence of adequate amounts of vitamin D, stimulating the absorption of calcium from the small intestine; and (4) lowering levels of plasma inorganic phosphate by inhibiting renal reabsorption of phosphate.

Calcitonin, also a polypeptide, is secreted not only in response to calcium levels but also to gastrointestinal hormones such as a glucagon. It lowers plasma calcium and phosphate levels by inhibiting bone resorption; it also has some minor action on water and electrolytes and decreases gastric acid secretion.

Studies of structural changes in the aging human parathyroids are few, and studies from laboratory animals reveal only minor changes, such as the presence of degenerating cells containing colloid and mitochondria showing bizarre patterns. Structural changes of C cells are rare although, in old rats, the ratio of C cells to thyroid cells appears to increase.

A study of the immunoassyable PTH shows a decline after 60 years of age in white men but not white women, with variable effects depending on the race (Roof *et al.,* 1976), while in other studies the hormone levels increase with aging (Wiske *et al.,* 1979). In these experiments, some of the biologically inactive fragments of the hormone molecule may be responsible for the high immunoassyable levels.

Both PTH and CT are derived by the action of proteases from preprohormones, which are less active biologically but immunologically similar; with aging the cleavage of the precursor hormones may be altered, resulting in the secretion of the less active preprohormones.

Little is known of the changes with aging in CT and whether and how they affect the aging of bone. The decrease in CT has been reported in humans (Deftos *et al.,* 1979) and is greater in men than women. Since CT decreases bone resorption, its potential usefulness in the therapy of age-related demineralization and osteoporosis has been explored but without beneficial results (Jowsey *et al.,* 1971). Further discussion of the potential role of these and other hormones in aging of bone is presented in Chapter 22.

References

Bantle, J. P.; Dillman, W. H.; Oppenheimer, J. H.; Bingham, C.; and Runger, G. C.: Common clinical indices of thyroid hormone action: Relationships to serum free, 3,5,3'-triiodothyronine concentration and estimated nuclear occupancy. *J. Clin. Endocrinol. Metab.,* **50:**286–293, **1980.**

Bermudez, F.; Surks, M. I.; and Oppenheimer, J. H.: High incidence of decreased serum T_3 concentration in patients with nonthyroidal disease. *J. Clin. Endocrinol. Metab.,* **41:**27–32, **1975.**

Blichert-Toft, M.; Hummer, L.; and Dige-Petersen, H.: Human TSH level and response to TRH in the aged. *Gerontol. Clin.*, **17**:191–203, **1975**.

Burrow, G. N.: Thyroid hormone therapy in nonthyroid disorders. In Werner, S. C., and Ingbar, S. H. (eds.): *The Thyroid: A Fundamental and Clinical Text,* Harper & Row, Hagerstown, MD, **1978**.

Burrows, A. W.; Shakespear, R. A.; Kesch, R. D.; Cooper, E.; Aickin, C. M.; and Burke, C. W.: Thyroid hormones in the elderly sick "T4 euthyroidism." *Br. Med. J.*, **4**:437–439, **1975**.

Chopra, I. J.; Solomon, D. H.; Chopra, U.; Wu, S. Y.; Fisher, D. A.; and Nakamura, Y.: Pathways of metabolism of thyroid hormones. *Recent Prog. Horm. Res.*, **34**:521–567, **1978**.

Choy, V. J.; Klemme, W. R.; and Timiras, P. S.: Variant forms of immunoreactive thyrotropin in aged rats. *Mech. Ageing Dev.*, **19**:273–278, **1982**.

Cole, G. M.; Segall, P. E.; and Timiras, P. S.: Hormones during aging. In Vernadakis, A., and Timiras, P. S. (eds.): *Hormones in Development and Aging,* SP Medical & Scientific Books, New York, **1982**.

Crewe, F. A. E.: Rejuvenation of the aged fowl through thyroid medication. *Proc. Roy. Soc.*, **45**:252–260, **1924–1925**.

Davis, P. J., and Davis, F. B.: Hyperthyroidism in patients over the age of 60 years. *Medicine,* **53**:161–181, **1974**.

Deftos, L. J.; Burton, D.; Bone, H. G.; Catherwood, B. D.; Parthemore, J. G.; Moore, R. Y.; Minick, S.; and Guillemin, R.: Immunoreactive calcitonin in the intermediate lobe of the pituitary gland. *Life Sci.*, **23**:743–748, **1978**.

Denckla, W. D.: Role of pituitary and thyroid glands in the decline of minimal O_2 consumption with age. *J. Clin. Invest.*, **53**:572–581, **1974**.

Eberhardt, N. L.; Valcana, T.; and Timiras, P. S.: Triiodothyronine nuclear receptors: An in vitro comparison of the binding of triiodothyronine to nuclei of adult rat liver, cerebral hemisphere and anterior pituitary. *Endocrinology,* **102**:556–561, **1978**.

Everitt, A. V.: The thyroid gland, metabolic rate and aging. In Everitt, A. V., and Burgess, J. A. (eds.): *Hypothalamus, Pituitary and Aging,* Charles C Thomas, Springfield, IL, **1976**.

Finch, C. E.; Foster, J. R.; and Mirsky, A. E.: Aging and the regulation of cell activities during exposure to cold. *J. Gen. Physiol.*, **54**:690–712, **1969**.

Finch, C. E., and Landfield, P. W.: Neuroendocrine and autonomic functions in aging mammals. In Finch, C. E., and Schneider, E. L. (eds.): *Handbook of the Biology of Aging,* 2nd ed., Van Nostrand Reinhold, New York, **1985**.

Fleischmann, W. (ed.): *Comparative Physiology of the Thyroid and Parathyroid Glands,* Charles C. Thomas, Springfield, IL, **1951**.

Foster, K. G.; Ellis, F. P.; Dore, C.; Exton-Smith, A. N.; and Wiener, J. J.: Sweat responses in the aged. *Age Ageing,* **5**:91–101, **1976**.

Fujita, H.: Fine structure of the thyroid follicle. In Motta, P. M. (ed.): *Ultrastructure of Endocrine Cells and Tissues,* Martinus Nijoff, Boston, **1984**.

Gambert, S. R.: Atypical presentation of thyroid disease in the elderly. *Geriatrics,* **40**:63–65, **1985**.

Green, M. F.: The endocrine system. In Pathy, M. S. J. (ed.): *Principles and Practice of Geriatric Medicine,* John Wiley & Sons, Chichester, UK, **1985**.

Gregerman, R. I., and Davis, P. J.: Effects of intrinsic and extrinsic variables on thyroid hormone economy. Intrinsic physiologic variables and non-thyroidal illness. In Werner, S. C., and Ingbar, S. H. (eds.): *The Thyroid,* Harper & Row, New York, **1978**.

Gregerman, R. I., and Solomon, N.: Acceleration of thyroxine and triiodothyronine turnover during bacterial pulmonary infections and fever: Implications for the functional state of the thyroid during stress and in senescence. *J. Clin. Endocrinol. Metab.*, **27**:93–105, **1967**.

Hegedus, L.; Perrild, H.; Poulsen, L. R.; Anderson, J. R.; Holm, B.; Schnohr, P.; Jensen, G.; and Hansen, J. M.: The determination of thyroid volume by ultrasound and its relationship to body weight, age, and sex in normal subjects. *J. Clin. Endocrinol. Metab.*, **56**:260–263, **1983**.

Heikoff, L. E.; Luxenberg, J.; Feigenbaum, L. A.: Low yield of screening for hypothyroidism in healthy elderly. *J. Am. Geriatr. Soc.*, **32**:616–617, **1984**.

Herrmann, J.; Heinen, E.; Kroll, H. J.; Rudorff, K. H.; and Kruskemper, H. L.: Thyroid function and thyroid hormone metabolism in elderly people. Low T_3 syndrome in old age? *Klin. Wochenschr.*, **59**:315–323, **1974**.

Hruza, Z.: Effect of endocrine factors on cholesterol turnover in young and old rats. *Exp. Gerontol.*, **6**:199–204, **1971**.

Hurley, J. R.: Thyroid disease in the elderly. *Med. Clin. North Am.*, **67**:497–499, **1983**.

Ikejiri, K.; Yamada, T.; and Orgura, H.: Age-related glucose intolerance in hyperthyroid patients. *Diabetes,* **27**:543–549, **1978**.

Ingbar, S. H.: The influence of aging on the human thyroid hormone economy. In Greenblatt, R. B. (ed.): *Geriatric Endocrinology,* Raven Press, New York, **1978**.

Jowsey, J.: *Metabolic Diseases of Bone,* Saunders Publ., Philadelphia, PA, **1977**.

Keys, A.; Taylor, H. L.; and Grande, F.: Basal metabolism and age of adult man. *Metabolism,* **22**:579–587, **1973**.

Klein, I., and Levey, G. S.: Unusual manifestations of hypothyroidism. *Arch. Intern. Med.*, **144**:123–128, **1984**.

Klug, T. L., and Adelman, R. C.: Evidence for a large thyrotropin and its accumulation during aging in rats. *Biochem. Biophys. Res. Commun.*, **77**:1431–1437, **1977**.

Klug, T. L., and Adelman, R. C.: Altered hypothalamic-pituitary regulation of TSH in male rats during aging. *Endocrinology,* **104**:1136–1142, **1979**.

Larsen, P. R.; Dick, T. E.; Markowitz, B. P.; Kaplan, M. M.; and Gard, T. G.: Inhibition of intrapituitary thyroxine to 3,5,3'-triiodothyronine conversion prevents the acute suppression of thyrotropin release by thyroxine in hypothyroid rats. *J. Clin. Invest.*, **64**:117–128, **1979**.

Margarity, M.; Valcana, T.; and Timiras, P. S.: Thyroxine deiodination, cytoplasmic distribution and nuclear binding of thyroxine and triiodothyronine in liver and brain of young rats. *Mech. Ageing Dev.*, **29**:181–189, **1985**.

Masoro, E. J.: Metabolism. In Finch, C. E., and Schneider, E. L. (eds.): *Handbook of the Biology of Aging,* Van Nostrand Reinhold, New York, **1985**.

Meisami, E.: Complete recovery of growth deficits after reversal of PTU-induced postnatal hypothyroidism in the female rat: A model for catch-up growth. *Life Sci.*, **34**:1487–1496, **1984**.

Minaker, K. L.; Meneilly, G. S.; and Rowe, J. W.: Endocrine systems. In Finch, C. E., and Schneider, E. L. (eds.): *Handbook of the Biology of Aging,* Van Nostrand Reinhold, New York, **1985**.

Naidoo, S., and Timiras, P. S.: Effects of age on the metabolism of thyroid hormones by rat brain tissue *in vitro*. *Dev. Neurosci.*, **2**:213–224, **1979**.

Naidoo, S.; Valcana, T.; and Timiras, P. S.: Thyroid hormone receptors in the developing rat brain, *Am. Zool.*, **18**:522–545, **1978**.

Ohara, H.; Kobayaki, T.; Shiraishi, M.; and Wada, T.:

Thyroid function of the aged as viewed from the pituitary thyroid system. *Endocrinol. Jpn.*, **21**:377–386, **1974.**

Ooka, H.: Changes in extrathyroidal conversion of thyroxine (T4) to triiodothyronine (T3) *in vitro* during development and aging of the rat. *Mech. Ageing Dev.*, **10**:151–156, **1979.**

Ooka, H.; Fujita, S.; and Yoshimoto, E.: Pituitary-thyroid activity and longevity in neonatally thyroxine-treated rats. *Mech. Ageing Dev.*, **22**:113–120, **1983.**

Ooka, H., and Shinkai, T.: Effects of chronic hyperthyroidism on the lifespan of the rat. *Mech. Ageing Dev.*, **33**:275–282, **1986.**

Petersdorf, R. G.: Disturbances of heat regulation, and chills and fever. In Isselbacker, K. J.; Adams, R. D.; Braunwald, E.; Petersdorf, R. G.; and Wildon, J. D. (eds.): *Harrison's Principles of Internal Medicine*, McGraw-Hill, New York, **1980.**

Robertson, T. B.: The influence of thyroid alone and of thyroid administered together with nucleic acids upon the growth and longevity of the white mouse. *Aust. J. Exp. Biol. Med. Sci.*, **5**:69–88, **1928.**

Roof, B. S., and Gordan, G. S.: Hyperparathyroid disease in the aged. In Greenblatt, R. B. (ed.): *Geriatric Endocrinology*, Vol. 5, Raven Press, New York, **1978.**

Rosenbaum, R. L., and Barzel, U. S.: Levothyroxine replacement dose for primary hypothyroidism decreases with age. *Ann. Intern. Med.*, **96**:53–55, **1982.**

Ross, H.: Endocrinology. In Andrews, J. (ed.): *Geriatrics for Everyday Practice*, Karger, Basel, **1981.**

Sawin, C. T.; Castelli, W. P.; Hershman, J. M.; McNamara, P.; and Becherach, P.: The aging thyroid. Thyroid deficiency in the Framingham study. *Arch. Intern. Med.*, **145**:1386–1388, **1985.**

Segall, P. E., and Timiras, P. S.: Age-related changes in thermoregulatory capacity of tryptophan-deficient rats. *Fed. Proc.*, **34**:83–85, **1975.**

Segall, P. E., and Timiras, P. S.: Pathophysiologic findings after chronic tryptophan deficiency in rats: A model for delayed growth and aging. *Mech. Ageing Dev.*, **5**:109–124, **1976.**

Slack, J.; Noble, N.; Meade, J. W.; and North, W. R. S.: Lipid and lipoprotein concentrations in 1604 men and women in working population in northwest London. *Br. Med. J.*, **2**:353–357, **1977.**

Story, J. A., and Griffith, D. R.: Effect of exercise on thyroid hormone secretion rate in aging rats. *Horm. Metab. Res.*, **6**:403–406, **1974.**

Story, J. A., and Kritchevsky, D.: Age-related changes in cholesterol metabolism. In Kitani, K. (ed.): *Liver and Aging*, Elsevier/North, Amsterdam, **1978.**

Studer, H.; Riek, M. M.; and Greer, M. A.: Multi-nodular goiter. In De Groot, L. J.; Cahill, G. F.; and Odell, W. D. (eds.): *Endocrinology*, Grune & Stratton, New York, **1979.**

Tamasy, V.; Meisami, E.; Vallerga, A.; and Timiras, P. S.: Rehabilitation from neonatal hyperthyroidism: Spontaneous motor activity, exploratory behavior, avoidance learning and responses of pituitary-thyroid axis to stress in male rats. *Psychoneuroendocrinology*, **11**91–103, **1986a.**

Tamasy, V.; Meisami, E.; Du, J- Z.; and Timiras, P. S.: Exploratory behavior, learning ability, and thyroid hormonal responses to stress in female rats rehabilitating from postnatal hypothyroidism. *Dev. Psychobiol.*, **19**:537–553, **1986b.**

Timiras, P. S.: Physiology of ageing: Aspects of neuroendocrine regulation. In Pathy, M. S. J. (ed.): *Principles and Practice of Geriatric Medicine*, John Wiley & Sons, Chichester, UK, **1985.**

Tunbridge, W. M. G.; Evered, D. C.; Hall, R.; Appleton, D.; Brewis, M.; Clark, F.; Evans, J. G.; Young, E.; Brid, T.; and Smith, P. A.: The spectrum of thyroid disease in a community: The Whickham survey. *Clin. Endocrinol.*, **7**:481–493, **1977.**

Utiger, R. D.: Decreased extrathyroidal triiodothyronine production in nonthyroidal illness: Benefit or harm? *Am. J. Med.*, **69**:807–810, **1980.**

Walker, R. F., and Timiras, P. S.: Pacemaker insufficiency and the onset of aging. In Carpenter, D. (ed.): *Cellular Pacemakers*, vol. 2. John Wiley & Sons, New York, **1982.**

Walfish, P. G., and Gryce, C. E.: Testing your older patient's thyroid function. *Geriatrics*, **37**:135–150, **1982.**

Walton, K. W.; Scott, P. J.; Dykes, P. W.; and Davies, J. W. L.: Significance of alterations in serum lipids in thyroid dysfunction. 2. Alterations of metabolism and turnover of ^{131}I low-density lipoproteins in hypothyroidism. *Clin. Sci.*, **29**:217–238, **1965.**

Wiske, P. S.; Epstein, S.; Bell, N. H.; Queener, S. F.; Edmondson, J.; and Johnston, C. D.: Increases in immunoreactive parathyroid hormone with age. *N. Engl. J. Med.*, **300**:1419–1421, **1979.**

Wren, J. C.: Thyroid function and coronary atherosclerosis. *J. Am. Geriatr. Soc.*, **16**:696–704, **1968.**

Wollner, L., and Spalding, J. M. K.: The autonomic nervous system. In Brocklehurst, J. C. (ed.): *Textbook of Geriatric Medicine and Gerontology*, Livingston, Edinburgh, **1978.**

Young, R. E.; Jones, S. J.; Bewsher, P. D.; and Hedley, A. J.: Age and the daily dose of thyroxine replacement therapy for hypothyroidism, *Age Ageing*, **13**:299–303, **1984.**

CHAPTER

16 THE ENDOCRINE PANCREAS AND CARBOHYDRATE METABOLISM

The age-impaired ability to maintain glucose homeostasis after a glucose challenge has long been realized (Spence, 1920–1921). The mechanisms of this age-related reduction in carbohydrate economy have been extensively investigated and their elucidation is now emerging despite several confounding factors, including: differentiation of the effects of growth and development from those of aging; composition of the diet with the regard to both caloric and carbohydrate content; exercise; body composition with particular reference to body fat content; presence of pathologic conditions; role of medications and drugs. These considerations are also applicable to animal models, especially rodents, which may present multiple, but not all, signs of age-related carbohydrate alterations.

In this chapter, we shall examine first the aging of the endocrine function of the pancreas and, second, the effects of this aging on carbohydrate metabolism and lifespan.

AGING OF THE ENDOCRINE PANCREAS

Several hormones participate in the regulation of carbohydrate metabolism (Bailey and Flatt, 1982; Minaker *et al.*, 1985). Four of them are secreted by the cells of the islets of Langerans in the pancreas: two, insulin and glucagon, with major actions on glucose metabolism and two, somatostatin and pancreatic polypeptide, with modulating actions on insulin and glucagon secretion. Other hormones affecting carbohydrate metabolism include: epinephrine, thyroid hormones, glucocorticoids, and growth hormone. Some of their actions have been discussed in the respective chapters (12 and 15).

Structure and Function of the Pancreas. The pancreas lies inferior to the stomach, in a bend of the duodenum. It is both an endocrine and an exocrine gland. The exocrine functions are concerned with digestion. The endocrine function consists primarily of the secretion of the two major hormones, insulin and glucagon.

These hormones are secreted by acinar cells grouped into islets, the so-called islets of Langerhans. Four cell types have been identified in the islets each producing a different hormone with specific actions: A cells produce glucagon, B cells produce insulin, D cells produce somatostatin, and F or D1 cells produce pancreatic polypeptide. These hormones are all polypeptides. Insulin is secreted only by the B cells of the islets of Langerhans whereas the other hormones are also secreted by the mucosa of the gastrointestinal tract and somatostatin is also found in the brain (Chapter 12).

Two of these hormones, insulin and glucagon, are important in the regulation of carbohydrate, protein, and lipid metabolism. Somatostatin may regulate, locally, the secretion of the other pancreatic hormones; in brain (hypothalamus) and spinal cord it may act as a neurohormone and neurotransmitter (Chapter 12). The function and origin of the pancreatic polypeptide are still uncertain although the hormone may influence gastrointestinal function and promote intraislet homeostasis.

A diagram of an islet of Langerhans is presented in Figure 16–1 and a list of the pancreatic hormones in Table 16–1.

With aging, few morphologic changes have been reported in the endocrine pancreas. Among these, a certain degree of atrophy, an increased incidence of tumors, and deposition of amyloid material and lipfuscin granules have been described in humans (Andres and Tobin, 1977). In rats, a decrease in the proportion of large to small islets and an increase in B cells have been interpreted as a possible compensatory mechanism for the decreased responsiveness of tissues to insulin (Reaven *et al.*, 1983). Somatostatin levels also increase with aging, and treatment of islets with antisomatostatin antibodies may partially reverse impairments of the glucose-stimulated insulin response (Chaudhuri *et al.*, 1983). The totality of these changes is, in most cases, minor and does not produce significant cellular alterations, except per-

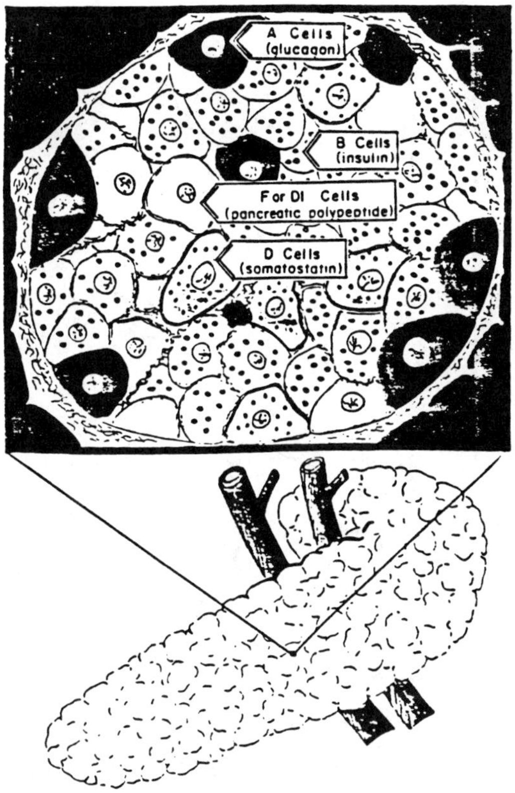

Figure 16–1. *Diagrammatic Representation of the Pancreas with Pancreatic Cells.*

haps for decreased cAMP activity (Lipson *et al.*, 1981).

Secretion and Actions of Insulin and Glucagon. Insulin is synthesized in the B cells as part of a larger preprohormone—preproinsulin—which includes a 23-amino-acid leader sequence that is attached to proinsulin; this leader sequence is lost upon entrance of the molecule into the endoplasmic reticulum leaving the proinsulin molecule. Kallikrein, an enzyme present in the islets, aids in the conversion of proinsulin to insulin. In this conversion, a C-peptide chain is removed from the proinsulin molecule producing the disulfide-connected A and B chains that are insulin. Once in the circulation, insulin is degraded within 5 minutes in the liver and kidneys. C peptide and kallikrein are also present in the circulation, having been secreted with the insulin.

Antibodies to components of islet cells have been detected in a high proportion of patients with insulin-dependent diabetes, that is, diabetes due to insulin deficiency. In these conditions, antibody attack on B cells leads to extensive loss of these cells, characteristic of insulin-dependent diabetes and perhaps initiated by genetic mechanisms.

Table 16–1. MAJOR PANCREATIC HORMONES

PANCREATIC SITE	HORMONE	ALTERNATE SOURCE
B cells	Preproinsulin Proinsulin Insulin (+ connecting C peptide)	—
A cells	Proglucagon Glucagon (+ glicentin)	GI mucosa
D cells	Somatostatin	GI mucosa CNS
F or D cells	Pancreatic Polypeptide	GI mucosa

GI = gastrointestinal; CNS = central nervous system.

Table 16–2. MAJOR ACTIONS OF INSULIN

Facilitates glucose transport through certain cell membranes
Stimulates enzyme systems for conversion of glucose to glycogen
Slows gluconeogenesis
Regulates lipogenesis
Promotes protein synthesis and growth

At the target cells, insulin binds with specific membrane receptors forming an insulin-receptor complex, which is taken into the cell by endocytosis. The complex enters the lysosomes where it is cleaved, the hormone internalized, and the receptor recycled. Increased circulating levels of insulin reduce the number of receptors—down-regulation of receptors—and decreased insulin levels increase the number or affinity of receptors. The number of receptors per cell is also decreased in obesity and acromegaly, and receptor affinity is decreased by excess glucocorticoids.

Glucagon, a product of the A-cell, derives, like insulin, from a larger polypeptide precursor (proglucagon) and, like insulin, is degraded in the liver. The A cell also produces a large molecule, glicentin, with some glucagon activity. In the A-cell granule, glucagon is located in the center and glicentin in the periphery. Both glucagon and glicentin can also be found in cells of the intestinal mucosa. Little is known of the exact function of glicentin or its relation to glucagon.

The major actions of insulin as listed in Table 16–2 are: (1) facilitation of glucose transport through certain membranes; (2) stimulation of the enzyme system for conversion of glucose to glycogen; (3) slowdown of gluconeogenesis; (4) regulation of lipogenesis; and (5) promotion of protein synthesis and growth.

These actions of insulin are mediated by the binding of the hormone to membrane receptors to trigger several simultaneous actions. A major effect of insulin is to promote the entrance of glucose into the cell in muscle, adipose tissue, and connective tissue.

Glucose enters the cell by facilitated diffusion

along an inward gradient created by low intracellular free glucose and is limited by the availability of a specific carrier. In the presence of insulin the rate of movement of glucose into the cell is greatly stimulated in a selective fashion.

In the liver, insulin does not affect the movement of glucose across membranes directly but facilitates glycogen deposition and decreases glucose output. Consequently, there is a net increase in glucose uptake. Insulin induces or represses the activity of many enzymes; however, if these actions are direct or indirect is not known. For example, insulin suppresses the synthesis of key gluconeogenic enzymes and induces the synthesis of key glycolytic enzymes such as glucokinase. Glycogen synthetase activity is also increased. Insulin likewise increases the activity of enzymes involved in lipogenesis.

GLUCOSE TOLERANCE TEST

Despite the paucity of the morphologic changes, a number of functional tests of glucose metabolism suggest impaired competence with aging (Andres and Tobin, 1975; Jackson, 1985; Cole *et al.*, 1982; Minaker *et al.*, 1985; Davidson, 1979, 1981; DeFronzo, 1979, 1981; Timiras, 1985). Many clinical studies indicate a very slight (about 1 mg/dl/decade) age-related increase in fasting blood glucose levels in healthy individuals—not significantly affected by sex or adrenal steroids (Davidson, 1979; Andres and Tobin, 1977). However, this modest age-related increase in fasting blood glucose levels is associated with striking changes in response to a glucose challenge. For example, more than 50 percent of randomly selected subjects over 60 years of age have significantly altered glucose tolerance tests when compared with younger individuals. A typical oral glucose tolerance test measures the response to a standard oral test dose of glucose; the variables are represented by the fasting (preglucose) levels, the time and magnitude of the peak blood glucose after administration, and the time required for blood glucose levels to return to normal or to the preglucose levels. In young adults, fasting blood glucose levels range from 76 to 110 mg/dl after oral administration of glucose (40 mg/m^{2}body surface); glucose levels rise to a peak of about 120 mg/dl after 30 minutes but have returned to preglucose levels within 1 hour. In diabetes mellitus, fasting glucose is greater than 115 mg/dl and the 1-, 1.5-, and

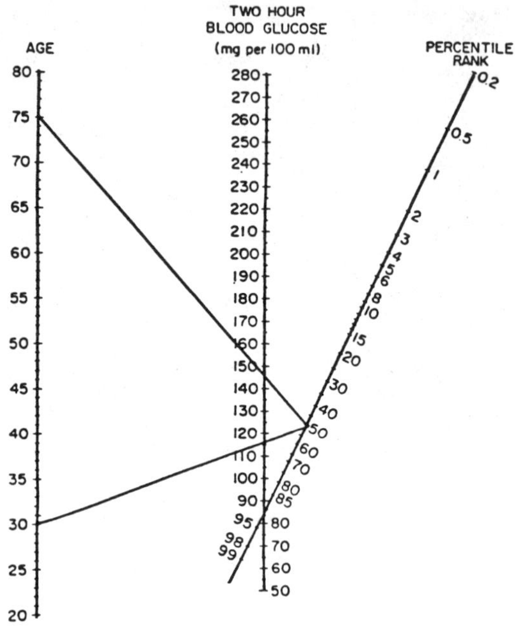

Figure 16–2. *Oral Glucose Tolerance Test Nomogram.*

To note, that a 30-year-old individual has a 2-hour blood test concentration of about 115 mg/100 ml and a 70-year-old has 145 mg/100 ml; but both intersect at the same percentile rank. While the nomogram serves well as a model for an approximate comparison of values among individuals, the tremendous individual variability makes this model questionable for a more precise evaluation.

2-hour postglucose values are greater than 185, 165, and 140 mg/dl, respectively. In the elderly, blood glucose levels are higher and take longer to return to normal compared to the younger individual.

These findings have led to hundreds of publications and considerable controversy has resulted from the apparent need to label more than half of the older population as diabetic. This clinical dilemma may be neatly resolved by introducing age-corrected nomograms for the glucose tolerance test (Figure 16–2) or by substituting higher fasting glucose, rather than decreased glucose tolerance, as the principal criterion for diagnosis. The progressive increase in glucose intolerance with age cannot, however, be denied. It remains to establish whether physiologic or pathologic factors underlie the increased glucose intolerance with aging.

Table 16–3. MECHANISMS OF LOSS OF GLUCOSE TOLERANCE WITH AGING

	Pancreatic Level
Reduced insulin secretion	Depressed initial response to glucose (Normal late response to glucose)
	Increased ratio of circulating proinsulin to insulin
	Peripheral Level
Tissue insulin resistance	Reduced tissue uptake of glucose
	Reduced postreceptor response
	Reduced hepatic glucogenesis
	Loss of lean body mass with increase in adipose tissue

MECHANISMS OF DECREASED GLUCOSE TOLERANCE IN THE ELDERLY

What is the mechanism of the loss of glucose tolerance with age? The answer has been sought either at the pancreas level, where insulin secretion may be depressed, or at the peripheral level, where *resistance of target tissues to insulin* may be increased (DeFronzo, 1979, 1981; Rowe *et al.*, 1983) (Table 16–3). With regard to the first possibility, some investigators have shown that the initial response to glucose—that is, the initial insulin rise—is depressed but not the late response. However, even if an altered responsiveness to glucose exists, it is minor and insufficient to contribute significantly to the observed impairment in glucose tolerance. Indeed, insulin secretion itself and its metabolism, hepatic extraction of insulin, insulin half-life, insulin clearance, and so forth are not significantly changed in the elderly. In fact, in some cases, the higher blood glucose levels prevailing in the elderly are associated with higher insulin levels than in younger subjects.

A corollary to the decreased insulin secretion hypothesis is a proportional increase in the secretion of proinsulin, which, we have noted, has considerably less biologic activity than insulin. Proinsulin levels in the basal state do not differ significantly in the elderly as compared to younger controls, but after glucose loading, the amount of proinsulin relative to that of insulin is greater in some older individuals. Considerable attention has been directed to the enzymes that cleave prohormones (Marx, 1987). It is possible that the enzyme for cleaving proinsulin to insulin and C peptides may become less efficient with aging, hence the high levels of the prohormone (Gold *et al.*, 1981). Alternatively, the increased resistance of peripheral tissues to insulin with aging may create a greater demand for insulin with consequent insufficient time for cleaving the prohormone and, therefore, the increased release of the prohormone rather than the hormone. Irrespective of its causes, the elevation of proinsulin to insulin ratio with aging is too small to account for the alterations in glucose tolerance.

If insulin secretion and metabolism are normal even in advanced age, then insulin resistance must be responsible for the observed alterations. According to some, peripheral glucose uptake in the elderly is only one-third that in the young and has been associated with a marked decrease in the number of insulin receptors (Pagano *et al.*, 1981). Others do not find any difference in the number and affinity of insulin receptors between young and old. If this were the case, then the defect or defects in peripheral uptake are likely to reside at the postreceptor level and may involve a number of cytoplasmic processes such as receptor-mediated phosphorylation/dephosphorylation events or the generation of intracellular mediators following receptor-ligand interactions. Clarification of these intracellular events awaits further study both in adult and in aged cells.

In conclusion, the mechanism for glucose intolerance of aging is still a subject of debate; the prevalent view is that it reflects a major reduction in peripheral tissue responsiveness to glucose and insulin (Rowe *et al.*, 1983; Fink *et al.*, 1983). While this reduced responsiveness has been associated with alterations in receptors, current data remain controversial and the possibility of a postreceptor defect is being actively investigated.

OTHER MECHANISMS RESPONSIBLE FOR GLUCOSE INTOLERANCE IN THE ELDERLY

A number of other factors that may be responsible for or related to glucose intolerance with aging are: (1) loss of hepatic sensitivity to insulin and thereby reduced glycogenesis; (2) increased glucagon levels; (3) changes in diet and exercise regimen; (4) loss of lean muscle mass and increase in adipose tissue. The latter factor—that is, increase in adipose tissue—illustrates the complexity of the regulation of glucose and insulin sensitivity and is discussed below.

Insulin resistance with aging has been associated with the well-documented increase in body fat (Crepaldi *et al.*, 1983; Borkan *et al.*, 1982; Runcie, 1985). With aging, adipose tissue cells, the adipocytes, increase in number and in size. Enlargement reduces the concentration of receptors on the cell surface (Olefsky and Reaven, 1975). This relative reduction, coupled with a possible reduction in the absolute number of receptors suggested by some investigators, would lead to reduced insulin binding and decreased cell response to the hormone (Bolinder *et al.*, 1983).

However, whether adipocyte size or adipocyte aging is primarily responsible for the increased insulin resistance remains unresolved. Attempts to clarify this controversy have managed to further confuse the issue: for example, caloric (food) restriction in rats reduces adipose tissue and adipocyte size and maintains responsiveness to insulin and glucagon into old age, suggesting a cause—small adipocyte size—and effect—high insulin sensitivity—relationship. However, caloric restriction retards the aging process, in general, and persistence of normal insulin response may merely reflect this antiaging affect, also reflected in the maintenance of small-size adipocytes.

With regard to insulin resistance and obesity in humans, not only the amount but the distribution of adipose tissue may be important (Ostman *et al.*, 1979; Maugh, 1982; Runcie, 1985). When obese women are divided into those with upper-body obesity and those with lower-body obesity; the former show diabetic symptoms, and biopsy of adipose tissue in these women shows normal number of adipose cells of greatly increased size. Adipose tissue from the diabetes-free lower-body obese shows increased number of adipocytes of normal size. An appropriate diet reduces body size more easily in the upper-body obese, probably by reducing adipocyte size, and reestablishes normal insulin sensitivity and disappearance of diabetic symptoms. In the lower-body obese, weight loss is more difficult to achieve for it is possible only by reducing adipocyte number, and diabetic symptoms, rarely found, are difficult to control. These studies may be valuable in identifying the at-risk population for the type of insulin-resistant diabetes that becomes manifest at a late age; they may also provide some better understanding of aging-related insulin resistance.

MULTIPLE ENDOCRINE CAUSES OF ALTERED CARBOHYDRATE METABOLISM WITH AGING

It must be kept in mind that, besides alterations of the endocrine pancreas, obesity and hyperglycemia may be caused by a number of endocrine disorders. This multifactorial etiology may be profitably studied in animal models such as the ob/ob mouse, which is obese and shows hyperinsulinemia and insulin resistance. The etiology of the syndrome has been related to a number of neuroendocrine defects involving the hypothalamic satiety center, the neurotransmitter serotonin, temperature regulation, and alterations in glucocorticoid and thyroid hormones. Despite these metabolic and endocrine disorders, the lifespan is little affected, and as the animal ages, there is a remission of symptoms. Spontaneous remission with aging of diabetic or prediabetic symptoms is also a common finding in humans.

Despite the close relationship between aging and obesity and insulin resistance, it must be realized that adipose tissue is responsible for the removal of less than 5 percent of injected glucose in both humans and rats. Since the primary sites of glucose uptake are the liver and muscles, it is in these tissues that the age-related defect in transport must develop. This conclusion is supported by the observation of maturation-associated low insulin binding in hepatic and muscle cells in rats (Bonen *et al.*, 1981; Gold *et al.*, 1976; Goodman *et al.*, 1983). Since the decline in glucose disposal and the development of insulin resistance often begin before 50 years of age in humans, it is unlikely that the age-related increase in adipose tissue or loss of lean tissue could play a major role. Rather several factors must intervene simultaneously to explain the increased insulin resistance of the elderly.

GLUCAGON CHANGES IN THE ELDERLY

The actions of glucagon are, in general, antagonistic to those of insulin. Glucagon promotes glycogen and lipid breakdown and conversion of nonglucose molecules to glucose and ketone bodies. It raises blood sugar because it stimulates adenylate cyclase in liver cells. While insulin serves as a hormone of fuel storage, glucagon serves as a hormone of fuel mobilization through glycogenolysis and gluconeogenesis. Following a meal, stimulation of B-cell secretion of insulin and suppression of A-cell secretion of glucagon serve to store fuels in liver, muscle, and adipose tissue. Conversely, during starvation, stimulation of glucagon secretion and suppression of insulin secretion direct the breakdown of fuels stored intracellularly—as reflected in lipolytic and ketogenic actions—to meet the energy needs of the brain and other tissues (Table 16–4). A related role for glucagon as the hormone of injury and insult has been proposed. For example, impaired glucose tolerance and hyperglycemia noted with infections, trauma, burns, and myocardial infarctions are all associated with increased plasma glucagon. The significance of this increase is still unclear but may have some relevance to glucagon secretion in aging.

Few detailed studies have been conducted on the secretion and metabolism of glucagon in the elderly and those available do not indicate any abnormality. However, after glucose administration, an apparently paradoxic rise in glucagon has been reported in experimental animals as well as in patients with insulin-resistant diabetes (Simonson and DeFronzo, 1983). This paradoxic increase may be triggered by the injury action of the hormone and may contribute to the defect in glucose metabolism. Other still little-known actions of glucagon on motor, vascular, and secretory functions in the intestinal tract are relatively unstudied in the elderly.

Table 16–4. GLUCAGON IN AGING

Anti-insulin Effect
Gluconeogensis
Glycogenolysis
Lipolysis
Ketogenesis
Anti-injury Effect
Gluconeogenesis
In Aging
Paradoxic increase despite glucose intolerance and hypoglycemia
Anti-injury effect

ACCELERATED AGING AND DIABETES MELLITUS

Diabetes mellitus is a health problem common in humans. It affects almost 5 percent of the population in the United States, and the number of those affected is rapidly rising with the increasing elderly population. In the United States and Western Europe, the disease affects about 16 percent of the aged 65 and over, and the size of the diabetic population is likely to double in 15 years (West, 1978; Jackson, 1985). In countries (with more limited food availability) the number of diabetics is much lower (as low as 2 percent); the low rates have been related to a variety of factors among which the diet is most important, but also exercise, lifestyle, and heredity may all contribute to the low risk and reduced severity of the disease.

In all cases, when the disease is present, it has a tremendous impact not only on the immediate health but also on the long-term viability of the individuals who are often disabled by it (Andres, 1981; Blumenthal, 1983). A variety of "diseases of old age" (e.g., coronary heart disease, glomerulonephrosis, retinopathy, limb gangrene, stroke, cataract) are consequences or complications of diabetes and a major cause of ill health and mortality. While some diabetics live long lives with little indisposition, in general the rate of disability of diabetics is two to three times greater than in nondiabetics (Jackson, 1985). For example, in diabetics, blindness is about 10 times and

Table 16–5. CHARACTERISTICS OF DIABETES MELLITUS

Decreased glucose uptake	Hyperglycemia Decreased glycogenesis Increased hepatoglucogenesis Glycosuria Polyuria Polydipsia Polyphagia
Increased protein catabolism	Increased plasma amino acid Increased gluconeogenesis Weight loss, growth inhibition Negative nitrogen balance
Increased lipolysis	Increased free fatty acids Ketosis Acidosis
Vascular changes	Microangiopathies

gangrene about 20 times more common, and 14 percent of diabetics (usually the elderly) are bedridden for an average of 6 weeks per year (Jackson, 1985).

Insulin Deficiency, Diabetes Mellitus, and Abnormalities of Carbohydrate Metabolism. The impact of insulin action is most easily explained by observing the metabolic disturbances that occur in the event of insulin deficiency such as with diabetes mellitus (Table 16–5). Major signs of this disease characterized by severe metabolic alterations are:

1. hyperglycemia or high blood sugar due to reduced glucose uptake by cells, together with increased hepatic glucogenesis;
2. glycosuria (glucose in urine) and diuresis (increased urinary excretion); as a consequence of the hyperglycemia, the threshold for glucose reabsorption by the kidney is exceeded, and glucose and accompanying water are excreted;
3. hunger symptoms, due to low intracellular glucose, lead to increased food intake or polyphagia. Despite polyphagia, there is weight loss due to inability to assimilate glucose and lack of growth due to reduced cellular uptake of amino acids.

In addition, protein and lipid metabolism are affected in liver, muscle, and adipose tissue with the following alterations:

4. decreased entry of amino acids into muscle and decreased protein synthesis in liver with consequent loss of weight and impairment of growth in children;
5. increased lipolysis together with reduced lipogenesis. Insulin is necessary for glucose uptake in adipose tissue and for lipogenesis; it also controls the release of free fatty acids into the circulation, which is increased;
6. increased ketone body production in the liver due to increased circulating fatty acids. As a consequence of the ketone bodies, the pH of body fluid is decreased. Acidosis, following pH fall and dehydration, following diuresis will combine to lead to loss of consciousness or coma;
7. vascular complications superimposed on aging-induced vascular changes.

Table 16–6. DIABETES AND ACCELERATED AGING

DIABETES	AGING
Microangiopathy	—
Cataracts	Cataracts
Neuropathy	Neuropathy
Accelerated atherosclerosis	Atherosclerosis
Early decreased fibroblast proliferation	Decreased fibroblast proliferation
Autoimmune involvement	Autoimmune involvement
Skin changes	Skin changes

While historically the majority of authors have been concerned with the increased incidence of diabetes with aging, in recent years a growing number of investigators have reversed this focus to ask whether there might not be an acceleration of aging in diabetes (Table 16–6). Patients with diabetes display an increased incidence of several features commonly associated with aging: cataracts, microangiopathy, neuropathy, dystrophic skin changes, and accelerated atherosclerosis (Levine, 1979). Accelerated atherosclerosis is a major feature of the various genetic syndromes reported to resemble premature aging, and all of these syndromes include abnormal glucose tolerance (Goldstein, 1978). Further, in normal aging, in patients with progeria, and in diabetics, there is a reduction in the proliferative capacity of cultured fibroblasts (Goldstein *et al.*, 1969; Vracko and Benditt, 1975; Goldstein, 1978). Vracko and Benditt have evoked this reduced proliferative capacity as a causal explanation of microangiopathy. This finding may also be related to a reduced response to insulin and to growth factors, such as nonsuppressible insulinlike activity (NSILA). Insulin resistance has been reported in cells from patients with Werner's syndrome (Kissebah *et al.*, 1979), and a decreased response to NSILA has been reported in normal aging and progeria (Goldstein, 1978). In addition, in both juvenile-onset and maturity-onset diabetics, preliminary results have indicated an accelerated rate of collagen aging (the aging of collagen having been represented as the fundamental aging process) (Chapter 23), which may be linked to certain clinical symptoms of diabetes associated with aging (Kohn, 1978, 1979). Finally, the putative autoimmune etiology of juvenile-onset diabetes, observations of immune dysfunction in aging and in diabetes, and the reports of increased pancreatic amyloidosis in senile humans and animals have excited the interest of proponents of an immunogenesis of aging (Walford *et al.*, 1978). Collectively, these studies point to the possibility of an intriguing relationship between diabetes and aging.

MICROANGIOPATHY

A widening of the capillary basement membrane thickness (CBMT) is one of the important pathologic changes in diabetic patients (Siperstein *et al.*, 1968; Williamson and Kilo, 1977) and has been implicated in retinopathy, renal failure, and limb gangrene, depending on the primary tissue affected. Whether or not such basement membrane thickening also occurs in normal human aging is currently a matter of controversy. Siperstein and co-workers (1968) report no change in muscle CBMT with age in normal controls, while other authors report a progressive increase in muscle CBMT with age (Jordan and Perley, 1972; Kilo *et al.*, 1972; Camerini-Davalos *et al.*, 1979). An increase in CBMT with age has also been reported to occur in the rat kidney (Yagihashi *et al.*, 1978). The etiology of CBMT is also disputed (Osterby, 1976; Wolf and Berle, 1974).

PATHOLOGIC VERSUS PHYSIOLOGIC CONSIDERATIONS

The relationship between pathologic and aging processes is complicated by several issues. There is obviously a great deal of genetic variability in human populations with respect to both lifespan and predisposition to diabetes. Twin studies have demonstrated a high degree of concordance in late-onset diabetics that would make the incidence of a putative recessive diabetic gene greater than 40 percent. However, genetic factors in diabetes are at present poorly understood, probably owing to the considerable heterogeneity in this difficult-to-define disorder (Cruetzfeldt, 1976). Juvenile-onset diabetes has recently been linked to several specific major histocompatibility complex (HLA) phenotypes that may predispose selected individuals to viral infection or autoimmune reactions (Chapter 8), but the basis of genetic factors in late-onset diabetes remains obscure. The apparent high heritability of late-onset diabetes may indicate a pathology complicated by the effects of "normal aging," or alternatively, "diabetes" may represent an acceleration of basic aging processes in a large, genetically predisposed percentage of the population.

Not all members of a population or even all populations can be demonstrated to develop coronary heart disease, yet this pathology is clearly age-related, and remains the largest single cause of death in the elderly in the industrialized nations. Similarly, while diabetes (or abnormal glucose tolerance) may not be demonstrable in all aging individuals or populations, it remains unequivocally age-related and ranks as the sixth largest killer in the United States (Department of Health, Education and Welfare, 1978). Whatever genetic and pathologic components ultimately prove to underlie selected specific manifestations of aging or the evident heterogeneity in diabetes and atherosclerosis, it is perhaps significant in this regard to note that the currently recommended treatment for late-onset diabetes mellitus is carefully restricted diet and regular exercise, and both are commonly considered to be the normal healthy individual's best defenses against atherosclerosis and senility, while the best assurance of a long lifespan remains the thoughtful choice of long-lived parents.

References

Andres, R.: Aging and diabetes. *Med. Clin. North America,* **55**:835–846, **1981.**

Andres, R., and Tobin, J. D.: Aging and the disposition of glucose. *Adv. Exp. Biol. Med.,* **61**:239–249, **1975.**

Andres, R., and Tobin, J. D.: Endocrine systems. In Finch, C., and Hayflick, L. (eds.): *Handbook of the Biology of Aging,* Van Nostrand Reinhold, New York, **1977.**

Bailey, C. J., and Flatt, P. R.: Hormonal control of glucose homeostasis during development and aging in mice. *Metabolism,* **31**:238–246, **1982.**

Blumenthal, H.: Diabetes mellitus as a disorder of information flow. In Blumenthal, H. (ed.): *Handbook of the Diseases of Aging,* Van Nostrand Reinhold, New York, **1983.**

Bolinder, J.; Kager, L.; Ostamn, J.; and Arner, P.: Differences at the receptor and postreceptor levels between human omental and subcutaneous adipose tissue in the action of insulin on lipolysis. *Diabetes,* **32:**117–123, **1983.**

Bonen, A.; Tan, M. H.; and Watson-Wright, W. M.: Insulin binding and glucose uptake differences in rodent skeletal muscles. *Diabetes,* **30:**702–704, **1981.**

Borkan, G. A.; Gerzof, S. G.; Robbins, A. H.; Hults, D. E.; Silbert, C. K.; and Silbert, J. E.: Assessment of abdominal fat content by computerized tomography. *Am. J. Clin. Nutr.,* **36:**172–177, **1982.**

Camerini-Davalos, R. A.; Oppermann, W.; Rebagliati, H.; Glasser, M.; and Bloodworth, J. M. B.: Muscle capillary basement membrane width in genetic prediabetes. *J. Clin. Endocrinol. Metab.,* **48:**251–259, **1979.**

Chaudhuri, M.; Sartin, J. L.; and Adelman, R. C.: A role for somatostatin in the impaired insulin secretory response to glucose by islets from aging rats. *J. Steroid Biochem.,* **38:**431–435, **1983.**

Cole, G. M.; Segall, P. E.; and Timiras, P. S.: Hormones during aging. In Vernadakis, A., and Timiras, P. S. (eds.): *Hormones in Development and Aging,* SP Medical & Scientific Books, New York, **1982.**

Crepaldi, G.; Lefebvre, P. J.; and Galton, D. J. (eds.): *Diabetes, Obesity and Hyperlipidemias,* Academic Press, New York, **1983.**

Creutzfeldt, W.: Etiological and promoting factors in the pathogenesis of diabetes mellitus. In Creutzfeldt, W.; Kobberling, J.; and Neel, J. V. (eds.): *The Genetics of Diabetes Mellitus,* Springer-Verlag, Berlin, **1976.**

Davidson, M. B.: The effect of aging on carbohydrate metabolism: A review of the English literature and a practical approach to the diagnosis of diabetes mellitus in the elderly. *Metabolism,* **28:**688–705, **1979.**

Davidson, M. B.: *Diabetes Mellitus, Diagnosis and Treatment,* John Wiley & Sons, New York, **1981.**

DeFronzo, R. A.: Glucose intolerance and aging: Evidence for tissue insensitivity to insulin. *Diabetes,* **28:**1095–1101, **1979.**

DeFronzo, R. A.: Glucose intolerance and aging. *Diabetes Care,* **4:**493–501, **1981.**

Department of Health, Education and Welfare (HEW) Facts of life and death. HEW publication #PHS79-1222, National Center for Health Statistics, Hyattsville, MD, November **1978.**

Fink, R. I.; Kolterman, O. G.; Griffin, J.; and Olefsky, J. M.: Mechanisms of insulin resistance in aging. *J. Clin. Invest.,* **71:**1523–1535, **1983.**

Gold, G.; Karoly, K.; Freeman, C.; and Adelman, R. C.: A possible role for insulin in the altered capability for hepatic enzyme adaptation during aging. *Biochem. Biophys, Res. Commun.,* **73:**1003–1009, **1976.**

Gold, G.; Reaven, G. M.; and Reaven, E. P.: Effect of age on pro-insulin and insulin secretory patterns in isolated rat islets. *Diabetes,* **30:**77–82, **1981.**

Goldstein, S.: Human genetic disorders that feature premature onset and accelerated progression of biological aging. In Schneider, E. L. (ed.): *The Genetics of Aging,* Plenum Press, New York, **1978.**

Goldstein, S.; Littlefield, J. W.; and Soeldner, J. S.: Diabetes mellitus and aging: diminished plating efficiency of cultured human fibroblasts. *Proc. Natl. Acad. Sci. USA,* **64:**155–160, **1969.**

Goodman, M. N.; Dluz, S. M.; McElaney, M. A.; Beber, E.; and Ruderman, N. B.: Glucose uptake and insulin sensitivity in rat muscle: Changes during 3–96 weeks of age. *Am. J. Physiol.,* **244:**E93–100, **1983.**

Jackson, R. A.: Diabetes. In Pathy, M. S. J. (ed.): *Principles and Practice of Geriatric Medicine,* John Wiley & Sons, London, UK, **1985.**

Jordan, S. W., and Perley, M. J.: Microangiopathy in diabetes mellitus and aging. *Arch. Pathol.,* **93:**261–265, **1972.**

Kilo, V.; Vogler, N. J.; and Williamson, J. R.: Muscle capillary basement membrane changes related to aging and diabetes mellitus. *Diabetes,* **21:**881–905, **1972.**

Kissebah, A. H.; Tulloch, B.; and Vydelingum, N.: Insulin resistance in Werner's syndrome, a postreceptor defect. American Diabetes Association, Abstract 177, 39th Annual Meeting, July **1979.**

Kohn, R. R. (ed.): *Principles of Mammalian Aging,* 2nd ed., Prentice-Hall, Englewood Cliffs, NJ, **1978.**

Kohn, R. R.: The question of accelerated collagen aging in diabetes mellitus. In Korenman, S. G. (ed.): *Endocrine Aspects of Aging,* Summary of papers presented at a conference jointly sponsored by the National Institute of Aging and the Endocrine Society, Bethesda, MD, Oct. 18–20, **1979.**

Levine, R.: Relation of diabetes to aging and atherosclerosis. In Cherkin, A. (ed.): *Physiology and Cell Biology of Aging,* Raven Press, New York, **1979.**

Lipson, L. G.; Bobrycki, V. A.; Bush, M. J.; Tietjen, G. E.; and Yoon, A.: Insulin values in aging: studies on adenylate cyclase, phosphodiesterase, and protein kinase in isolated islets of Langerhans in rats. *Endocrinology,* **108:**620–624, **1981.**

Maugh, T. H.: A new marker for diabetes. *Science,* **215:**651, **1982.**

Marx, J. L.: A new wave of enzymes for cleaving prohormones. *Science,* **235:**285–286, **1987.**

Minaker, K. L.; Rowe, J. W.; Pallotta, J.; and Sparrow, D.: Clearance of insulin: influence of steady state insulin level and age. *Diabetes,* **31:**132–135, **1982.**

Minaker, K. L.; Meneilly, G. S.; and Rowe, J. W.: Endocrine systems. In Finch, C. E., and Schneider, E. L. (eds.): *Handbook of the Biology of Aging,* Van Nostrand Reinhold, New York, **1985.**

Olefsky, J. M., and Reaven, G. M.: Effects of age and obesity on insulin binding to isolated adipocytes. *Endocrinology,* **96:**1486–1498, **1975.**

Osterby, R.: Microangiopathy in diabetics of different etiologies. In Creutzfeldt, W.; Hobberling, J.; and Neel, J. V. (eds.): *The Genetics of Diabetes Mellitus,* Springer-Verlag, Berlin, **1976.**

Ostman, J.; Arner, P.; Engfeldt, P.; and Kager, L.: Regional differences in the control of lipolysis in human adipose tissue. *Metabolism,* **28:** 1198–1204, **1979.**

Pagano, G. N.; Casadar, N.; Diana, A.; Psue, E.; Bozzo, C.; Ferrero, F.; and Lenti, G.: Insulin resistance in the aged: the role of peripheral insulin receptors. *Metabolism,* **30:**46–49, **1981.**

Reaven, E. P.; Wright, E.; Mondon, C. E.; Solomon, R.; Ho, H.; and Reaven, G. M.: Effect of age and diet on insulin secretion and insulin action in the rat. *Diabetes,* **32:**175–180, **1983.**

Rowe, J. W.; Minaker, K. L.; Paollotta, J.; and Flier, J. S.: Characterization of the insulin resistance of aging. *J. Clin. Invest.,* **71:**1581–1587, **1983.**

Runcie, J.: Obesity. In Pathy, M. W. S. J. (ed.): *Principles and Practice of Geriatric Medicine,* John Wiley & Sons, London, UK, **1985.**

Simonson, D. C., and DeFronzo, R. A.: Glucagon physiology and aging: evidence for enhanced hepatic sensitivity. *Diabetologia,* **25:**1–7, **1983.**

Siperstein, M. D.; Unger, R. H.; and Madison, L. L.: Studies of muscle capillary basement membranes in normal subjects, diabetic and prediabetic patients. *J. Clin. Invest.,* **47:**1973–1999, **1968.**

Spence, J. C.: Some observations on sugar tolerance with special reference to variations found at different ages. *Q. J. Med.,* **4:**314–326, **1920–1921.**

Timiras, P. S.: Physiology of ageing: aspects of neuroendocrine regulation. In Pathy, M. S. J. (ed.): *Principles and Practice of Geriatric Medicine,* John Wiley & Sons, Chichester, UK, **1985.**

Vracko, R., and Benditt, E. P.: Restricted replicative lifespan of diabetic fibroblasts *in vitro*: its relation to microangiopathy. *Fed. Proc.,* **34:**68–70, **1975.**

Walford, R. L.; Smith, G. S.; Meredith, P. J.; and Cheney, K. E.: Immunogenetics of aging. In Schneider, E. L. (ed.): *The Genetics of Aging,* Plenum Press, New York, **1978.**

West, K. M.: *Epidemiology of Diabetes and Its Vascular Complications,* Elsevier, New York, **1978.**

Williamson, J. R., and Kilo, C.: Current status of capillary basement-membrane disease in diabetes mellitus. *Diabetes,* **26:**65–73, **1977.**

Wolf, S., and Berle, B. B. (eds.): *Dilemmas in Diabetes,* Plenum Press, New York, **1974.**

Yagihashi, S.; Goto, Y.; Kakizaki, M.; and Kaseda, N.: Thickening of glomerular basement membrane in spontaneously diabetic rats. *Diabetologia,* **15:**309–312, **1978.**

CHAPTER

17 CARDIOVASCULAR ALTERATIONS WITH AGE

Atherosclerosis, Coronary Heart Disease, Hypertension

Cardiovascular disease continues to be the major cause of death in the United States and other industrialized, socioeconomically advanced countries. Indeed, cardiovascular disease associated with advancing age remains the most important single worldwide cause of death in old age in both sexes. This is, in part, because people are living longer and are more susceptible to the occurrence of degenerative diseases. It is also due to some unknown aspects of modern life that are increasing the incidence of atherosclerosis. This chapter will attempt, first, to define different types of arterial pathology and illustrate highlights of arterial structure. It will review some of the major lesions of atherosclerosis and their etiopathogenesis. Taking coronary heart disease and hypertension as examples, it will also briefly examine some of the clinical consequences of atherosclerosis, the chronic arterial disorder that is the major cause of heart attacks and strokes.

DEFINITIONS

Arteriosclerosis is a generic term for any vascular degeneration that leads to progressive thickening and loss of resiliency of the arterial wall. One type of arteriosclerosis is *atherosclerosis,* which refers to specific vascular alterations, such as atheromas or plaques characterized by a combination of fatty accumulation in the intima and an increase in connective tissue in the subintimal layers of the arterial wall (*Arteriosclerosis,* 1981). This form of arteriosclerosis is the most widespread and, at the same time, the most threatening, inasmuch as it affects vessels such as the aorta, the coronary, and the cerebral arteries that are extremely important in providing the necessary blood supply for the heart, brain, and other vital organs. Atherosclerosis, then, is the vascular disorder that underlies most arteriosclerotic heart disease or coronary heart disease and also plays a major role in cerebrovascular disease. Atherosclerosis dwarfs all other single causes of mortality in the United States and represents by far the major cause of death from cardiovascular diseases.

Arterial diseases may also arise from congenital structural defects, from inflammatory diseases (e.g., syphilitic aortitis), from hypersensitivity or autoimmune diseases that principally affect the smaller vessels and may lead to thromboangiitis obliterans, and from specific capillary lesions as in diabetic angiopathy.

PROGRESSIVENESS AND UNIVERSALITY OF ATHEROSCLEROSIS

Atherosclerosis, characterized by its progressive onset culminating in overt manifestations in old age, its widespread distribution throughout the arterial tree, and its consequences leading to severe disability or death, has been studied as a prototype of cardiovascular changes with age (Bierman, 1985; Lee, 1985; Kottke, 1985). In this respect, atherosclerosis must be viewed as a disease that, sooner or later, affects all of us. Working silently over the years from early childhood, it gradually destroys the arteries, ultimately preventing the exchanges of gases and nutrients necessary to keep organs, tissues, and cells alive and functioning normally.

Although a scourge of modern civilization and often discussed in relation to the pressures of an urban technocratic society, atherosclerosis has been with us from ancient times; the disease has been detected in Egyptian mummies and described in early Greek writings. There are several ways in which atherosclerosis impairs the normal function of the arteries: it may corrode the arterial walls to such a degree that they suddenly yield to the pressure of the blood inside and explode in a massive hemorrhage; in reaction to its destructive processes, it may set off a secondary proliferation of the tissues, thereby leading to a gradual blockage of the arterial lumen; or the changes induced in the arterial wall may induce clotting of the blood within the diseased artery and, in this way, obstruct blood flow. Thus, while atherosclerosis is a progressive disease that develops slowly over years or decades, the final "accidents" attributable to atherosclerotic alterations (hemorrhage, thrombosis) may be initiated within only a few seconds.

One of the characteristics of atherosclerosis is its universality in almost all animal species and throughout all populations within a species. So insistent and progressive is its onslaught with advancing age that it is generally considered to be an inevitable manifestation of aging—a "wearing out" of the arteries. In statistical terms, the accidents induced by atherosclerotic arterial disease, associated with high blood pressure, have been found responsible for more deaths in middle-aged and elderly persons than all other diseases put together—at least in North America and Europe. Indeed, death by heart attack or stroke is now so common that we have come to regard it as a natural end of the lifespan; at the same time, however, much of the gravity of atherosclerosis is the accepted conviction that it kills us prematurely, in the sense that alterations in the arteries are capable of irreparably damaging such vital organs as the heart and brain at a time when the functional competence of these structures is otherwise sound. From the analogy of the heart or brain as a motor and the arteries as the pipes that convey the fuel to the motor comes the idea that if the motor is deprived of fuel because of a breakdown in the pipe system, it will stop working, even though the motor itself is without defect (Constantinides, 1965).

The question of how long we might live were it possible to prevent atherosclerosis remains unanswered; it would seem that complete prevention of atherosclerosis would add several years to life (Gresham, 1980; Morrison and Schjeide, 1984). Scientists throughout the world representing many disciplines are now attacking the problem of atherosclerosis both to understand the nature of the disease and to find means of preventing or curing it. The vast literature available on the subject attests to the enormity of interest and research effort that have been and continue to be devoted to the problems of atherosclerosis.

ETIOPATHOGENESIS

COURSE OF ATHEROSCLEROSIS

Although the consequences of atherosclerotic lesions become manifest clinically in the fourth decade of life and thereafter, atherosclerosis is not exclusive to advanced age but, rather, represents the culmination of progressive changes in the arterial wall from childhood (Lee, 1985). Vascular changes that occur in infancy and childhood are clearly identifiable microscopically. They consist of intimal thickening, cell proliferation, accumulation of proteoglycans, and formation of fibrous matrix. Some, but not all, contain lipids and, in this case, can be readily observed as fatty streaks.

The general pattern of the lesions varies from one individual to another and among different populations throughout the world. The approximate time sequence involved in the development of atherosclerotic lesions with respect to specific pathologic changes has been generally established (at least in North America) to proceed in the following order (Figure 17–1): the fatty streaks appear in the arteries during the first decade of life (as early as the first years or even months or days of life) and continue into the second decade, and in the cerebral arteries in the third decade. The fibrous or "pearly" plaques appear from the second decade on; clinical consequences (e.g., cardiac infarct, stroke, gangrene, and aneurysm) occur from the fourth decade on (McGill *et al.*, 1963).

Atherosclerosis seems to develop in several "waves" throughout the lifespan, inasmuch as early and late stages of the lesions can be found side by side in the same vessel or in different vessels of the same person. However, this view assumes that the early stage is represented by the fatty

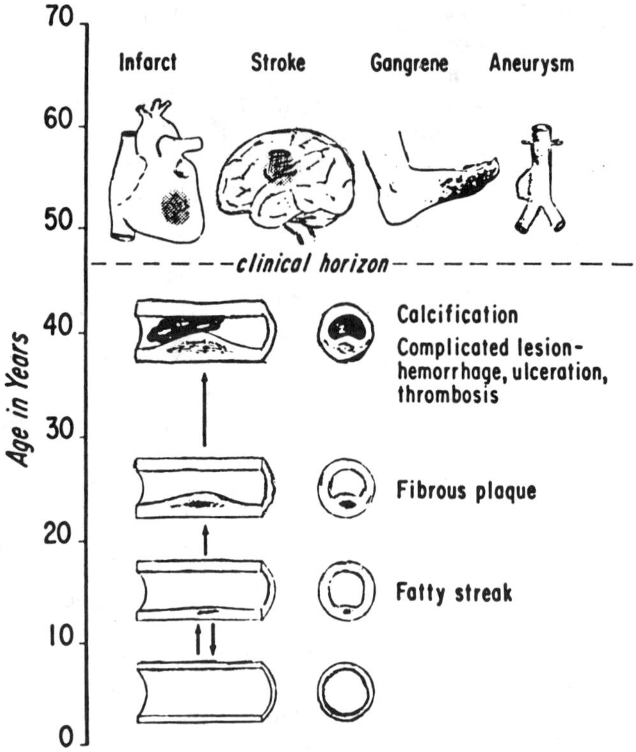

Figure 17–1. *Natural history of atherosclerosis shown in this diagrammatic concept of the pathogenesis of human atherosclerotic lesions and their clinical manifestations* (From McGill *et al.*, 1963).

streaks and advanced stages of the same lesion by the appearance of plaques, a concept that is negated by the observation that the two types of lesions are often found in different locations and that some populations with a fair amount of fatty streaks do not subsequently develop a commensurate number of plaques. That the lesions are distinct and independent is supported by the fact that all lesions do not progress to the same degree in all individuals and that it is possible for the two types of lesions to coexist.

From a morphologic and biochemical point of view, the natural history of the disease remains a subject of controversy. It has been traditionally accepted, for example, that atherosclerosis is primarily an alteration of the intima and that atherosclerotic lesions start in the innermost layers where they can be confined for a long time, and eventually spread to the entire arterial wall. The question of the primary site of the lesions, however, loses some of its importance in the light of the current concept that the entire arterial wall represents a functioning unit.

So far, the study of atherosclerosis has been approached from two main directions: (1) the study of atherosclerotic lesions in humans, i.e., the analysis of the various morphologic and biochemical components of the lesions, the timetable of their appearance, their location, their consequences, and their relationship to the normal and external environment of the body; and (2) the attempts to reproduce the human disease in animals to discover the factors that may be capable of preventing or curing such lesions. However, it is recognized that, in general, animal observations are not always referrable to humans and that atherosclerotic lesions, in particular, differ in different species; nevertheless, experimentally induced atherosclerotic lesions represent a useful model of the study of human disease.

Types and Structure of Arteries. In its journey from the heart to the tissues, the blood passes through channels of six principal types: elastic arteries, muscular arteries, arterioles, capillaries, venules, and veins. In this system, the arteries show a progressive diminution in diameter as they recede from the heart, from about 25 mm in the aorta to 0.3 mm in some arterioles. The reverse is true for the veins; the diameter is small in the venules and progressively increases as the veins approach the heart. All arteries are comprised of three distinct layers, intima, media, and adventitia, but the proportion and structure of each varies with the size and function of the particular artery.

The morphology of the arteries is illustrated in Figure 17–2 and represented diagramatically in Figure 17–3. A large artery, like the aorta, is comprised of the following layers, going from the lumen to the most external layers:

1. The intima, or innermost layer, consists of a layer of endothelial cells separated from the inner layer by a narrow layer of connective tissues that anchors the cells to the arterial wall.
2. A large layer of elastic fibers forms the internal layer.
3. Below this layer are concentric waves of smooth muscle cells intermixed with elastic fibers—elastic lamellae and smooth muscle cells are embedded in a ground substance rich in proteoglycans. Proteoglycans are formed of disaccharides bound to protein and serve as binding or "cement" material in the interstitial spaces. The outer layer of the media is penetrated by branches of the vasa vasorum.
4. Between the smooth muscle layer and the adventitia, there is another layer of elastic fibers, the elastica externa. Layers 2, 3, and 4 form the media.
5. The outer layer or adventitia is formed of irregularly arranged collagen bundles, scattered fibroblasts, a few elastic fibers, and blood vessels, which, because of their location, are called vasa vasorum or vessels of the vessels.

This structure of the aorta and large arteries corresponds well with their function, which serves as a blood reservoir and to stretch or recoil with the pumping action of the heart. The wall of the arterioles contains less elastic fibers but more smooth muscle cells than that of the aorta. The arterioles represent the major site of the resistance to blood flow, and small changes in their caliber cause large changes in total peripheral resistance. Muscle cells are innervated by noradrenergic nerve fibers, which are constrictor in function, and in some cases, by cholinergic nerve fibers, which dilate the vessels.

The capillary structure shows a diameter just large enough to permit the red blood cells to squeeze through in single file. In the same manner as the intima of the arteries, the capillary wall is formed of a layer of endothelial cells resting on a basement membrane. The major function of the capillaries is to promote exchange of nutrients and metabolic end-products between the blood and the interstitial tissues. Such exchanges are facilitated by the presence of specialized junctions, gaps, or fenestrations.

Some Characteristics of Blood Flow and Arterial Function. The arterial system provides not only for circulation of the blood as a whole but, when necessary, for the special needs or functions of a particular organ. Certain organs—brain, heart, kidney—receive a larger proportion of blood than others, and within the same organ, blood flow varies considerably depending on the degree of activity, as dramatically evidenced in the 30-fold increase in blood flow to the exercising muscle. The velocity of blood flow declines gradually, from approximately 8 cm/second in the medium-sized arteries to 0.3 cm/second in the arterioles; pressure, on the other hand, remains high in the large and medium-sized arteries but falls rapidly in the small arteries to low levels of 30 to 40 mm Hg; the magnitude of the drop varies depending on the degree of arteriolar constriction. The mechanisms that regulate arteriolar diameter and hence blood flow through the arteries involve both local factors (e.g., release of chemical substances into tissue) and systemic factors (e.g., stimulation of the baroreceptors and the vasomotor center) (Table 17–1).

The arterial system as a whole is never static but continuously undergoes structural changes and adaptations that permit the organism to respond to changing requirements for blood supply. Even at birth, arteries vary in structure and in distribution depending on the hemodynamic conditions under which they operate. Arteries continue to change with maturation and advancing age of the individual, changes that are continuously affected by extrinsic as well as intrinsic factors; in the process of adapting to environmental stimuli, structural changes occur at particular sites, and the gross pattern of vascular distribution to an organ or part may undergo considerable change, as in the development of collateral circulation.

Evidence from human and experimental observations suggests that the rigid classification of the various elements that form the arterial wall into definite "species" of cells has to be abandoned in favor of a far more versatile view of the cellular configuration of the arteries. It seems that these cells are not irrevocably specialized but, rather, that they can assume more than one function when the need arises. For example, a muscle cell will not only contract upon stimulation but, under certain conditions, it could also phagocytize lipid and even produce collagen or elastic fibers—a potential that might have a bearing on the formation of atherosclerotic lesions.

BLOOD SUPPLY TO THE ARTERIAL WALL AND METABOLIC EXCHANGES

Blood supply of a nonfunctioning organ or part of an organ can be diminished and, conversely, blood supply of an actively functioning part can be increased by three basic elements: (1) arteriovenous anastomoses, i.e., short channels that connect arterioles to venules, bypassing the capillaries; (2) specialized muscular arrangements in the walls of arteries, as in the sphincters

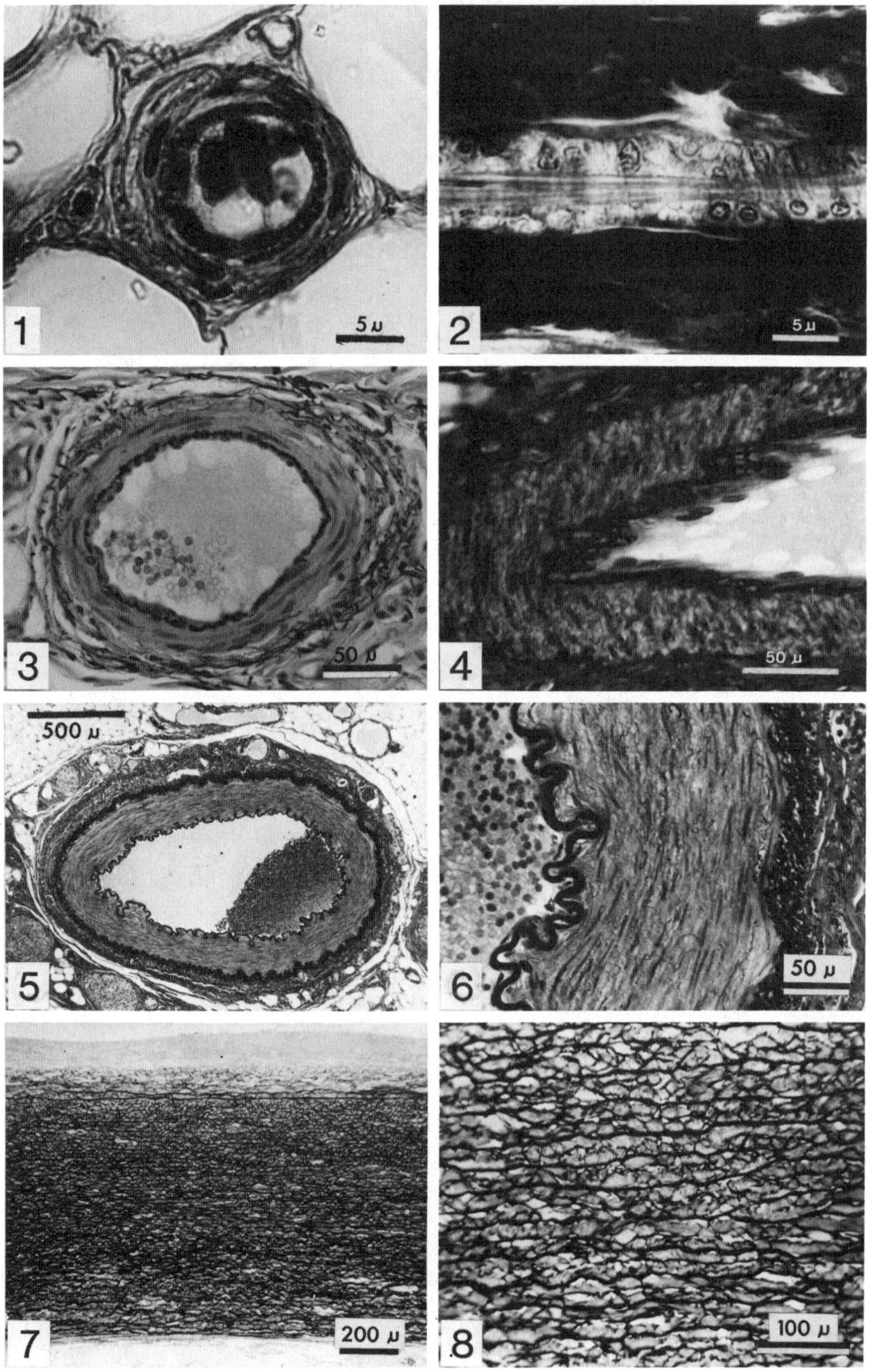

Figure 17–2.

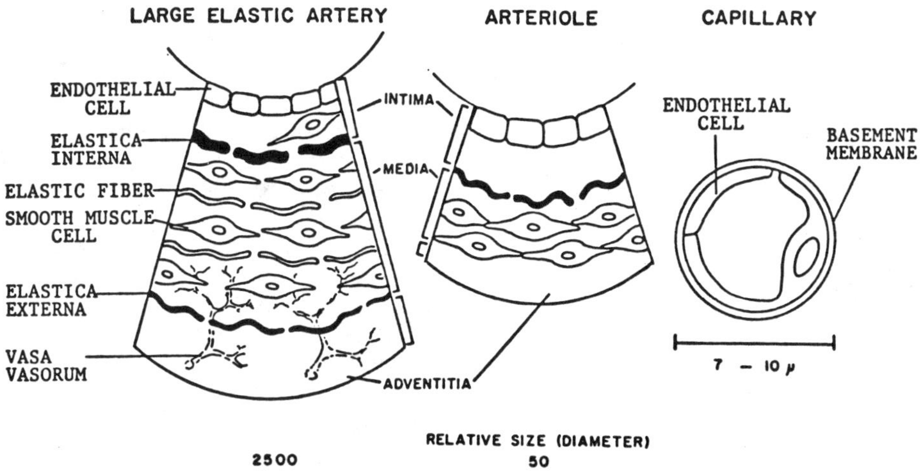

Figure 17–3. *Diagrammatic representation of the arterial wall illustrating a large (elastic) artery, an arteriole and a capillary.* (Drawing by S. Oklund).

of hepatic and splenic arteries; and (3) arrangement of the capillaries in the capillary bed in such a manner that there is a preferential capillary channel from arteriole to venule (a controversial assumption that presupposes contractile structures in the capillaries). One of the best examples of how blood circulation adjusts to hemodynamic requirements is represented by the establishment of a collateral circulation (i.e., circulation that is carried on through secondary channels) when the main arterial supply to a specific organ or tissue is cut off. Adequate blood supply to the heart is generally assured at all times by the presence of a rich system of anastomoses not only between the two main coronary arteries, but also between the coronary arteries and arteries from the pericardium, lungs, thorax, and diaphragm. Thus, in the case of thrombosis of one of the coronaries, provided that the process of occlusion is sufficiently slow, competent collateral circulation can be established.

The extent of vascularization of the arterial wall varies from species to species: for example, vascularity is less well developed in humans, rabbit, and chicken (spe-

◄ **Figure 17–2.** *Morphology of normal arterial vessels.*

(1) Arteriole-cross section (human mesentery). Stain: iron hematoxylin-aniline blue. Note: Red blood cells in lumen, endothelial nucleus, internal elastic membrane, smooth muscle cells with elongate nuclei. (2) Arteriole—longitudinal section (cat ileum submucosa). Stain: Mallory-Azan. Note: Smooth muscle cells coiling around endothelial tube which contains the nucleus of an endothelial cell. (3) Small artery—cross section (human external ear, subcutaneous tissue). Stain: Verhoeff and Van Gieson. Note: Distinct internal elastic membrane and smooth muscle of media; elastic fibers are beginning to accumulate to form an external layer. (4) Small artery—tangential section showing fenestrated internal elastic membrane (human external ear, subcutaneous tissue). Stain: as in (1). Note: All elastic membranes in the arterial tree bear fenestrae (window-like openings). (5) Medium-artery—cross section, low power (human mesenteric artery). Stain: as in (1). Note all layers of the wall, intima (with internal elastica), media and adventitia (with externa elastica) are distinct. (6) Medium artery—cross section, high power. Stain: as in (1). Note: Internal elastic membrane, well-developed muscular media, adventitia with external elastic tissue disposed as coarse fibers in helices, hence, cut tangentially. (7) Large artery—cross section, low power (human aorta). Stain: as in (3). Note: thick intima and high content of elastic tissue (appearing as black lines). (8) Large artery—cross section, high power (human aorta). Stain as in (3). Note: multiple thick membranes forming concentric tubes interconnected by finer cross membranes. The interstices are filled mainly with collagenous connective tissue and sparse smooth muscle. (Courtesy of Dr. E.S. Evans).

Table 17–1. SUMMARY OF FACTORS REGULATING ARTERIOLAR DIAMETER

VASODILATOR	VASOCONSTRICTOR
Reduced oxygen tension	Norepinephrine
Reduced pH	Epinephrine
Increased CO_2	Angiotensin II
Increased temperature	Vasopressin
Lactic acid	
Histamine release	
Potassium ions	
Adenosine-adenosine nucleotides	
Kinins	

With aging: reduced capacity for arteriolar dilation or constriction because of:
reduced elasticity
collagen cross-linkage
calcification
adrenergic receptor sensitivity
atherosclerosis

Table 17–2. LOCALIZED FACTORS CONTRIBUTING TO ATHEROSCLEROTIC LESIONS

Marginal vascularization of arterial wall
Relative ischemia
Limited metabolic exchange
Blood turbulence and mechanical stress

cies highly susceptible to atherosclerosis) than in the horse, goat, and cow (species less susceptible to the disease) (Schlichter and Harris, 1949). The type and amount of the blood supply to the vascular wall may represent a central problem of angiopathy (Gozna *et al.*, 1974; Ross, 1981); that is, the lack of adequate vascularization would represent a major cause of arterial disease (Table 17–2). As stated above, the intima and inner media purportedly obtain their nutrition by diffusion from the lumen; thus, any process that causes a thickening of the intima, as well as any process that damages the vasa vasorum, might be expected to cause an ischemic type of injury to the arterial tissue (i.e., due to blood insufficiency). Conversely, when the atherosclerotic lesion has reached the stage of plaque, regardless of the causes of plaque formation (e.g., lipid infiltration, thrombosis), the lesion becomes vascularized. Thus, although an inadequacy of blood supply to the arterial walls has been implicated in the initial stages of atherosclerosis, the increased vascularization that is associated with further development of the lesion has been viewed as an aggravating factor in advanced stages of the disease (Jellinek *et al.*, 1983). Increased vascularization may also be responsible, at least in part, for the sudden accidents such as hemorrhage, with or without thrombosis, that are characteristic of these advanced stages.

Connected with the problem of vascularization and likewise involved with the special structure of the arterial wall, are the exchanges of metabolic products between the vessel wall and lumen and vice-versa. Diffusion, which normally regulates nutritional exchanges between blood and tissues varies, with the layer of the arterial wall. In the intima, for example, because of its proximity to the blood stream, nutrients diffuse from the blood and products of arterial tissue metabolism are discharged into the lumen in the reverse direction. The other layers are too thick to be nourished by diffusion; in the adventia and outer media, metabolic needs are supplied by the vasa vasorum, leaving the inner portion of the media metabolically undersupplied and therefore, at risk. Hence, any change in thickness of the tissue layer that the metabolic substances must cross to and from the lumen or any alterations in the circulation of the vasa vasorum, will lead to alterations in metabolic exchanges, accumulation of metabolic by-products and, once the lesion has been established, will aggravate the lesion and impair eventual recovery processes (Patel and Vaishnaw, 1980).

LOCALIZATION OF LESIONS

It must be kept in mind that atherosclerotic lesions are focal; that is, they have preferred sites of occurrence and sites where they are seldom found. Thus, other factors to be considered in evaluating the etiology and progression of the atherosclerotic lesion is their location along the arterial wall and the influence of blood turbulence. Preferred sites are around the orifices of arteries branching off a major artery, such as the intercostal arteries from the descending aorta. Another preferred site is at the bifurcation of a large artery into two smaller ones such as the abdominal aorta bifurcating into the two iliac arteries. It is at these preferred sites that the lesion begins and progresses rapidly. One of the reasons for these preferential locations is that in these regions—orifices and bifurcations—blood flow increases in velocity, exceeds critical velocity and become turbulent. It is this turbulence, that is, increased velocity and more erratic flow, that creates a mechanical stress at the orifice or bifurcation favoring the onset and progression of the lesion (Patel and Vaishnaw, 1980).

STRUCTURAL CHANGES IN ATHEROSCLEROTIC LESIONS

As mentioned above, atherosclerotic lesions begin at an early age and progress continuously throughout life. The localization, rate of progression, or type of lesion varies widely depending on several factors related to the structure and function of the vessel considered, specific hemodynamic physiologic requirements, and a number of associated pathologic conditions—either local (e.g., hemorrhages, thrombi) or systemic (e.g., hypertension, diabetes) (Table 17–3) (Moore, 1981; Vikhert and Zhdanov, 1981). In all cases, atherosclerosis occurs fundamentally as a localized lesion of the wall. Although its diffusion—in the vessel itself, in the area of the vessel, and throughout the whole body—may be considerable, the steadily progressing pathologic process is always confined to one focal point, the form and size of which depends on both local and generalized conditions. The atherosclerotic plaque or atheroma represents the characteristic site at which the histogenesis of the disease can best be analyzed (Woolf, 1982). Although it has not yet been possible to detect the precise beginning of an atherosclerotic lesion, there are a sufficient number of characterizing features in those lesions to assign them the descriptive terms "early" and "advanced" (Figures 17–4 and 17–5).

Table 17–3. GENERAL CHARACTERISTICS OF ATHEROSCLEROTIC LESIONS

Early onset—progressive
Focal lesions
Early lesions
Advanced lesions
Damage
Repair
Localized-type lesions, progression influenced by:
Local factors—vessel structure and metabolism, blood turbulence
Systemic factors—diabetes, hypertension, stress

EARLY LESIONS

For large elastic arteries like the aorta, lesions usually begin in the form of scattered foci in which the innermost layers of the vascular wall show signs of damage accompanied by the growth of repair tissue. In the smaller arteries, the progression of events is less easily identifiable, but damage and repair processes still represent the most important characteristics of the early lesion in these structures.

The intima thickens as a result of an increase in tissue fluid in the intimal ground substance. At the same time, there is a disruption and disintegration of the innermost elastic lamellae, followed first by moderate influx and then swelling and flooding of the area with amorphous materials, primarily proteins and sulfated proteoglycans. The proteins seem to derive from the blood, perhaps as a consequence of the increased permeability of the damaged endothelium (as in all inflammatory edemas) and are often coupled with lipids, which become visible when uncoupled. The origin of proteoglycans is uncertain; they may derive from the blood or they may be formed *in situ*; in any case, they are very similar to the materials that accumulate in most young repair tissues of the body where they help to build collagen fibers, the principal component of scars.

Other studies of experimentally-induced atherosclerosis suggest that the initial lesion consists of proliferation of muscle cells in the media where their multiplication gives rise to a cell mass impinging into the intima. These muscle cells degenerate and accumulate lipids and the resulting mass will be invaded by macrophages and connective tissue in an attempt to circumscribe and encapsulate. This view of the early lesions, forms the basis of the muscle monoclonal hypothesis (Benditt, 1977; Ross and Glomset, 1973), which identifies the abnormal proliferation of muscle cell clones as the first event in atherosclerosis pathogen-

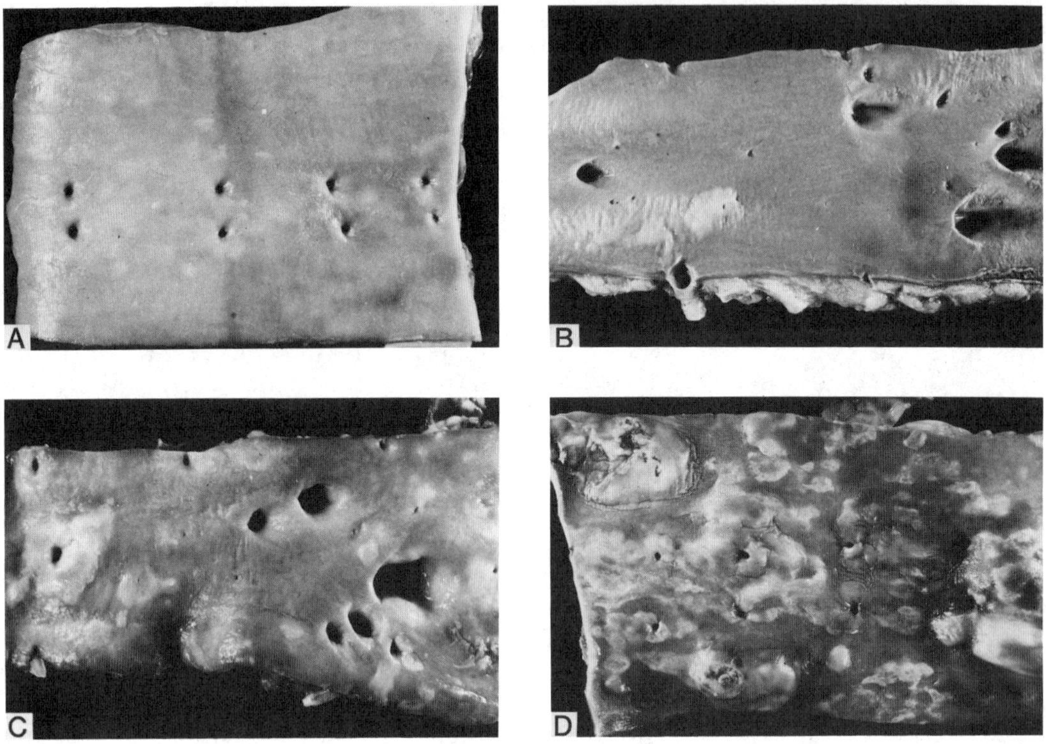

Figure 17–4. *Progression of morphologic changes in human aorta from early to advanced atherosclerosis.*

Aortas were split open and the intima exposed for photography. A. Aorta (thoracic) of a 32-year-old male showing early fatty plaques (represented by lighter coloration) localized mainly around the orifices of the intercostal arteries. As discussed in the text, because of the contribution of hemodynamic factors in the genesis of the atherosclerotic lesion, orifices of collateral arteries are frequently the site at which lesions first appear. B. Aorta of a 24-year-old female showing early fatty plaques, also around the orifices of collateral arteries. C. Aorta of a 55-year-old male showing advanced plaques characterized not only by a greater amount of fatty material but also by fibrotic thickening of the wall. D. Aorta of a 65-year-old male showing large, complicated and calcified plaques. (Courtesy of Dr. O.N. Rambo).

esis; this proliferation would be triggered by a variety of toxic substances, dietary habits, changes in blood lipids and hypertension.

The next phases of the atherosclerotic lesion involve the repair processes that work to circumscribe or eliminate the production of masses of new fibers—mostly collagen but also elastic fibers—within and above the area of injury. One of the consequences of these processes is the further aggravation of intimal hyperplasia or thickening. These initial lesions contain very little abnormal fat, if any, and, appropriately, some investigators have classified this period as the "prelipid" stage of atherosclerosis. Sooner or later, lipid does appear in some of these lesions, mostly in their basal portions and not only within the cells themselves but also in the intercellular spaces and on the disintegrating elastic lamellae. The lipid material, first in the form of small droplets, gradually fills up the cells imparting a "foamy" appearance in histologic section. With the increase in the number of foam cells and the amount of extracellular lipid, this fat accumulation becomes visible to the naked eye as tiny yellow spots or streaks in the inner lining of the arteries, the so-called "fatty spots" or "fatty

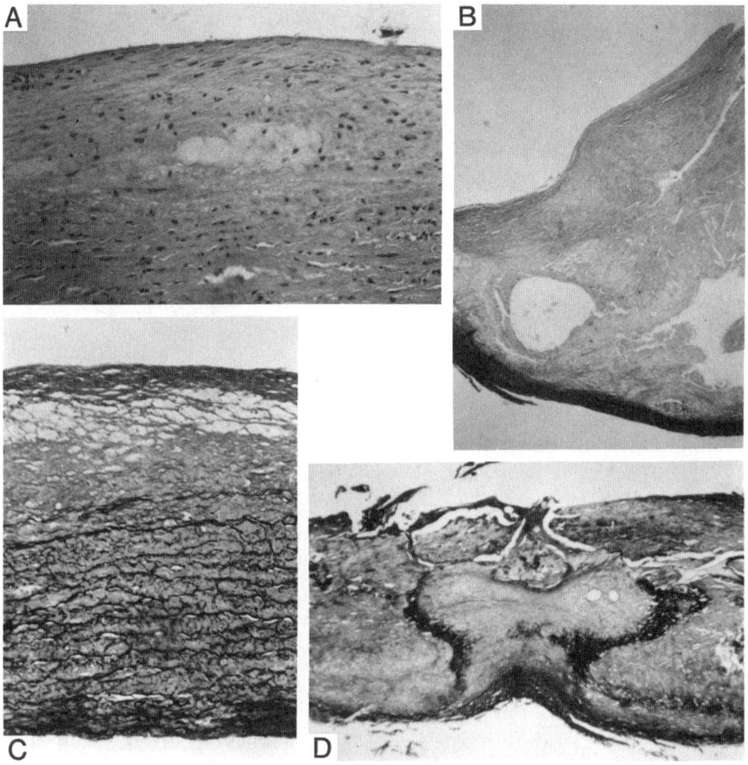

Figure 17–5. *Progression of microscopic changes in human arteries from early to advanced atherosclerosis.*

A. Earliest fatty plaque in fibrous intima (aorta from 24-year-old male: hematoxylin-eosin stain; ×224). B. Large, atheromatous cystic plaque (carotid artery from a 65-year-old male; Verhoeff and Van Gieson stain; ×35). C. Atheromatous plaque showing both fatty infiltration and alterations of elastic tissue (carotidendarterectomy in 68-year-old male; stain as in B; ×140). D. Large ulcerated calcified plaque with metaplastic bone (carotid artery with occlusion in 79-year-old male; stain as in B; ×35). (Courtesy of Dr. O.N. Rambo).

streaks." Taken as evidence of lesion, these fatty streaks are most commonly found in the aorta of children and younger individuals although similar foci have been described in octogenarians and centenarians who showed a so-called "juvenile" atherogenic index.

Ground Substance. Studies of the ground substance (extracellular matrix) and its major constituents, the proteoglycans, show progressive quantitative and qualitative changes of these substances as the atherosclerotic lesion progresses. Alone, as part of the larger group of glucosaminoglycans, and in combination with other components of the ground substance, such as hyaluronic acid and embedded substances such as collagen and elastin, the proteoglycans regulate some important visco-elastic and water-binding properties of tissues, including those of the arterial wall (Table 17–4). Impairment of these properties with aging would result in alterations of the ground substance with reduction of its functions of mechanical support and hydration. Such alterations would translate into a weakening of the arterial wall with inability to support compressive

Table 17–4. PROBABLE ROLE OF GROUND SUBSTANCE IN EARLY ATHEROSCLEROTIC LESIONS

MAJOR COMPONENTS	PROPERTIES
Glucosaminoglycans (proteoglycans) Hyaluronic acid Collagen Elastin	Viscoelastic (impaired with aging, reduced mechanical support) Water-binding (with aging, reduced hydration, altered transport)

Table 17–5. PERCENTAGE OF TOTAL LIPIDS IN HUMAN AORTIC INTIMA AT DIFFERENT AGES AND IN DIFFERENT TYPES OF LESIONS[a]

	AGE (YEARS)		TYPE OF LESION		
LIPID GROUP	15	65	FATTY STREAK	FIBROUS PLAQUE	CALCIFIED FIBROUS PLAQUE
Cholesterol ester	12.5	47.0	59.7	54.1	56.3
Free cholesterol	20.8	12.2	12.7	18.4	22.4
Triglycerides	24.8	16.6	10.0	11.1	6.5
Phospholipids	41.9	24.2	17.6	16.6	14.8

[a]Adapted from Smith, E.B.: The influence of age and atherosclerosis on the chemistry of aortic intima. Part 1. The lipids. *J. Atheroscl. Res.*, 5:224–240, 1965.

load of normal blood pressure; it would also result in chemical alterations of transport and binding of water-soluble substances. Thus, this hypothesis emphasizes the role of proteins and carbohydrates in the early causes of the atherosclerotic lesion, in contrast to the emphasis on lipid alterations supported by other theories.

ADVANCED LESIONS

These lesions, found mainly in adults and elderly persons in whom autopsic examinations are conducted more frequently, have been studied more exhaustively than the early lesions typical of the first decade of life. Detailed morphologic descriptions of advanced human atherosclerosis can be found in most textbooks of pathology and in specific texts dealing with atherosclerosis. Only a very brief summary will be presented here.

With the passing of years, more and more lipids accumulate into the fatty streaks of the established lesion (Table 17–5); the foam cells increase in number to the extent that the cells in the center die—probably because of lack of oxygen supply and because the enormous amount of fat in their cytoplasm displaces or alters the organelles concerned with normal cellular function. The lipid released from the disintegrating foam cells, along with extracellular lipid, assembles in large pools, partly in the form of cholesterol crystals and partly as an amorphous mixture of triglycerides, phospholipids, and sterols. The whole material has the consistency of a soft paste or gruel (hence the term "atheroma" from the Greek "ather" indicating a gruel-like substance). An aorta that is riddled with atheromatous plaques may contain as many as 100 or more times its normal content in lipids.

The mass of extracellular lipid acts as an irritant to the arterial wall and provokes a proliferative reaction in the surrounding vascular tissue, similar to the inflammatory reaction that occurs in response to any foreign body encountered by the organism. The resulting scar develops like a sac, encapsulating the gruel, but remaining much thicker on the lumen side of the arterial wall where it forms a thick barrier between the blood stream and the gruel. At this stage, the atherosclerotic lesion has progressed considerably from its earlier manifestation as a fatty streak; not only is it larger and thicker, but it seems to rise above the inner surface of the artery like a cushion, resembling an encapsulated abscess. Because of its appearance, the lesion has been given the name "atheromatous abscess," but it is also called a "raised plaque" or a "fibrous plaque," and its characteristic pearly-white color resulting from the high content of collagen fibers in the capsule has given it also the name of "pearly plaque."

One of the main characteristics of the advanced atheroma is its progressiveness. As the plaque grows with fat, it consumes more and more of the arterial wall underneath it, transforming the cells into foam cells and disintegrating one elastic lamella after another. In this process, the entire media is destroyed and the atheroma invades the adventitia, which then reacts by setting up a series of inflammatory-like responses such as hyperemia (due to vascular invasion) and lymphocytic infiltration. Simultaneously, the capsule of the advanced atheroma, perhaps in a compensatory effort, thickens considerably, building a new arterial wall; however, containing neither muscle nor elastic fibers but rather almost exclusively scar (connective) tissue, this wall is functionally less efficient. As the pearly plaque becomes established, calcium deposits precipitate on the gruel, the capsule, or both, in the form of either fine granules, thin strips, or huge masses. In the coronaries, for example, with the accumulation of large amounts of calcium over the years, the arteries become exceedingly hard and brittle—hence the term "hardening" or "sclerosis" of the arteries.

Up to this stage, the changes in the atherosclerotic lesion have been counterbalanced by repair processes and, consequently, there has been no loss of tissue; indeed, in the sense that the lesion continues to form scar tissue, it can be viewed as "productive." In this respect, the function of the vessel, although impaired, is not drastically altered inasmuch as there is still a lumen and an intact, though thickened, wall with a relatively smooth lining permitting blood supply to the tissues. Some lesions can remain in this stage for an indefinite period of time, whereas others eventually undergo changes that cause the breakdown of the vessel, inviting the perils that have made atherosclerosis a deadly disease.

When the capsule of the atheroma breaks away, the plaque is transformed into an ulcer, part of the exposed gruel is carried away by the bloodstream, and the rest forms an uneven, abnormal surface over which the blood clots. In some cases, the ulceration is accompanied by varying degrees of hemorrhage into the gruel or under the lips of the ulcer; before the original arterial wall has been destroyed by the atheromatous process, the ulceration breaks through the remnant of the wall causing rupture of the artery and massive hemorrhage into the space outside. Although little is yet known of the precise factors that promote ulceration and hemorrhage in plaques, it has been suggested that they might be favored by certain local changes in the lesions (e.g., extensive cell necrosis in the capsule) as well as hemodynamic events (e.g., sudden rise in blood pressure).

Other complications of advanced atherosclerosis include narrowing or widening of the arterial lumen, thrombosis, and rupture of the arterial wall. The widespread view that atherosclerosis narrows and tends to shut down the arterial lumen is valid mainly for some arteries such as the coronaries, which are embedded into an unyielding environment. Arterial occlusion by stenosis (narrowing) of the lumen is usually a slow process, and collateral circulation, as previously described, frequently has time to establish itself so that a sufficient blood supply reaches the area normally serviced by the stenotic vessel. Large arteries, such as the aorta, are widened by the atherosclerotic process as a result of the progressive weakening of the wall by the formation of scar tissue, causing it to give way to the mounting pressure within. In these cases, the arteries not only widen but also tend to lengthen, bending and twisting in the process. Aneurysms, balloonlike bulges that press on neighboring structures and often explode, frequently occur in a given spot in the wall that is much weaker than the rest.

Thrombosis is the process by which a plug of clot (thrombus) is formed in a blood vessel (or in one of the heart cavities) by coagulation of the blood, remaining at the point of its formation (in this respect, it is distinguished from the "embolus," which is also a clot of coagulated blood but is carried in the blood current, and an "embolism," which represents the plugging of an artery by a clot [embolus] that has been brought to its place by the blood current). For reasons not yet fully understood, thrombi develop more frequently in atherosclerotic than in normal arteries, appearing particularly on the ulcerated plaques (Bang *et al.*, 1982) on the arterial wall or wherever there is a crack or fissure in the plaque. "Mural" thrombi, which are small and flat and develop over the surface of the wall of the large arteries, are relatively harmless inasmuch as they do not seriously impede the flow of blood through the vessel. When, however, the thrombus is large or develops in a small artery (such as a coronary artery or a cerebral vessel), it can fill its entire lumen and block all flow of blood, with disastrous results for the tissues that were supplied by the plugged vessel. Such an occlusion generally occurs suddenly, within minutes or hours, leaving little or no time for a collateral circulation to become established. In addition to its coincidence with atherosclerosis, the occurrence of thrombosis also has been related to blood chemistry (e.g., high blood lipids) and hemodynamic changes (e.g., hypertension).

Rupture of the arterial wall that has been weakened by atherosclerosis also can be triggered by hypertension. When the rupture occurs in the relatively small cerebral arteries, the result is a "stroke." When it occurs in the aorta, especially in the descending portion, the usual result is massive bleeding in the abdominal cavity (a consequence surgeons try to avoid by reconstruction of the artery).

ROLE OF PLATELETS

In the previous discussion we have emphasized the involvement of the arterial wall in the formation of the atherosclerotic lesion. Equally important is the participation of some of the blood components. Cholesterol and lipoproteins will be discussed in Chapter 18. Other blood constituents include the platelets, a type of blood cell, and the blood coagulation system. An example of this association—arterial wall and blood constituents—is represented by thrombus formation, one of the complications of the atherosclerotic process (Schwartz *et al.*, 1981; Zucker, 1980; Bang *et al.*, 1982; Widhalm and Sinzinger, 1983).

As already mentioned, fatty and fibrous plaques are more frequent and severe at the bifurcation of an artery. In this region, endothelial denudation, that is, ulceration or even minor loss of continuity of the endothelial surface overlying the atheroma, usually initiates the formation of the thrombus within the arterial wall.

Collagen from the subintimal layers causes platelets to adhere to the roughened surface. This surface adhesion is a normal function of platelets. The collagen causes hydrolysis of some of the constituents (phosphatidylinositol) of the platelet inner membrane and the consequent release of the contents of the granules that are abundant in these cells. The release is associated with calcium flux and the formation of thromboxane A2, a membrane lipid derivative, which further activates the release process. The substances released by the platelets are primary growth factors, which promote further aggregation of platelets and initiation of clotting mechanisms. It is to be noted here, that aspirin causes a moderate inhibition of thromboxane formation, an action that would be of value in reducing the incidence of recurrences in patients with some forms of stroke. Thus, by platelet aggregation and release, and by clotting stimulation, a fibrous platelet plug is formed and friable fibrinoplatelet material may break off and enter the circulation. Emboli circulate in the blood and may occlude some smaller artery, for example in the eye or brain. Alternatively, the thrombocytic process may completely occlude the artery at the level of the original plaque.

EXPERIMENTAL ATHEROSCLEROSIS

As we have indicated before, atherosclerotic lesions have been found in all animal species investigated. In addition, lesions resembling those occurring in humans can be produced in animals, particularly by manipulation of the diet, although other methods (e.g., trauma of the arterial wall) are also successfully used for these purposes (Table 17–6). The various aspects of atherosclerosis from onset to potential therapy are being actively studied by a variety of experimental *in vivo* and *in vitro* approaches. *In vivo* experiments consist of studies of naturally occurring and experimentally induced atherosclerosis (Sandler and Bourne, 1963; Constantinides, 1965; Liker and Robinson, 1985). Atherosclerotic lesions have been found in all animal species investigated but with specific characteristics for each species. Comparison of lesions among species may provide some interesting information, however, marred by the difficulty of extrapolating from one species to another and especially to humans.

Table 17–6. EXPERIMENTAL ATHEROSCLEROSIS

In Vivo
Interspecies studies
Dietary manipulation (lipids)
Trauma of arterial wall (mechanical, viral)
Alteration of clotting system
Hormones, stress
In Vitro
Culture of individual cell types
Effects of various factors (toxic substances) on cultured cells
Molecular studies of early lesion
Action of local growth-promoting factors

Lesions resembling those occurring in humans have been produced in animals by various methods based on the different theories of atherosclerosis. One method often used is manipulation of the diet to elevate plasma lipids, for example by increasing cholesterol content in particularly susceptible animals such as the rabbit. To accelerate the course of atherosclerosis and to induce lesions resembling more closely those of humans, other interventions have been associated with high-fat diet, as, for example, diets also rich in carbohydrates (or pancreatectomy of the animals, resulting in endogenous high levels of glucose); administration of hormones, such as adrenocorticoids (to mimic stimulation of the adrenal cortex by stress); alterations of the arterial wall, e.g., by mechanical injury or bacterial or viral infections; alterations of the clotting system and of the platelets. With respect to the platelets, it must be noted that in the past decade research has focused, largely through the application of cell techniques, on the behavior of the individual cell types, normal constituents of the arterial wall or migrating into the arterial wall. We now know that each of these cells, endothelial, muscle, monocyte/macrophage, as well as the blood platelets can produce growth factors and that these may contribute to the cell proliferation ultimately leading to atheroma formation. *In vitro* studies have contributed to our knowledge of how these cells interact with lipoproteins, including the several receptors involved, how muscle cells may be induced to proliferate by various mitogens, and how cross-linking of collagen may induce alterations in membrane permeability and ground substance viscous properties.

THEORIES OF ATHEROSCLEROSIS

From the description of atherosclerosis presented so far, it emerges clearly that the atherosclerotic lesion is a complex, multifactorial process. However, at the present state of our knowledge, our ability to understand the lesions may be better advanced by concentrating on studying simple parts of the process rather than trying to tie everything together into a single theory. In fact, this is just what is current today with three major theories, each dealing with different processes in the arterial wall. There are also several minor theories but we will address here only the major ones. They include:

- Lipid accumulation theory. According to most recent work, some kind of alteration of blood lipoproteins (to be discussed in Chapter 18) such as accumulation of low-density lipoprotein (LDL) or altered ability of the cell to interact with LDL would result in the accumulation of lipids in the arterial wall (Avogaro *et al.*, 1983). An example of this accumulation is represented by the foam cells, mentioned above. Lipid infiltration involves not only muscle cells, but also migrating monocytes; thus, our understanding should cover not only how lipid infiltrates the arterial wall, but also how monocytes accumulate in the lesion. While, at least in humans, lipid infiltration appears to be an early event, the open question is what effect does that lipid have on the subsequent stages leading to the advanced lesion and on the clinical effects of the disease?
- Smooth muscle cell proliferation. According to the original theory, the atherosclerotic lesion would begin as a mutagenic event in muscle cells triggered by mechanical, chemical, or viral injury (Benditt and Benditt, 1973; Benditt, 1977). Such an event would result in the transformation of the muscle cell from a normal to a replicating cell, and the proliferative state would lead to the formation of a benign tumor capable of inducing both damage and repair mechanisms of the lesion. In this sense, the atherosclerotic lesion would resemble a tumor and our understanding of its pathogenesis would depend a great deal on progress in tumor research.
- The thrombogenic theory states that the onset of the lesion may be related to early alterations of the endothelial cells of the intima (or the basement membrane) leading to a small hemorrhage and thrombus formation (Bang *et al.*, 1982). Current research in this area investigates the surface proteins of the platelets, the mechanisms of interaction of platelets with the con-

nective tissue of the arterial wall, the series of events leading to the activation of the platelet to release its granule content (possibly representing growth factors), and the role of the blood-clotting system in contributing to thrombosis.

The presence of at least three major theories of atherosclerosis indicates that none can explain satisfactorily the atherosclerotic process. However, they have opened the way to intensive experimentation *in vivo* and *in vitro,* which, with the current advances in molecular biology, will hopefully provide the necessary answers to begin effective prevention and therapy.

CORONARY HEART DISEASE

One of the major life-threatening consequences of atherosclerosis involves the coronary arteries, that is, the arteries that supply blood to the heart. Atherosclerosis of the coronaries leads to coronary heart disease (CHD), also called ischemic heart disease, which implies reduced blood flow to the heart and, consequently, both angina pectoris and myocardial infarction. Other possible consequences include arrhythmias due to defects of impulse conduction and electrocardiographic (ECG) changes. All these conditions lead to heart failure, severe disability, and death.

CHD continues to be the major cause of disability and death in the United States. Its prevalence increases with age and shows a significant sex difference, women having a much lower incidence than men; this sex difference disappears after 70 years of age. Stress is another significant contributing factor to the high CHD incidence in the elderly (Figure 17–6).

CHD MORTALITY DECLINING?

The prevalence of CHD is still high despite a steady decrease in mortality from this cause since the late 1960s. This decline includes all sectors of the adult population. In the 35-to-74-year age group, the rate of mortality due to CHD has fallen by 30 percent and is all the more remarkable because it turned around after a sustained period of rising CHD as far back as at least 1940. The current striking decline in the United States is greater than that observed in any other country, but let us not forget that the incidence there is among the highest. Apparently we have been doing the "right things" during the past 25 years in regard to CHD

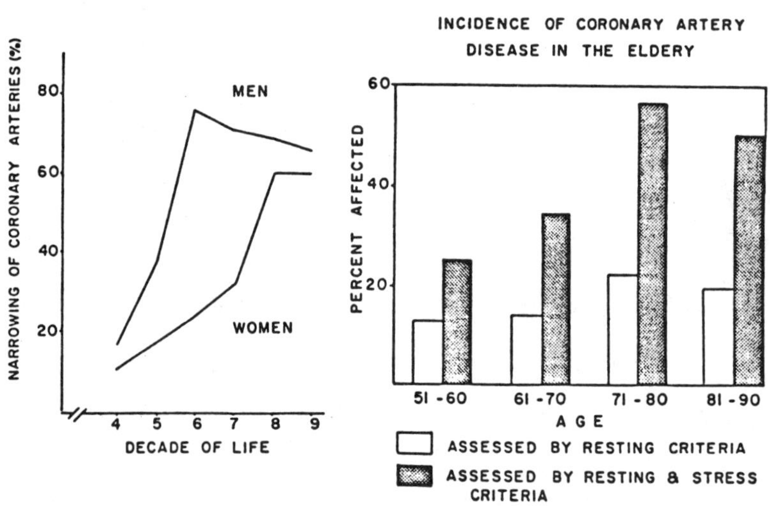

Figure 17–6. *Percentage narrowing of coronary artery lumen with aging (on the left); note sex differences with narrowing coronary artery occurring earlier and being more severe in men than women. Incidence of coronary artery disease with aging (on the right). Note the increase in incidence with age, particularly under conditions of stress. (Drawing by S. Oklund).*

and the major adult cardiovascular diseases, generally (Pell and Fayerweather, 1985; Stamler, 1985). Two major factors may account for this:

- the first, and most important, is the improvement in lifestyle, amelioration of the diet, increased physical exercise (see also Chapters 18, 22, 25, and 26), and cessation of cigarette smoking;
- the second factor is therapeutic improvement, including: better control of hypertension, better medical care in the hospital for patients with CDH, and more widespread use of coronary bypass surgery and other methods of coronary revascularization.

The right and left coronary arteries arising from the aorta as it emerges from the left ventricle are the major vessels supplying blood to the myocardium. Venous drainage is via a superficial system ending primarily in the coronary sinus, and via a deep system that drains the remainder of the heart and empties directly into the heart chambers.

Coronary flow at rest (250 ml/min) is 5 percent of the cardiac output. The heart extracts 70 to 80 percent of the oxygen, close to the maximum amount possible from this blood. Therefore, oxygen consumption can be significantly increased on demand only by increasing blood flow. Coronary flow is influenced by several local factors, which regulate flow through vasodilation or vasoconstriction (Table 17–7).

Major *vasodilators* include reduced oxygen and increased carbon dioxide concentration, increased products of metabolism (hydrogen ions, potassium, lactic acid), local agents (prostaglandins, adenine nucleotides, and adenosine) and neural stimulation (stimulation of parasympathetic innervation). Major *vasoconstrictors* include angiotensin II (Chapter 12) and neural stimulation of the sympathetic innervation. As for the brain, the cardiac circulation is preferentially preserved when that of other organs is compromised.

Table 17–7. LOCAL REGULATION OF CORONARY BLOOD FLOW

VASODILATION	VASOCONSTRICTION
↓ Oxygen	Angiotensin II
↑ CO_2	Sympathetic stimulation (direct)
↑ H+	
↑ K+	
↑ Lactic acid	
↑ Prostaglandins	
↑ Adenine nucleotides and adenosine	
Vagal stimulation	

Table 17–8. SYMPTOMS OF ANGINA PECTORIS AND ACUTE MYOCARDIAL INFARCTION IN THE ELDERLY

Angina Pectoris
Pain, less marked than in adult; may present as headache or epigastric distress
Myocardial Infarction
Variable presentation with chest pain, including breathlessness, confusion, fainting, GI symptoms, sweating, hypotension, etc.

CHD CONSEQUENCES

When progressive narrowing of the coronary lumen reduces flow through the coronary artery to the point that the myocardium becomes ischemic, angina pectoris develops. If the myocardial ischemia is severe and prolonged, irreversible changes occur in the cardiac muscle and the result is myocardial infarction.

Signs and Symptoms. The major sign of angina pectoris is squeezing or pressurelike pain, retrosternally, radiating to the left shoulder, arm, hand, neck, and jaw. The pain often appears with exertion, emotion, or a large meal. Anginal pain in the elderly is often less marked, possibly due to reduced activity or altered pain perception; it may be effort-induced or may occur at rest or in bed and may be present as headache or epigastric pain relieved by antacids (Table 17–8).

Major signs and symptoms of myocardial infarction are variable in the elderly, although chest pain remains the commanding feature in patients admitted to the coronary care units. Other symptoms include: breathlessness, confusion, behavior change, fainting, palpitations, vomiting, sweating, abdominal pain, hypotension. The pain may last over 30 minutes and is not relieved by multiple doses of nitroglycerine. Diagnosis is confirmed by EEG changes (Table 17–8). With the establishment of the infarct, irreversible changes occur in the myocardium: muscle cells first become leaky and the rise in serum enzymes and isoenzymes is a biochemical diagnostic sign of the infarct. The first enzyme to be elevated is serum glutamic oxaloacetic transaminase (SGOT) followed by creatinine phosphokinase (CPK) and lactic dehydrogenase (LDH).

RISK FACTORS IN CHD

CHD epidemiology, so important in identifying the causes and subsequent prevention and treatment, can best be studied by focusing on the consequences. Indeed, the decreased mortality from CHD may be ascribed primarily to identification of risk

Table 17–9. MAJOR RISK FACTORS IN CORONARY HEART DISEASE

Age
Genetic predisposition
Hypertension
Diabetes mellitus
Hypercholesterolemia
Cigarette smoking
Also:
Obesity
Poor physical fitness and lack of exercise
Personality type (?)

Table 17–10. MAJOR TYPES OF CORONARY HEART DISEASE TREATMENT

Medical treatment
Diet
Exercise
No smoking
Pharmacologic agents
Surgical treatment
Aortocoronary bypass graft
Percutaneous transluminal coronary angioplasty with streptokinase anticoagulant therapy

factors and to their prevention. Studies in various populations have identified the following risk factors that predispose to the development of CHD: age, genetic predisposition, hypertension, diabetes mellitus, hypercholesterolemia, cigarette smoking. Other risk factors include: obesity, poor physical fitness and lack of exercise, personality type (Table 17–9).

In a 1964–1972 study on a cohort of 7500 white Kaiser Permanente Medical Care Program members, initially free of CHD and ranging in age from 60 to 79 years of age, the following mortality risk factors until 1980 were: increasing age, high systolic blood pressure and moderate to high serum cholesterol, cigarette smoking, alcohol consumption, increased body weight, alterations of pulse and white blood count, high serum uric acid. For males, the most important risk factors were age, blood pressure, and body weight; and for females, age, blood pressure, cigarette smoking, cholesterol, uric acid, and nonconsumption of alcohol (no drinks versus 1 to 2 drinks per day) (Sidney, 1986).

These lists dictate specific preventive measures such as treatment of hypertension and diabetes, elimination of cigarette smoking, amelioration of dietary habits toward an optimal body weight, and encouragement of measures to improve physical fitness.

Management. The reduction of mortality due to CHD arises from the awareness of contributing factors and their alleviation or amelioration (Table 17–10). Therefore, medical treatment includes: (1) treatment of the underlying disease, if any (hypertension, diabetes mellitus, hyperlipidemias) (Harris, 1970), (2) nutritional therapy, cessation of smoking, behavioral therapy, and physical exercise, especially for cardiac rehabilitation (see Chapters 18, 22, and 26) (Bazan *et al.*, 1981; Feldman, 1983; Herd and Weiss, 1983; Case *et al.*, 1985; Fielding, 1985; Kushi *et al.*, 1985), (3) pharmacologic agents with the intention of increasing cardiac blood flow, reducing cardiac work, and preventing clotting (see Chapter 24). In addition, surgery has also been successful with aortocoronary bypass grafts and transluminal coronary angioplasty with streptokinase anticoagulant therapy (Gersh *et al.*, 1985; Kennedy *et al.*, 1985; Koren *et al.*, 1985; Mock *et al.*, 1985).

HYPERTENSION

Blood pressure depends on cardiac output and peripheral vascular resistance. The World Health Organization defines normal blood pressure as below 140 mm Hg for the systolic pressure and 90 mm Hg for the diastolic, and hypertension as a sustained elevation of the arterial pressure with a systolic blood pressure of 160 mm Hg or more and a diastolic of 95 mm Hg or more, or both. The condition is present in over 60 percent of people over 60 years of age. This is often a silent disease, that is, presenting no symptoms; therefore, the true incidence of hypertension is probably much higher (Horan *et al.*, 1986).

Hypertension is an important risk factor for cardiovascular morbidity and mortality in males and females at any age. The interaction of atherosclerosis and hypertension is complex but crucial in the progression of cardiac and cerebrovascular disease. Al-

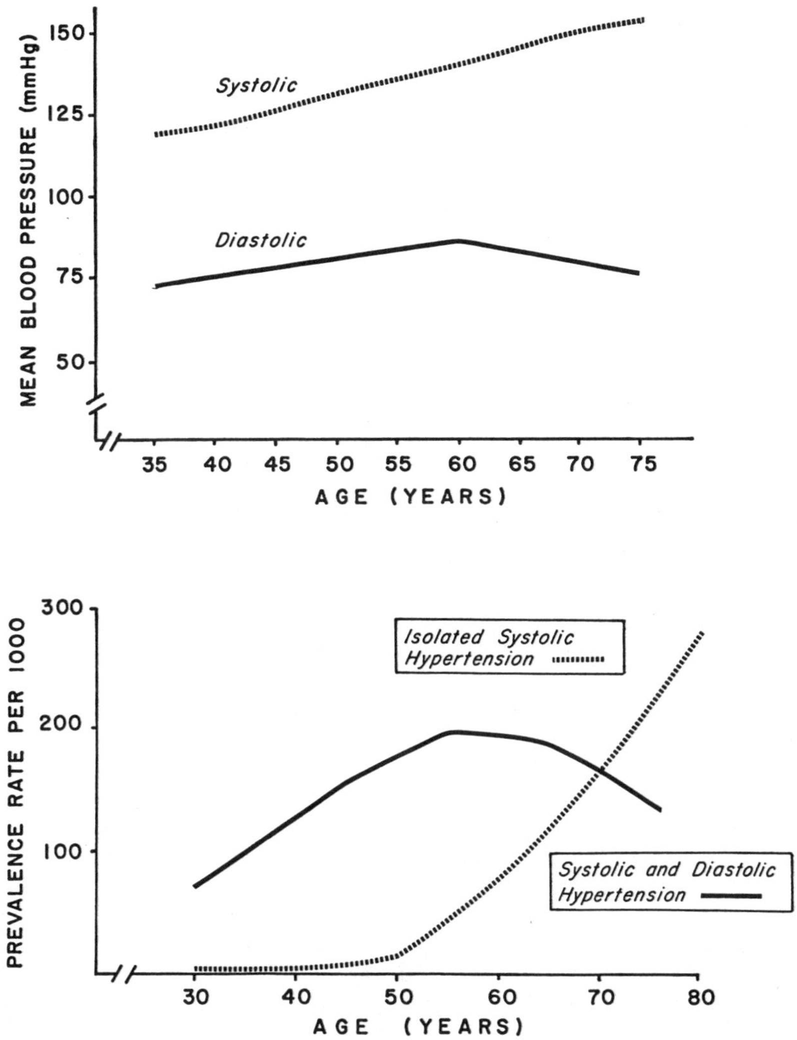

Figure 17–7.

A. Increase with aging in mean systolic blood pressure but not in diastolic pressure. B. Prevalence of isolated systolic hypertension continues to increase with aging whereas combined systolic and diastolic hypertension increases at a younger age but levels off after 60 years of age.

though it is unclear whether hypertension plays a greater role than any other of the risk factors discussed above in the etiology of CHD, or whether atherosclerosis is the major cause of hypertension, no one questions the existence of an interaction between the two. The importance of hypertension as the most prominent reversible risk factor for cardiovascular and cerebral complications in the elderly cannot be overemphasized.

Blood pressure increases with age, but the systolic and diastolic pressures behave differently over time. Systolic pressure rises slowly commencing in the early adult years and continuing on to old age. Diastolic pressure rises steadily in early adulthood but begins to decline at about age 60. This accounts for the high prevalence of isolated systolic hypertension in the elderly (Figure 17–7). The elderly with combined systolic and diastolic hypertension have

Table 17–11. CAUSES OF HYPERTENSION

Essential hypertension	Unknown
Renal hypertension	Glomerulonephritis Pyelonephritis Polycystic disease Renal artery narrowing
Endocrine	Hypo/hyperthyroidism Hypersecretion of aldosterone (Conn's syndrome) Hypersecretion of glucocorticoids (Cushing's syndrome) Congenital virilizing adrenal hyperplasia Adrenal medullary tumor (pheochromocytoma)
Coarctation of the aorta (narrowing)	
Polypharmacy	Sympathomimetic amines Steroids Nonsteroid analgesics Tricyclic antidepressants, etc.

Table 17–12. FACTORS THAT CONTRIBUTE TO HYPERTENSION IN THE ELDERLY

Atherosclerosis
Renal impairment
Hormonal defects
Blunted baroreceptor responses

disproportionately higher systolic pressures (Rowe, 1983).

ESSENTIAL HYPERTENSION

Most elderly patients with elevated blood pressure have essential hypertension, which, in fact, comprises 90 percent of the cases (Tables 17–11 and 17–12). Its etiology is unknown, but all of the affected elderly have increased peripheral resistance, probably related to atherosclerosis. Resistance to blood flow depends to a minor degree on blood viscosity but to a greater degree on the diameter of the vessels, primarily the arterioles. Reduction of the arteriolar diameter increases resistance and increased resistance results in increased diastolic pressure. Increased rigidity of the larger arteries contributes to the increase in systolic pressure.

The remaining 10 percent of elevated blood pressure cases are due to other factors, including chronic renal and endocrine diseases and polypharmacy. Renal hypertension may be due to kidney damage secondary to infections, glomerulonephritis and pyelonephritis, to polycystic disease, or to narrowing of the renal artery, primarily due to atherosclerosis. Hypertension of endocrine origin may be due to alterations of thyroid function or to increased secretion of adrenal steroids, as in Conn's syndrome (with aldosterone hypersecretion), virilizing hyperplasia (with increased mineralocorticoids), or Cushing's syndrome (with glucocorticoid hypersecretion) (Laragh, 1985). Tumors of the adrenal medullary tissue, generally outside the adrenal, are called pheochromocytomas. They induce a type of hypertension that is often episodic (but may be sustained) and is characterized by very high systolic pressure. Coarctation of the aorta is a congenital narrowing of the thoracic aorta, producing severe hypertension in the upper part of the body.

Numerous drugs, alone or in combination, may also induce hypertension as a side effect. Singling out steroids, one can speak of "pill hypertension." This refers to hypertension in women or women who are chronic users of oral contraceptives; however, there is evidence that these women are predisposed to hypertension in any case.

HYPERTENSION IN THE ELDERLY

Hypertension is characterized in the elderly by marked lability (Niarchos and Laragh, 1980; Tuck and Sowers, 1982; Franklin, 1983; Gavras and Gavras, 1983; Kannel, 1985; Williams, 1985) (Table 17–13). Therefore, casual measurements of blood pressure can be particularly unreli-

Table 17–13. CLINICAL MANIFESTATIONS OF HYPERTENSION IN THE ELDERLY

Lability of blood pressure
Prevalence of orthostatic hypotension
Presence of an auscultatory gap

able, and several readings should be taken over an interval of time. The measurement should also be taken with the individual in different positions, sitting, reclining, standing, for orthostatic hypotension (occurs upon standing and produces syncope) due to reduced autonomic responsiveness is prevalent in the elderly.

Orthostatic (postural) hypotension consists in a fall in blood pressure upon moving suddenly from the supine to the standing position. It occurs in some young and adult individuals and in many elderly. The hypotension causes a transitory cerebral ischemia (reduced blood flow) with dizziness, dimness of vision, and even fainting or syncope (loss of consciousness). The fall in blood pressure is due to inability to compensate rapidly for the gravitational changes in blood pools that occur with standing, depriving the brain of the required amounts of blood.

The major compensation on assuming the upright position is triggered by the drop in blood pressure in the baroreceptors (carotid sinus and aortic arch) with consequent increase in cardiac rate, venoconstriction, and increased levels of renin and aldosterone. All these responses induce peripheral vasoconstriction and increased cardiac output with normalization of the blood pressure and decreased cerebral vascular resistance with increased blood flow.

Failure or slowing down of all these compensatory mechanisms results in hypotension. This abnormality is quite frequent in the elderly because of autonomic insufficiency, abnormal baroreceptors, myocardial arrhythmias, and impaired cerebral vascular adjustments (Weisfeldt, 1980). It is also often the consequence of various medications to which the elderly may be particularly sensitive.

The blood pressure must be taken in both arms and peripheral pulses examined to exclude coarctation of the aorta. General physical examination must exclude endocrine disorders, and abdominal examination may reveal an enlarged polycystic kidney. Auscultation of abdominal bruits is of little diagnostic help in the elderly. With the auscultatory method of measuring blood pressure, the first sounds heard (after releasing pressure in the inflatable cuff) represent the systolic pressure (as read in mm Hg on the sphygmomanometer): these are followed by the so-called sounds of Korotkoff, and the disappearance of these sounds corresponds to the diastolic pressure (as read in mm Hg). In some elderly patients, there is an auscultatory gap, which consists of a silent interval below the beginning of the sounds of Korotkoff at systole. In this case, blood pressure must first be measured by palpation to avoid missing a very elevated systolic blood pressure, as may occur by auscultation alone.

Table 17–14. GENERAL GUIDELINES FOR TREATMENT OF HYPERTENSION IN THE ELDERLY

Use nonpharmacologic maneuvers when possible
Use pharmacologic therapy cautiously
Avoid sudden changes in blood pressure
Watch for orthostatic hypotension

The majority of elderly hypertensives are asymptomatic, i.e., have no apparent subjective symptoms.

Signs of hypertensive end-organ damage include left ventricular enlargement, cardiac failure, and retinal changes. Malignant hypertension, that is, a type of severe hypertension with an accelerated course of 1 to 2 years, is rare but not unknown in the elderly and may or may not be associated with very high levels of blood pressure. Fundoscopy, examination of the blood vessels of the fundus of the eye, will show evidence of hemorrhages and soft exudates with or without edema of the papilla. Proteinuria is often present.

MANAGEMENT

Hypertension of specific origin is curable by eliminating the cause; therefore, the cause must be sought out and the appropriate treatment initiated whether by surgery, hormonal suppression, or drug administration (O'Malley and O'Brien, 1980). However, the likelihood of detecting a treatable cause of hypertension in the elderly patient is small, and more specialized investigation is justified only if there is any clear evidence of a primary underlying cause. In the absence of such specific cause, treatment consists primarily in keeping the blood pressure within normal limits with the help of single or combined antihypertensive drug treatment (see Chapter 24).

References

Arteriosclerosis. Report of the Working Group on Arteriosclerosis of the NHLBI, U.S. Department of Health and Human Services, Washington, DC, NIH Publication no. 81-2034, **1981.**

Avogaro, P.; Bittolo-Bon, G.; Cazzolato, G.; Belussi, F.; and Pontoglio, E.: Lipids and proteins of lipoproteins in human atherosclerosis. *Przegl. Lek.*, **40:**713–718, **1983.**

Bang, N. U.; Tessler, S. U.; Heidenreich, R. O.; Marks, C. A.; and Mattler, L. E.: *Thrombosis and Atherosclerosis*. Year Book Medical Publishers, Chicago, **1982.**

Bazan, N. G.; Paoletti, R.; and Iacono, J. M. (eds.): *New Trends in Nutrition, Lipid Research, and Cardiovascular Disease,* Current Topics in Nutrition and Disease, Vol. 5, Alan R. Liss, New York, **1981.**

Benditt, E. P.: The origin of atherosclerosis. *Sci. Am.*, **236:**74–85, **1977.**

Benditt, E. P., and Benditt, J. M.: Evidence for a monoclonal origin of human atherosclerotic plaques. *Proc. Natl. Acad. Sci. USA,* **70**1753–1756, **1973.**

Bierman, E. L.: Arteriosclerosis and aging. In Finch, C. E., and Schneider, E. L. (eds.): *Handbook of the Biology of Aging,* Van Nostrand Reinhold, New York, **1985.**

Case, R. B.; Heller, S. S.; Case, N. B.; and Moss, J. A.: Type A behavior and survival after acute myocardial infarction. *N. Engl. J. Med.*, **312:**737–741, **1985.**

Constantinides, P.: *Experimental Atherosclerosis,* Elsevier, Amsterdam, **1965.**

Feldman, E. B.: *Nutrition and Heart Disease,* Churchill Livingston, New York, **1983.**

Fielding, J. E.: Smoking: Health effects and control. *N. Engl. J. Med.*, **313:**491–498 (part I) and **313:**555–561, **1985.**

Franklin, S. S.: Geriatric hypertension. *Med. Clin. North Am.*, **67:**395–417, **1983.**

Gavras, H., and Gavras, I.: *Hypertension in the Elderly,* John Wright PSG, Boston, **1983.**

Gersh, B. J.; Kronmal, R. A.; Schaff, H. V.; Frye, R. L.; Ryan, T. J.; Mock, M. B.; Myers, W. D.; Atheara, M. W.; Gosselin, A. J.; Kaiser, G. C.; Bourasse M. G.; and Fillip, T.: Comparison of coronary bypass surgery and medical therapy in patients 65 years of age or older. *N. Engl. J. Med.*, **313:**916–919, **1985.**

Gresham, G. A.: *Reversing Atherosclerosis,* Charles C Thomas, Springfield, IL, **1980.**

Gozna, E. R.; Marble, A. E.; Shaw, A.; and Holland, J. G.: Age-related changes in the mechanics of the aorta and pulmonary artery of man. *J. Appl. Physiol.*, **36:**407–410, **1974.**

Harris, R.: *The Management of Geriatric Cardiovascular Disease,* J. B. Lippincott, Philadelphia, **1970.**

Herd, J. A., and Weiss, S. M.: *Behavior and Atherosclerosis,* Plenum Press, New York, **1983.**

Horan, M. J.; Steinberg, G. M.; Dunbar, J. B.; and Hadley, E. C. (eds.): *NIH Blood Pressure Regulations and Aging,* Biomedical Information Corporation, New York, **1986.**

Jellinek, H.; Detre, Z.; and Veress, B.: *Transmural Plasma Flow in Atherogenesis,* Akademiai Kiado, Budapest, **1983.**

Kannel, W. B.: Hypertension and aging. In Finch, C. E., and Schneider, E. L. (eds.): *Handbook of the Biology of Aging,* Van Nostrand Reinhold, New York, **1985.**

Kennedy, J. W.; Ritchie, J. L.; Davis, K. B.; Stadius, M. L.; Maynard, C.; and Fritz, J. K.: The Western Washington randomized trial of intracoronary streptokinase in acute myocardial infarction. *N. Engl. J. Med.*, **312:**1073–1078, **1985.**

Koren, G.; Weiss, A. T.; Hasin, Y.; Appelbaum, D.; Welber, S.; Rozenman, Y.; Lotan, C.; Mosseri, M.; Sapoznikov, D.; Luria, M. H.; and Gotsman, M. S.: Prevention of myocardial damage in acute myocardial ischemia by early treatment with intravenous streptokinase. *N. Engl. J. Med.*, **313:**1384–1389, **1985.**

Kottke, B. A.: Disorders of the blood vessels. In Pathy, M. S. J. (ed.): *Principles and Practices of Geriatric Medicine,* John Wiley & Sons, New York, **1985.**

Kushi, L. H.; Lew, R. A.; Stare, F. J.; Ellison, C. R.; Lozy, M.; Bourke, G.; Daly, L.; Graham, I.; Hickey, N.; Mulcahy, R.; and Kerancy, J.: Diet and 20-year mortality from coronary heart disease. *N. Engl. J. Med.*, **312:**811–818, **1985.**

Laragh, J. H.: Atrial natriuretic hormone, the renin-aldosterone axis, and blood pressure-electrolyte homeostasis. *N. Engl. J. Med.*, **313:**1330–1340, **1985.**

Lee, K. T. (ed.): Atherosclerosis. *Ann. NY Acad. Sci.*, **454, 1985.**

Liker, I. N., and Robinson, R. W.: Atherosclerosis: Cattle as a model for study in man. *Monographs on Atherosclerosis,* Vol. 12, Karger, Basel, **1985.**

McGill, H. C.; Geer, J. C.; and Strong, J. P.: Natural history of human atherosclerotic lesions. In Sandler, M., and Bourne, G. H. (eds.): *Atherosclerosis and Its Origin,* Academic Press, New York, **1963.**

Mock, M. B.; Reeder, G. S.; Schaff, H. V.; Holmes, J. R.; Vlietstra, R. E.; Smith, H. C.; and Gersh, B. J.: Percutaneous transluminal coronary angioplasty versus coronary artery bypass. *N. Engl. J. Med.*, **312:**916–919, **1985.**

Moore, S. (ed.): Vascular injury and atherosclerosis. In *The Biochemistry of Disease,* Vol. 9, Marcel Decker, New York, **1981.**

Morrison, L. M., and Schjeide, O. A.: *Arteriosclerosis: Prevention, Treatment and Regression,* Charles C Thomas, Springfield, IL, **1984.**

Niarchos, A. P., and Laragh, J. H.: Hypertension in the elderly. *Modern Ger. Cardiov. Dis.*, **49:**45–54, **1980.**

O'Malley, K., and O'Brien, E.: Management of hypertension in the elderly. *N. Engl. J. Med.*, **302:**1397–1404, **1980.**

Patel, D. J., and Vaishnaw, R. N.: *Basic Hemodynamics and Its Role in Disease Process,* University Park Press, Baltimore, **1980.**

Pell, S., and Fayerweather, W. E.: Trends in the incidence of myocardial infarction and in associated mortality and morbidity in a large employed population. *N. Engl. J. Med.*, **312:**1005–1011, **1985.**

Roberts, J. C., Jr., and Strauss, R. (eds.): *Comparative Atherosclerosis,* Harper & Row, New York, **1965.**

Ross, R.: Atherosclerosis: A problem of the biology of the arterial wall cells and their interactions with blood components. *Arteriosclerosis,* 1293–311, **1981.**

Ross, R., and Glomset, J. A.: Atherosclerosis and the arterial smooth muscle cell. *Science,* **180:**1332–1339, **1973.**

Rowe, J. W.: Systolic hypertension in the elderly. *N. Engl. J. Med.*, **309:**1246–1247, **1983.**

Sandler, M., and Bourne, G. H.: Histochemistry of atherosclerosis in the rat, dog and man. In Sandler, M., and Bourne, G. H. (eds.): *Atherosclerosis and Its Origin,* Academic Press, New York, **1963.**

Schlichter, J., and Harris, R.: The vascularization of the aorta. A comparative study of the aortic vascularization of several species in health and disease. *Am. J. Med. Sci.*, **218:**610–615, **1949.**

Schwartz, S. M.; Gajdusek, C. M.; and Selden, S. C.: Vascular wall growth control, the role of the endothelium. *Arteriosclerosis,* **1:**107–106, **1981.**

Sidney, S.: Risk factors for coronary heart disease in the elderly. American Heart Association 26th Annual

Conference on Cardiovascular Disease Epidemiology, San Francisco, March 3–5, **1986.**

Smith, E. B.: The influence of age and atherosclerosis on the chemistry of aortic intima. Part 1. The lipids. *J. Atheroscl. Res.,* 5:224–240, **1965.**

Stamler, J.: Coronary heart disease: Doing the "right things." *N. Engl. J. Med.,* **312:**1053–1055, **1985.**

Tuck, M., and Sowers, J.: Hypertension and aging. In Koreman, S. G. (ed.): *Endocrine Aspects of Aging,* Elsevier Biomedical, New York, **1982.**

Vikhert, A. M., and Zhdanov, V. S.: *The Effects of Various Diseases on the Development of Atherosclerosis,* Pergamon Press, New York, **1981.**

Weisfeldt, M. L. (ed.): *The Aging Heart—Its Function and Response to Stress,* Raven Press, New York, **1980.**

Widhalm, K., and Sinzinger, H.: Current aspects of atherosclerosis lipids, lipoproteins, platelets, prostaglandins and experimental findings. *Atherogenesis,* Vol. 5, M. Maudrich, Wein, **1983.**

Williams, B. H. O.: The cardiovascular system. In Pathy, M. S. J. (ed.): *Principles and Practice of Geriatric Medicine,* John Wiley & Sons, New York, **1985.**

Woolf, N.: *Pathology of Atherosclerosis,* Butterworth Scientific, London, **1982.**

Zucker, M. B.: The functioning of blood platelets. *Sci. Am.,* **242:**86–103, **1980.**

CHAPTER

18 AGING OF THE CARDIOVASCULAR SYSTEM

Lipoproteins

Trudy M. Forte

As discussed in the previous chapter, the cause of cardiovascular disease, primarily atherosclerosis, is complex, and many factors can contribute to the development of premature atherosclerosis. Factors that singly or in combination are contributors to the premature manifestation of the disease and early death include: hypercholesterolemia; hypertension; diabetes mellitus; smoking; genetic predisposition; obesity; and stress. As this list of offenders implies, plasma cholesterol and, by extension, plasma lipoproteins have a significant role in the process of atherogenesis. The structure, synthesis, and metabolism of plasma lipoproteins are reviewed in this chapter and their role as either positive or negative risk factors in premature atherosclerosis presented.

LIPOPROTEIN NOMENCLATURE, STRUCTURE, AND COMPOSITION

Specific lipid-containing macromolecules in the plasma, the *lipoproteins,* have an important role in the development of the atherosclerotic lesion (see Steinberg, 1983). Certain lipoproteins predispose to premature atherosclerosis, while others have a protective role. Lipids circulating in the plasma include free fatty acids, which are bound to albumin, and cholesterol, triglyceride, and phospholipids, which are bound to specific proteins, the apolipoproteins, to form lipoprotein complexes. There are five major classes of lipoproteins, which are recognizable on the basis of size and lipid content. The density of these lipoproteins is inversely proportional to their lipid content so that high-density lipoproteins have the lowest total lipid and the highest protein content. The major lipoproteins from least dense to most dense are: chylomicrons, very-low-density, intermediate-density, low-density, and high-density lipoproteins.

Generally, one thinks of lipoproteins in terms of pathologic conditions such as coronary artery disease, but in fact they are molecules that are necessary for the maintenance of overall body functions. They are extremely important in the body since the lipids they carry, especially the triglycerides, are a major source of energy for cells. Fat-soluble vitamins are also transported by lipoproteins. Cholesterol transported by these macromolecules is utilized by the cells for cell division, cell growth, and membrane repair; cholesterol is also essential for the production of steroid hormones, both adrenocortical hormones, discussed in Chapter 12, and sex hormones, in Chapters 13 and 14. An overabundance of lipoproteins, however, particularly those carrying cholesterol, can be deleterious, particularly by predisposing to premature cardiovascular disease.

As mentioned previously, lipoproteins are protein-lipid complexes that transport insoluble lipids, principally cholesterol and triglyceride, in the blood and interstitial fluids. A schematic of a generic lipoprotein is illustrated in Figure 18–1. The lipoprotein particle is essentially an oil droplet (hence, globular in shape) stabilized by a surface coat of hydrophilic (water-loving) molecules, including proteins and phospholipids. The core of the particle consists of the highly insoluble lipids, cholesteryl ester, and triglyceride. Free cholesterol may also be associated with the surface components, as indicated in the illustration. As total protein (the apolipoproteins) on the particles increases, the particles become smaller and denser. The difference in densities of the particles is the fundamental basis for the nomenclature used for de-

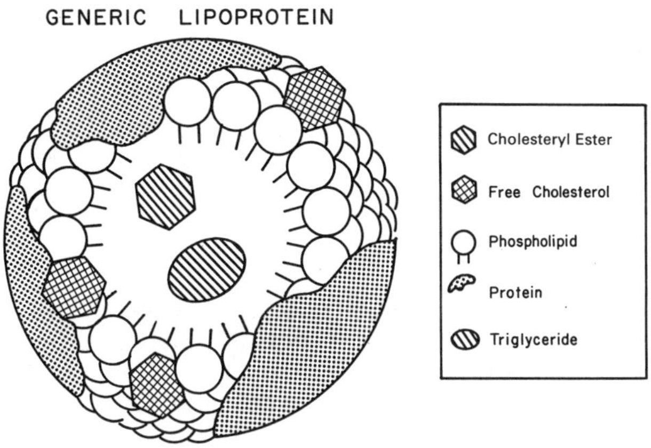

Figure 18–1. *Generalized organization of mature plasma lipoproteins.*

Particles are overall globular in morphology with polar (water soluble) components on the surface to stabilize the particle in the aqueous plasma environment. The polar constituents are primarily protein (apolipoprotein) and phospholipid. Some free cholesterol may also be on the surface. The core of the particle consists of the non-polar (highly insoluble in an aqueous enviornment) components, cholesteryl ester or triglyceride. (Drawing by S. Oklund)

fining lipoproteins, i.e., very-low-density (VLDL), intermediate-density (IDL), low-density (LDL), and high-density (HDL) lipoproteins.

Major Classes of Lipoproteins. The major lipoprotein classes and their composition are summarized in Table 18–1. Essentially, lipoproteins are grouped in three major categories:

1. *Chylomicron (CM) and very-low-density lipoprotein (VLDL).* These are relatively low in protein, phospholipid, and cholesterol, but high (55 to 95 percent) in triglyceride. In more general terms, these particles are referred to as triglyceride-rich lipoproteins.
2. *Intermediate-density lipoproteins (IDL) and low-density lipoproteins (LDL).* These are characterized by high levels of cholesterol, mainly in the form of cholesteryl esters. The latter form of cholesterol is highly insoluble. Since up to 50 percent of the LDL mass is cholesterol, it is not surprising that LDL has a significant role in the development of atherosclerotic disease.
3. *High-density lipoprotein (HDL).* The hallmarks of these particles are their high protein content (50 percent) and relatively high phospholipid content (30 percent). HDL are generally divided into two important subclasses, HDL_2, and HDL_1; of the two, HDL_2 are larger and less dense, while HDL_3 are smaller and more dense.

PLASMA LIPOPROTEIN CONCENTRATIONS

The most commonly used clinical indicator for measuring potential risk of premature cardiovascular disease is the level of plasma lipids. Fasting levels of triglyceride, cholesterol, and HDL cholesterol can often be used to identify possible abnormalities. The expected normal adult plasma lipid levels are shown in Table 18–2. Females characteristically have lower triglyceride (80 mg/dl; dl = 100 ml plasma) than males (120 mg/dl) and have higher HDL cholesterol (55 mg/dl versus 43 mg/dl for males). For comparison, the lipid levels from normal, full-term neonates are also provided. The newborn has triglyceride and total cholesterol levels one-half to one-third those of the adult. The HDL cholesterol levels are relatively high (35 mg/dl) in the newborn, where the ratio of total cholesterol to HDL cholesterol is 2 compared with the adult values of 3.5 for females and 4.6 for males. HDL are considered beneficial; that is, they are protective against atherosclerosis, whereas LDL are positive risk factors. Therefore, the lipid levels in infants are perhaps the most "ideal," for at birth

Table 18–1. NOMENCLATURE AND COMPOSITION OF PLASMA LIPOPROTEINS

NOMENCLATURE	WEIGHT (PERCENT)			
	PROTEIN	PHOSPHOLIPID	CHOLESTEROL	TRIGLYCERIDE
Chylomicron (CM)	1–2	3–6	2–7	80–95
Very-low-density lipoprotein (VLDL)	5–10	15–20	10–15	55–65
Intermediate-density lipoprotein (IDL)	19	19	38	23
Low-density lipoprotein (LDL)	20–25	22	45	10
High-density lipoprotein (HDL)	45–50	30	20	5

Table 18–2. NORMAL PLASMA LIPID LEVELS

	TRIGLYCERIDE	TOTAL CHOLESTEROL (MG/DL)	HDL CHOLESTEROL
Adult female	80	190	55
Adult male	120	200	43
Neonate	38	70	35

plasma total cholesterol is low while HDL cholesterol is relatively high. Except for genetic abnormalities (such as homozygous familial hypercholesterolemia, to be discussed below), the vascular walls of neonates are free of fatty streaks. Fat accumulation appears in the first years of life, indicating that dietary input and environmental factors probably influence the initiation and progression of atherosclerosis. At birth, no distinction can be seen between male and female infants since sex hormones are low in levels and apparently have little metabolic influence at this stage of development.

Factors Influencing Lipoprotein Levels

In the adult, *sex* differences have a definite effect on plasma lipid levels, as shown by the higher levels of triglyceride and total cholesterol and the lower levels of HDL cholesterol in the males as compared to the females. Indeed, females, before menopause, tend to have lower total cholesterol than males, but the most functionally significant difference is the *higher* HDL cholesterol in females, that is, 55 mg/dl in females versus 43 mg/dl in males. This increase in HDL cholesterol is in a specific subclass of HDL, the HDL_2. As already mentioned, HDL_2 are larger and less dense—that is, lighter—than HDL_3, which represent the primary HDL subclass in men. Epidemiologic studies suggest that HDL_2 play a protective role in atherogenesis. In women, the hormone estrogen has an important role in elevating HDL_2 and, thus, tends to protect premenopausal women from early onset of atherosclerosis. Indeed, we have discussed in Chapter 13, incidence of cardiovascular disease increases after menopause.

HDL_2 levels can also be increased by *physical exercise*. It is now known that male marathon runners have HDL patterns similar to those of females. An obvious conclusion is that exercise is beneficial in maintaining healthy HDL levels. *Cigarette smoking*, on the other hand, decreases HDL levels, while cessation of smoking reverses the effect.

Differential Role of Lipoproteins in Atherosclerosis

As already mentioned, HDL have been termed beneficial or "good" lipoproteins, inasmuch as high plasma HDL levels correlate with decreased risk of cardiovascular disease. Conversely, LDL have been labeled "bad" lipoproteins since increases in LDL cholesterol are directly linked with increased risk of cardiovascular disease. However, even with the LDL class, one can distinguish specific subclasses such as LDL-I and LDL-II, which are larger and less dense, and LDL-III and LDL-IV, which are smaller and more dense. The latter particles increase risk to atherosclerosis because their increased number parallels a decrease in HDL cholesterol, particularly HDL_2. Indeed, high levels of these small LDL and the concomitant decrease in HDL levels suggest a double-jeopardy risk for cardiovascular disease.

The plasma triglyceride and cholesterol levels discussed in Table 18–2 are those of young adults; these levels tend to increase with advancing age. The effect of aging on plasma total cholesterol levels is shown in Figure 18–2. The age-related increase in total plasma cholesterol is less marked between 20 and 40 years in women than in men; however, females show a distinct upward trend at approximately 55 years, an age that coincides with menopausal events such as decreased estrogen levels.

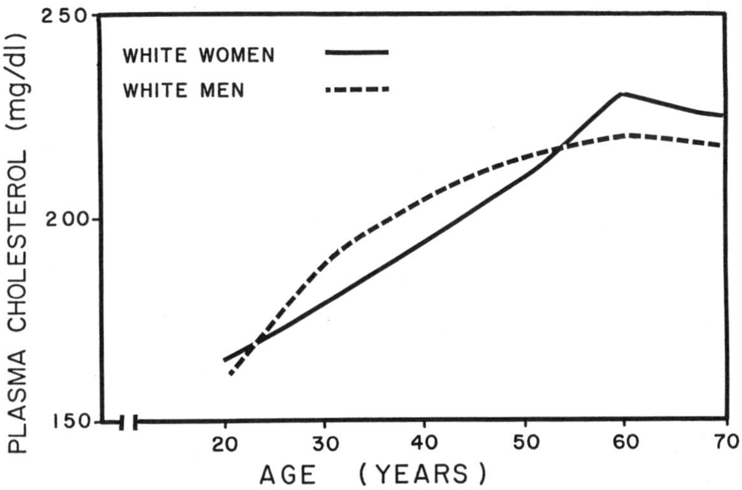

Figure 18–2. *Plasma cholesterol levels in women versus men from age 20 to 70.*

White women (———) during the premenopausal period have lower total cholesterol levels than corresponding males (----). After menopause (between 50–60 years) there is a distinct increase in total cholesterol in women. Figure derived from data published by NIH [The Lipid Res. Clin. Population Studies Data Book, DHEW, 1980] (Drawing by S. Oklund).

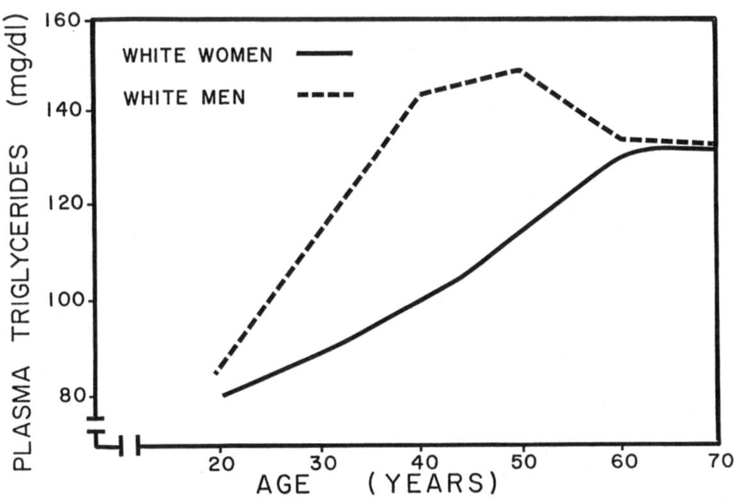

Figure 18–3. *Plasma triglyceride levels in women (———) versus men (----).*

White males have higher levels between 20–50 years of age, while both sexes are quite comparable after age 50. Figure derived from data in reference 2. (Drawing by S. Oklund)

The increase in levels of plasma lipids with aging is also evident with respect to triglycerides (Figure 18–3). These lipids increase very noticeably with age; in men, the increase is already significant at 40 years, while in women the levels increase significantly between 50 and 60 years.

SYNTHESIS OF LIPOPROTEINS

The vital effects of the lipoproteins in well-being and survival and their implication in the etiopathology of cardiovascular disease necessitates a close consideration of the metabolism of these macromole-

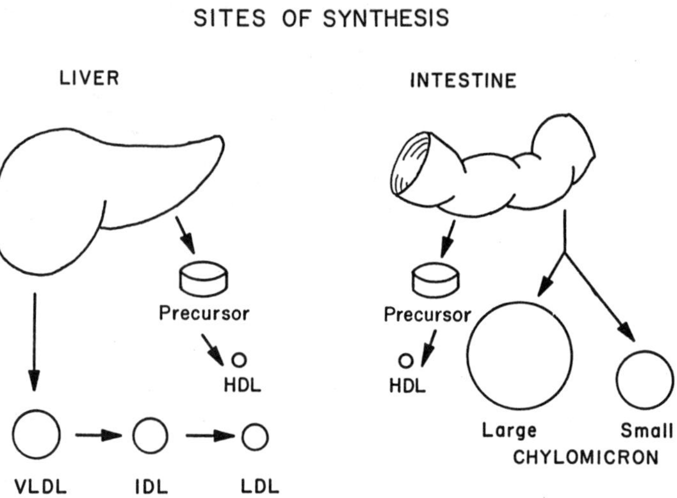

Figure 18–4. *Sites of synthesis of the major plasma lipoproteins.*

Liver secretes VLDL which during lipolysis generates smaller, denser particles including intermediate density (IDL) and low density (LDL) lipoprotein particles. High density lipoproteins are also secreted by the liver; however, as indicated on the schematic, the nascent or precursor particle is discoidal in shape rather than spherical. These nascent particles are subsequently transformed in the plasma to the mature, spherical forms. The small intestine secretes mainly triglyceride-rich particles in the form of large and small chylomicrons. The intestinal cells also secrete nascent HDL which are similar in their chemical characteristics to those secreted by the liver. (Drawing by S. Oklund)

cules. Indeed, in recent years, the wealth of research is providing a clearer understanding of their synthesis, distribution, and catabolism, as well as their binding to cell receptors and intracellular metabolism.

There are two major sites of synthesis of lipoproteins: the liver and the small intestine (Figure 18–4). The liver is the major organ regulating cholesterol homeostasis. Parenchymal liver cells secrete VLDL, which are large molecules rich in triglycerides. VLDL loses core lipid, mainly triglyceride, through lipolysis and gives rise to IDL and LDL. The generally accepted mechanism for the formation of LDL is by way of this precursor-product relationship wherein large triglyceride-rich VLDL is the precursor and the smaller, cholesteryl ester-rich particle, LDL, is the final product. The liver is also the site of synthesis for HDL. Newly secreted HDL, however, is chemically and structurally different from circulating HDL. The newly secreted particles, like membranes, possess mainly phospholipid and free cholesterol organized as a bilayer, are discoidal in shape, and contain little or no core lipids. Such discoidal HDL are "immature" forms of HDL whereas the spherical ones are mature HDL. Discoidal HDL have been termed "nascent" or precursor HDL, and normally they are rapidly converted to mature HDL by the plasma enzyme lecithin:cholesterol acyltransferase (LCAT) discussed below.

Lipoprotein secretion by the intestine is regulated to a great extent by what we eat. Dietary lipids are secreted in the form of large and small chylomicrons. The intestine, like the liver, also secretes an HDL (Figure 18–4), which is discoidal in shape. This intestinal precursor of HDL must also undergo transformation via the LCAT enzyme reaction in order to assume the morphology and chemistry of normal circulating plasma HDL.

Apolipoproteins: Their Role in Lipoprotein Metabolism

Although the lipid moiety in lipoproteins is involved in processes of growth and survival as well as development of disease, it is the proteins associated with the lipids that direct the metabolism and ultimate fate of lipoproteins (see Jackson *et al.*, 1976). Lipoprotein proteins, or apolipoproteins, are important constituents that impart specific properties and functions to the molecule. The major apolipoproteins (apo) are: apoAI, apoAII, apoB, apoCI, apoCII, apoCIII, and apoE. Their molecular weights vary from 8000 daltons for apoCI to 540,000 for apoB, as shown in Table 18–3.

The function and origin of apolipoproteins are summarized in Table 18–4. ApoAI is the major protein of HDL and is synthesized in both the liver and the intestine. The levels of plasma apoAI may turn out to be a better indicator of atherosclerotic risk than plasma cholesterol or even HDL cholesterol. This apolipoprotein is the major activator of the enzyme LCAT, which, as indicated, is necessary for transformation of the discoidal precursor of HDL to the spherical mature HDL.

ApoAII is the second most abundant apolipoprotein on HDL and, like apoAI, is produced by both liver and intestine. Its functional significance is not completely understood, although it is thought that it may inhibit LCAT and thereby modulate plasma HDL by indirectly influencing the conversion of free cholesterol to cholesteryl ester.

ApoB is an extremely important protein that is associated with the less dense lipoproteins including chylomicrons, VLDL, and LDL. It is the sole protein of LDL, the low-density lipoprotein. It originates from both the intestine and the liver. ApoB has two important functions:

1. it is necessary for the secretion of triglyceride-rich particles from both the liver and intestine. In a rare genetic disease where apoB is not synthesized, the intestinal cells absorb lipids but are unable to repackage and secrete the lipids as chylomicrons. Steatorrhea, that is, the presence of excess lipids in stools, and diarrhea ensue, along with malnutrition. Since the liver is also a site of apoB synthesis, this organ is affected and becomes fatty because of the intracellular accumulation of triglycerides. The lack of apoB has broader implications since degradation of VLDL and chylomicrons normally produces LDL. In turn, LDL are important transporters of cholesterol, required for normal growth and development.
2. ApoB is also a ligand, i.e., a substance that binds to specific membrane receptors. The receptor that recognizes apoB is called the LDL receptor or the B-E receptor; its function is to internalize LDL into the cell, thereby delivering cholesterol for various cellular functions. All cells possess LDL receptors to a greater or lesser degree. Clearly, receptors are functionally necessary to mediate normal cell metabolism; however, an overabundance of LDL and apoB can lead to saturation of the receptors with a consequent accumulation of excess cholesterol in the plasma and initiation of the atherosclerotic process. The levels of apoB in plasma are good indicators of atherosclerotic risk, for elevated apoB levels correlate with elevated levels of circulating cholesterol.

ApoE is another apolipoprotein that is recognized by the B-E receptor. It plays a particularly important role in targeting VLDL remnants to the liver where they are catabolized. VLDL remnants are the smaller, denser particles enriched in cholesteryl ester, which are formed following hydrolysis of triglyceride. It is thought that apoE may also play a role in promoting the efflux of excess cholesterol *from* cells; in other words, it plays a role in *reverse cholesterol transport* (see Roheim, 1986). This reverse transport is probably important in decreasing the burden to cholesterol for the cell, particularly the cell membrane. A family has recently been described that has a genetic de-

Table 18–3. CLASSIFICATION OF MAJOR APOLIPOPROTEINS

APOLIPOPROTEIN	MOLECULAR WT. (DALTONS)
ApoAI	28,000
ApoAII	17,000
ApoB	540,000
ApoCI	8,000
ApoCII	10,000
ApoCIII	12,000
ApoE	34,000

Table 18–4. PROPERTIES OF MAJOR APOLIPOPROTEINS

APOLIPOPROTEIN	FUNCTION	ORIGIN
ApoAI	Activator of LCAT[a]	Intestine, liver
ApoAII	Inhibitor of LCAT	Intestine, liver
ApoB	Recognition of cell receptor, triglyceride transport from cell	Intestine, liver
ApoE	Recognition of cell receptor	Liver
ApoCI	Activator of LCAT	Liver
ApoCII	Activator of lipoprotein lipase	Liver
ApoCIII	Modulated apoE uptake Lipoprotein lipase inhibitor	Liver

[a]LCAT = lecithin:cholesterol acyltransferase.

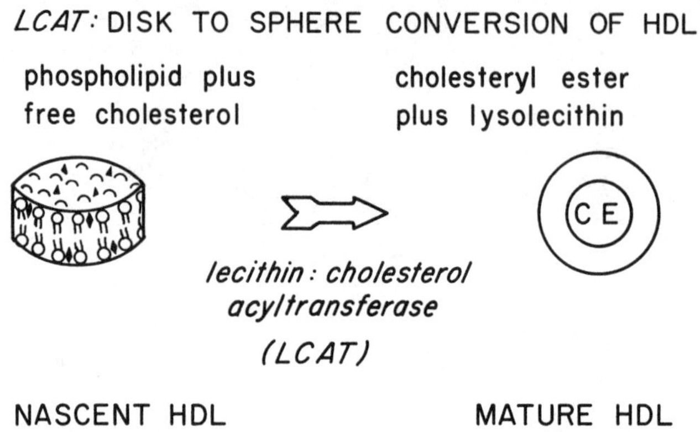

Figure 18–5. *Lecithin:cholesterol acyltransferase (LCAT) activity and transformation of nascent discoidal HDL to mature plasma HDL.*

Nascent HDL secreted either by the intestine or the liver consist of bilayers of phospholipid and free cholesterol stabilized by protein. In the presence of the enzyme LCAT, free cholesterol is esterified to cholesteryl ester with the concomitant production of lysolecithin. Cholesteryl ester is highly non-polar and hence moves to the interior of the HDL, thus forming a core and converting a disk to a sphere. Lysolecithin, the other product of the reaction, is bound to albumin. (Drawing by S. Oklund)

fect whereby apoE is not synthesized. Homozygous family members have premature coronary artery disease and elevated plasma cholesterol and triglyceride levels, thus suggesting that apoE plays a significant role in human lipid metabolism.

The apoC proteins are often referred to as the "small" proteins. They are synthesized in the liver and function principally as required cofactors in the enzyme systems that hydrolyze lipoproteins (Table 18–4). ApoCI acts as an activator of LCAT and, in this respect, is functionally similar to apoAI. ApoCI levels in plasma are extremely low compared with apoAI, which suggests that apoCI may have other as yet unidentified function(s). ApoCII is a cofactor in lipoprotein lipase activation; the protein is essential for degradation of chylomicrons and VLDL whereby core triglyceride are hydrolyzed to free fatty acids. The absence of plasma apoCII leads to gross elevation of plasma triglyceride levels.

ApoCIII has a functional role in two areas of lipoprotein metabolism: it acts as an inhibitor of lipoprotein lipase activity and hence modulates triglyceride hydrolysis, and it also modulates the cellular uptake of apoE-containing lipoprotein particles.

ENZYMES IN LIPOPROTEIN METABOLISM

Lecithin:Cholesterol Acyltransferase (LCAT). This enzyme, synthesized by the liver and secreted into the plasma, is involved in the maturation of HDL, and it plays a crucial, albeit indirect, role in removal of excess cholesterol from cells and tissues (*reverse cholesterol transport*). The proposed role of LCAT in the transformation of immature or nascent HDL is illustrated in Figure 18–5. Newly formed or nascent precursor HDL consist of small bilayers of phospholipids stabilized on their rim by HDL apolipoproteins. Free cholesterol is inserted between the phospholipids in a fashion similar to that in cell membranes. In the plasma compartment where LCAT is present, the disks are rapidly converted into spheres upon the formation of cholestryl ester by the following reaction: phospholipid + free cholesterol $\xrightarrow{\text{LCAT}}$ cholesteryl ester + lysophospholipid. The major phospholipid in lipoproteins is lecithin. The fatty acid in the second position on lecithin is removed and added to cholesterol at the position of the hydroxyl group; this then gives rise to cholesteryl ester (highly insoluble) and lysolecithin. Lysolecithin formed in the reaction rapidly binds to plasma albumin. Cholesteryl ester is extremely nonpolar and moves into the core, thus inducing the structural change from disk to sphere.

LCAT is also responsible for enlarging the size of mature, circulating HDL (Figure 18–6). Small HDL can pick up excess cholesterol from cells, and in the presence of LCAT, the added cholesterol is esterified. This mechanism of loading circulating HDL with cholesterol is extremely important for it allows for efflux of excess cholesterol

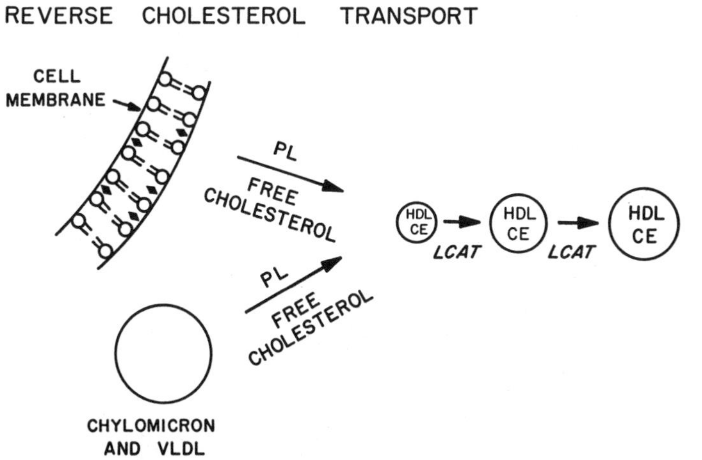

Figure 18–6. *The role of HDL in removal of excess cholesterol from cell membranes and triglyceride-rich lipoprotein surfaces.*

Small HDL can incorporate free cholesterol and phospholipid from both these sources. In the presence of LCAT, the newly accrued cholesterol is esterified producing a particle with a larger core. The cholesteryl ester associated with the large HDL is transferred to IDL and LDL which are subsequently taken up by the liver and cholesterol excreted as bile salts. The removal of excess cellular and plasma cholesterol via the HDL mechanism is called reverse cholesterol transport. (Drawing by S. Oklund)

from cells—the so-called reverse cholesterol transport described earlier. Reverse transport may represent an important step in preventing atherosclerosis. The cholesteryl ester in HDL is eventually taken up by the liver, where it is excreted in the form of bile acids.

HDL also has an integral role in the normal catabolism of chylomicrons and VLDL. During lipolysis of these triglyceride-rich particles, excess surface material, including protein, phospholipid, and free cholesterol, is generated. Such excess surface material is removed by uptake into HDL, as suggested in Figures 18–6 and 18–7.

The critical role of LCAT in maintaining HDL function and structure is dramatically illustrated by a rare disease, familial LCAT deficiency. In these patients, LCAT is not synthesized and secreted by the liver; as a consequence HDL levels are extremely low and the circulating form of HDL is *discoidal* in shape. Free cholesterol levels in almost all cells are elevated, and life-threatening sequelae include: fatty liver, degenerative kidney disease, and premature coronary artery disease. This disease demonstrates without a doubt that HDL cholesterol esterification is necessary for reverse cholesterol transport and the prevention of premature atherosclerosis.

Lipoprotein Lipase (LPL). This enzyme is important for the metabolism of triglyceride-rich lipoproteins. LPL is synthesized by adipocytes, heart, and kidney, but migrates from the sites of synthesis to the capillary endothelium, where it is bound to the cell surface. LPL is responsible for catabolism of the large, triglyceride-containing lipoproteins, principally chylomicrons and VLDL. It catalyzes the hydrolysis of triglyceride to free fatty acids and glycerol and requires the presence of apoCII, which is an activator of the enzyme. The action of LPL in the degradation of chylomicrons and VLDL is illustrated in Figure 18–7. VLDL and chylomicrons interact with LPL at the endothelial cell surface where hydrolysis occurs. The triglyceride core of these large particles is removed, thus generating fatty acids, excess surface material, and remnants.

The fatty acids are utilized by cells for energy. Chylomicrons and VLDL remnants that are generated during lipolysis are rich in cholestryl ester and contain apoE, as well as apoB, on their surfaces; they are rapidly cleared from the plasma through re-

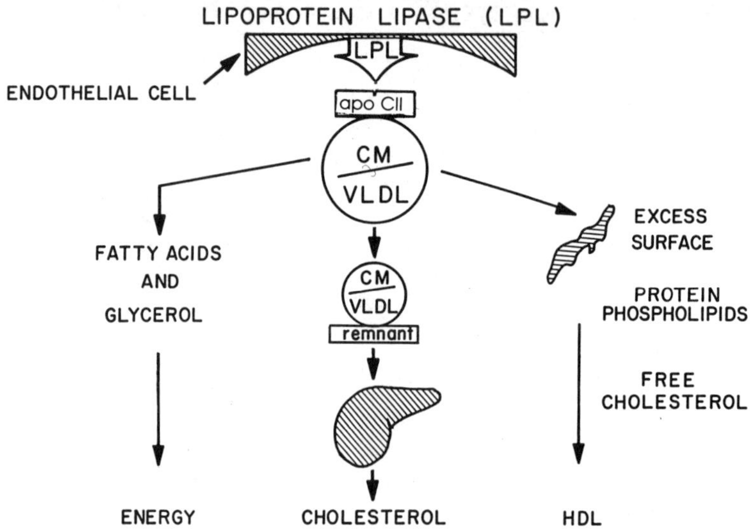

Figure 18–7. *A schematic diagram of the physiological function of lipoprotein lipase.*

The enzyme is found on the lumenal surfaces of capillary endothelium and requires apolipoprotein (apo) CII as an activator. Triglyceride-rich particles including chylomicrons (CM) and very low density lipoprotein (VLDL) carry apoCII and activate the enzyme; in so doing, the triglyceride core is hydrolized and constitutive parts of triglyceride free fatty acids and glycerol, are liberated. Removal of core triglyceride creates a remnant particle which is smaller and denser and contains a high proportion of cholesterol. Most of the remnants are removed by the liver. Excess surface components (protein, phospholipid, and free cholesterol) generated by shrinking of the core are taken up by HDL. This enzyme is a key one in clearing triglyceride-rich lipoproteins. (Drawing by S. Oklund).

ceptor-mediated uptake and degradation by the liver. This degradation step is vital for normal cholesterol metabolism. It is now known that some individuals possess apoE protein that has a single amino acid substitution, which leads to loss of recognition of the protein by the receptor. In this disease the remnants accumulate in the plasma and are directly linked with an increased risk to premature atherosclerosis.

Excess surface components will also be produced when the triglyceride core in chylomicrons and VLDL shrinks. These components, especially phospholipids and free cholesterol, are incorporated into HDL (Figure 18–6).

INTERACTION OF LIPOPROTEINS WITH CELLS

The LDL Receptor. As we have inidicated previously, lipoproteins interact with cells and are responsible for delivery of cholesterol to both hepatic and nonhepatic tissues. LDL are the major transporters of cholesterol in the body; cholesterol in the form of cholesteryl ester is delivered to cells by uptake of LDL by a *specific receptor mechanism, the apoB-E receptor,* also called the *LDL receptor.* Although all cells possess apoB-E receptors to a greater or lesser degree, the liver, based on total mass, contains the largest number of apoB-E receptors. This receptor is functionally extremely important in the regulation of intracellular cholesterol synthesis and flux, and in addition, it regulates further synthesis of the receptor. The function of the high-affinity apoB-E receptor is outlined in Figure 18–8 and is based on the work of Brown and Goldstein (1984, 1986). Essentially, liver and peripheral cells possess high-affinity specific receptors that recognize LDL (or apoE-containing remnant). LDL (or remnant) binds to the receptor and is internalized in a structure referred to as the endosome. The endosome is converted into a lysosomal body wherein hydrolysis and degradation of the internalized lipoprotein

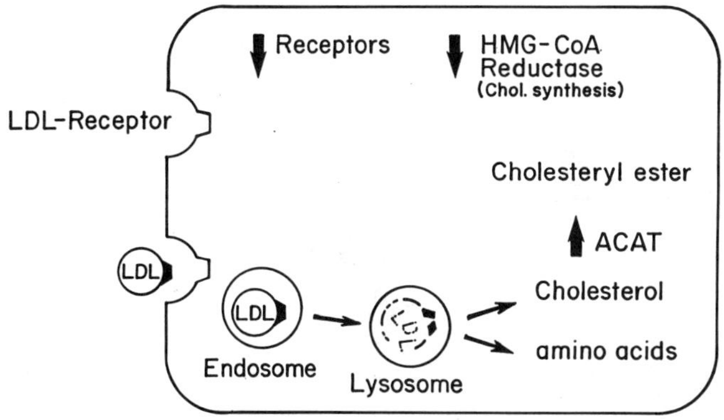

Figure 18–8. *Schematic outline of the function of the LDL (also called B-E) receptor.*

This receptor plays an important role in catabolism of cholesterol-containing lipoproteins. Lipoproteins carrying apolipoproteins (apo) B or E are recognized by the receptor and bound. The bound particles are internalized in a membrane-bound sac, the endosome. Hydrolytic enzymes invade the vesicle which becomes a lysosome in which proteins and lipids are broken down to amino acid and free cholesterol. In the cytosol, cholesterol is esterified to cholesteryl ester by the cellular enzyme, acyl coenzyme A:cholesterol acyltransferase (ACAT). Cholesterol coming into the cells down-regulates, or decreases, the activity of the cell's own cholesterol-making machinery. The rate-limiting step in *de novo* synthesis of cell cholesterol is 3-hydroxy-3-methylglutaryl coenzyme A (HMGCoA) reductase; therefore, this enzyme is the one regulated by receptor-mediated cholesterol accumulation. In addition to a decrease in HMGCoA reductase, accumulation of cellular cholesterol also decreases the number of LDL receptors on the cell surface. Overall, the receptor-mediated process is a finely tuned system in the regulation of cholesterol metabolism. (Drawing by S. Oklund).

takes place. The LDL is broken down into its molecular constituents, amino acids and cholesterol.

In the cell, catabolism of LDL results in the activation of several self-regulatory processes. Accumulation of free cholesterol *up-regulates,* that is, stimulates, the enzyme acyl-coenzyme A:cholesterol acyltransferase (ACAT), which reesterifies cholesterol. The accumulation of cellular cholesterol, then *down-regulates,* that is, decreases, the enzyme 3-hydroxy-3-methylglutaryl coenzyme A (HMGCoA) reductase, which is the rate-limiting step in cellular cholesterol synthesis. In other words, the cell slows down its own machinery for synthesizing cholesterol when adequate amounts are being delivered to it by the lipoproteins. In addition to down-regulating the HMGCoA reductase, degraded LDL down-regulates synthesis of the apoB-E receptor, and thus the cell reduces its uptake of cholesterol. The entire cell is finely tuned for an elegant maintenance of cholesterol homeostasis.

Receptor-mediated uptake and degradation of apoB- and apoE-containing lipoproteins is important in maintaining normal plasma cholesterol levels. Elevated levels of cholesterol-containing particles such as VLDL remnants and LDL could result in saturation of the apoB-E receptors and accumulation of excess cholesterol in the plasma, with the increased risk to cardiovascular disease. The risk to cardiovascular disease is also enormously increased when apoB-E receptors are defective or deficient. This does happen in certain genetic defects where either the receptor protein is not synthesized or the synthesized protein is defective. Patients with such receptor defects are hypercholesterolemic and their condition is called familial hypercholesterolemia. In the homozygous form, patients can have staggeringly high plasma cholesterol levels, as high as 1000 mg/dl as compared to the normal 150–200 mg/dl. These patients have precocious atherosclerosis and, unless managed extremely carefully, will not survive the second decade of life. The disease state is a clear case of overproduction and underutilization of LDL. Heterozygotes for

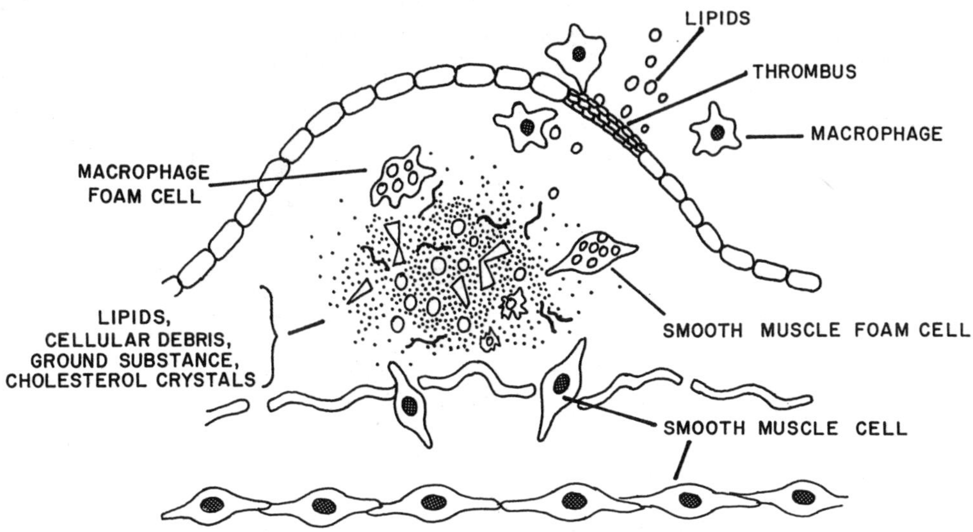

Figure 18–9. *Schematic of the role of the macrophage in cholesterol catabolism.*

Macrophages accumulate cholesterol by means of the scavenger receptor; however, the internalized cholesterol is not reutilized and it accumulates within the cell in the form of lipid droplets or foam cells. The macrophage/foam cell in the artery wall ultimately dies and releases its residue of cholesterol which accumulates in the lesion. The macrophage also releases factors which stimulate smooth muscles to proliferate and accumulate lipids, thus further augmenting and atherosclerotic process. (Drawing by S. Oklund).

the disease have decreased numbers of functional receptors and, therefore, have elevated plasma cholesterol and premature coronary artery disease.

The Scavenger Receptor. In addition to the apoB-E receptor, another receptor, the *scavenger receptor,* is functionally important; the scavenger pathway for lipoprotein uptake is functional in *macrophages*. This receptor is a high-affinity, non-LDL receptor that recognizes modified LDL and actively removes it. Modified lipoproteins may accumulate in the plasma because of altered apoB structure or because normal B-E receptors are defective. In the latter case, lipoprotein residence time in the plasma is increased, thus increasing the likelihood of protein alterations, particularly by oxidation reactions. Altered lipoproteins are bound and internalized by the macrophage scavenger receptor. A current theory on the development of the atherosclerotic lesion involves this pathway (Figure 18–9) (Mahley, 1981; Ross, 1986). As we have previously discussed, macrophages enter the arterial intima in regions of endothelial damage. The macrophages accumulate lipids by scavenging lipoproteins present at the injury site. This is probably a protective function of mopping up LDL; however, if the insult continues, more macrophages accumulate at the site and LDL are accumulated in great abundance. The macrophage cannot, however, utilize the extra burden of cholesterol, which accumulates within the cell in the form of lipid droplets, the so-called foam cells. These cells eventually die. It is believed that the lipids released from the cells may be taken up by the smooth muscle cells, which also become lipid-laden, the smooth muscle foam cells. In addition, the macrophage releases factors that act as mitogens to increase smooth muscle cell division, which in turn adds to the mass of the plaque (Chapter 17).

DISEASES RELATED TO LIPOPROTEINS

Hyperlipoproteinemia. When the concentration of plasma lipoproteins exceeds an arbitrary normal value, which is typically defined as the 95th percentile of a ran-

Table 18–5. DISEASES RELATED TO LIPOPROTEINS

DISORDER	CLINICAL FINDINGS
Secondary Hyperlipoproteinemias	
Diabetes mellitus	Atheromas Pancreatitis Xanthomas
Hyperthyroidism	Atheromas
Alcohol excess	Pancreatitis Xanthomas
Estrogen excess (oral contraceptives)	Pancreatitis Xanthomas
Primary Hyperlipoproteinemias	
Single gene	Atheromas Pancreatitis Xanthomas
Multiple genes	Atheromas

dom population, the condition is designated hyperlipoproteinemia. This value varies with age and sex. Clinical concern arises because an elevated concentration of lipoproteins can accelerate the development of atherosclerosis. Not only may atheromas form, but deposition of cholesterol may also occur in tendons and skin, producing raised nodules called *xanthomas*; these are overt manifestations of severe hypercholesterolemia. Severe hypertriglyceridemia, e.g., elevated triglycerides (levels above 2000 mg/dl), predisposes for pancreatitis.

Hyperlipoproteinemias are designated either primary or secondary (Table 18–5). Secondary hyperlipoproteinemias are complications of more generalized disturbances such as diabetes mellitus, hypothyroidism, excessive intake of ethanol, or the intake of high doses of estrogen. Primary hyperlipoproteinemias may be due to a single gene defect or to a combination of genetic factors; in addition, genetic factors may be exacerbated by environmental or dietary factors. The incidence of the different primary hyperlipoproteinemias ranges from 1 in 250 in the population to 1 in 1 million.

Knowledge of the plasma concentrations of cholesterol and triglycerides usually reveals the class of lipoprotein that is high, and this is useful in making a diagnosis and in designing proper drug therapy.

Treatment protocol for hyperlipoproteinemias is summarized in Table 18–6. Basic to the treatment of all hyperlipidemias is a diet that maintains normal body weight and that minimizes the plasma lipid concentration. If the patient is overweight, weight loss should be attempted and then maintained on a diet low in cholesterol and saturated animal fats, and relatively high in polyunsaturated vegetable oils. These polyunsaturated fats improve the palatability when saturated fats are restricted and also reduce the concentrations of plasma LDL cholesterol. Only rare individuals require a diet severely reduced in total fat.

Table 18–6. TREATMENT OF HYPERLIPOPROTEINEMIAS

Correct underlying metabolic disturbance
Diet: low cholesterol and animal fat; relatively high polyunsaturated fats (vegetable oils)

Drug therapy:
- Nicotinic acid—reduces synthesis of VLDL, lowers LDL
- Clofibrate—reduces synthesis and increases catabolism of VLDL (raises LPL activity)
- Mevinolin—reduces cholesterol synthesis, increasing LDL receptors, lowers LDL
- Cholestyramine colestipol—binds and removes bile acids, increases cholesterol conversion to bile acid, lowers body cholesterol

Patients with secondary hyperlipidemia require treatment of the underlying disorder (diabetes, hypothyroidism, excess alcohol consumption, estrogen excess, etc.) and should reduce all other risk factors, such as smoking and hypertension, and maintain physical fitness.

Primary hyperlipoproteinemia requires more aggressive treatment; in addition to a proper diet, drugs that lower plasma lipoprotein concentrations are used (Oliver, 1985). These drugs function either by diminishing the production of lipoproteins or by increasing the efficiency of their removal.

Nicotinic acid (niacin) has long been used to reduce the production of VLDL, and in so doing it also lowers LDL. Nicotinic acid does produce cutaneous flush and pruritus (itching) involving the face and upper body, but this does subside with continued use. It may, however, interfere with compliance, that is, the patient's willingness to continue with the drug.

Another drug effective in decreasing the synthesis of VLDL and increasing VLDL catabolism (by increasing the activity of LPL) is Clofibrate. Clofibrate appears to have specific efficacy in a distinct type of genetic hyperlipoproteinemia.

The most encouraging new drug in treating these disorders is Mevinolin. Mevinolin is a competitive inhibitor of the rate-controlling enzyme in the production of cholesterol, HMGCoA reductase. To compensate for a reduction in cholesterol synthesis in the liver, the number of hepatic receptors for LDL increases, and this brings about a reduction in plasma LDL. Again, this may be more effective in certain types of hyperlipoproteinemias, such as familial hypercholesterolemia.

Normally, cholesterol in the liver is converted to bile acids, which are delivered to the small intestine lumen where some of the cholesterol in the form of bile acid is ultimately excreted and some is reabsorbed. Normally, formation of bile acids has a negative-feedback effect on further production of bile acids. Removing the bile acids so that they no longer exert negative feedback speeds up the conversion of cholesterol to bile acids and reduces body pools of cholesterol, including xanthomas. Resins such as cholestyramine and colestipol have such an effect; they readily bind bile acids and increase the flux of cholesterol from cells.

Both nicotinic acid and Mevinolin may be used in combination with one of the bile acid-binding resins, and these combinations are usually synergistic, allowing the doses of both substances to be lowered. It is thus apparent that drugs utilized in treating dysfunctions of lipid metabolism must be selected and tailored according to the individual condition.

References

Brown, M. S., and Golstein, J. S.: How LDL receptors influence cholesterol and atherosclerosis. *Sci. Am.*, **251**:58–66, **1984.**

Brown, M. S., and Goldstein, J. S.: A receptor-mediated pathway for cholesterol homeostasis. *Science*, **232**:34–47, **1986.**

Jackson, R. L.; Morrisett, J. D.; and Gotto, A. M., Jr.: Lipoprotein structure and metabolism. *Physiol. Rev.*, **56**:259–316, **1976.**

Mahley, R. W.: Cellular and molecular biology of lipoprotein metabolism in atherosclerosis. *Diabetes*, **30** (Suppl. 2):60–65, **1981.**

Oliver, M. F.: Strategy, yield and risks of controlling plasma lipids in the primary prevention of CHD. In Kritchevsky, D.; Holmes, W. L.; and Paoletti, R. (eds.): *Drugs Affecting Lipid Metabolism*, Plenum Press, New York, **1985.**

Roheim, P. S.: Atherosclerosis and lipoprotein metabolism: Role of reverse cholesterol transport. *Am. J. Cardiol.*, **57**:3C–10C, **1986.**

Ross, R.: The pathogenesis of atherosclerosis—An update. *N. Engl. J. Med.*, **314**:488–500, **1986.**

Steinberg, D.: Lipoproteins and atherosclerosis: A look back and a look ahead. *Arteriosclerosis*, **3**:283–301, **1983.**

The Lipid Research Clinics Population Studies Data Book, Vol. 1. The Prevalence Study, Washington, DC, Government Printing Office, **1980** DHEW Publication no. (NIH) 80-1527.

CHAPTER 19 AGING OF RESPIRATION

The Lung, a Battered Organ

Respiratory function includes both an external process—oxygen (O_2) absorption and carbon dioxide (CO_2) removal from the body—and an internal metabolic process—cellular gaseous exchanges. This chapter is concerned with the former, that is, the uptake of O_2 and excretion of CO_2 through the lungs and their transport by erythrocytes to and from the tissues.

In the respiratory system, (a) the lungs represent the gas-exchange organ; (b) the chest wall, with the respiratory muscles (that increase or decrease the size of the thoracic cavity), the brain centers, and nerve tracts (that control the muscles) represent the pump that ventilates the lungs. In addition to gaseous exchange, the lungs perform other functions. They participate in the immunologic defenses of the body (by phagocytizing particles from the inspired air and from the blood), in metabolic functions (by synthesizing, storing, or releasing into the blood such substances as surfactant and prostaglandins), and in endocrine functions (by transforming angiotensin I into angiotensin II, a powerful vasoconstrictor and stimulus for aldosterone secretion, Chapter 12). A few specialized lung cells contain biologically active peptides, some with pressor (e.g., vasoactive intestinal peptide [VIP]) and some neuronal (e.g., opioid peptides) activity.

The respiratory system in humans is mature by age 20 (Polgar and Weng, 1979). Pulmonary function begins to gradually decline in healthy subjects after the age of 25 (Masoro, 1981). This decline is linked to progressive deleterious changes that occur in respiratory structures including the lung, the thoracic cage, and respiratory muscles as well as the respiratory center in the CNS. These changes, however, are minor compared to the constant effects of the environment and other insults to the respiratory system—infections, pollution, cigarette smoking, disordered immune responses, unfavorable working conditions—to which the organism is exposed throughout the lifespan (Cander and Moyer, 1964; Muiesan *et al.*, 1971; Shephard, 1978, 1982; Smith and Serfass, 1981; Buskirk, 1985; Davies, 1985). Although the major function of the lungs is to ensure the efficient exchange of air (oxygen) with the environment, this very function is performed at the peril of contamination from the many toxic substances transported in the air. Indeed, the degree and the rate of age-related changes in structure and function of the lungs are variable and dependent on the habits of the individual (particularly smoking, physical exercise), the environment in which he/she lives (urban versus rural), and disease (infections, industrial diseases). The lungs are "battered" not only by external insults, but also by formation of oxygen radicals, so deleterious to tissues, in the pulmonary cells in immediate contact with the gaseous environment rich in O_2. The toxic effects of O_2 are discussed in Chapter 7.

NORMAL AGE-ASSOCIATED CHANGES IN THE LUNG

Air passes first through the nasal passages (nares) where it is filtered of the larger contaminants, enters the pharynx where it is warmed and absorbs water vapor, flows down the trachea and through the bronchi and bronchioles, and proceeds through the respiratory bronchioles and the aveolar ducts to the alveoli. The alveoli are the functional units of the lungs.

Alveolar Structure and Function. The major structural characteristic of the alveolus is the close proximity of the capillary blood and the alveolar air, separated only by the capillary endothelium and the thin basement membrane supporting the alveolar cells. This arrangement facilitates gas exchanges between blood and air.

Two types of epithelial cells (pneumocytes)

line the alveolus. Type I cells are extremely thin with few intracellular organelles and are designated agranular pneumocytes. Type II cells contain many organelles and lipid droplets and are designated granular pneumocytes. These type II cells produce surfactant, a proteolipid that coats the alveolar cells and lowers the surface tension at the air-fluid interface.

Another, less frequent cell type in the lung is the alveolar macrophage. These cells are loaded with digestive enzymes and can ingest foreign materials, as do white blood cells. They migrate from the blood stream and patrol the tissues of the lung on the alveolar side, gliding on the surfactant.

STRUCTURAL CHANGES

The architecture of the lung is altered in aging (Liebow, 1964). The alveolar ducts and respiratory bronchioles are enlarged while the alveoli become shallower and flatter with loss of septal tissue (Table 19–1). These changes do not appreciably affect total lung capacity (the maximum volume of air in the lungs and airways) when this volume is corrected for the age-related decrease in height (Figure 19–1). However, air distribution is altered with an increase in alveolar duct air but a decrease in alveolar air and, therefore, a decrease in optimal transport surface. The amount of elastic tissue, abundant in the lung and partly responsible for the stretchability of this organ, is decreased with age (Turner *et al.*, 1968) while fibrous tissue is increased (Pierce and Ebert, 1965). The decrease in elastic tissue is associated with an increase in elastin, a major protein of this tissue. This apparently paradoxic increase has been explained as the consequence of structural changes in elastin with age: the "old" elastin undergoes a number of cross-linkages (as do other connective tissue fibers, Chapter 23), which decrease its extensibility and increase its resistance to solution during purification. The importance of lung elasticity is illustrated by the condition of emphysema in which the lungs lose their elasticity owing to disruption of elastic tissue. The nature of the exact changes in the elastic fibers during aging is unclear, but it is likely that alteration in the distribution of elastic tissue is more functionally significant than changes in amounts. With aging, abnormal location or structure of the fibers may be responsible for impairments of ventilation and perfusion of the lungs.

Table 19–1. MORPHOLOGIC CHANGES IN THE THORAX AND LUNG WITH AGE[a]

MORPHOLOGIC CHANGE	FUNCTIONAL SIGNIFICANCE
Thorax	
Calcification of bronchial and costal cartilage	↑ resistance to deformation of chest wall (↑ elastic work)
↑ stiffness in costovertebral vertebral joints	↑ use of diaphragm in ventilation
↑ rigidity of chest wall	
↑ anterior-posterior diameter (kyphosis)	↓ tidal volume response to exercise hyperpnea
Wasting of respiratory muscles	↓ maximal voluntary ventilation
Lung	
Enlarged alveolar ducts	↓ surface area for gas exchange
↓ supporting duct framework, enlarged alveoli	
Thinning, separation of alveolar membrane	↑ physiologic dead space
↑ mucous gland	
↓ number, thickness of elastic fibers (?)	↓ lung elastic recoil
↓ tissue extensibility (alveolar wall)	↓ VC, RV/TLC, and[b]
	↓ ventilatory flow rate
	↓ ventilation distribution
	↑ resistance to flow in small airways
↓ pulmonary capillary network	
↑ fibrosis of pulmonary capillary intima	↓ ventilation: blood flow equality

[a]Modified from Reddan, 1981, in Everett L. Smith and Robert C. Serfass, 1981. Copyright by Enslow Publishers, Inc. Reproduced with permission of Enslow Publishers, Inc., Hillside, N.J.

[b]VC = vital capacity; RV = residual volume; TLC = total lung capacity.

The net effect of these structural alterations is a decreased alveolar surface area, which is 75 m^2 at 30 years and decreases by 4 percent per decade thereafter (Niewoehner and Kleinerman, 1964; Thurlbeck and Angus, 1975; Mauderly, 1978). The configuration and mechanical properties of the chest wall also change with aging, owing to increased curvature of the spine and calcification of the intercostal cartilage (Pump, 1971). All these changes resemble those found in emphysema (Reid, 1967).

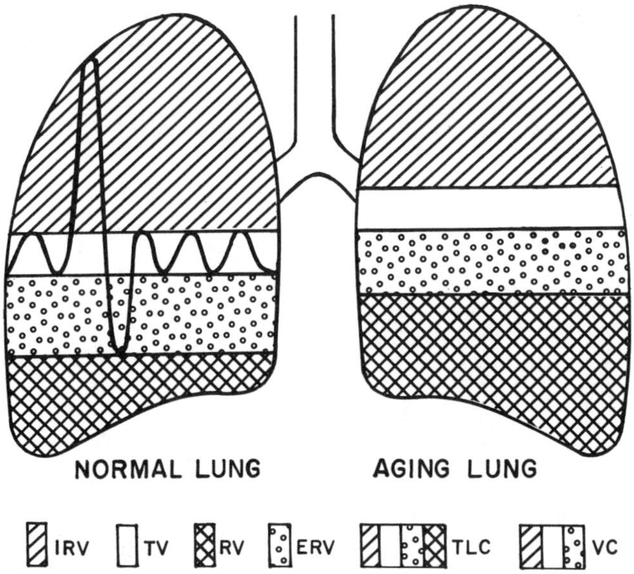

Figure 19–1. *Changes in Lung Volumes with Aging.*

With aging, note particularly the decrease in VC and the increase in RV. IRV, inspiratory reserve volume; TV, tidal volume; RV, residual volume; ERV, expiratory reserve volume; TLC, total lung capacity; VC, vital capacity.

CHANGES IN LUNG VOLUMES

Lung volume and pressure characteristics change dramatically from birth to death, with major and rapid changes during childhood and adolescence and slower but progressive alterations with increasing age. These changes involve both the lungs and chest wall and are often divergent (Reddan, 1981) (Table 19–1). The chest becomes stiffer because of calcification of costal cartilages, while the lungs become more distended because of a slightly increased compliance (i.e., stretchability) and decreased recoil (Mittman *et al.*, 1965). Consequently, lung volumes are altered and ventilation rate at rest and especially, during physical exercise, is decreased.

Lung Volumes and Measurements. Total lung capacity (TLC) is 6 L in men (4.2 L in women) distributed in the following volumes (in men):

tidal volume: amount of air that moves into and out of the lungs with each quiet inspiration and expiration (=0.5 L);

inspiratory reserve volume (=3.3 L) and *expiratory reserve volume* (1 L): amount of air that moves into or out of the lungs following maximal inspiration or expiration;

residual volume: air left in the lungs after maximal expiration (=1.2 L);

dead space: air in the airways (=150 ml);

vital capacity: the greatest amount of air that can be expired after a maximal inspiration. It is frequently taken as an index of pulmonary function and ranges from 3 to 4 L in adult females to 4.5 to 5.5 L in adult males. A more precise index is to measure vital capacity per unit of time: for example, in asthma, vital capacity appears normal, but when timed, it shows a significantly prolonged time because of bronchial constriction.

pulmonary ventilation rate (or respiratory minute volume) is normally 6 L/breath × 12 breaths/minute and *maximal voluntary ventilation* is the largest volume of air that can be moved into and out of the lungs in 1 minute by voluntary effort; it may be as high as 125 to 180 L/minute.

With aging, vital capacity decreases to approximately 75 percent of its value in the 7th decade as compared to that at the age of 17 years (taken as men/women average of 4.8 L). Residual volume increases nearly 50 percent during this time. However, total lung capacity remains unchanged (Jones *et al.*, 1978) (Table 19–2 and Figure 19–1). Other measures of ventilatory mechanics decline as well: these include forced expiratory volume/second, which decreases by 32 ml/year in males and 25 ml/year in females starting from the age of 25 years (Morris *et al.*, 1971), and specific airway conductance, which also progessively slows with aging.

CHANGES IN ARTERIAL PO_2

As with many other functions, not all parameters of pulmonary function follow a similar timetable of decline (Edelman *et al.*,

Table 19–2. LUNG VOLUMES AND VENTILATION VARIABLES IN 20- AND 60-YEAR-OLD INDIVIDUALS MATCHED FOR HEIGHT AND WEIGHT[a]

	MEN		WOMEN	
VARIABLE	20 YEARS	60 YEARS	20 YEARS	60 YEARS
Total lung capacity (TLC) (L)[b]	7.20	6.90	5.10	4.70
Vital capacity (L)	5.20	4.00	4.17	3.29
Functional residual capacity (L)	2.20	3.50	2.40	2.50
Residual volume (% TLC)	25	40	28	40
Forced expiratory volume in 1 second				
(a) L/BTPS	4.45	3.17	3.26	2.26
(b) % VC	81	71	80	70
Maximum voluntary ventilation (L/min)	150	99	110	77
Maximal expiratory flow at 50% VC (liters/sec^{-1})	5.00	3.80	4.40	2.70
Closing volume (% VC)	8	25	8	25
Recoil pressure of lung at 60% TLC (cm H_2O)	7.8	4.4	7.8	4.4
Recoil pressure of chest wall at 60% TLC (cm H_2O)	−6.0	−4.0	−6.0	−4.0

[a]Modified from Reddan, 1981, in Everett L. Smith and Robert C. Serfass, *Exercise and Aging,* 1981. Copyright by Enslow Publishers, Inc. Reproduced with permission of Enslow Publishers, Inc., Hillside, NJ.
[b]L = liter; BTPS = body temperature and pressure saturated with water vapor.

1968). For example, expiratory flow rates begin to decline at an age when vital capacity is still intact (Hurwitz *et al.,* 1980). This early decrease in expiratory rate may reflect the reduced elastic recoil in the elderly; it may cause a premature closure, during expiration of some regions of the lungs, with trapping of air in sites distal to the closure and, consequently, poor mixing of inspired air (Anthonisen *et al.,* 1969; LeBlanc *et al.,* 1970). This abnormality is responsible, at least in part, for the age-related changes in arterial Po_2 and arterial-alveolar Po_2 differences (Davis *et al.,* 1980).

Among the most important physiologic changes with aging is the progressive reduction in arterial Po_2 due to premature airway closure and loss of elastic recoil. The latter two conditions result in an imbalance of lung ventilation and gas perfusion, and these, combined with decreased cardiac output, lead to lowered O_2 uptake and pressure (Astrand *et al.,* 1973). As a nomogram has been adopted in the case of the age-related increase in fasting blood glucose (Chapter 16), similarly a nomogram has been proposed to calculate the expected arterial O_2 tension in relation to age, with the arterial O_2 tension falling to 75 mm Hg in the 7th decade (Morris *et al.,* 1971). In contrast, Pco_2 remains remarkably constant throughout life despite a reduction in CO_2 sensitivity in most tissue, possibly including the brain.

CONTROL OF VENTILATION

Control of ventilation by brain centers (chemoreceptors in medulla and pons) and by peripheral (carotid and aortic bodies) chemoreceptors is markedly altered in the elderly (Levitsky, 1985). It is unclear whether this is due to intrinsic alteration of neural control, such as decreased sensory perception of Pco_2, pH, and Po_2, or loss of synchrony of higher CNS inputs, or to alterations of mechanical factors, such as stiffness of chest wall and reduced neuromuscular competence and responsiveness to neural inputs. Neither of these hypotheses is presently substantiated and further research is needed in this area (Peterson *et al.,* 1981). Responses to hypercapnia (increased Pco_2) and hypoxia (reduced Po_2) are reduced by 50 percent in the aged as compared to the young (Kronenberg and Drage, 1973; Dill *et al.,* 1980).

RESPONSES TO EXERCISE

Physical exercise stimulates the active tissue to utilize more O_2 and to eliminate more CO_2, which requires coordinated cardiovascular and respiratory adjustments. Circulatory changes increase blood flow to the exercising muscle. Respiratory adjustments include increased ventilation—to provide more O_2, eliminate more CO_2, and dissipate heat—and increased extraction of O_2 from the blood in the exercising muscle—by increased blood flow and shift in the O_2 dissociation curve. With aging, lung ventilation, already impaired under quiet conditions, is inadequate to muster the necessary adjustments to meet the increased demands of exercise (Hartley *et al.*, 1969; Muiesan *et al.*, 1971; Assmussen *et al.*, 1975). The loss of elastic recoil and decreased functional residual capacity (i.e., gas volume remaining in lungs at the end of quiet expiration) inhibit the effective range of tidal volume; the early closure of the airways similarly inhibits the expiratory flow. Consequently the ventilatory response to exercise is less efficient in older (69 years of age) than younger men (deVries and Adams, 1972). Dyspnea, or shortness of breath, ensues and necessitates the early cessation of exercise. The loss of vital capacity with aging restricts the potential tidal volume that may be reached during maximal exercise. At rest, only a minor fraction of the potential lung volume and flow changes is used, and even during maximum exercise, the maximal inspiratory and expiratory flow rates and volumes are not usually reached. With increasing age, during moderate to heavy exercise the ability to reach maximal rates and volumes is severely curtailed, and therefore, ventilation cannot increase sufficiently to provide for the increased metabolic demands (Shephard, 1978).

This impaired efficiency of the lungs in the aged individual to shift from resting to maximal function also depends on the decline in the strength and endurance of the respiratory muscles. Although the diaphragm is the predominant muscle to drive ventilation at rest, during increasing exercise, the rib cage and abdominal muscles assist the diaphragm in augmenting ventilation rates (Edge *et al.*, 1964). Because of the increased stiffness with aging of the rib cage, the diaphragm takes over a higher proportion of the mechanical effort needed for increasing ventilation (Rizzato and Marrazini, 1970; Roussos and Macklem, 1977). The diaphragm is a muscle not easily fatigued; therefore, whether it becomes fatigued in old age together with the other accessory respiratory muscles (abdominal and intercostal) during increasing ventilatory activity needs further investigation. Exertional dyspnea (i.e., shortness of breath after exercise) is common among the elderly when exercising. Yet the respective roles of decrements in muscle strength, increase in thoracic stiffness, and loss of lung compliance remain to be elucidated. Inasmuch as fatigue after muscular exercise has a strong CNS component, other factors besides muscular decrements, such as impaired coordination, insufficient motivation, arthritic involvement of the joints, and others, may also play an important role in limiting the adaptive competence of the elderly in undertaking physical exercise.

In addition to difficulty in adjusting ventilatory responses to exercise, the elderly have an earlier onset of the shift from aerobic (requiring O_2) to anaerobic (independent of O_2) metabolism (Shock, 1964; Tlusty, 1969a,b). Both the time required to reach steady-state level at the onset of exercise and the time required to return to preexercise resting levels are prolonged with age after moderate to heavy exercise. Alveolar-capillary gas exchange is reduced and alveolar-arterial Po_2 differences are increased with exercise in middle-aged men. Nevertheless, gas diffusion capacity at 65 years is comparable to that at younger ages (Donevan *et al.*, 1955; Shephard, 1982).

Despite the overall decline in performance during exercise, the elderly can and should undertake a regimen of physical exercise adequate to their capabilities and needs. Discussion of such regimens is presented in Chapter 25. Age-related respiratory changes during sleep are discussed in Chapter 10.

LIFE CYCLE OF ERYTHROCYTES*

The major function of red blood cells (erythrocytes) is to carry oxygen (O_2) and carbon dioxide (CO_2) to and from the tis-

---

*This section (pp. 307–310) contributed by R. W. Atherton, Ph.D., Department of Zoology and Physiology, University of Wyoming, Laramie, WY.

sues. This function is made possible by the presence in the cell of the pigment hemoglobin, which binds to O_2 and CO_2. The erythrocytes are biconcave disc-like cells produced in the bone marrow. In mammals they lose their nuclei before leaving the bone marrow; they survive 120 days in the circulation. Because of their gas-carrying capacity they can be viewed as an extension of the lungs.

The study of blood and blood cells is the object of continuing research, with a wealth of literature available on the contributing role of the hemopoietic system to the functional integrity of the organism. The collection of blood is easy compared to the collection of other tissues *in vivo,* and alterations in the entire organism or in specific organs or tissues are often reflected in alterations of the blood. Furthermore, information both practical and theoretical has accumulated on the preservation and storage of blood and plasma for purposes of transfusion, and, thus, a substantial amount of knowledge is available, indirectly, on the aging of blood and blood cells. In this respect, the erythrocyte represents one of the most thoroughly studied cell types in this category, and its particular life cycle has been well delineated. In addition, as a cell that undergoes continual renewal in the life of the organism, the erythrocyte has been studied as an example of how aging in general may affect cell turnover. Similar studies undertaken in epithelial cells of the intestinal mucosa (Chapter 21), cells that are also continuously replaced during the lifespan of the organism, have demonstrated, with the aid of tritiated thymidine autoradiography, that the variability from cell to cell within a cell population is increased gradually with aging; cell turnover is also accomplished in a progressively longer period of time (Lesher *et al.,* 1961). It has been suggested further that this phenomenon is related mainly to the lengthening of the "interphase" (G1) portion of the DNA cycle, that is the phase that precedes DNA synthesis, and is presumably related to the accumulation of necessary precursors (Thrasher and Greulich, 1965).

The cause of the interphase lengthening is not known, but it may make a cell more susceptible to damage. For example, it has been demonstrated that DNA damage occurs in older cells (Price *et al.,* 1971). Following this observation, Karran and Ormerod (1973) demonstrated an increase in single-strand breaks with erythrocytes from aged chickens. However, it is not clear, as the authors note, whether these changes were truly reflective of *in vivo* aging or a result of the preparative alkaline sucrose sedimentation technique employed. Since changes in the circulating erythrocyte reflect studies on an already aged cell, it may be more important to investigate age-dependent changes in erythropoietic stem cells. When old rodents (mice and rats) are exposed to hypoxia or bleeding, the erythropoietic response is slower than that observed in younger animals (Garcia, 1957; Grant and LeGrand, 1964; Harrison, 1975a). A series of creative experiments addressed this question. Both young and old erythropoietic stem cells served as donor tissue to genetically anemic host mice. Both donors, regardless of age, cured the anemia (Harrison, 1972). Furthermore, anemic mice with old donor erythropoietic grafts responded as well as normal young mice to erythropoietic stimuli (Harrison, 1973, 1975a). These studies are of particular importance to geriatric medicine. For example, in a comprehensive mouse study analyzing 16 hematologic parameters, only hematocrit decreased as a function of age and not of disease (Finch and Foster, 1973). When evaluating the human literature, it is not uncommon to identify an elderly patient with "old-age anemia." However, in the "Framingham study" no decrease in hematocrit was observed in elderly individuals when controlled for health (Gordon and Shurtleff, 1973). Thus, what appears to be a disease of old age should be reevaluated to determine whether other factors, e.g., endocrine, could be the cause of anemia in older patients (Rowe and Minaker, 1985; Timiras and Brownstein, 1987).

The Erythrocyte as a Model of Cellular Aging. The following discussion will deal primarily with the erythrocyte as a prototype of a cell in which the life cycle is telescoped—developing, acquiring specific functional competence, aging, and dying within a relatively short period of time, an average of 120 days in man—a process that is repeated in countless millions of such cells throughout the human lifespan. Indeed, when one studies the changes in erythrocyte structure and function with age, one must consider not only the life cycle of each cell but also the modifications that are associated with the development and aging of the total organism. Recently an entire volume has been devoted to the red cell as a suitable model for aging (Eaton *et al.*, 1985). In this book, cellular aspects, hemoglobin, membrane activation, metabolism, and comparative aspect of erythrocyte aging are discussed by authors of numerous chapters.

In most vertebrates, including humans, the primitive and embryonic erythrocyte is characteristically different from the adult type in its morphologic, functional, and biochemical properties (Lucas and Jamroz, 1961; Hollan *et al.*, 1968; Ceresa-Castellani and Leone, 1969). Typical of these cells at all age periods, however, is that their lifespan is set; even during embryogenesis, erythrocytes are studied as models of "programmed cell death." Although no differences are observed in the lifespan of mature erythrocyte population whether the individual is 18 or 80, total red cell mass, as a proportion of body weight, shows a diminution in the elderly (Woodford-Williams *et al.*, 1962).

The changes characteristic of the aging erythrocyte involve a diminished cell size and increased cell density (probably owing to a decrease in lipid content), a relative decrease in intracellular potassium, and an increase in sodium (probably owing to permeability changes of the cell membrane), a reduction in the activity of certain enzymes (e.g., glucose-6-phosphate dehydrogenase) but not all, a reduction of surface charge and increase in fragility, a less reversible deformability, and an increased agglutinability. These abnormalities might explain the increased binding of the older red blood cell by the reticuloendothelial cells implicated in the removal from the circulation and destruction of the old erythrocytes (Prankerd, 1958; Danon, 1968; Bishop and Van Gastel, 1969). Indeed, it appears that in the older erythrocytes "loss of elasticity" and "deformity" associated with a "geometric restriction" during circulation may represent one of the major causes of cell removal and cell death (Canham and Burton, 1968). Of current interest is the senescent cell antigen (Kay, 1985), which appears on aged cells such that binding of IgG autoantibodies aids in the removal of erythrocyte by macrophages. Also hemoglobinopathies may serve as a genetic marker for erythrocyte removal from the circulation (Steinberg, 1984). Furthermore, with the influx of data on posttranslational modification of proteins, it is not surprising that glycosylation (Winterhalter, 1985) and methylation of erythrocyte membranes may be an issue relevant to red cell removal (Clark, 1985). In elderly humans, biochemical changes in the erythrocyte membrane have been reported. Specifically, phosphatidylcholine decreases while phosphatidylethanolamine increases (Gold and Altschuler, 1972). In addition, phospholipid content in human erythrocyte membranes may decline (Hegner *et al.*, 1979) or may remain unchanged (Araki and Rifkind, 1980).

CHANGES IN HEMOGLOBIN

Whether alterations also occur in the content, structure, and function of hemoglobin within the aging erythrocyte remains to be clarified. In general, gross alterations have not been observed with the aging of the cell, but it is entirely possible that subtle functional modifications do occur, especially in response to abnormal (increased) functional requirements. Studies of the incorporation of ^{51}Cr in young and old erythrocytes have shown a preferential labeling of the younger cell, but whether this is due to differences in cell size, permeability, metabolism, or aging of the hemoglobin itself has not been established (Schapira *et al.*, 1962). Hemoglobin, like collagen (see Chapter 23), may undergo specific changes with age, the "old hemoglobin" differing from the "young hemoglobin" in a number of physiochemical properties (in the same manner as embryonic and fetal hemoglobin differs from the adult form) (Schapira *et al.*, 1962; Walter *et al.*, 1965). Inasmuch as the main function of hemoglobin is to carry O_2, O_2 dissociation curves of young and old erythrocytes also have been compared and generally reveal that old erythrocytes exhibit a significantly greater oxyhemoglobin saturation than young erythrocytes—a finding that perhaps may be attributable to macromolecular changes with age in the structure of the hemoglobin (Edwards *et al.*, 1961).

AGING OF THE HEMOPOIETIC SYSTEM

Inasmuch as the erythrocytes are formed in the hemopoietic system and primarily in the bone marrow, the function of this system has been studied to determine whether it undergoes functional impairment with aging. In general, few changes have been reported with respect to either stem cell kinetics, bone blood flow, bone marrow cellularity, or erythropoiesis *per se* (Coggle and Provkakis, 1964; Roylance, 1968; Little, 1969). Similarly, when the erythropoietic function was stimulated by hypoxia, hemorrhagic anemia, and cobalt feeding, no deterioration could be detected in the physiologic adjustments involving increased erythrocyte formation (Grand and LeGrande, 1964).

One of the primary observations drawn from studies of the aging red blood cell is that despite the specific changes that characterize its life cycle, the effects of aging, in general, on cell turnover, cell renewal, and cell function appear to be minimal, at least under steady-state conditions (Das, 1969). In addition, it seems that the capacity of the hemopoietic system to respond to increased functional demand, such as imposed by hypoxia, is not impaired by aging. For example, both young and old rats when exposed to low oxygen pressure respond with a comparable increase in hematocrit value, total circulating hemoglobin, and number of erythrocytes as well as total red cell volume and total blood volume (Garcia, 1957). Thus, it has been concluded that the homeostatic function of the blood, vital to the regulation of bodily function, is not significantly affected by aging. The regenerative potential of the erythrocyte, seemingly inexhaustible *in vivo,* stands in contrast with studies *in vitro* that suggest, rather, that some cells (fibroblasts), despite their proliferative capacity, ultimately lose the ability to regenerate. The erythrocyte as a product of the erythron with a specific protein of paramount importance remains a most suitable model for aging; it may provide direction for some most interesting and profitable avenues for the study of aging (Swislocki, 1985).

SOME PULMONARY DISORDERS WITH AGING

The major respiratory disorders of the elderly include: chronic bronchitis (i.e., chronic infection or inflammation of the bronchi), often coexisting with emphysema (see below), neoplasia, and lung infections, particularly pneumonia. While some of these disorders, e.g., bronchitis and emphysema, are not necessarily life-threatening, they represent a considerable "burden" for the well-being of the elderly in terms of days of hospitalization, physician consultation, days of sickness, and almost continuous discomfort (Black and Pole, 1975). From the perspective of the entire lifespan, the proportion of deaths due to respiratory diseases (in Western countries) is highest (approximately 30 percent) in the first year of life, falling to lower values (approximately 5 percent) in late adolescence and early adulthood. From the fifth decade, the incidence of respiratory disease rises steadily and in those over 85 years of age accounts for 25 percent of all deaths. In the last 20 years, the death rate from respiratory disease has fallen with the exception of bronchiogenic carcinoma (still rising, especially in young women) and pneumonia (remaining constantly high) (Davies, 1985). Of the respiratory diseases, emphysema and pneumonia will be considered briefly.

Oxygen Toxicity in Lungs. The overall effects of oxygen-free radicals in tissues and cells have been presented in Chapter 7. In the lungs, these molecules may contribute both to the acute oxygen toxicity that occurs when individuals breathe higher-than-normal concentrations of oxygen, and to the chronic damage to elastic tissue that leads to emphysema.

The acute oxygen toxicity is of particular significance for critically ill patients who require respirators. Although the lowest possible doses of oxygen are given, the potential damage to the lung must always be considered. Sometimes it may be necessary to choose between "allowing a patient to die immediately and giving pure oxygen which may kill in days" (Marx, 1987). Indeed, experiments in rats show that breathing oxygen increases the production of free radicals in pulmonary epithelial cells and macrophages with consequent death of the animals within 3 days. If, however, animals are protected by the administration of the enzymes superoxide dismutase and catalase, death of the animal is prevented.

The chronic damage to lung tissue by oxygen is based on the inflammatory reaction that represents the first event in emphysema. The response to the phagocytic cells that infiltrate the inflamed tissue includes, not only the liberation of free radicals, but also the induction of enzymes such as elastase, which breaks down the elastic tissue of the lungs. Under normal conditions, elastase activity is controlled by inhibitors such as alpha$_1$-protease inhibitor. Thus emphysema would result from inactivation of this enzyme. Cigarette smoking would also stimulate free-radical formation, thereby further aggravating the cell damage.

Oxidants may cause lung tissue injury also by inhibiting the production of adenosine triphosphate (ATP) necessary for cell energy. ATP production is blocked by oxidants directly, through DNA strand breaks damage and, indirectly, through activation of the enzyme poly-ADP ribose polymerase that suppresses a cofactor needed for ATP production. Activation of this enzyme may also lead to cancer development with DNA strand breaks acting as tumor promoters. Oxygen free radicals may convert exogenous chemicals to active carcinogens. This mechanism may be operative in the lungs where cancer incidence is high and increasing in some sections (young women) of the cigarette-smoking population.

EMPHYSEMA

This disorder, together with chronic bronchitis, represents an often intolerable burden for the elderly (Black and Pole, 1975; Bignon and Scarpa, 1981; Snider, 1983; Sterling, 1983). In the United Kingdom, more than 40,000 patients, 60 years of age and older, require help with some aspects of daily living as a result of this disease. In the United States, 3.3 percent of disabilities are ascribed to this disease. These numbers are only estimations, as age alone is associated with a significant increase in the prevalence of morning cough, even in nonsmokers, and decline in respiratory competence (Gulsvik, 1979).

Etiopathogenesis of Emphysema. This respiratory disease is characterized by: (1) diffuse distention and overaeration of the alveoli; (2) disruption of intraalveolar septa; (3) loss of pulmonary elasticity; (4) increased lung volume; and (5) associated impairment of pulmonary function. Functional impairment leads to: (1) disturbed ventilation; (2) altered air and blood flow; and (3) frequently partial obstruction of bronchi.

Causes of emphysema range from an inherent defect of elastic tissue to association with fibrotic pulmonary diseases such as silicosis, to consequences of chronic diffused bronchitis due to age and aggravated by cigarette smoking.

Emphysema and Cigarette Smoking. Heavy cigarette smoking is the most common cause of emphysema. Smoking increases the number of pulmonary alveolar macrophages, which release a chemical substance that attracts leukocytes to the lungs. Leukocytes in turn release proteases such as elastase, which attacks the elastic tissue in the lungs. Normally, a plasmaprotein alpha$_1$-antitrypsin inactivates elastase and other proteases. In emphysema, the activity of this enzyme is decreased. This inactivation of the enzyme may be promoted by oxygen radicals, which are released by the leukocytes (Chapters 7 and 8). Thus, with smoking, there is both an increased production of elastase and a decreased activity of the inactivating enzyme with the resulting destruction of elastic fibers.

A hereditary association has been noted with the affected individuals characterized by an alpha$_1$-antitrypsin deficiency. In the homozygous individuals, emphysema develops early in life (about 20 years of age) even in the absence of cigarette smoking.

The most frequent manifestations of emphysema are exertional dypsnea and chronic cough with mucus. Minor respiratory infections, which would be of no consequence in young individuals with normal lungs, can produce fatal and near-fatal disturbances of respiratory function in elderly individuals with emphysema. Loss of elasticity and restructuring of alveoli by large air sacs results in poor and uneven alveolar ventilation and inadequate perfusion of the underventilated alveoli. The result is hypoxia (low O_2 levels) and hypercapnia (high CO_2 levels). Lung compliance is increased. Inspiration and expiration are labored (as manifested by wheezing) and more work is required for breathing. Because of increased lung volume and increased use of accessory (shoulder and abdominal) muscles, the chest becomes enlarged and barrel-shaped as the chest wall expands. Hypercapnia induces acidosis, at first compensated by urinary retention of bicarbonate. When this compensatory mechanism fails, especially in the aged in whom renal competence is marginal (Chapter 20), the ensuing respiratory acidosis represents a medical emergency and must be treated accordingly. Hypoxia stimulates production of red blood cells, which are increased in number (polycythemia). This contributes to hypertension, which causes the right side of the heart to enlarge, and then to cardiac failure (the so-called "cor pulmonale" or congestive right heart failure) (Murphy and Bone, 1984).

Management. Given the burden inflicted by the disease and its frequency, treatment and prevention are still inadequate. Emphasis on prevention with cessation of cigarette smoking continues to yield only slow responses despite extensive efforts to counsel and educate. Treatment is essentially symptomatic and includes the use of (1) pharmacologic agents such as bronchodilators (to relieve bronchial spasm), mucus liquefiers (to thin the mucous secretions), and antibiotics (to control potential infections); (2) administration of O_2 to be used cautiously to prevent acidosis; and (3) exercise to strengthen abdominal muscles and diaphragm to aid in lung ventilation. The use of respiratory aids in the form of aerosols, sprays, etc., may also be of benefit (Petty and Nett, 1984).

PNEUMONIA

Pneumonia is an inflammatory process of the lung parenchyma most commonly caused by infection. The infectious agent (often the Bacillus pneumococcus) is frequently present among the normal flora of the respiratory tract. The development of pneumonia is, therefore, usually attributed to an impairment of natural resistance. Indeed, the decline of immune competence with aging (Chapter 8) may explain why pneumonia remains, despite the availability of antibiotics, a serious, life-threatening problem with the elderly.

In most cases of community-based epidemics of pneumonia, the elderly are more susceptible with respect to severity and complications (e.g., lung abscess, bacteremia) as well as mortality (as high as 80 percent in those aged 60 and older) (Macfarlane *et al.,* 1982). The rise in pneumonia after the seventh decade registered in several Western countries, including the United States, may simply reflect the type of death certification, pneumonia being the terminal expression of other diseases. However, studies of hospitalized elderly suggest a true increase (Mylotte and Bearn, 1981). While the true cause may be failure of immunologic competence, the immediate cause has been ascribed to aspiration in the lungs of oropharyngeal flora during sleep (Huxley *et al.,* 1978). This is a common occurrence in the elderly in whom the mucobronchial defense barrier is impaired owing to deficient ciliary activity, mucus production, and mechanical reflexes.

Presentation and Management. The diagnosis of pneumonia in the elderly is more difficult than in the young because of the atypical presentation. The classic features of chest pain, cough, and purulent or blood-stained sputum (spit) are uncommon. There is a lack of cough, toxic confusion predominates, and dehydration occurs early. Progression of the disease may produce further lung damage (e.g., abscess) or aggravate extrapulmonary manifestations, such as the confusional state, or induce additional damage, such as pericarditis (inflammation of the pericardium, the sac surrounding the heart), ischemic heart disease, and meningitis (inflammation of the membranes surrounding the brain).

Treatment involves the use of antimicrobial agents, primarily antibiotics, the correction of dehydration, and ultimately the treatment of the underlying disease. Prevention includes the use of anti-influenza vaccination and perhaps pneumococcal vaccination (still under investigation).

Rehabilitation after recovery is important both physiologically and psychologically and requires the use of an individually tailored program, based on exercise, oxygen therapy, and coordinated support of family and health providers.

References

Anthonisen, N. R.; Danson, J.; Robertson, P. C.; and Ross, W. R. D.: Airway closure as a function of age. *Resp. Physiol.,* **8:**58–65, **1969.**

Araki, K., and Rifkind, J.: Erythrocyte membrane cholesterol: An explanation of the aging effect on the rate of hemolysis. *Life Sci.,* **26:**2223–2230, **1980.**

Assmussen, E.; Fruensgaard, K.; and Norgaard, S.: A followup longitudinal study of selected physiologic functions in former physical education students after forty years. *J. Am. Geriatr. Soc.,* **23:**442–450, **1975.**

Astrand, I.; Astrand, P. O.; Hallback, I.; and Kilbom, A.: Reduction in maximal oxygen uptake with age. *J. Appl. Physiol.,* **35:**649–654, **1973.**

Bignon, J., and Scarpa, G. L. (eds.): *Biochemistry, Pathology, and Genetics of Pulmonary Emphysema,* Pergamon Press, New York, **1981.**

Bishop, C., and Van Gastel, C.: Changes in enzyme activity during reticulocyte maturation and red cell aging. *Haematologia,* **3:**29–41, **1969.**

Black, D. A. K., and Pole, J. D.: Priorities in biochemical research: Indices of burden. *Br. J. Prev. Soc. Med.,* **29:**222–227, **1975.**

Buskirk, E. R.: Health maintenance and longevity: Exercise. In Finch, C. E., and Schneider, E. L. (eds.): *Handbook of the Biology of Aging,* Van Nostrand Reinhold, New York, **1985.**

Cander, L., and Moyer, J. H. (eds.): *Aging of the Lung,* Grune & Stratton, New York, **1964.**

Canham, P. B., and Burton, A. C.: Distribution of size and shape in populations of normal human red cells. *Cir. Res.,* **22:**405–422, **1968.**

Ceresa-Castellani, L., and Leone, V. F.: The primitive erythropoietic series in the chick embryo: Studies with the electron microscope. *Anat. Rec.,* **165:**453–465, **1969.**

Clark, S.: The role of aspartic acid and asparagine residues in the aging of erythrocyte membranes: Cellular metabolism of racemized and isomerized forms by methylation reactions. In Eaton, J. W.; Knozen, D. K.; and White, J. G. (eds.): *Cellular and Molecular Aspects of Aging. The Red Cell as a Model,* Alan R. Liss, New York, **1985.**

Coggle, J. E., and Provkakis, C.: The effect of age on the bone marrow cellularity of the mouse. *Dev. Biol.,* **10:**191–201, **1964.**

Danon, D.: Biophysical aspects of red cell ageing. *Bibl. Haematol.,* **15:**275–287, **1969.**

Das, B. C.: An examination of variability of blood chemistry, hematology, and proteins in relation to age. *Gerontologia,* **15:**275–287, **1969.**

Davies, B. H.: The respiratory system. In Pathy, M. S. J. (ed.): *Principles and Practice of Geriatric Medicine,* John Wiley & Sons, Chichester, UK, **1985.**

Davis, C.; Campbell, E. J. M.; Openshaw, P.; Pride, N. B.; and Woodruff, G.: Importance of airway closure in limiting maximal expiration in normal man. *J. Appl. Physiol.,* **48:**695–701, **1980.**

deVries, H. A., and Adams, G. M.: Comparison of exercise responses in old and young men. II. Ventilatory mechanics. *J. Gerontol.,* **27:**349–352, **1972.**

Dill, D. B.; Hillyard, S. D.; and Miller, J.: Vital capacity, exercise performance and blood gases at altitude as related to age. *J. Appl. Physiol.,* **48:**6–9, **1980.**

Donevan, R. E.; Palmer, W. H.; Varvis, C. J.; and Bates, D. V.: Influence of age on pulmonary diffusing capacity. *J. Appl. Physiol.,* **14:**783–792, **1955.**

Eaton, J. W.; Konzen, D. K.; and White, J. G.: *Cellular and Molecular Aspects of Aging. The Red Cell as a Model,* Alan R. Liss, New York, **1985.**

Edelman, N. H.; Mittman, C.; Norris, A. H.; and Shock, N. W.: Effects of respiratory pattern on age differences in ventilation uniformity. *J. Appl. Physiol.,* **24:**59–63, **1968.**

Edge, J. R.; Millard, F. J. C.; Reid, L.; and Simon, G.: The radiographic appearance of the chest in persons of advanced age. *Br. J. Radiol.,* **37:**769–774, **1964.**

Edwards, M. J.; Koler, R. D.; Rigas, D. A.; and Pitcairn, D. M.: The effect of *in vivo* aging of normal human erythrocytes and erythrocyte macromolecules upon oxyhemoglobin dissociation. *J. Clin. Invest.,* **40:**636–642, **1961.**

Finch, C. E., and Foster, J. R.: Hematological and serum electrolyte values of the C57BL/6J male mouse in maturity and senescence. *Lab. Anim. Sci.,* **23:**339–349, **1973.**

Garcia, J. F.: Erythropoietic response to hypoxia as a function of age in the normal male rat. *Am. J. Physiol.,* **190:**25–30, **1957.**

Gold, M., and Altschuler, H.: Red blood cells and plasma phospholipids in aged humans. *J. Gerontol.,* **27:**444–450, **1972.**

Gordon, T., and Shrutleff, D.: Means at each examination and inter-examination variation of specific characteristics: Framingham study exams 1–10. In Kannel, W. B. (ed.): *The Framingham Study: An Epidemiological Investigation of Cardiovascular Disease,* U.S. Dept. of Health, Education & Welfare, NIH #74-618, Bethesda, MD, **1973.**

Grant, W. C., and LeGrande, M. C.: The influence of age on erythropoiesis in the rat. *J. Gerontol.,* **19:**505–509, **1964.**

Gulsvik, A.: Prevalence of respiratory symptoms in the City of Oslo. *Scand. J. Respir. Dis.,* **60:**275–285, **1979.**

Harrison, D. E.: Normal function of transplanted mouse erythrocyte precursors for 21 months beyond donor life spans. *Nature New Biol.,* **237:**220–221, **1972.**

Harrison, D. E.: Normal production of erythrocytes by mouse marrow continuous for 73 months. *Proc. Natl. Acad. Sci. USA,* **70:**3184–3188, **1973.**

Harrison, D. E.: Normal function of transplanted marrow cell lines from aged mice. *J. Gerontol.,* **30:**279–285, **1975a.**

Harrison, D. E.: Definitive erythropoietic responses of aged mice not improved by young marrow. *J. Gerontol.,* **30:**286–288, **1975b.**

Hartley, L. H.; Grimby, G.; Kilbom, A.; Nilsson, N. J.; Astrand, I.; Bjure, J.; Ekblom, B.; and Saltin, B.: Physical training in sedentary middle-aged and older men. III. Cardiac output and gas exchange at submaximal and maximal exercise. *Scand. J. Clin. Lab. Invest.,* **24:**335–344, **1969.**

Hegner, D.; Platt, D.; Heckers, H.; Schloeder, V.; and Breuninger, V.: Age-dependent physiological and biochemical studies of human red cell membranes. *Mech. Ageing Dev.,* **10:**117–130, **1979.**

Hollan, S. R.; Szelenyi, J. G.; Breur, J. H.; Medgyesi, G. A.; and Soter, V. N.: Differences between the structure and function of human adult and foetal erythrocytes. *Folia Haematol.,* **90:**125–133, **1968.**

Hurwitz, J. A.; Liben, A.; and Becklak, M. R.: Lung function in young adults—Evidence for differences in the chronological age at which various functions start to decline. *Thorax,* **35:**615–619, **1980.**

Huxley, E. J.; Vinslov, J.; Gray, W. R.; and Pierce, A. K.: Pharyngeal aspiration in normal adults and patients with depressed consciousness. *Am. J. Med.,* **64:**564–568, **1978.**

Jones, R. L.; Overton, T.; Hammerlindel, D.; and Sproule, B. J.: Effects of age in regional residual volume. *J. Appl. Physiol.,* **44:**195–199, **1978.**

Kanber, G. J.; King, F.; Eschar, Y.; and Sharp, J. T.: The alveolar arterial oxygen gradient in young and elderly men during air and oxygen breathing. *Am. Rev. Respir. Dis.,* **97:**376–381, **1968.**

Kay, M. M. B.: Senescent cell differentiation antigen. In Eaton, J. W.; Knozen, D. K.; and White, J. G. (eds.): *Cellular and Molecular Aspects of Aging. The Red Cell as a Model,* Alan R. Liss, New York, **1985.**

Karran, P., and Ormerod, M. G.: Is the ability to repair damage to DNA related to the proliferative capacity of a cell? The rejoining of X-ray-produce strand breaks. *Biochim. Biophys. Acta,* **299:**54–64, **1973.**

Kronenberg, R. S., and Drage, C. W.: Attenuation of the ventilatory and heart rate responses to hypoxia and hypercapnia with aging in normal men. *J. Clin. Invest.,* **52:**1812–1819, **1973.**

LeBlanc, P.; Ruff, F.; and Milic-Emili, J.: Effects of age and body position on "airway closure" in man. *J. Appl. Physiol.,* **28:**448–451, **1970.**

Lesher, S.; Fry, R. J.; and Kohn, H. I.: Age and generation time of the mouse duodenal epithelial cell. *Exp. Cell Res.,* **24:**334–343, **1961.**

Levitsky, M. G.: Effects of aging on the respiratory system. *Physiologist,* **27:**102–107, **1985.**

Liebow, A. A.: Biochemical and structural changes in the aging lung. Summary. In Cander, L., and Moyer, J. H. (eds.): *Aging of the Lung,* Grune & Stratton, New York, **1964.**

Little, K.: Bone marrow and aging. *Gerontologia,* **15:**155–170, **1969.**

Lucas, A. M., and Jamroz, C.: *Atlas of Avian Hematology,* Monograph No. 25, US Department of Agriculture, Washington, DC, **1961.**

Macfarlane, J. T.; Finch, R. G.; Ward, M. J.; and Nourae, A. D.: Hospital study of adult community acquired pneumonia. *Lancet,* **2:**255–257, **1982.**

Marx, J. L.: Oxygen free radicals linked to many diseases. *Science,* **235:**529–531, **1987.**

Masoro, E. J. (ed.): *CRC Handbook of Physiology in Aging,* CRC Press, Boca Raton, FL, **1981.**

Mauderly, J. L.: Effect of age on pulmonary structure and function of immature and adult animals and man. *Fed. Proc.,* **38:**173–177, **1978.**

Mittman, C.; Edelman, N. H.; Norris, A. H.; and Shock, N. W.: Relationship between chest wall and pulmonary compliance and age. *J. Appl. Physiol.,* **20:**1211–1216, **1965.**

Morris, J. F.; Mosk, A.; and Johnson, L. C.: Spirometric standards for healthy non-smoking adults. *Am. Rev. Respir. Dis.,* **103:**57–67, **1971.**

Muiesan, G.; Sorbini, C. A.; and Grassi, V.: Respiratory function in the aged. *Bull. Physio-Pathol. Resp.,* **7:**973–1009, **1971.**

Murphy, M. L., and Bone, R. C.: *Cor Pulmonale in*

Chronic Bronchitis and Emphysema, Futura, Mount Kisco, NY, **1984.**

Mylotte, J. M., and Bearn, T. R.: Comparison of community acquired and nosocomial pneumococcal bacteraemia. *Am. Rev. Respir. Dis.,* **123:**265–268, **1981.**

Niewoehner, D. E., and Kleinerman, J.: Morphologic basis of pulmonary resistance in the human lung and effects of aging. *J. Appl. Physiol.,* **36:**412–418, **1964.**

Peterson, D. D.; Pack, A. I.; Silage, D. A.; and Fishman, A. P.: Effects of aging on the ventilatory and occlusion pressure responses to hypoxia and hypercapnia. *Am. Rev. Respir. Dis.,* **124:**387–391, **1981.**

Petty, T. L., and Nett, L. M. (eds.) *Enjoying Life with Emphysema,* Lea & Febiger, Philadelphia, **1984.**

Pierce, J. A., and Ebert, R. V.: Fibrous network of the lungs and its change with age. *Thorax,* **20:**469–476, **1965.**

Polgar, G., and Weng, T. R.: The functional development of the respiratory system: From the period of gestation to adulthood. *Am. Rev. Respir. Dis.,* **120:**625–695, **1979.**

Prankerd, T. A. J.: The aging of red cells. *J. Physiol. (London),* **143:**325–331, **1958.**

Price, G. B.; Modak, S. P.; and Makinodan, T.: Age associated changes in DNA of mouse tissue. *Science,* **171:**917–920, **1971.**

Pump, K. K.: The aged lung. *Chest,* **60:**571–577, **1971.**

Reddan, W. G.: Respiratory system and aging. In Smith E. L., and Serfass, R. C. (eds.): *Exercise and Aging,* Enslow Publishing, Hillside, NJ, **1981.**

Reid, L.: The aged lung. In *The Pathology of Emphysema,* Lloyd-Luke, London, **1967.**

Rizzato, G., and Marrazini, L.: Thoracoabdominal mechanics in elderly men. *J. Appl. Physiol.,* **28:**457–460, **1970.**

Roussos, C. S., and Macklem, D. T.: Diaphragmatic fatigue in man. *J. Appl. Physiol.,* **43:**189–197, **1977.**

Rowe, J. W., and Minaker, : Geriatric medicine. In Finch, C. E., and Schneider, E. L. (eds.) *Handbook of the Biology of Aging,* Van Nostrand Reinhold, New York, **1985.**

Roylance, P. J.: An evaluation of erythropoiesis in the young rat. *Cell Tiss. Kinet.,* **1:**299–308, **1968.**

Schapira, G.; Labie, D.; Rosa, J.; and Dreyfus, J. C.: Evidence for a distinct fraction of hemoglobin, specifically associated with the young erythrocytes. *Biochem. Biophys. Res. Commun.,* **9:**167–172, **1962.**

Shephard, R. J. (ed.): *Physical Activity and Aging.* Croom Helm Ltd., London, **1978.**

Shephard, R. J. (ed.): *Physiology and Biochemistry of Exercise,* Praeger, New York, **1982.**

Shock, N. W.: An essay on aging. In Cander, L., and Moyer, J. H. (eds.): *Aging of the Lung,* Grune & Stratton, New York, **1964.**

Smith, E. L., and Serfass, R. C. (eds.): *Exercise and Aging,* Enslow Publishers, Hillside, NJ, **1981.**

Snider, G. L.: *Symposium on Emphysema,* Clinics in Medicine, W. B. Saunders, Philadelphia, **1983.**

Steinberg, M. H.: Role of hemoglobin instability in premature red cell destruction. In Eaton, J. W.; Knozen, D. K.; and White, J. G. (eds.): *Cellular and Molecular Aspects of Aging. The Red Cell as a Model,* Alan R. Liss, New York, **1984.**

Sterling, G. M. (ed.): *Respiratory Disease,* William Heinesman Medical Books, London, **1983.**

Swislocki, N. I.: Impromptu discussion of comparative aspects of red cell aging. In Eaton, J. W.; Knozen, D. K.; and White, J. G. (eds.): *Cellular and Molecular Aspects of Aging. The Red Cell as a Model,* Alan R. Liss, New York, **1985.**

Thrasher, J. D., and Greulich, R. C.: The duodenal progenitor population. I. Age related increase in the duration of the cryptal progenitor cell. *J. Exp. Zool.,* **159:**39–46, **1965.**

Thurlbeck, W. M., and Angus, G. E.: Growth and ageing of normal human lung. *Chest,* **67:**3s–7s, **1975.**

Timiras, M. L., and Brownstein, H.: Prevalence of anemia and correlation of hemoglobin with age in a geriatric screening clinic population. *J. Am. Geriatr. Soc.,* **35:**639–643, **1987.**

Tlusty, L.: Physical fitness in old age. I. Aerobic capacity and other parameters of physical fitness followed by means of exercise in ergometric examination of elderly individuals. *Respiration,* **26:**161–181, **1969a.**

Tlusty, L.: Physical fitness in old age. II. Anaerobic capacity, anaerobic work in graded exercise, recovery after maximum work performance in elderly individuals. *Respiration,* **26:**287–299, **1969b.**

Turner, J. M.; Mead, J.; and Wohl, M. E.: Elasticity of human lungs in relation to age. *J. Appl. Physiol.,* **25:**664–671, **1968.**

Walter, H.; Brake, J. M.; and Selby, F. W.: Aspects of the aging of the avian (nucleated) red blood cell *in vivo. Exp. Cell Res.,* **37:**420–428, **1965.**

Winterhalter, K. H.: Nonenzymatic glycosylation of proteins. In Eaton, J. W.; Knozen, D. K.; and White, J. G. (eds.): *Cellular and Molecular Aspects of Aging. The Red Cell as a Model,* Alan R. Liss, New York, **1985.**

Woodford-Williams, E.; Webster, D.; Dixon, M. P.; and MacKenzie, W.: Red cell longevity in old age. *Gerontol. Clin.,* **4:**183–1983, **1962.**

CHAPTER

20 THE KIDNEY, THE LOWER URINARY TRACT, AND BODY FLUIDS

Mary L. Timiras

As with other systems, the urinary tract is both directly and indirectly affected by aging. Direct effects are exemplified by intrinsic cellular changes involving the nephron as well as the muscles of the bladder or the prostate. Indirect effects may be secondary to cardiovascular, endocrine, or metabolic alterations occurring with aging that have vital repercussions on urine formation and excretion. Reciprocally, physiologic decrements in renal function and disturbances of the lower urinary tract may not only alter the elimination of end-products of metabolism, but also impair other functions such as regulation of body fluids, acid-base balance, and blood pressure. The latter has been discussed in Chapter 17. Finally, given the metabolic and excretory functions of the kidney with respect to drugs of environmental, recreational, and therapeutic nature, the decline of renal function with aging can modify the renal handling of drugs and thereby alter drug pharmacokinetics, including toxicity and therapeutic effectiveness. Such drug-related considerations are important at any age but are particularly so in the elderly to whom multiple drugs are simultaneously prescribed, increasing dangers of polypharmacy and iatrogenicity (Chapter 24).

In the present chapter, the following aging-related changes will be reviewed: (1) changes in renal function, including considerations of drug excretion; (2) changes in the lower urinary tract, including the problems of urinary incontinence and prostatic hypertrophy; and (3) changes in body fluids and acid-base balance.

AGING-RELATED CHANGES OF RENAL FUNCTION

All parameters of renal function are affected by aging, but the age of onset, rate and course of changes, and consequences vary. Thus, glomerular filtration, closely dependent on the efficiency of the renal blood flow and the integrity of the glomerular basement membrane, appears affected at an earlier age and more severely than tubular reabsorption and secretion. After the age of 30, in humans, renal function as measured by several fuctional tests (see below) gradually decreases and by 60 years has been further reduced to half. This decline has been ascribed to a gradual loss of nephrons and diminished enzymatic and metabolic activity of tubular cells as well as an increased incidence of pathologic processes, primary atherosclerosis (see Chapter 17), which involves the renal blood circulation, an essential factor in determining renal competence. Likewise, a number of experimental animal studies show an overall decline of renal competence involving glomerular and tubular functions. A discussion of declining renal function is preceded by a brief summary of renal structure and function.

Some Gross Structural Characteristics and Major Functions of the Kidney. The kidneys are paired organs lying on either side of the descending (abdominal) aorta and receive their blood via the renal arteries, two main collaterals of the aorta. A smooth outer capsule covers the cortex, which contains the majority of the glomerular portion of the individual nephron (Figure 20–1). The nephron represents the functional unit and grossly is formed of the glomerulus, in the cortex, and the renal tubule, which dips down and occupies the medulla, the inner portion of the renal parenchyma. Running parallel to the tubules in the medulla is a network of blood vessels, the vasa recta, which participate, with the tubular loop of Henle, in controlling the osmolality of the medulla through a countercurrent mechanism. The urine formed in the nephron flows into collecting ducts and out through the calyces and the pelvis to the ureter.

The glomerulus is formed by a tuft of capillaries between the entering, afferent, and the exiting, efferent, arterioles. Filtration is through a fenestrated glomerular endothelium, which is separated by a basal lamina from the interdigi-

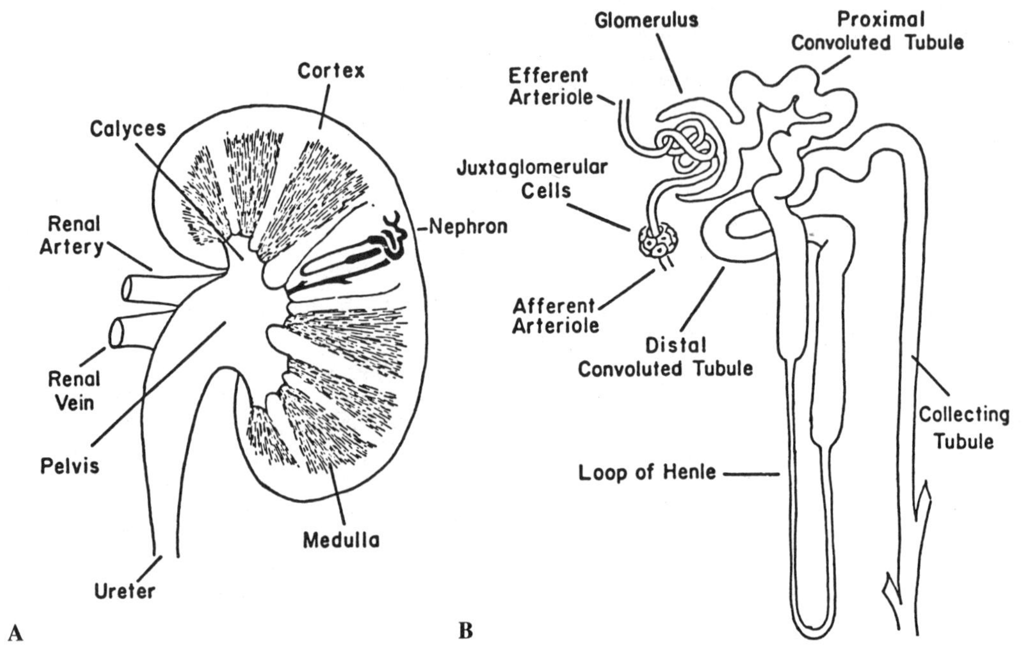

Figure 20–1. *Diagram of the kidney (A) and of a nephron (B).* (Drawing by S. Oklund)

tated epithelial cells, the so-called podocytes, of the tubular epithelium. The filtrate has the same composition as plasma, except for the absence of proteins. The epithelial cells lining the various segments (proximal tubule, loop of Henle, distal tubule, collecting duct) of the renal tubule have been divided into types and subtypes on the basis of minor differences in histologic structure; there is some evidence that these differences correlate with differences in function, which is either reabsorption or secretion. Cells of the afferent arteriolar wall and the abutting distal tubule form the juxtaglomerular apparatus, site of the formation and release of renin. Cells of the distal convoluted tubule and the collecting duct are sensitive to hormones, aldosterone for sodium reabsorption and antidiuretic hormone (ADH) for water reabsorption.

The kidneys adjust the amount of water and electrolytes excreted in order to keep the body fluid relatively constant in volume and composition as well as maintain blood pH through the secretion of H^+, that is, maintain fluid and acid-base balance and homeostasis. Kidneys also excrete end-products of metabolism. They have certain endocrine functions: they are responsible for the secretion of renin, hence regulate the renin-angiotensin system and, indirectly, blood pressure (see Chapter 17) and aldosterone secretion (see Chapter 12); they activate vitamin D and thereby play a role in Ca^{2+} metabolism; they secrete erythropoietin and maintain the hemoglobin level (Table 20–1).

Table 20–1. MAJOR FUNCTIONS OF THE KIDNEY

Water and electrolyte regulation
Metabolic products excretion
Hydrogen ion excretion and maintenance of blood pH
Endocrine functions
Renin-angiotensin (blood pressure)
Vitamin D activation (Ca^{2+} metabolism)
Erythropoietin (hemoglobin levels)

Tests of Renal Function. At all ages, the competence of renal function is assessed by a number of tests among which the most routinely used are: urine volume (per 24 hours), analysis of urine constituents, and urine concentration and dilution tests. Other measures of renal function include: clearance tests, that is, clearance of a substance from the plasma during passage through the kidney (for example, inulin to measure glomerular filtration rate and para-aminohippuric acid [PHA] to measure renal blood flow). Radiologic, isotopic, ultrasonic, magnetic resonance spectroscopy and imaging, and tomographic imaging as well as biopsies and other less common tests represent more laborious and expensive means of assessing specific conditions.

GLOMERULAR FUNCTION

The function of the glomerulus is to selectively filter plasma to produce a glomerular filtrate that, under normal healthy conditions, is practically free of proteins. Glomerular filtration is determined by mea-

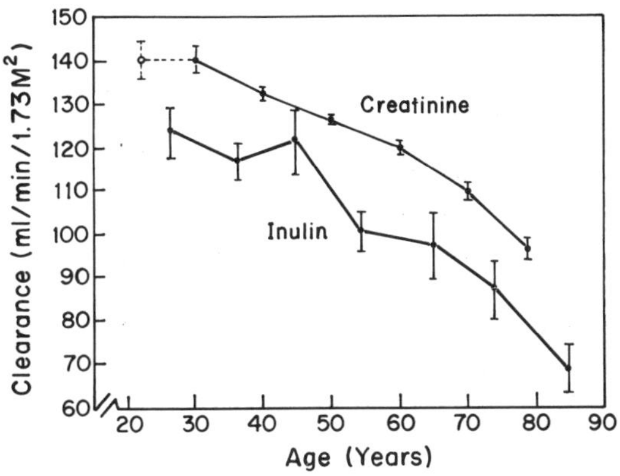

Figure 20–2. *Glomerular Filtration Rate With Age.*

Decrease in glomerular filtration rate with age as measured by creatinine and inulin clearance. Creatinine is a normal endogenous metabolic product and inulin a polymer of fructose.

suring the clearance of plasma and the excretion in the urine of a substance such as inulin or creatinine, which is freely filtered through the glomeruli but not secreted or reabsorbed by the tubule. This technique establishes the filtration rate in a normal average young man as approximately 125 ml/min. With aging, commencing as early as 30 years, the glomerular filtration rate decreases progressively and significantly (Shock, 1946; Davies and Shock, 1950; Rowe *et al.*, 1976) (Figure 20–2).

Creatinine Clearance. Both inulin, a polysaccharide administered intravenously, and creatinine, a normal endogenous product of protein metabolism, are usually utilized to assess glomerular function. Creatinine clearance, which does not involve any drug administration, is most frequently used and is calculated by the following formula:

$$\text{Creatinine clearance} = \frac{(140 - \text{age}) \times \text{body weight (in kg)}}{72 \times \text{serum creatinine (in mg\%)}}$$

A 20-year-old individual, with a serum creatinine of 1 mg% and a body weight of 72 kg, has a creatinine clearance of 120 mg% whereas a 90-year-old with the same body weight and serum creatinine has a creatinine clearance of 50 mg%, a greater than 50% reduction. The reduction with aging in the urinary output of creatinine, a muscle-specific metabolite, has been interpreted as reflecting a reduction in lean body mass as demonstrated to occur in old age by loss of radioactively labeled potassium, the major intracellular electrolyte.

The above equation is valid only with the assumption that renal function decreases with age at a rate of 1 ml/min/year after age 40. Although this provides a better estimate than no correction at all, recent studies have shown great variation in the rate of decline of renal function. In some individuals, no decrease in renal clearance can be detected with advancing age (Lindeman *et al.*, 1985).

Creatinine clearance is often measured in elderly individuals not merely as a test of renal function, but as a guide to drug administration so that dosage can be adjusted depending on age, serum creatinine, and creatinine clearance (see Chapter 24).

Of the factors that affect the glomerular filtration rate, the most important are characteristics of the glomerular wall and renal blood flow. Studies in humans show that the decrease in glomerular function may be due primarily to a loss or alteration of glomeruli and secondarily to alterations in blood flow, although the reverse sequence may also be true. Irrespective of the primary site of the lesion, studies in rats show a 30 percent incidence of necrotic glomeruli with age while, after food restriction, the incidence is reduced to 2 percent (Durakovic and Mimica, 1983).

Microscopic and ultramicroscopic studies of the glomerulus in rats reveal a progressive thickening (from 1300 Å, neonatally, to 4800 Å, at the old age of 2 years) of the basement membrane in some areas (focal or segmental thickening) and collapse (with loss of distinct layers) in others. Podocytes are lost or undergo swelling or atrophy. Proliferation of interstitial collagen leads to progressive sclerosis. As a consequence of these alterations in the glomerular structure, abnormal proteinuria appears in about 25 percent of male rats at a young age, and its incidence and severity increases progressively with age, although less so in female animals (Bolton and Sturgill, 1981).

In humans, widespread glomerular necrosis is rare. However, even in humans, histologic studies show a thickening of the glomerular basement membrane with concomitant biochemical alterations such as a progressive decrease (e.g., 3.7 percent reduction per decade) in some amino acids suggesting a diminution of the collagenous component (Smalley, 1980). In humans, however, alterations of renal blood flow appear to be primarily responsible for the glomerular alterations, and age-related decreases in blood flow have been reported (Brod, 1968; Rowe, 1976); moreover, these changes are potentially reversible (McDonald *et al.,* 1951).

Aging-Related Changes in Day/Night Urine Excretion. In the normal adult, urine flow and electrolyte excretion follow a day/night pattern with higher levels in the daytime. This pattern may have evolved to permit undisturbed sleep. In the elderly, the rhythm is shifted, with increased water and electrolyte excretion during the night. This shift may involve the glomerular filtration along with hormonal control of urine concentration and may be regulated by extrarenal, hypothalamic factors (Kirkland *et al.,* 1983).

GLOMERULAR FUNCTION AND DIETARY PROTEINS

Changes with aging in glomerular function do not pose any threat by themselves to well-being; likewise, renal function is not seriously compromised with aging, even in octagenerians. If, however, intrinsic renal disease or surgical loss of renal tissue or other factors, such as diet, add to the glomerular burden of age, then the course of glomerular sclerosis and reduced glomerular filtration rate may be hastened appreciably. Under normal conditions, very little protein is filtered in the glomeruli and excreted in the urine. One manifestation of impairment in glomerular filtration is altered permeability with consequent proteinuria, that is, more than the usual trace amounts of protein in the urine. In addition, high-protein diets make it more difficult to prevent filtration of protein. Experiments show that dietary proteins may induce glomerular damage and that reduction of dietary protein intake reduces this damage. For example, feeding rats a diet low in protein or restricted in total calories reduces age-related proteinuria. A similar beneficial effect has been demonstrated after long-term administration of the adrenal steroid dehydroepiandrosterone, which would act by reducing weight gain and/or oxidative processes or by some still unclear hormonal action (Pashko *et al.,* 1986). Dietary restriction seems to extend the life of laboratory animals and such extension may involve the beneficial effects of a low-protein diet on renal function (Everitt *et al.,* 1982). Thus, rats consuming 75 kcal of food per day, a really large quantity, show high protein excretion throughout life from 4 mg/day at 70 days, just after sexual maturation, to 88 mg/day at the old age of 900 days. The normal food consumption is more in the range of 50 to 65 kcal/day, and with this diet, protein excretion is halved. If food is severely restricted to 12.5 kcal/day, the rise in proteinuria with age is abolished. The same modification is apparent even with short-time food restriction in old animals. When the diet is reduced from 60 to 25 kcal/day, protein excretion decreases by 40 percent in 1 week and continues at this level for the next week, even after discontinuation of the restricted diet (Figure 20–3).

In humans, the current diet offers sustained (three meals a day) rather than intermittent (feast or famine of animals in the wild) intake of protein. Such sustained "excess" would impose rigorous demands on glomerular filtration rate and renal blood flow, thereby contributing to the decline of these functions with aging. It may also be responsible for the inexorable progressiveness of the renal deficits and the greater incidence of renal pathology in the elderly. Calorie or protein restriction fairly early in the course of renal disease slows the rate of decline in glomerular filtration. This is true not only for aging, but also for metabolic and renal disorders; this is the case, for example, of obesity in which diet modification leading to body weight loss reduces the often present proteinuria associated with glomerular sclerosis (Brenner *et al.,* 1982).

TUBULAR FUNCTION

The aged kidney is unable to concentrate urine as does the young kidney, and because of this, water and electrolyte metabolism are potentially critical in the elderly, even among those who have no overt signs or laboratory tests indicating renal dysfunction.

The ability to concentrate or dilute urine is gradually lost, with the result that the elderly individual is unable to cope optimally with either dehydration or water load (Phillips *et al.,* 1984). This inability is manifested after both stimulation and inhibition of antidiuretic hormone (ADH) secretion (Helderman *et al.,* 1978). Administration of ethanol, a drug that is a known ADH inhibitor, reduces circulating ADH levels up to

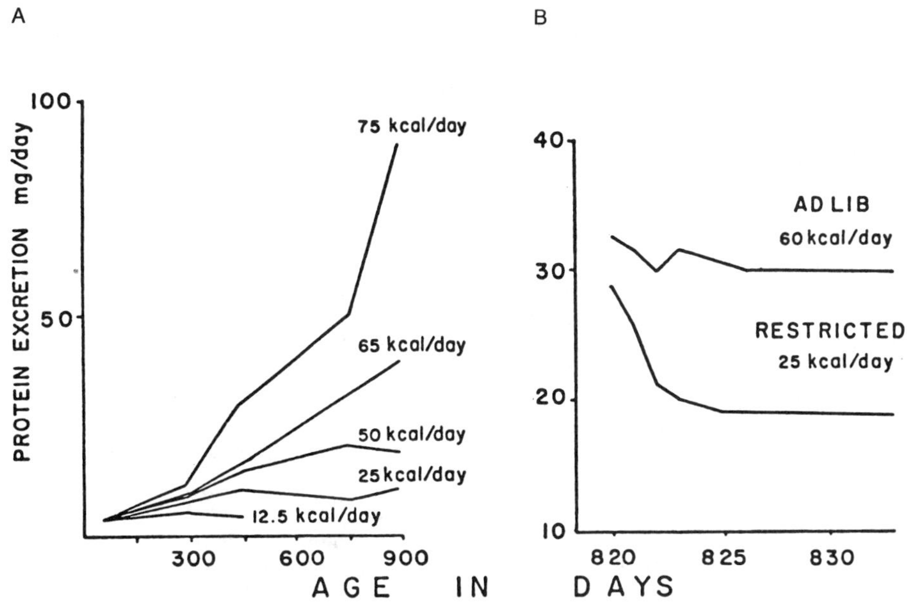

Figure 20–3. *Dietary caloric restriction reduces aging-related proteinuria in male rats.*

A. Proteinuria is reduced proportionately to the severity of the caloric restriction: severe food restriction (12.5 kcal/day) initiated at a young age (70 days) abolishes the steep rise in protein excretion with aging (but is not compatible with long life) and a less severe restriction (25 or 50 kcal/day) markedly inhibits it. B. This effect of caloric restriction is also observed in old (820 days) rats in which about one-week restriction was sufficient to reduce significantly proteinuria.

120 minutes after administration in young individuals. In old subjects, ADH levels are decreased immediately after alcohol ingestion, but increase thereafter as shown at 120 minutes (Figure 20–4). In the young individual, low ADH levels are associated with the expected diuresis or increased water clearance. In old individuals, ADH inhibition occurs early after alcohol administration and then disappears; concomitantly diuresis does not occur or is only minimal.

As for ADH inhibition, ADH stimulation induces different responses in the elderly as compared to the young. In response to the same osmotic challenge, ADH levels increase, but more in old subjects than in young. Thus, administration of a hypertonic sodium chloride solution increases ADH levels much more in the elderly than in the young, but this increase in ADH levels is not accompanied in the elderly by the expected increase in water retention observed in the young (Figure 20–4). Attempts to identify the site(s) of the decreasing function, either renal or extrarenal, have not yet led to definitive conclusions. Administration of a standardized dose of ADH to young and old individuals shows a decline in the ability of the tubules to perform osmotic work and increase water retention in old individuals (Miller and Shock, 1953). However, further studies suggest that decrements in the ability of cellular membranes in the collecting duct to become more water permeable under ADH influence occur primarily in old individuals with renal infections or hypertension; these decrements should not, therefore, be viewed as the usual accompaniment of aging (Lindeman *et al.*, 1966). Further experiments show that, in aged rats, decreased responsiveness of collecting tubular epithelium to ADH is the most likely explanation for the impairment of urine-concentrating ability (Bengele *et al.*, 1981), while reduced secretion and levels of ADH would not play an important role in this impairment. Whether the defect in renal regulation of

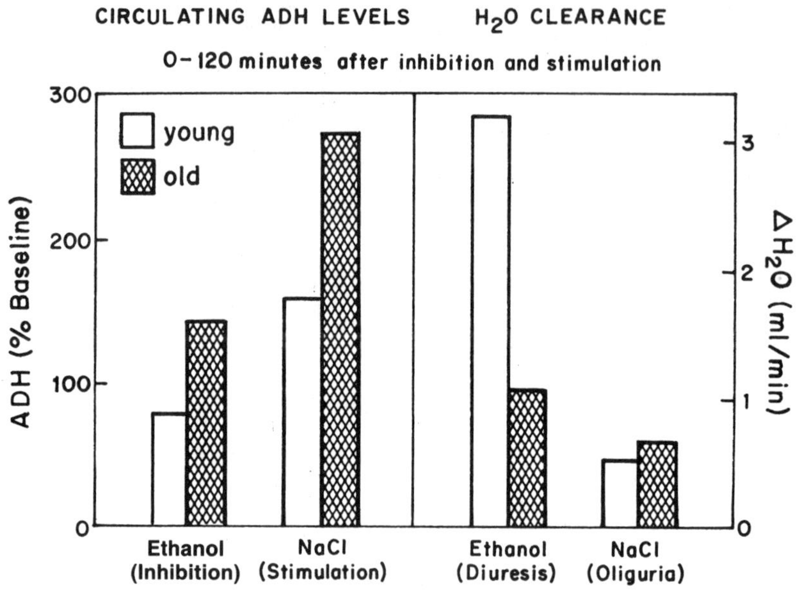

Figure 20–4. *Age related changes in tubular responses to antidiuretic hormone (ADH).*

Ethanol inhibits ADH and is less efficient in this inhibition in the elderly as reflected in the diuresis which ensues. Hypertonic sodium chloride increases ADH more in the elderly than the young, however the expected increase in water retention does not occur.

water excretion lies in the hypothalamus, the pituitary, or the kidney, there is no doubt about the relative inability of the aged kidney to concentrate or dilute urine and the consequent ease with which the elderly person may develop acute or chronic renal failure. As long as the total water intake is adequate—2.5 to 3.0 liters/day—renal function will be adequate. Crises will arise when water intake is diminished due to loneliness, immobility, confusion, fear of incontinence, etc. This may also occur with unnecessary use of diuretics.

Failure to concentrate urine may also be related to sodium loss, particularly in the distal nephron (Nunez *et al.,* 1978). Elderly persons are more prone to develop hyponatremia and hypokalemia during diuretic therapy or due to an inadequate diet. Body potassium content is less in the elderly than the young (Cox and Shalaby, 1981) even when measured in terms of lean (fat-free) body weight and this lower content may be due to renal loss as well as poor intake.

Blood urea and blood creatinine are usually unchanged in aged, healthy individuals, even though, as in the case of creatinine, their urinary excretion may be altered. Normal serum creatinine, despite decreased excretion, may reflect low production, perhaps related to reduced muscle mass and function. Blood urea may be reduced owing to diminished protein intake, often present in the elderly or, more rarely, to liver disease and insufficient urea production.

Renal Aging in Laboratory Animals. A number of experimental animal studies show an overall renal functional decline, as illustrated in the following examples; reduced proliferative (compensatory) growth of remaining kidney after unilateral nephrectomy (Phillips and Leong, 1967); reduced rate of oxidative processes in homogenate of renal cortex from aged rats (Barrows *et al.,* 1960); reduced Na^+, K^+-ATPase activity and decreased PHA accumulation by aged rat kidney slices (Beauchene *et al.,* 1965); reduced urine concentration ability in aged rats in response to ADH (Bengele *et al.,* 1981); and potentially damaging effect of a high-protein, high-calorie diet on renal aging and eventual preventive success with dietary restriction (Everitt *et al.,* 1982).

RENAL DISEASE IN THE ELDERLY

Compounding the relatively minor impairment of renal function in the healthy elderly is the increased incidence of renal dis-

Table 20–2. COMMON RENAL PROBLEMS IN THE AGED

Renal failure
Impaired drug excretion
Urinary tract infections
Hypertension
Miscellaneous disorders
Tuberculosis
Nephritis
Diabetes, etc.

eases and the reduced ability to handle the excretion of drugs. The major renal disorders of the young and middle aged—acute nephritis, collagen disorders, and malignant hypertension—are uncommon in old age. If they occur, they present and are treated, as in the young, with caution to protect water and electrolyte balance.

In the aged population, the common problems affecting renal function are related to damage induced by infections or drugs or by hypertension or they are consequent to miscellaneous disorders such as tuberculosis, nephritis, diabetes mellitus, amyloidosis, collagen disorders, and so forth (Table 20–2). If untreated, these disorders may lead, perhaps more easily than in the young and with more life-threatening consequences, to impairment and, finally, to failure of renal function (Frocht and Fillit, 1984).

FAILURE OF RENAL FUNCTION: PATHOGENESIS AND MANAGEMENT

Renal failure refers to the inability of the kidneys to handle electrolytes and other substances that must be excreted. Normally one-third of the nephrons can eliminate all of the normal waste products from the body and prevent their accumulation in body fluids. When the number of functioning nephrons falls to 10 to 20 percent of normal, urinary retention and death follow.

Clinically, urinary failure is designated as either acute or chronic. The acute form is the most frequent in the elderly. In both cases, the consequences depend to a great extent on the food and water intake of the individual. With moderate intake, the most important signs are: (1) generalized edema, resulting from salt and water retention; (2) acidosis, resulting from failure to excrete normal acidic products; (3) high concentration of nonprotein nitrogens, especially urea, resulting from failure to excrete metabolic end-products; (4) high concentration of other urinary products, including creatinine, uric acid, phenols, etc. This condition of failing excretion is called *uremia* because of the high concentrations of normal urinary excretory products that collect in the body fluids (Table 20–3).

Table 20–3. SIGNS OF RENAL FAILURE

Generalized edema
Acidosis
Increased circulating nonprotein nitrogens (urea)
Increased circulating urinary retention products

Table 20–4. SELECTED CAUSES OF ACUTE RENAL FAILURE

Prerenal
Loss of body fluids
Inadequate fluid intake
Surgical shock or myocardial infarction
Renal
Drug toxicity
Immunologic reactions
Infectious diseases
Thrombosis
Postrenal
Intravascular hemolysis
Urinary tract obstruction

Acute renal failure refers to a sudden cessation of renal function following various insults to the normal kidney. The causes of acute renal failure are numerous and are divided into prerenal, renal, and postrenal depending on whether they are traced to alterations of the kidney itself or to extrarenal alterations (Table 20–4). Prerenal causes most likely to be found in the aged include: loss of body fluids (e.g., vomiting, diarrhea); inadequate fluid intake (often associated with the overuse of diuretics and laxatives); and surgical shock or myocardial infarction.

Renal causes are relatively rare in the elderly; they include: drug toxicity due to certain antibiotics (sulfonamides, aminoglycosides, amphoteracin B); x-ray contrast materials (in a rather dehydrated individual); drug-induced immunologic reactions (Bennett *et al.,* 1980); infectious diseases; gram-negative bacteremia with shock or peritonitis; thrombosis and other circulatory alterations due to atherosclerosis; and intravascular hemolysis such as may follow transurethral resection of the prostate.

Postrenal causes are due primarily to urinary tract obstructions, such as occurs with prostatic enlargement.

Chronic renal failure results from slow, progressive renal dysfunction. It is more often a disease of young and middle-aged individuals, as survival is reduced in the major instances such as in glomerulonephritis and polycystic disease. The most common causes in the elderly are: (1) progressive renal sclerosis (due to atherosclerosis); (2) chronic pyelonephritis; and (3) slow but progressive enlargement of the prostate.

When urine output is acutely reduced to 20 to 200 ml/day (oliguria) following any of the foregoing events, the patient is in acute renal failure. Renal tubular necrosis is the characteristic finding and scattered basement membrane disruption occurs. The urine contains protein, red cells, epithelial cells, and characteristic dirty-brown casts. Rate of protein catabolism in the body governs the rate of accumulation of metabolic products in body fluids, and the signs of uremia appear with nausea, vomiting, diarrhea, lethargy, and hypertension.

Acute renal failure may be resolved, spontaneously, in a few days or up to 6 weeks (Oliveria and Winearls, 1984). Management depends on the mechanism that is responsible for the failure. Therefore, the initial step involves differentiation between a prerenal oliguric state versus an intrinsic renal state. This is important because the treatment for a hypovolemic—reduced blood volume—prerenal state consists of fluid and intravascular volume replacement; such treatment can lead to a dangerous fluid overload in a patient with intrinsic renal disease such as acute tubular necrosis. Examination of the urine for the fractional excretion of sodium is the safest and most reliable method for making this differentiation.

Fractional sodium excretion measures the kidney capacity to conserve sodium and excrete creatinine. Fractional excretion of sodium (FE_{Na}) is determined according to the following formula:

$$FE_{Na} = \frac{U_{Na} \div P_{Na}}{U_{cr} \div P_{cr}} \times 100 \quad \begin{array}{l} < 1 \longrightarrow \text{prerenal} \\ > 1 \longrightarrow \text{intrinsic renal} \end{array}$$

The urine sodium concentration is divided by the plasma sodium concentration, and this is then divided by the urine creatinine concentration over the plasma creatinine concentration. When this value, multiplied by 100, is less than 1, then prerenal azotemia—high blood nitrogen—is responsible for the renal failure. When the fractional excretion of sodium is greater than 1, this indicates intrinsic renal failure.

Another method, simpler but more dangerous, especially for the elderly, is to administer a fluid challenge of either isotonic saline or mannitol together with a potent diuretic such as furosemide. A response to these maneuvers may indicate that one is dealing with prerenal azotemia.

Management of acute renal failure includes: (1) treatment of the underlying cause, for example, the discontinuation of nephrotoxins should any be implicated; (2) careful fluid monitoring to avoid fluid overload and congestive failure; (3) electrolyte monitoring such as hyperkalemia and acidosis; (4) prevention of infection as this is the major cause of mortality in patients with acute tubular necrosis; (5) alteration of the diet to limit sources of nitrogen, potassium, phosphorus, and sulfate. This involves limiting protein to no more than 40 gm per day and supplying sufficient calories (at least 3000) to prevent endogenous protein catabolism.

Dialysis Treatment and Kidney Transplantation in the Elderly. The question often arises to what extent "heroic interventions" are justifiable and advisable in the elderly. In the case of renal failure, dialysis and kidney transplantation represent interventive measures that are widely utilized with considerable success in the young and adult. Evidence for their rational use with a favorable outcome in the elderly has been shown from the relatively few cases treated so far and from animal experimentation. Clearly, while all contraindications and immediate and long-term risks of these measures must be taken carefully into consideration, as they may be magnified in the elderly, age alone should not deter one from their appropriate use (Nicholls *et al.*, 1984). Dialysis is indicated on an emergency basis in the following situations: (1) blood volume overload leading to congestive heart failure; (2) hyperkalemia, that is high blood potassium, which is refractory to medical management; (3) severe acidosis; (4) neurologic abnormalities resulting from a rapid increase in azotemia; and (5) severe hyponatremia, that is low sodium blood levels. Dialysis should not be withheld from an elderly patient in acute renal failure merely on the basis of his/her age. It is not usually easy to accurately determine the patient's prognosis at the onset of the acute illness, and therefore, major decisions in management, such as the use of dialysis, should be initially made with the assumption that a positive outcome will occur. Thus, aggressive dialysis in acute renal failure should be the rule rather than the exception.

Indication for and success of transplantation of organs such as the kidney depend on several criteria such as normal function and competency of the organ to be transplanted and the age (young) and health (good) of the donor. With respect to age, although the use of kidneys from older donors is controversial, a number of data suggest that age alone should not eliminate using older kidney donors when their renal function and tissue matches are good (Matus *et al.*, 1976). Pregnancy puts a strain on kidney function, but a report of a successful pregnancy in a renal transplant recipient with a kidney from a 75-year-old donor supports the view that an old kidney may function normally (Coulam and Zincke, 1981). Systematic studies in young adult rats, bilaterally nephrectomized and receiving kidneys transplanted from animals of progressive ages, until quite advanced age, show a good recipient survival, but old kidneys functioned less well than young on the average (Van Bezooijen *et al.*, 1974). It is possible that the kidneys from old donors are more susceptible to the hypoxia induced by surgery or age-related renal metabolic changes. Reciprocally, kidney transplants in older individuals (with young kidney donors) seem to fare as well as in the young once the surgical and pharmacologic measures appropriate to the age of the individuals are taken into account.

It is to be recalled here that, in addition to the practical applicability of these studies, it is of interest that old tissues and organs may continue to function in younger individuals beyond their normal survival time. Such a survival contradicts some of the aging somatic mutation theories (see Chapter 4) that claim intrinsic aging of all tissues in all individuals. Of equal interest is the length and success of survival of tissues and organs from young individuals when transplanted in an elderly subject. In view of the many advances in organ transplantation and the increasing number of successful transplants, more valuable data are expected on this subject in the near future.

DRUGS AND THE AGING KIDNEY

Just at an age when renal function may be reduced, the elderly individual is receiving multiple and long-term drug therapy. This so-called polypharmacy is discussed in Chapter 24. Changes in renal function represent one variable in drug excretion, and an understanding of this variable as well as the mechanism of action will provide the basis for a sound therapeutic regimen. The kidney is the major route of drug elimination. Questions that should always be posed, and are perhaps more crucial in the elderly, are (Table 20–5): (1) Is the major route of excretion of a given drug via the kidney? (2) How competent are the kidneys of the individual to be receiving the drug? (3) What are the side effects of the drug?

Table 20–5. DRUGS AND AGING KIDNEYS

Questions:
Is the drug excreted primarily by the kidney?
How competent are the kidneys?
What are the side effects?
What are the consequences of drug toxicity when the kidney is impaired?

The effects of drugs and their relationship to the kidney may be considered in two ways: (1) What problems may arise from potentially toxic effects of certain drugs on the kidney? (2) What are the properties of the prescribed drug when renal function is diminished?

KIDNEY SUSCEPTIBILITY TO DRUGS

The kidneys are particularly susceptible to the toxic effects of drugs and other chemical agents because: (1) blood flow to the kidney is high, 20 percent of cardiac output; (2) drugs tend to accumulate in the renal medulla as water is removed from the glomerular filtrate; (3) drug accumulation increases when renal function is impaired; (4) reduced hepatic enzyme activity in the elderly increases circulating drug levels and renal toxicity; and (5) incidence of autoimmune disorders increases with aging with consequent hypersensitivity reactions in the kidney (Table 20–6).

The manifestations of renal drug intoxication are not unique to the aged kidney; they are, however, more frequent, and when they occur, they may be more severe than in the adult. In the aged kidney, toxic effects are seen with lower doses than in the adult and the consequences are more dangerous, taking into account the multiplicity of drugs taken by the elderly, the generally long duration of treatment, and the often impaired condition of the kidney.

Examples of drugs and the mechanisms whereby they induce renal damage include: (1) dehydration-induced uremia due to use of diuretics and laxatives; (2) obstruction of urinary tract due to deposition of crystalline matters such as calcium from excessive

Table 20–6. ETIOPATHOLOGY OF RENAL DRUG TOXICITY

High renal blood flow
Increased drug concentration and accumulation in kidney
Increased hepatic enzyme inhibition in the elderly
Increased autoimmune disorders in the elderly

Table 20–7. SOME EXAMPLES OF DRUG TOXICITY IN ELDERLY INDIVIDUALS WITH DIMINISHED RENAL FUNCTION

DRUGS	RESPONSE
Aminoglycosides	Deafness and kidney toxicity
Nitrofurantoin	Neuropathy
Oral antidiabetics	Hypoglycemia
Digoxin	Vomiting and irregular heartbeat
Nonsteroidal antiinflammatory agents	Renal failure
Anticholinergics	Confusional states

administration of vitamin D; (3) vascular lesions produced by thiazide diuretics; (4) glomerular damage by penicillinlike antibiotics; (5) interstitial and tubular damage from radiologic contrast media; and (6) papillary necrosis due to analgesics.

CONSEQUENCES OF AGE-RELATED DECLINE IN RENAL FUNCTION ON DRUG KINETICS

A standard dose of a drug, normally cleared through the kidney, when given to an elderly individual, is likely to accumulate in blood and tissue. This accumulation can be much higher than necessary for therapeutic benefit and may certainly produce side effects, forerunners of iatrogenic disease. Common examples of this toxicity in the elderly are (Table 20–7): (1) deafness and kidney toxicity with aminoglycosides such as the antibiotic streptomycin; (2) neuropathy with nitrofurantoins to treat urinary tract infections; and (3) hypoglycemia with some oral antidiabetic drugs.

A particularly important and interesting drug with reference to the elderly is digoxin, which is used to treat congestive heart failure. Digoxin is a digitalis glycoside that increases the strength of cardiac contraction and slows conduction. High levels induce vomiting, irregular pulse, and other effects. Because the drug, once prescribed, may be administered for the duration of life and because it is excreted through the kidney, the dosage in the elderly is about half that in the adult to avoid toxicity. The toxicity is enhanced by low serum potassium, which, again, occurs frequently in the elderly, owing to the vigorous use of the antihypertensive diuretics or to poor diet. Another prominent example comes from the use of over-the-counter analgesics, which are more likely to produce renal damage than aspirin. Yet another example are the anticholinergic agents used in treating Parkinsonism, depression, and also urinary incontinence. These cannot be readily handled by the aged kidney, they accumulate and produce severe side effects such as confusional states.

To minimize the consequence of drug toxicity in the elderly, one should assess renal competence before prescribing a drug treatment. Simultaneously, the dose should be appropriately adjusted, and/or the frequency of administration should be lowered or enhanced. The blood levels of the drug should be measured at frequent intervals both to establish optimal dose and to monitor and avoid possible toxicity throughout administration.

AGING-RELATED CHANGES IN THE FUNCTION OF THE LOWER URINARY TRACT

It has been written that the major health problems of the elderly can be easily recalled by listing them under five words *I*nstability, *I*mmobility, *I*ncontinence, *I*mpaired cognition, and *I*atrogenic diseases, all starting with the letter "I" (Feigenbaum, 1984). Of these, one of the most embarrassing and distressing is urinary incontinence. Failure of urinary continence often results from alterations in the function of some of the structures of the lower urinary tract, and in fact it may sometimes involve all these structures; it will, therefore, be one of the major topics to be discussed in this section.

Recent surveys show that incontinence occurs in 10 to 15 percent of community-dwelling elderly and in 50 to 60 percent of those living in institutions. However, statistics are not accurate inasmuch as people often fail to disclose the condition.

Many consider it inevitable and many refuse to admit to it. Normal control of bladder and urethral function is taken for granted by the majority of individuals and, in fact, remain efficient in most individuals well into old age. However, when it occurs, failure of this control is often considered a main threat to the welfare of those affected; it conjures up fears of rejection, which are often real and further restrict the social interactions of the elderly. Urinary incontinence may result not only from aging of the urinary tract, but may also reflect disorders of locomotion and of cognitive function and, as such, may be viewed as an indicator of overall decline of physiologic competence.

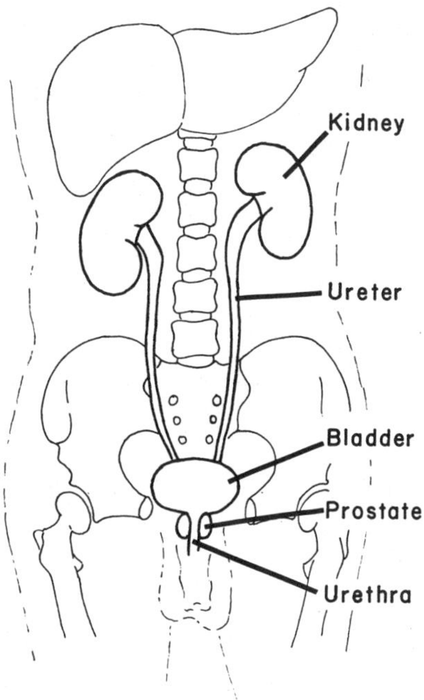

Figure 20–5. *Diagram of the major components of the urinary tract in man.* (Drawing by S. Oklund).

Structure and Function of the Lower Urinary Tract. The structures involved in transfer, storage, and excretion of urine are the ureter, the bladder, and the urethra (Figure 20–5). These retroperitoneal and pelvic organs are similar in both sexes except for the urethra and associated structures, such as the prostate, which are sex-specific.

All these structures consist essentially of smooth muscle lined by a mucosa. The largest is the bladder, which is a smooth muscle chamber comprised of a body, formed of the detrusor muscle with a weblike structure, a neck, and a trigone near the neck through which the ureters and urethra pass. The detrusor muscle, by contraction, is mainly responsible for emptying the bladder. Release of urine from the bladder is controlled by internal and external sphincters. The internal sphincter responds to pressure built up in the bladder by stimulation of stretch receptors; the external sphincter, composed of striated muscle, is under voluntary control (Figure 20–6). The main function of these structures is micturition, that is the process by which the bladder empties when it becomes filled with urine. The physiology of micturition and its disorders is still unclear.

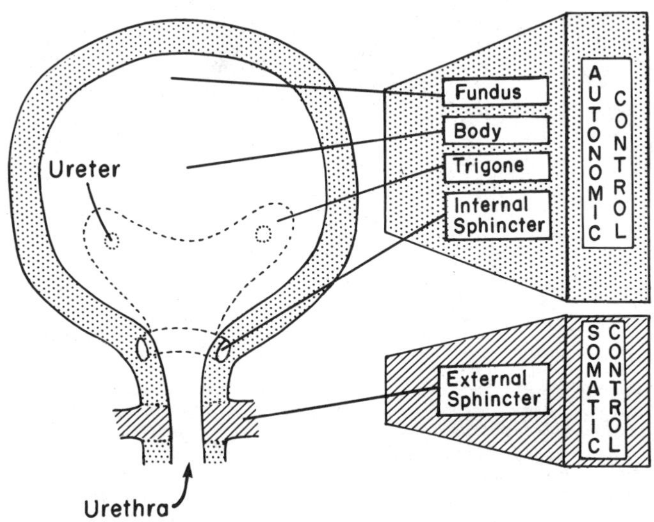

Figure 20–6. *Schematic of urinary bladder with structures under autonomic and somatic nervous control.* (Drawing by S. Oklund.)

Basically, micturition may be considered a special reflex, stimulated or inhibited by higher brain centers. Like defecation, it is subject to voluntary facilitation or inhibition. The events of micturition consist of progressive filling of the bladder with urine from the kidneys through the ureters. Once the bladder is filled, there is a tension threshold, which initiates a reflex to micturate, or, at least, a conscious desire to urinate.

The innervation of the bladder consists of three components, the two branches of the autonomic nervous system and the somatic nerves, which align with the type of muscle, smooth or striated. The autonomic fibers, both sympathetic and parasympathetic, act on smooth muscles (detrusor, trigone, internal sphincter) and the somatic fibers travel to the skeletal (striated) muscle (external sphincter). The act of micturition involves a complex coordination of neural and muscular responses leading to: (1) relaxation of the internal sphincters under parasympathetic control and of the external sphincter under somatic control; (2) constriction of the ureteral sphincters under sympathetic control; and (3) contraction of the detrusor muscle, under parasympathetic control. The entire sequence is under voluntary control and can be initiated or inhibited at will. In the absence of inputs from the cerebral cortex and other high brain centers, spinal reflexes may take over control and induce automatic emptying of the bladder whenever the retained volume of urine reaches a critical level. When the voluntary system is active, the desire to urinate becomes apparent after approximately 150 to 300 ml of fluid has collected.

URINARY CONTINENCE

In view of the complexity of the mechanisms regulating micturition, the high prevalence of incontinence in the elderly should not be surprising (Williams and Pannill, 1982). Continence depends on a long list of physiologic requirements, several of which undergo changes with aging (Table 20–8). These include: motivation to be continent, adequate cognitive function to understand the need for continence, mobility and dexterity to find and utilize the appropriate sanitary facilities. Normal urinary tract function, another necessary requirement for continence, depends on appropriate storage and emptying of the bladder; urine storage in the bladder depends, in turn, on its relaxation (absence of involuntary contractions, accommodation of increased urine volume under low presure, closure of sphincters, etc.) as well as its contraction (normal contractile mechanisms, absence of anatomic obstruction, sphincter relaxation, etc.). Physical and environmental barriers (e.g., bed rails, distant toilet location) must also be considered as possible causes of incontinence. Finally, the administration of drugs for a variety of ills and their effects, particularly on cognitive functions, may also contribute to incontinence.

Table 20–8. PHYSIOLOGIC REQUIREMENTS FOR CONTINENCE

Motivation to be continent
Adequate cognitive function
Adequate mobility and dexterity
Normal lower urinary tract function
- Storage
  - No involuntary bladder contractions
  - Appropriate bladder sensation
  - Closed bladder outlet
  - Low-pressure accommodation of urine
- Emptying
  - Normal bladder contraction
  - Lack of anatomic obstruction
  - Coordinated sphincter relaxation and bladder contraction

Absence of environmental or iatrogenic barriers

CAUSES AND COURSE OF URINARY INCONTINENCE IN THE ELDERLY

Urinary incontinence can be defined as the involuntary loss of urine sufficient in amount and frequency to be a social/health problem. It is most frequent in the elderly. It is stressful not only for those affected but also for their family and caregivers and can play a decisive role in the decision to place an elderly subject in a nursing home (Brocklehurst, 1982; Freed, 1982; Williams, 1983).

Although, urinary incontinence is not an inevitable consequence of aging, certain aging-related changes may contribute to the etiology of incontinence (Table 20–9). For example, in postmenopausal women, the

Table 20–9. AGE-RELATED CHANGES CONTRIBUTING TO INCONTINENCE

In Females

Estrogen deficiency
- Weak pelvic floor and bladder outlet
- Decreased urethral muscle tone
- Atrophic vaginitis

In Males

Increased prostate size
- Impaired urinary flow
- Urinary retention
- Detrusor instability

reduction in estrogen levels weakens the tissues around the pelvic floor and bladder outlet, decreases the tone of urethral smooth muscle, and causes atrophic vaginitis, all of which contribute to the decrease in urethral contractility and pressure with aging. In elderly men, hypertrophy (benign or malign) of the prostate represents one of the major causes of incontinence as it leads to a decline in urinary outflow rate, increased risk of urine retention, and increased instability of the detrusor muscle. Other causes include: delirium, effects of drugs such as anticholinergics (inducing urinary retention) and diuretics (inducing polyuria), diseases such as infections and diabetes. A mnemonic device to remember the major causes of acute incontinence is the word DRIP, where *D* stands for delirium, *R* for urinary retention due to anticholinergic drugs and restricted motility, *I* for infection, and *P* for polyuria due to diuretics or diabetes (Figure 20–7).

Many of the causes of acute incontinence may be easily diagnosed and reversed. However, when they have been addressed without any significant improvement, the incontinence is considered persistent and its management is considerably more difficult than the acute form. Persistent urinary incontinence is categorized into four types with corresponding specific etiologies and interventions:

Stress incontinence, due to increased intraabdominal pressure as in coughing and laughing, is caused by weakness of the pelvic floor musculature and is common in multiparous women:

Urge incontinence, due to inability to delay voiding after perception of bladder fullness, may be caused by mild outflow obstruction or by a central nervous system disorder such as stroke;

Overflow incontinence, due to a leakage of urine resulting from mechanical forces of an overdistended acontractile bladder, may be due to prostatic obstruction or to neurogenic disturbances such as neurogenic acontractile bladder; and

Functional incontinence, due to inability or psychologic unwillingness to get to the toilet, is caused by cognitive deficits, psychologic conditions, or unavailability of caretakers.

Differential diagnosis of incontinence types is based not only on the urinary symptoms but also on a complete history and physical examination including evaluation of mental status, physical activity, and ambulation. An abdominal examination should look for signs of bladder distention; a rectal examination for prostate size, rectal sphincter tone, and the presence of fecal impaction; a pelvic examination for uterine prolapse or atrophic vaginitis. Laboratory tests should include a urinalysis, a urine culture, and postvoid residual. This is a simple test to determine how much urine remains in the bladder after voiding. A catheter is placed in the bladder after the subject has voided and the volume of urine is measured. If the volume of urine is greater than 100 ml, then a more complete urologic or gynecologic evaluation is warranted.

MANAGEMENT OF INCONTINENCE

Management varies with the type of incontinence (Resnick, and Yalla, 1985) (Table 20–10) and includes strengthening of abdominal and pelvic muscles by exercise (Kegel's exercises) (Kegel, 1948; Kegel and

CAUSES OF ACUTE URINARY INCONTINENCE

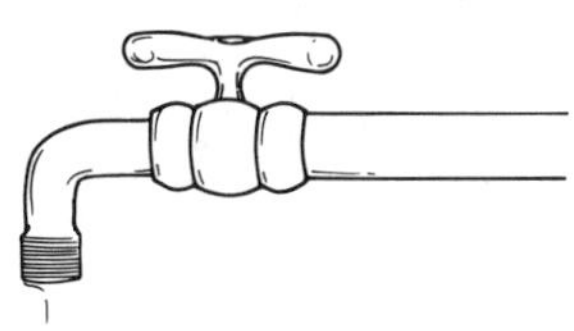

D elirium
R etention, Restricted mobility
I nfection, Inflammation, Impaction
P olyuria

Figure 20–7. *Mnemonic device for the major causes of acute urinary incontinence.*

Table 20–10. MANAGEMENT OF URINARY INCONTINENCE

TYPE	MANAGEMENT
Stress	Exercises Alpha-adrenergic agonists Estrogen Surgery
Urge	Bladder relaxants Surgery
Overflow	Surgery Catheterization
Functional	Habit training Scheduled toileting Hygenic devices

Powell, 1950); administration of estrogen; surgical bladder neck suspension for stress incontinence; administration of bladder relaxants for urge incontinence; intermittent catheterization or removal of the prostate, for overflow incontinence; habit training, scheduled toileting, undergarment devices, and indwelling catheterization (taking into account the risks involved, such as danger of infection) for functional incontinence.

As indicated above, urinary incontinence is a widespread problem among the elderly. Yet, despite its prevalence and its serious consequences for those affected, it receives little or no attention because of social taboos and ignorance of its physiologic and pathologic causes. Few of the health care providers are aware and knowledgeable of the problem. The assumption that once urinary incontinence occurs in an elderly individual it is to be accepted as an inevitable consequence of aging is false.

Urinary incontinence in the elderly can and must be treated in every case. Specific questioning as to urinary continence must be carried out in all routine evaluations of elderly patients, and in this, as in all disorders, an understanding of the physiopathology is essential for a rational diagnostic evaluation and treatment.

The Lower Urinary Tract and the Excretion and Action of Drugs. Dysfunction of the lower urinary tract amenable to pharmacologic intervention is rare, except for infections. Urinary retention, secondary to surgery or spinal cord injury, may also be relieved pharmacologically, but this and infections, although quite frequent in the elderly, are not exclusive of this age group. Infections are treated with antimicrobial agents and urinary retention with cholinergic agonists. The characteristics of neural control of micturition are presented in Table 20–11. Both parasympathetic and sympathetic impulses control bladder emptying, with cholinergic fibers inducing contraction of the detrusor muscle and relaxation of the internal sphincter muscle and thereby promoting emptying, and adrenergic fibers having the opposite effects. Somatic nerves also influence micturition by regulating the contraction/relaxation of the external sphincter. Cholinergic agonists (such as the drugs bethanecol and oxybutinin) are used to facilitate bladder emptying. While these drugs may act on other parasympathetic targets as well and, therefore, induce side effects, they are preferred to bladder catheterization with its attendant danger of infection.

In addition to being the target of specific drugs administered for therapeutic affects, the lower urinary tract, particularly the bladder, may bear the consequences or side effects of many prescribed as well as over-the-counter drugs. Thus, the bladder may become a victim of polypharmacy. Drugs in this category include decongestants, antihistamines, antidiarrheals, antipsychotics (such as phenothiazines), and tricyclic antidepressants. Even if they are taken as prescribed, their usage may add up to increasing toxicity. Most of these drugs have some autonomic activity. And most have anticholinergic actions; that is, they block the parasympathetic responses. For example, over-the-counter sleeping, asthma, and antidiarrheal medicines contain the belladonna alkaloids such as atropine or scopolamine or synthetic substitutes. They block the parasympathetic responses, inhibit micturition, and induce a degree of urinary retention (Table 20–12).

Table 20–11. NEURAL CONTROL OF MICTURITION

MUSCLE (TYPE)	PARASYMPATHETIC NERVES (CHOLINERGIC)	SYMPATHETIC NERVES (ADRENERGIC)	SOMATIC NERVES
Detrusor (smooth)	Contraction +++	Relaxation +	No effect
Trigone, internal sphincter (smooth)	Relaxation ++	Contraction ++	No effect
External sphincter (striated)	No effect	No effect	Relaxation

Table 20–12. DRUGS SECONDARILY AFFECTING THE LOWER URINARY TRACT

AUTONOMIC ACTION	DRUG TYPE	
Anticholinergic	Antidiarrheals Sedatives Antiasthmatics Antihistamines Antipsychotics (phenothiazines) Tricyclic antidepressants	Belladonna Alkaloids (over-the-counter)
Adrenergic	Decongestants	
Adrenergic block	Antihypertensives	

Acting on the other branch of the autonomic nervous system are the sympathetic or adrenergic drugs. Sympathomimetics, such as some decongestants and alpha-adrenergic blockers, relax the detrusor muscle, constrict the sphincters, and promote urine retention. Some of the alpha-adrenergic blockers, extensively utilized as antihypertensive drugs (see Chapter 24), have some additional side effects that are distressing in the older male, for they also prevent contraction of the vas deferens and inhibit ejaculation (Table 20–12).

AGING OF THE PROSTATE

Changes with aging in the prostate have already been briefly discussed in Chapter 14 together with the aging of the male reproductive function. The changes considered here are those affecting the function of the lower urinary tract, particularly the bladder—the neck of which is encircled by the prostate—and the urethra (Figure 20–8).

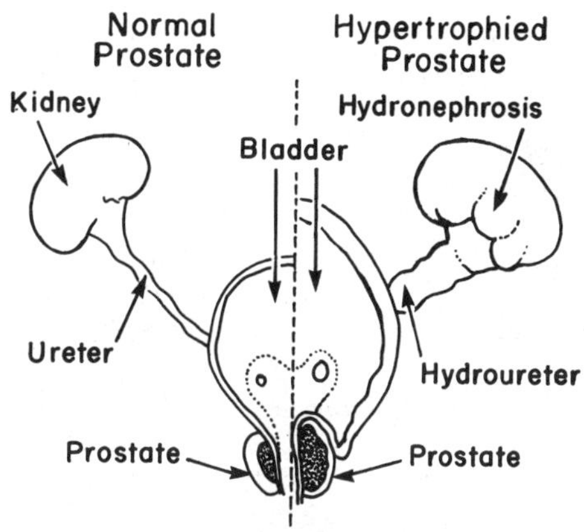

Figure 20–8. *Consequences of prostate hypertrophy.*

The enlarged prostate constricts the urethra with consequent difficulties in bladder emptying and the occurrence of retrograde filling of the ureters and of the renal pelvis (hydronephrosis). (Drawing by S. Oklund).

Structure. In the adult, the prostate, weighing about 20 g, consists of three to five lobes, which have distinct significance in the development of benign enlargement or tumors. Histologically, it is a tubuloalveolar gland with epithelial secretory cells distributed along a basement membrane and separated by an abundant fibromuscular stroma. The secretory product of the gland contributes not only fluid to the semen, but also several enzymes and constituents that stimulate the motility and viability of sperm.

Aging changes can be detected after the age of 40 years. Between 40 and 60 years, a series of alterations have been described that are classified as presenile. They consist essentially of atrophy of smooth muscle and proliferation of fibrous tissue and are associated with a flattening of the secretory epithelium. However, these changes are not uniform nor are they distributed throughout the gland; in fact, these presenile atrophic changes appear prominent in the outer regions while the inner mass undergoes hyperplasia. After the age of 60, the entire prostate undergoes a slower but more uniform atrophy with the accumulation of small concretions that represent residual secretory products.

While, with aging, there is an overall atrophy of the prostate, one-third or more of males over the age of 60 have a so-called benign prostatic hyperplasia (also referred to as hypertrophy), characterized by a nodular enlargement of prostatic tissue, particularly the inner portion of the gland, leading to significant obstruction of the urethra and urine outflow from the bladder (Glynn *et al.,* 1985; Hieble and Caine, 1986). The etiology of this enlargement is still obscure but has been ascribed, in addition to hormonal factors, to heredity, infection, atherosclerosis, sexual activity, etc. (Mawhinney, 1985). The incidence of the hypertrophy is extremely low in some Oriental races, reflecting, perhaps, a hereditary factor. The presence of functioning testes is necessary for the development of hyperplasia, as no cases have been found in eunuchs.

The prostatic enlargement is most frequently adjacent to the neck of the bladder and the urethra, where it obstructs urine outflow. This obstruction results in profound changes in the bladder, ureters, and kidneys. Micturition requires increased pressure of the detrusor muscle, producing hypertrophy and thickening of the bladder wall.

As the prostate continues to enlarge, the bladder finally reaches the limits of compensatory hypertrophy, after which there is a gradual decompensation and, eventually, complete failure to contract and to void with urinary retention.

The most serious consequence of prostatic enlargement is progression of obstruction to the point of retrograde filling of the ureters and renal pelvis, with eventual hydronephrosis and infection (pyelonephritis). If the obstruction is not relieved, renal failure with uremia and death follow (Figure 20–8).

DIAGNOSIS AND MANAGEMENT OF PROSTATIC ENLARGEMENT

Benign prostatic enlargement can be detected by palpation on rectal examination and by urinary signs, including hesitancy and straining to initiate micturition and reduced force and caliber of urinary stream. In most serious cases, the above signs are associated with hematuria, hydronephrosis, and pyelonephritis with attending signs and symptoms. In the absence of appropriate treatment, there is anura and uremia. All these signs and symptoms may be related to failure to empty the bladder. They can be relieved by the administration of alpha-adrenoreceptor antagonists (Caine, 1985; Hieble *et al.,* 1986) and catheterization of the bladder. The treatment of choice is surgical removal of the prostate and results in complete disappearance of all symptoms (Muir Gray, 1985; Farrar, 1985). In the case of prostatic carcinoma the treatment includes not only surgical removal, irradiation, and chemotherapy, but alteration of the sex hormone environment (Hammond *et al.,* 1978; Chlebowski and Brosman, 1982) (Table 20–13).

Table 20–13. THERAPEUTIC INTERVENTIONS FOR PROSTATIC ENLARGEMENT

Benign prostatic hyperplasia
Bladder catheterization
Surgical resection
Prostatic carcinoma
Castration
Estrogen administration
Antiandrogenic progestins
Surgery, irradiation, and chemotherapy

Hormonal Involvement in Prostatic Enlargement. The prostate is a target for androgens, the male sex hormones; as such it contains hormone receptors, particularly for the testosterone metabolite dihydrotestosterone, the most functionally active androgen. The testes secrete primarily androgens, but also small amounts of estrogens, which secretion, contrarily to the ovary, increases with aging. It has been suggested that prostatic enlargement and, possibly, prostate carcinoma are the consequence of the continuing levels of androgens as the reawakening of inductive stroma-epithelial influences (Neubauer *et al.,* 1985).

It is on this endocrinologic basis that prostatic carcinoma is treated either by decreasing the levels of androgens by castration or by administration of antiandrogens or estrogens. Such a hormonal treatment, while not particularly effective in benign prostatic hyperplasia, controls prostatic cancer in 70 to 80 percent of cases. Indeed, hormonal treatment is attempted first in incipient carcinomas and eventually associated with surgical resection, radiation, and chemotherapy. Of the hormonal treatment—castration, estrogens, or antiandrogenic progestins—it is still undecided which is preferable and, in fact, the best approach may vary with the type of cancer and the extent of metastases. For example, attempts have been made to classify prostatic carcinomas by androgen receptor analysis and to charter treatment accordingly (Trachtenberg *et al.,* 1982). But, unfortunately, data suggesting that dehydrotestosterone content and number of receptors of the primary tumor may predict the effectiveness of the antiandrogen treatment are still preliminary and need further clinical and experimental confirmation. Nevertheless the anticarcinogenic effectiveness of changing the androgenic environment on prostatic cancer represents a striking example of how changes in the hormonal environment may intervene in the course of malignant changes in a hormone target organ.

WATER AND ELECTROLYTE DISTRIBUTION AND ACID-BASE BALANCE

The kidney of the normal, healthy, older individual is well capable of maintaining water and electrolyte distribution and acid-base balance within homeostatic limits. This is remarkable as some changes do occur in body composition. With aging there is generally a loss of fat-free body weight and tissue mass, a reduction in body minerals, and a gain in body fat (Allen *et al.*, 1960; Forbes and Reina, 1970; Shukla *et al.*, 1973; Steen *et al.*, 1977). These age differences carry over to sex differences, with women showing a greater increase in total body weight owing to increased body fat and men maintaining their body weight. This maintained body weight is due to reciprocal changes in lean body mass (decreased) and body fat (increased) (Figure 20–9). Some gross comparisons in "reference man" between 25 and 70 years show the following percent changes, at age 25: fat, 14 percent; water, 61 percent; cell solids, 19 percent; and bone mineral, 6 percent; and at age 70: 30 percent, 53 percent, 12 percent, and 5 percent, respectively.

These changes in body composition may vary based on several factors related either to the individual or to the methodology. For example, gain in body fat often increases into the 60s but declines thereafter and, at all ages, depends on a number of variables among which the degree of physical activity is most consistent. In contrast, lean body mass or body cell mass (as measured by body density through water displacement or helium dilution) continues to decrease with aging, more in males than in females (Forbes and Reina, 1970). Some studies show a 3.6 percent decrease per decade from age 30 to 70 and, thereafter, 9 percent per decade. If nonfat mass is measured by

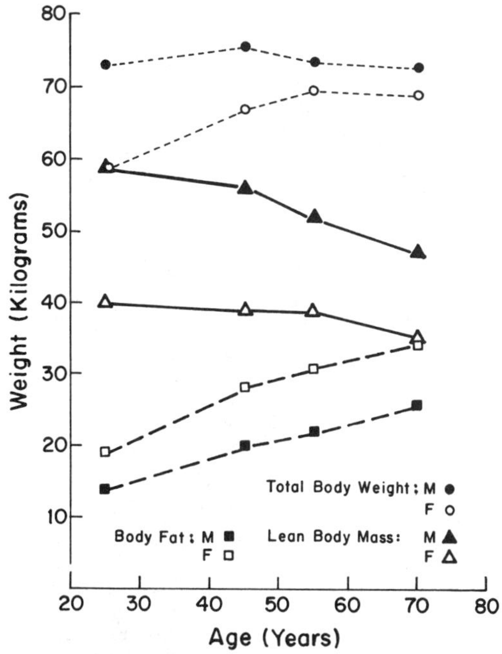

Figure 20–9. *Age-related weight changes in body composition of males and females.*

Males maintain overall body weight despite a decrease in lean body mass and an increase in body fat. Females not only have an increase in body weight, but this is mostly due to the increase of body fat.

total body potassium, one observes that potassium decreases with aging as does lean body mass early, but with advancing age, after 70 years, potassium decrease is more pronounced than lean body mass (Cox and Shalaby, 1981). It has been suggested that at older ages, the degenerative loss of lean tissue is in part replaced by other tissue that is low in potassium (Behnke and Myhre, 1982) and has a lower metabolic rate (Allen *et al.*, 1960). An alternative explanation with respect to regression of metabolic rate with aging is that the oxygen uptake of cells in old individuals is not significantly different than in young; rather there are fewer functioning cells (Shock *et al.*, 1963).

For example, while total body water is diminished with age, extracellular water remains unchanged and intracellular water decreases. The reduction in total body and intracellular water in the absence of change in extracellular water can be taken as further support for a loss of functioning cells with increasing age (see also Chapter 5).

References

Allen, T. H.; Anderson, E. C.; and Langham, W. H.: Total body potassium and gross body composition in relation to age. *J. Gerontol.*, **15**:348–357, **1960.**

Barrows, C. H.; Falzone, J. A.; and Shock, N. W.: Age difference in the succinoxidase activity of homogenates and mitochondria from the livers and kidneys of rats. *J. Gerontol.*, **15**:130–133, **1960.**

Beauchene, R. E.; Fanestil, D. D.; and Barrows, C. H.: The effects of age on active transport and sodium-potassium-activated ATPase activity in renal tissue of rats. *J. Gerontol.*, **20**:306–310, **1965.**

Bengele, H. H.; Mathias, R. S.; Perkins, J. H.; and Alexander, E. A.: Urinary concentrating defect in the aged rat. *Am. J. Physiol.*, **240**:147–150, **1981.**

Behnke, A. R., and Myhre, L. G.: Body composition and aging: A longitudinal study spanning four decades. In Loeppky, J. A., and Riedesel, M. L. (eds.): *Oxygen Transport to Human Tissues*, Elsevier, New York, **1982.**

Bennett, W. M.; Luft, F.; and Porter, G. A.: Pathogenesis of renal failure due to aminoglycosides and contrast media used in roentgenography. *Am. J. Med.*, **69**:767–774, **1980.**

Bolton, W. K., and Sturgill, B. C.: Ultrastructure of the aging kidney. In Johnson, J. E., Jr. (ed.): *Aging and Cell Structure*, Vol. 1, Plenum Press, New York, **1981.**

Brenner, B. M.; Meyer, T. W.; and Hostetter, T. H.: Dietary protein intake and the progressive nature of kidney disease: The role of hemodynamically mediated glomerular injury in the pathogenesis of progressive glomerular sclerosis in aging, renal ablation and intrinsic renal disease. *N. Engl. J. Med.*, **307**:652–659, **1982.**

Brocklehurst, J. C.: Incontinence. In Ham, R. J. (ed.): *Geriatric Medicine Annual*, Medical Economics Books, Oradell, NJ, **1982.**

Brod, J.: Changes of renal function with age. *Scripta Medica*, **41**:223–229, **1968.**

Caine, M.: Clinical experience with adrenoceptor antagonists in benign prostatic hypertrophy. *Fed. Proc.*, **45**:2604–2607, **1985.**

Chlebowski, R. T., and Brosman, S. A.: Diagnosis and treatment of genitourinary malignancy. In Block, J. B. (ed.): *Oncology*, John Wiley & Sons, New York, **1982.**

Coulam, C. B., and Zincke, H.: Successful pregnancy in a renal transplant patient with a 75-year-old kidney. *Surg. Forum*, **32**:457–459, **1981.**

Cox, J. R., and Shalaby, W. A.: Potassium changes with age, *Gerontology*, **27**:340–344, 1981.

Cox, J. R., and Shalaby, W. A.: Renal disease. In Pathy, M. S. J. (ed.): *Principles and Practice of Geriatric Medicine*, John Wiley & Sons, Chichester, UK, **1985.**

Davies, D. F., and Shock, N. W.: Age changes in glomerular filtration rate, effective renal plasma flow, and tubular excretory capacity in adult males. *J. Clin. Invest.*, **29**:496–507, **1950.**

Durakovic, Z., and Mimica, M.: Proteinuria in the elderly. *Gerontology*, **29**:121–124, **1983.**

Everitt, A. V.; Porter, B. D.; and Wyndham, J. R.: Effects of caloric intake and dietary composition on the development of proteinuria, age-associated renal disease, longevity in the male rat. *Gerontology*, **28**:168–175, **1982.**

Farrar, D. J.: The bladder and urethra. In Pathy, M. S. J. (ed.): *Principles and Practice of Geriatric Medicine*, John Wiley & Sons, Chichester, UK, **1985.**

Feigenbaum, L.: Geriatric medicine and the elderly patient. In Krugg, M. A., and Chatton, M. Y. (eds.): *Current Medical Diagnosis and Treatment*, Lange, Los Altos, CA, **1984.**

Forbes, G. B., and Reina, J. C.: Adult lean body mass declines with age: Some longitudinal observations. *Metabolism*, **19**:653–663, **1970.**

Freed, S. Z.: Urinary incontinence in the elderly. *Hosp. Pract.*, **17**:81–94, **1982.**

Frocht, H., and Fillit, H.: Renal disease in the geriatric patient. *J. Am. Geriatr. Soc.*, **32**:28–43, **1984.**

Glynn, R. J.; Campion, E. W.; Bouchard, G. R.; and Silbert, J. E.: The development of benign prostatic hyperplasia among volunteers in the normative aging study. *Am. J. Epidemiol.*, **121**:78–90, **1985.**

Hammond, G. L.; Kontturi, M.; Vihko, P.; and Vihko, R.: Serum steroids in normal males and patients with prostatic diseases. *Clin. Endocrinol.*, **9**:113–121, **1978.**

Helderman, J. H.; Vestal, R. E.; Rowe, J. W.; Tobin, J. D.; Andres, R.; and Robertson, G. L.: The response of arginine vasopressin to intravenous ethanol and hypertonic saline in man: The impact of aging. *J. Gerontol.*, **33**:39–47, **1978.**

Hieble, J. P.; Boyce, A. J.; and Caine, M.: Comparison of the α-adrenoceptor characteristics in human and canine prostate. *Fed. Proc.*, **45**:2609–2614, **1986.**

Hieble, J. P., and Caine, M.: Etiology of benign prostatic hyperplasia and approaches to its pharmacological management. *Fed. Proc.*, **45**:2601–2603, **1986.**

Kegel, A. H.: Progressive resistance exercise in the functional restoration of the perineal muscles. *Am. J. Obstet. Gynecol.*, **56**:238–248, **1948.**

Kegel, A. H., and Powell, T. O.: The physiologic treatment of urinary stress incontinence. *J. Urol.*, **63**:808–814, **1950.**

Kirkland, J. L.; Lye, M.; Levy, D. W.; and Banerjee, A. K.: Patterns of urine flow and electrolyte excretion in healthy elderly people. *Br. Med. J.*, **287**:1665–1667, **1983.**

Lindeman, R. D.; Lee, T. D.; Yiengst, M. J.; and Shock, N. W.: Influence of age, renal diseases, hypertension, diuretics and calcium on antidiuretic responses to suboptimal infusion of vasopressin. *J. Lab. Clin. Med.*, **68**:206–223, **1966.**

Lindeman, R. D.; Tobin, J.; and Shock, N. W.: Longitudinal studies on the rate of decline in renal function with age. *J. Am. Geriatr. Soc.*, **33**:278–285, **1985.**

Mawhinney, M. G.: Etiological considerations for the growth of stroma in benign prostatic hyperplasia. *Fed. Proc.*, **45**:2615–2617, **1985.**

McDonald, R. K.; Solomon, D. H.; and Shock, N. W.: Ageing as factor in renal hemodynamic changes induced by standardized pyrogen. *J. Clin. Invest.*, **30**:457–462, **1951.**

Miller, J. H., and Shock, N. W.: Age differences in renal tubular response to antidiuretic hormone. *J. Gerontol.*, **8**:446–450, **1953.**

Matus, A. J.; Simmons, R. L.; Kjellstrand, C. M.; Buselmeier, T. J.; and Najarian, J. S.: Transplantation of the aging kidney. *Transplantation*, **21**:160–161, **1976.**

Muir Gray, J. A.: Incontinence in the Community. In Pathy, M. S. J. (ed.): *Principles and Practice of Geriatric Medicine*, John Wiley & Sons, Chichester, UK, **1985.**

Neubauer, B. L.; Best, K. L.; Hoover, D. M.; Slisz, M. L.; Van Frank, R. M.; and Goode, R. L.: Mesenchymal-epithelial interactions as factors influencing male accessory sex organ growth in the rat. *Fed. Proc.*, **45**:2618–2626, **1985.**

Nicholls, A. J.; Waldek, S.; Platts, M. M.; Moorhead, P. J.; and Brown, C. B.: Impact of continuous ambulatory peritoneal dialysis on treatment of renal failure in patients aged over 60. *Br. Med. J.*, **13**:304–307, **1984.**

Nunez, M.; Iglesias, C. G.; Roman, A. B.; Commes, J. L. K.; Becerra, L. C.; Rome, J. M. T.; and Del Pozo,

S. D.: Renal handling of sodium in old people. A functional study. *Age Ageing,* **7**:178–181, **1978.**

Oliveria, D. B. G., and Winearls, C. G.: Acute renal failure in the elderly can have a good prognosis. *Age Ageing,* **13**:304–407, **1984.**

Pashko, L. L.; Fairman, D. K.; and Schwartz, A. G.: Inhibition of proteinuria development in aging Sprague-Dawley rats and C57BL/6 mice by long-term treatment with dehydroepiandrosterone. *J. Gerontol.,* **41**:433–438, **1986.**

Phillips, T. L., and Leong, G. F.: Kidney cell proliferation after unilateral nephrectomy as related to age. *Cancer Res.,* **27**:286–292, **1967.**

Phillips, T. L.; Rolls, B. J.; Ledingham, J. G. G.; *et al.*: Reduced thirst after water deprivation in healthy elderly men. *N. Engl. J. Med.,* **311**:753–759, **1984.**

Resnick, N. M., and Yalla, S. V.: Management of urinary incontinence in the elderly. *N. Engl. J. Med.,* **313**:800–805, **1985.**

Rowe, J. W.; Andres, R.; Tobin, J. D.; Norris, A. H.; and Shock, N. W.: The effect of age on creatinine clearance in men: A cross-sectional and longitudinal study. *J. Gerontol.,* **31**:155–163, **1976.**

Shock, N. W.: Kidney function tests in aged males. *Geriatrics,* **1**:232–239, **1946.**

Shock, N. W.; Watkin, D. M.; Yiengst, M. J.; Norris, A. H.; Gaffney, G. W.; Gregerman, R. I.; and Falzone, M. D.: Age differences in the water content of the body as related to basal oxygen consumption in males. *J. Gerontol.,* **18**:1–8, **1963.**

Shukla, K. K.; Ellis, K. J.; Dombrowski, C. S.; and Cohn, S. H.: Physiological variation of total-body potassium in man. *Am. J. Physiol.,* **224**:271–274, **1973.**

Smalley, J. W.: Age related changes in the amino acid composition of human glomerular basement membrane. *Exp. Gerontol.,* **15**:43–52, **1980.**

Steen, B.; Bruce, A.; Isaksson, B.; Lewin, T.; and Svanborg, A.: Body composition in 70-year-old males and females in Gothenburg, Sweden. A population study. *Acta. Med. Scand.,* **611**:87–112, **1977.**

Trachtenberg, J.; Bujnovsky, P.; and Walsh, P. C.: Androgen receptor content of normal and hyperplastic human prostate. *J. Clin. Endocrinol. Metab.,* **54**:17–21, **1982.**

Van Bezooijen, K. F. A.; deLeeuw-Israel, F. R.; and Hollander, C. F.: Long-term functional aspects of syngeneic orthotopic rat kidney grafts of different ages. *J. Gerontol.,* **29**:11–19, **1974.**

Williams, M. E.: A critical evaluation of the assessment technology for urinary continence in older persons. *J. Am. Geriatr. Soc.,* **31**:657–664, **1983.**

Williams, M. E., and Pannill, F. C.: Urinary incontinence in the elderly. *Ann. Intern. Med.,* **97**:895–907, **1982.**

CHAPTER

21 AGING OF THE GASTROINTESTINAL TRACT AND LIVER

The study of the aging of the gastrointestinal system discloses few alterations in gastrointestinal function, although cellular changes occur and involve secretory activity and motility of the major structures. Such changes are similar to those elsewhere in the body, but in the absence of localized disease, function is usually maintained in line with or even above requirements. Disorders and diseases, however, become more common with advancing age and involve all levels of the gastrointestinal tract, starting with the mouth and extending to the rectum, anus, and pelvic floor musculature (Figure 21–1).

Of the two major appendices of the gastrointestinal tract, the liver, the largest gland in the body, and the pancreas, with both endocrine and exocrine functions, the liver appears to be severely affected by aging. Given the numerous functions of this organ, alterations with aging have widespread repercussions for the well-being of the entire organism. However, in the liver as in the whole organism, not all functions are affected simultaneously or with equal severity. The bile, produced in the liver for optimal digestion and absorption of lipids, is important at all ages and is particularly crucial in the elderly, whose poor diet may be deficient in several essential elements (e.g., lipid-soluble vitamins); bile formation remains quite stable in healthy individuals well into old age. Another important hepatic function, the detoxification of many (therapeutic and recreational) drugs, is progressively restricted with advancing age and contributes, with the increased use of drugs (polypharmacy), to the greater susceptibility of the elderly to the potential toxicity of excessive or incorrect medication (Chapter 24). In the pancreas, the changes with aging of endocrine functions have been discussed in Chapter 16. Changes with aging of the exocrine functions, which involve powerful protein-splitting (proteolytic) enzymes, may lead to impaired digestion and absorption.

In this chapter, aging of the gastrointestinal tract will be presented first, followed by a brief discussion of the aging pancreas and liver. While in this chapter the focus will be on how late and how well digestion and absorption are retained, it must be kept in mind that limiting food intake may have beneficial effects. Since early studies, more than 40 years ago, evidence has been accumulating steadily that a dietary reduction of caloric intake or of specific food constituents will prolong life significantly in rodents (McCay *et al.*, 1935). The earlier the restriction begins, the more successful is the subsequent retardation of growth and prolongation of life (Segall and Timiras, 1976; Segall *et al.*, 1978, 1983). Such dietary effects have also been demonstrated in other species. It will always remain unthinkable to perform such restrictive experiments in humans. However, encouragement to limit caloric intake and to prevent or treat obesity is easily justified. Not only is life prolonged, but frequency and severity of a variety of pathologic changes are reduced in experimental animals (Chapter 25).

AGING OF THE GASTROINTESTINAL TRACT

The major function of the gastrointestinal (GI) system is to provide the organism with nutritive substances, vitamins, minerals, and fluids. The elderly are a heterogeneous group of individuals in many important aspects of nutrition. This is true in relation not only to age, but also to degree of health and disease, degree of physical activity, as well as psychologic and socioeconomic characteristics. Thus, "young elderly" (aged 65 to 75 years) are distinguished from "old elderly" (over 75 years). However, the latest edition of the American Recom-

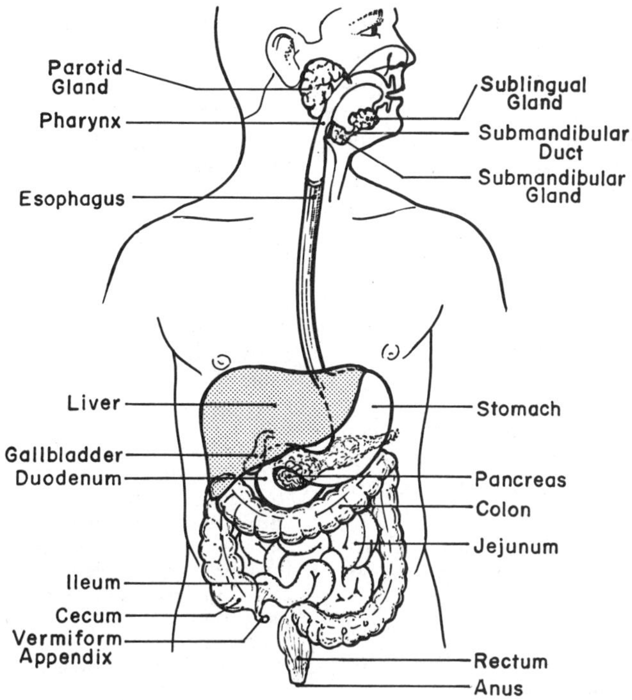

Figure 21–1. *Schematic representation of the gastrointestinal tract, with the liver and pancreas.*

mended Dietary Allowances (Food and Nutrition Board, 1980) groups individuals aged 51 years and older together into a single age group. Nevertheless, the elderly display a wide variety of individual differences, none better described than the aging-related changes in the mouth.

TEETH, GUMS, AND ORAL MUCOSA

In the mouth, food is mixed with saliva, chewed, and propelled into the esophagus. Chewing (mastication), a matter of breaking down large food particles, is a function of the teeth. The saliva contains the digestive enzyme ptyalin, which plays a minor role in starch digestion. It also contains mucin, a glycoprotein that lubricates the food and facilitates its passage through the esophagus on the way to the stomach.

With aging, the teeth undergo characteristic changes: they acquire a yellowish-brown discoloration from staining by extrinsic pigments from beverages, tobacco, and oral bacteria. The pulp recedes from the crown, the root canal becomes narrow and threadlike, and the roots become brittle and fracture easily during extractions. The odontoblast layer lining the pulp chamber becomes irregular and discontinuous and the pulp undergoes fibrosis and calcification (Walker, 1985). Concomitantly, with faster destruction than reconstruction of the dentin, the mandibular and maxillary bones in which the teeth are embedded undergo the same aging processes as all other bones (Tonna, 1979) (Chapter 22). Osteoporotic changes (i.e., increased bone loss) (Chapters 13 and 22) result in looser teeth, contributing ultimately to tooth loss.

The surfaces of the teeth involved in chewing become progressively worn down throughout life. This attrition is not only a consequence of chewing but also, in some individuals, of the habit of grinding or clenching the teeth together (so-called bruxism), often during REM sleep (Chapter 10). Abrasion (sometimes due to improper brushing) and erosion (often aggravated by the demineralizing action of soft drinks) are frequent. Although new caries (i.e., cavities with decay) are uncommon in the elderly, loss of interest in dental hygiene and a decline in dexterity needed for toothbrushing may lead to plaque accumulation and caries (Baum, 1981). These can be prevented by restoring appropriate hygienic measures self-managed or provided by a dental hygienist.

Recession of the gingivae (gums) occurs in all elderly. The epithelial attachment that forms a cuff around the tooth at the interface with the gums recedes and opens the way to accumulation of particulate material with bacteria (i.e., plaque), swelling, inflammatory hyperplasia, or low-grade infection. Whether such a gum recession is a physiologic process or the result of chronic peridontitis (i.e., inflammation of the periodontal membrane) due to a variety of local irritative factors remains to be clarified. Indeed, after the age of 40, chronic periodontitis is the major cause of tooth loss (Allen, 1944). Periodontal disease is not only common in aging humans, but it is usually found in aging experimental animals (e.g., mice, rats, dogs, monkeys, baboons). In both humans and experimental animals, the disease is due to local factors as well as some systemic predisposing disease (e.g., diabetes) or stress (e.g., cold exposure) (Toga *et al.*, 1979). Indeed, in germ-free animals, recession of gums does not occur with age (Amstad-Jossi and Schroeder, 1978).

With aging, the epithelium of the oral mucosa becomes relatively thin and atrophic. Specialized structures, such as the papillae of the tongue, also become atrophic (Chapter 11); others, like the palatal mucosa, undergo edema and keratinization (i.e., accumulation of a highly insoluble protein, keratin), a condition that seems to be delayed or prevented by the wearing of dentures. Keratin, also a normal component of the skin, is the product of epidermal cells (Skerrow, 1986) and undergoes characteristic changes with development (Fuchs and Hanukoglu, 1986) as well as extensive cross-linking with age and a number of conditions. The oral epithelium also exhibits increasing amounts of glycogen and alterations in collagen (Shklar, 1979).

Oral Diseases in the Elderly. While the above changes in oral structures with aging are gradual and relatively benign, they may predispose the involved tissues to a variety of pathologic conditions. Although very few oral diseases are characteristic of old age, many pathologic states are seen with greater frequency than in younger individuals. Among these, chronic periodontal disease (discussed above), xerostomia, mucositis and mucosal atrophy, leukoplakia, and malignant neoplasia (the latter beyond the scope of the present discussion) are the most common (Walker, 1985).

Xerostomia, or dry mouth, may be due to a large variety of factors in the elderly: primarily atrophy of the salivary glands and decline of salivary secretion. It may also be due to systemic disease (e.g., diabetes) or to heavy cigarette smoking or be a symptom of anxiety and depression. Several medications (antihypertensives, antidepressants, antihistamines) also affect salivary flow and may induce xerostomia, depending on the dose, in a smaller or larger number of patients. In this condition, the oral cavity is extremely dry; the mucosa appears red dry, fissured, and often coated with food particles and sloughed-off cells. Therapy involves cessation of the underlying cause (e.g., smoking) or treatment of the underlying systemic disease (diabetes) or the use of artificial saliva (Shannon, 1979). The decrease in salivary volume is associated with enzymatic changes, such as reduction in amylase activity and in electrolytes (Grad, 1954; Garrett, 1962).

Mucositis and *mucosal atrophy* are frequent occurrences in elderly individuals in whom the oral mucosa has become atrophic and less resistant to the irritation of oral noxious stimuli such as trauma, hot foods, smoking, to infections, and to chemotherapeutic agents or radiation therapy. These stimuli result in a chronic inflammatory process (mucositis) and, in more severe cases, in ulceration with pain.

Leukoplakia, or keratosis, is hyperplasia of the mucosa with accumulation of keratin, hence, the name "white patch." It is rarely seen in young individuals but is frequent after 60 years. It may be caused by pipe or cigarette smoking, by ill-fitting dentures, or by infections (e.g., candidiasis). It is associated with precancerous histologic alterations, in which case it must be treated as if it were a carcinoma (Waldron and Shafer, 1975).

SWALLOWING AND PHARYNGOESOPHAGEAL FUNCTION IN THE ELDERLY

Dysphagia, or difficulty in swallowing, is a common complaint of elderly individuals. It can result from alteration of any of the components of deglutition, a very complex motor activity, involving the mouth, the esophagus, and several levels of nervous control.

Deglutition, or swallowing, is a reflex response that pushes the contents of the mouth into the esophagus. The afferent stimuli are generated by the voluntary collection of the oral contents on the tongue and their propulsion backward into the pharynx and are carried by several nerves to the medulla oblongata, where they are integrated. The efferent fibers are carried also by several nerves to the pharyngeal musculature and the tongue. Inhibition of respiration and closure of the glottis are part of the reflex. Swallowing is impossible when the mouth is open; it is very rapid during eating but continues at a slower rate between meals.

Upon swallowing, the upper portion of the esophagus relaxes to permit entrance of the swallowed material, which then progresses through the esophagus to the stomach by peristaltic movements (circular waves). In the standing position liquids and semisolid foods may fall by gravity to the lower esophagus where the musculature relaxes upon swallowing and permits the passage of food in the stomach.

If the act of swallowing is divided, as it was more than a century ago by the French Magendie (1824), into three stages, it can be seen that all stages are affected by aging (Patel *et al.*, 1983). The first stage, in which the material to be swallowed is passed from the mouth to the pharynx, is a voluntary act, mediated through stimulation of skeletal muscles. These undergo aging-related changes with atrophy and increasing weakness common to all skeletal muscles (Chapter 22). The second stage, reflex in nature, is very short in duration but very complex in its neural control and involves the relaxation of the sphincter between pharynx and esophagus. In the third stage, reflex transport sweeps the contents onward through smooth muscle peristalsis. All these stages, which require a precisely timed contraction/relaxation sequence, are affected; they may become desynchronized and result in less efficient deglutition. Dysphagia of varying degrees of severity is a common complaint. In the most severe cases, dysphagia is associated with symptoms of choking and drowning with aspiration or regurgitation of food, while mild dysphagia may be found in otherwise healthy elderly. Severe dysphagia is always a symptom of a systemic disease, either of the muscle or of the nervous system. In addition to being an uncomfortable and unpleasant symptom, dysphagia leads to reduced and altered nutritional intake, particularly in the elderly. Malnutrition, weight loss, and dehydration are common features of this condition (Hellemans *et al.*, 1984).

Presbyesophagus (or old esophagus) is the most common disorder of the esophageal motility associated with old age (Soergel *et al.*, 1964; Hollis and Castell, 1974). Radiologic and manometric studies reveal an increased incidence of nonperistaltic contractions (with failure of the lower esophageal sphincter to relax), a reduced amplitude of peristaltic contractions, and a decreased responsiveness to cholinergic stimulation.

Other motor disorders of the esophagus in addition to those mentioned above and occurring at all ages, including old age, are: achalasia, in which food accumulates in the esophagus and the organ becomes extremely dilated; sphincter incompetence, which permits reflux of acid from the stomach; aerophagia, or ingestion of air, which can be regurgitated or absorbed in the intestine or expelled as flatus.

THE STOMACH AND DUODENUM: AGE-RELATED PHYSIOLOGIC AND PATHOLOGIC CHANGES

The stomach serves as a food reservoir and, by its churning movements (due to the presence of three smooth muscle layers), breaks down ingested food. It secretes the gastric juice, which contains a variety of substances: digestive enzymes (e.g., pepsin), mucus (which lubricates the food), hydrochloric acid (which destroys the ingested bacteria, aids in protein digestion, and is necessary for the transformation of iron for the synthesis of hemoglobin), hormones (gastrin, glucagon, somatostatin), and special peptides (VIP, substance P).

In addition, the cells of the gastric mucosa secrete an intrinsic factor (a glycoprotein) necessary for the absorption of vitamin B_{12} from the small intestine. Vitamin B_{12} is necessary for the maturation of red blood cells, and deficiency of the vitamin or intrinsic factor leads to a severe type of anemia (pernicious anemia).

With aging, some of the major changes in the stomach and neighboring duodenum involve the hydrochloric acid and pepsin secretions, which are decreased, under basal conditions, in the normal elderly (Figure 21–2). Changes with aging in some of the

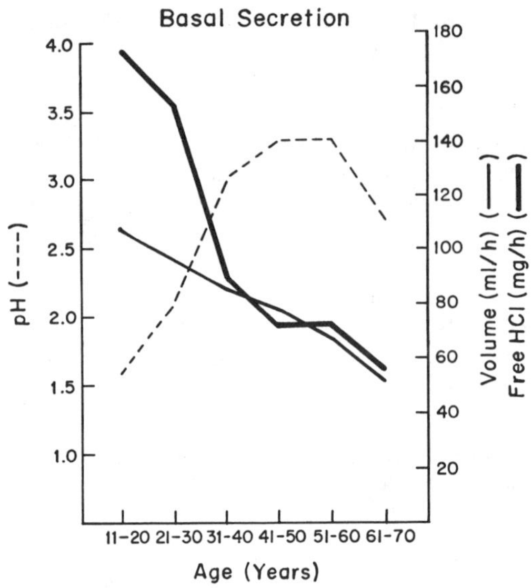

Figure 21–2. *Changes with age, under basal (pre-prandial) conditions of gastric secretion.*

Note, with advancing years, the moderate decrease in total volume and the greater decrease in free hydrochloric acid (HCl). As the free HCl decreases, pH increases.

digestive enzymes may be consequent directly to changes in the enzyme-secreting cells and organs or indirectly to hormonal and neural regulatory alterations (Table 21–1). The direct changes may involve cellular or enzymatic reduction (Chapters 5 and 6). More likely, the failure lies in alterations in the regulatory mechanism of enzyme synthesis and release due either to a change in the hormonal or neural stimuli or to a change in response (altered receptors).

However, with increasing age, the incidence of peptic ulcers is a common condition of Western society. Increased acid secretion is the major feature of gastric and duodenal ulcers. The number of parietal cells is increased, perhaps because of genetic predisposition or as a result of increased stimulation. Vagal overactivity has also been demonstrated. Acid production is inhibited in normal aged subjects by low intragastric pH, but in duodenal ulcer, this inhibition fails.

Regulation of Gastric and Duodenal Acidity. The hydrochloric acid secreted by the parietal cells in the body of the stomach is concentrated enough to produce tissue damage. However, in the normal adult, the mucosa of the stomach and the duodenum (the first part of the small intestine in proximity of the stomach) does not become irritated or digested. The gastric mucus was once thought to serve as a protective layer, but now the surface membranes of the mucosal cells and the tight junctions between the cells are considered the main barrier to acid damage. It appears that the stomach also has an alkaline secretion, which may play a role in protecting the stomach. In the duodenum, cells from the Brunner's glands secrete a thick alkaline mucus that probably helps protect the duodenal mucosa from the gastric acid. Independent of the Brenner's cells, duodenal cells secrete appreciable amounts of bicarbonate, which contribute to this protection.

A number of substances (aspirin, ethanol, caffeine, bile salts) tend to disrupt this barrier and cause gastric irritation. Disruption of the barrier may be severe enough to induce ulcers, i.e., loss of cells with bleeding and necrosis of tissues. These ulcers, called peptic ulcers (for their relation to digestion), may be situated in the stomach (usually near the pylorus, the region close to the duodenum) or the duodenum and will then be designated as gastric or duodenal ulcers.

Excessive acid production plays a major role in the pathogenesis of these ulcers. Gastrin, one of the gastrointestinal hormones, secreted by the gastric mucosal cells as well as the pituitary, pancreas (fetal), and brain, also stimulates gastric acid and pepsin secretion. In this manner, increased secretion of gastrin would contribute to the genesis of peptic ulcers. On the other hand, gastrin might also participate to some degree in regenerating processes inasmuch as it stimulates mucosal growth and gastric motility. The growth-promoting action may occur through stimulation of the epidermal growth hormone, secreted by the duodenal Brunner's glands.

Table 21–1. POSSIBLE MECHANISMS OF AGING-RELATED CHANGES IN DIGESTIVE ENZYME SECRETION

Enzyme-Secreting Organs	
Reduction in:	Number of cells Enzyme concentration Enzyme synthesis and release
Hormonal and Neural Regulation of Enzyme-Secreting Organs	
Reduction in:	Number of gastrointestinal endocrine cells Hormone concentration
Impairment of:	Sensitivity of endocrine cells to digestive stimuli
Alteration of:	Distribution and metabolism of gastrointestinal hormones Number and affinity of endocrine or neural receptors

The incidence of peptic ulcer is on the rise in developing countries, particularly India and Africa. In Western countries, including the United States, it is decreasing in the overall population (perhaps reflecting advances in treatment) but increasing in the elderly group. In this group not only is the incidence on the rise, but the severity of the disease and its consequences are also greater than in younger individuals (Marks, 1984).

Elderly patients tend to predominate among those admitted to hospitals for peptic disease, and patients over 60 years of age account for nearly 50 percent of those with gastric and 40 percent of those with duodenal ulcers (Morris and Dew, 1985). In these individuals, age is the major mortality risk. While, in many cases, the causes of the disease are unknown, drugs (aspirin, alcohol) and cigarette smoking may be important factors in the pathogenesis of the disease.

Management of Peptic Ulcer. Procedures used in the treatment of ulcers include dietary, pharmacologic, and surgical interventions. Pharmacologic interventions are aimed at inhibiting acid secretion and enhancing mucosal resistance to acid. A variety of antacids, most of which contain aluminum and magnesium hydroxide or calcium carbonate, are available. Inhibition of parasympathetic inputs (which stimulate acid secretion) by atropine gives variable responses and has many undesirable side effects. Hydrogen receptor blockers, such as cimetidine (the most commonly prescribed drug in the United States) and ranitidine, are also often used. Drugs capable of inhibiting $Na^{+}K^{+}$-ATPase and epidermal growth hormone are at the experimental stage. A number of substances increase the resistance of mucosal cells to acid by forming adherent protein complexes at the ulcer site. Usually the pharmacologic treatment is associated with special diets and cessation of cigarette smoking, inasmuch as healing rates of duodenal ulcer are probably adversely affected by cigarette smoking and the incidence of ulcers is higher in smokers than in nonsmokers (Sonnenberg *et al.*, 1980). If pharmacologic, dietary, and hygienic measures fail, surgical intervention is advisable, keeping in mind the special caution necessary in the older patient.

In addition to ulcers, disruption of the protective mucosal barrier may frequently occur with aging as a consequence of a variety of factors and contribute to gastric pathology. Whether alterations in the mucosal cells are spontaneous or secondary to chronic toxicity of drugs and alcohol or to mucosal ischemia due to hypotension remains unanswered. Disruption of the barrier allows luminal hydrogen ions to diffuse into mucosal cells causing damage. Gastrointestinal bleeding is often a consequence of duodenal and gastric ulcers (Kumpuris, 1983); it may also be associated with less severe mucosal alterations such as *gastritis* and gastric erosion, a form of gastric irritation and inflammation. The incidence of these alterations increases with aging. For example, the incidence of chronic and acute gastritis increases with age so that evidence of it is found in 50 percent of individuals over the age of 60 years. In view of the overall declining physiologic competence of the elderly and the debilitating nature of the disease, mortality rises rapidly with advancing age.

Vascular Alterations. As indicated above, gastrointestinal bleeding in the elderly presents a special problem—both incidence and mortality are high after the age of 60. Another cause of bleeding in the elderly are vascular malformations (ectasias) of the intestinal vessels, which are easily subject to bleeding. These ectasias occur throughout the GI tract, particularly the small bowels (40 percent), stomach (30 percent) and colon (25 percent). They are associated with aortic stenosis, age-related degenerative changes in tissues, and inherited collagen or ground substance defects (McGinty *et al.*, 1983).

Circulatory alterations are not confined to bleeding but also encompass ischemia, which can lead to mesenteric infarction. Ischemia may produce symptoms of varying severity from transient intestinal discomfort, to abdominal angina, infarction or, in cases of segmental ischemia, to ischemic colitis (Tune *et al.*, 1983; Tytgat and van Dongen, 1984).

ABSORPTION OF NUTRIENTS AND MALABSORPTION

Adequate nutrition is indispensable at all ages but especially in the young, who must provide extra calories for growth, and in the old, whose gastrointestinal function is only marginal. Indeed, dietary interventions to ensure a long and vigorous life have been popular for many centuries. Once achieved, old age has been recognized as a period requiring special attention to dietary habits (Beaumont and James, 1985).

In the intestine, primarily the small intestine, the intestinal contents are mixed with mucus, pancreatic juice, and bile. Digestion, which begins in the mouth and stomach, is completed in the lumen and mucosal cells of the small intestine. Digestion depends on a number of enzymatic processes under neural and hormonal stimuli, which can be affected in the elderly (Table 21–1). The products of digestion are then absorbed, along with vitamins and fluid in the small intestine (water also in the colon), and carried to the liver by the portal blood. The small intestine, with its many folds, finger-shaped villi, and array of microvilli on the luminal side of the cells, is particularly well designed for this function of absorption. The rate of nutrient transport by the intestine is related primarily to the surface area that is functionally exposed to the luminal contents. Several factors are important for the maintenance of optimal function of the small intestine (Table 21–2) and may be affected by aging. Thus, any change in intestinal architecture or diffusion barrier of the mucosal cells greatly affects transport. With aging some anatomic changes have been described in animals and in apparently healthy aged individuals (Webster, 1984, 1985).

Structure of the Intestinal Mucosa. Throughout the length of the small intestine, the mucosa displays many folds and is covered with villi formed of a single layer of columnar epithelium and containing a network of capillaries and one lymphatic vessel. The free edges of the mucosal cells are divided into microvilli, which form a "brush border." Folds, villi, and microvilli augment considerably the absorptive surface. The mucosal cells are formed from mitotically active undifferentiated cells located at the bottom of the villi (in the so-called crypts of Lieberkühn). They migrate up to the tips of the villi where they are sloughed into the intestinal lumen. The average life of these cells is 2 to 5 days, thereby representing a potential model (still little utilized) for the study of cellular aging. The crypts are also the site of active secretion of water and electrolytes.

Table 21–2. IMPORTANT FACTORS FOR THE MAINTENANCE OF OPTIMAL SMALL INTESTINE FUNCTION

A. The anatomic integrity of the absorbing small intestine
   1. By light and electron microscopy
   2. Normal intestinal mucosal cell replication
B. Normal gastrointestinal secretions
   Including basal and postprandial secretions from salivary, gastric, pancreatic, and hepatic cells
C. Coordinated gastrointestinal motility
D. Normal intestinal uptake and transintestinal transport, including adaptation to intraluminal substrates
E. Adequate intestinal blood supply
   1. To maintain cell oxygenation
   2. To maintain cell nutrient supply
F. Normal defense mechanisms against toxic injurious agents from the intestinal lumen
   1. Normal clearance of bacteria in the intestinal lumen
   2. Immunologic response to injury
   3. Mucosal cell wall integrity to prevent macromolecular uptake
   4. Mucosal cell detoxification of toxic absorbed materials

Studies in humans have reported, with aging, a reduced height and a frequent convoluted pattern of villi; changes were not observed in villus width, cell height, or mucosal thickness (Webster and Leeming, 1975; Warren *et al.*, 1978). However, in these studies, the nutritional status was not rigorously controlled and several individuals suffered minor deficiencies. In a number of animal species, advancing age is accompanied by alterations involving one or several of the following: changes in the overall shape of the villus, increase in collagen, mitochondrial changes, lengthening of the crypts, and prolonged replication time of the crypt stem cells (Fry *et al.*, 1962; Holt, 1983). All these changes are minor and none appears sufficient to explain the impaired absorption often found in the elderly. Other factors may intervene: altered villus motility limiting functional surface area; inadequate intestinal blood supply (due to atherosclerotic involvement of major intestinal vessels) (Tytgat and van Dongen, 1984); impaired water "barrier" restricting diffusion and transport.

Research concerning absorption of nutrients and vitamins is sparse in humans and even in laboratory animals. There are, however, with increasing age, reports of reduced absorption of several substances (e.g., sugar, calcium, iron) while digestion and motility remain relatively unchanged (Holt, 1983; Webster, 1985). Among the substances for which absorption has been studied in the elderly, calcium probably presents the best evidence for a gradual reduction with increasing age (Table 21–3). In addition to changes in bone calcium, with aging, calcium absorption and transport are altered. Calcium balance studies in humans reveal a significant drop in absorption with

Table 21–3. MECHANISMS OF REDUCED INTESTINAL CALCIUM ABSORPTION WITH AGING

↓ Intake of vitamin D (poor nutrition)
↓ Vitamin D conversion in skin (reduced sunlight exposure)
↓ Intestinal absorption
↓ Vitamin D metabolism (hepatic) and activation (renal)
↓ Cellular calcium binding (↓ receptors)

aging, starting at about age 60 (Nordin *et al.,* 1976). When young and old subjects were compared, the young individuals were capable of responding to a low-calcium diet by increasing intestinal calcium absorption, a response no longer found in the elderly (Ireland and Fordtran, 1973). Mechanisms responsible for this reduced calcium absorption included decreased intake or malabsorption of vitamin D, lack of sunlight and conversion (hydroxylation) in the skin, altered hepatic and/or renal hydroxylation of vitamin D, or impaired cellular binding of calcium (Table 21–3). There is conflicting evidence for other substances such as dextrose, xylose, iron, vitamin B_{12}, and fats, which may be reduced or may be absorbed normally at all ages.

Increased general frailty and weight loss may occur in the old, without evidence of any specific underlying cause, in the presence of a well-maintained appetite and a known and balanced diet. However, a relatively high percentage of old individuals suffer from malabsorption; at least 7 percent of residents in nursing homes are likely to have impaired absorptive ability.

Malabsorption and Disease. Many generalized conditions, such as rheumatoid arthritis (Chapter 22), afflicting the elderly may have some detrimental affects on absorption (Pettersson *et al.,* 1970). A number of small bowel disorders may be suggested as a cause of malabsorption, but their incidence is low and symptomatology vague. Other frequent causes of malabsorption include: infections (e.g., after gastrointestinal surgery, diarrhea), small intestine diverticula (i.e., small dilatations or pockets leading off from the intestinal tube); pancreatic insufficiency (rare); celiac disease (alterations of mucosa and cell transport); mental disorders (e.g., dementia) (McEvoy and James, 1984). Many old individuals with malabsorption are severely undernourished, weak, and debilitated. Management, therefore, includes both treatment of the specific underlying disease and appropriate diet. With energetic treatment, even severely ill patients have a good prognosis.

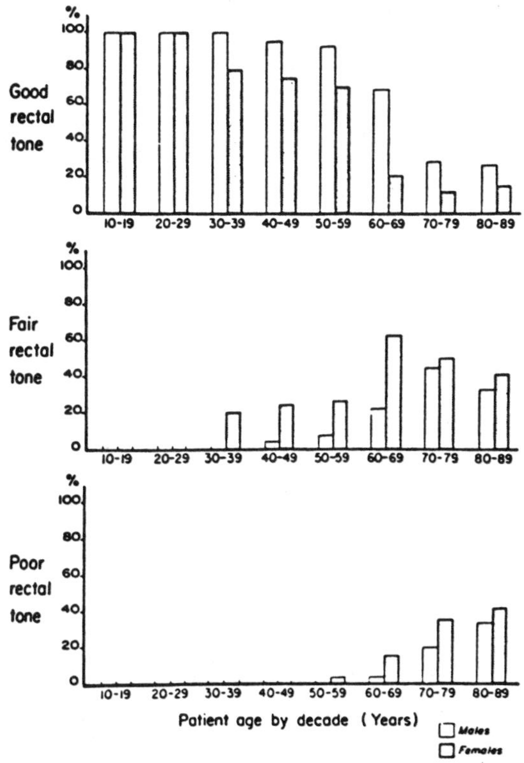

Figure 21–3. *Relationship of sphincter tone to age.*

Reproduced with permission from Stewart and Dodds, 1979.

INCONTINENCE

As discussed in Chapter 20, urinary incontinence is one of the major afflictions of old age. The same tragic consideration applies to fecal incontinence (Figure 21–3). The maintenance of normal control on fecal evacuation is regulated by complex neuromuscular functions (Figure 21–4). Should any physiologic decrement occur in the activity of the intestine itself, or in the muscles of the pelvic floor, or in the neural imputs, then the control of defecation may break down. A person with efficient sphincters may find control impossible during an attack of severe diarrhea. In the elderly, loss of sphincter muscle strength (Figure 21–5), merely as a consequence of aging, creates a more difficult problem when confronted with diarrhea. Certain neurologic

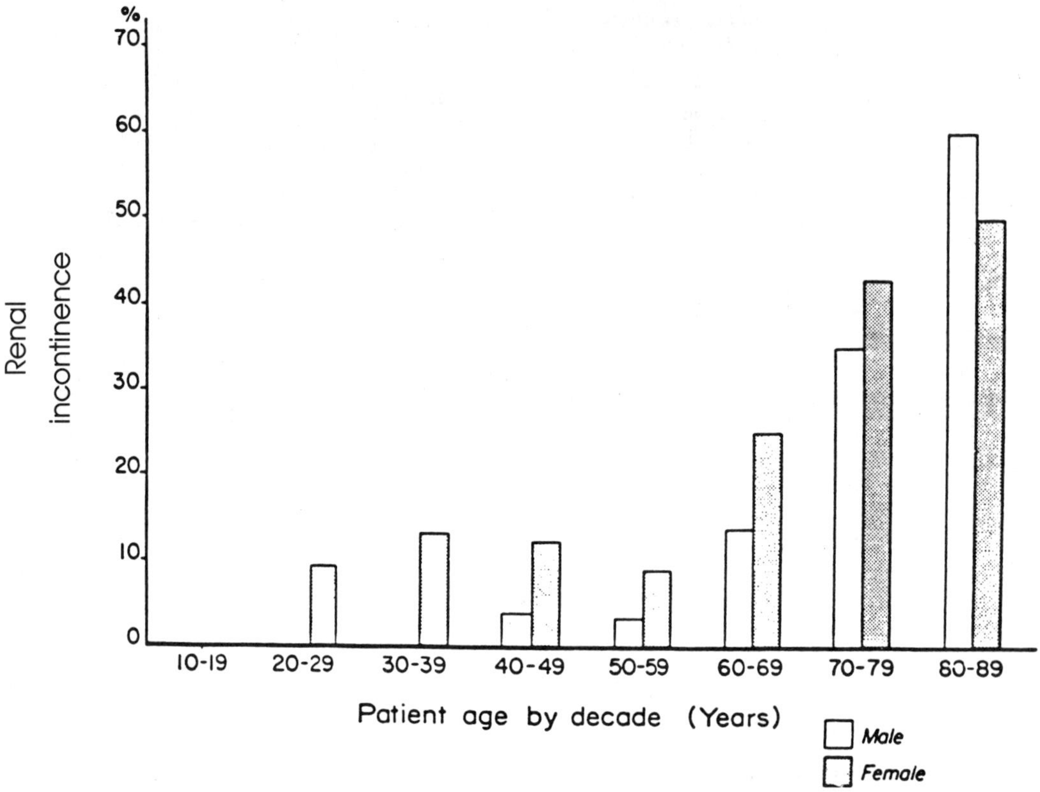

Figure 21–4. *Relationship of age and sex to fecal incontinence.* (Reproduced with permission from Stewart and Dodds, 1979.)

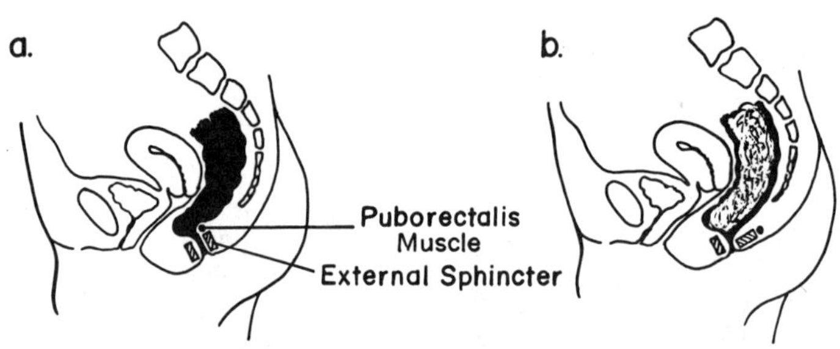

Figure 21–5. *Diagrammatic representation of some of the structures involved in defecation (here, in women).*

Note, that the external sphincter and the puborectalis muscle play an important role in maintaining normal fecal continence: *a.* When the rectum is empty and the sphincter is closed and *b.*, when it is full, and the sphincter is relaxed and displaced. Note, that one important action of the puborectalis muscle is to maintain angulation (bend) between the lower rectum and anal canal, upon which continence is largely dependent. Also note that, with increased rectal pressure, the activity of the sphincter increases, thereby protecting the individual from involuntary defecation. However, above a certain pressure (fecal volume) this protection is lost.

conditions affect the pelvic floor muscles, and these may be so severe that, even with a normal stool, continence cannot be preserved. At all ages, there may be organic deficiencies in the muscle ring due to trauma, and such deficiencies are more likely to occur in the elderly person.

Pelvic Structures and Defecation. Distention of the rectum, the last portion of the intestine, initiates reflex contractions of its musculature. In humans, the internal involuntary sphincter is excited by the sympathetic but inhibited by the parasympathetic nerve supply. The external sphincter (voluntary) is innervated by somatic nerves. The urge to defecate begins when the rectal pressure increases to a certain level (about 55 mm Hg), at which time both sphincters relax and the rectal contents are expelled. At a lower rectal pressure, defecation can be initiated by voluntary relaxation of the external sphincter and contraction of the abdominal muscles. Thus, defecation is a spinal reflex that can be voluntarily inhibited by contraction of the external sphincter or facilitated by its relaxation.

With aging, the rectal muscle mass is decreased in size and the sphincter is weakened. The external sphincter is always the most affected of the pelvic floor muscles. The high incidence of incontinence in the elderly makes it essential to exclude any possible underlying gastrointestinal infection or systemic disease. One classification is shown in Table 21–4 and may be compared with the causes of urinary incontinence (Chapter 20). Fecal incontinence may be caused by: (1) neurogenic alterations involving the cortex (e.g., dementia) or the spinal cord (e.g., failure to inhibit defecation upon entrance of feces into rectum); (2) muscle atrophy (due to trauma as in prolonged and difficult labor), a direct analogy to stress incontinence of urine (Chapter 20); (3) constipation (due to immobility, poor reflexes, difficulty in reaching the toilet); (4) diarrhea, which may cause incontinence at all ages but more frequently at older ages (Brocklehurst, 1984).

Table 21–4. CLASSIFICATION OF FECAL INCONTINENCE

CAUSE	CONSEQUENCE
Neurogenic	
Cortical	Loss of inhibition
Spinal	Reduced reflex activity
Muscle atrophy	"Stress" incontinence
Retention	Constipation
Overflow (bacteria, virus, allergies)	Diarrhea

Knowledge of the etiology of incontinence leads to some practical interventions. A first step is to rule out constipation or diarrhea and, if they are present, to treat them (Wienbeck and Erckenbrecht, 1984). If fecal incontinence persists, then other causes must be sought and appropriate management established.

AGING OF EXOCRINE PANCREAS

Besides its hormonal secretions, the pancreas produces a pancreatic juice containing enzymes (amylase, lipase, proteases) important for digestion. The enzymes are discharged by exocytosis and their secretion is controlled by a reflex mechanism and by the hormones secretin and cholecystokinin. The major enzyme is trypsin, which is secreted as an inactive proenzyme, trypsinogen. Some uncertainty exists regarding the effects of advancing age on pancreatic secretion (Laugier and Sarles, 1984). The senile gland is smaller, harder than normal (due to increasing fibrosis), and yellow-brown (due to accumulation of lipofuscin). Of the major enzymes, some (amylase) remain constant whereas others (lipase, trypsin) decrease dramatically (Meyer and Necheles, 1940). Secretin-stimulated pancreatic juice and bicarbonate concentration remain unchanged (Rosenberg *et al.*, 1966). Little is known so far about age-related changes in the hormones that regulate pancreatic function. While a decline in some functions of the pancreas occurs with aging, the genesis of this decline is unknown but has been related to diet (e.g., alcoholism), vascular sclerosis, general fibrosis, or lack of cell regeneration. However, as only one-tenth of pancreatic secretion is needed for normal digestion, it is not probable that age alone could lead to a significant pancreatic insufficiency capable of inducing severe digestive disorders.

In general, these age-related changes do not seriously compromise pancreatic function, but their presence may increase the incidence of pancreatic disease (acute and chronic pancreatitis, cancer) in the elderly.

AGING OF THE LIVER

Of the many functions of the liver—formation of bile, carbohydrate storage and metabolism, ketone body formation, reduction and conjugation of steroid hormones, inactivation of polypeptide hormones, detoxification of many drugs and toxins, manufacture of plasma proteins, urea formation, and regulation of lipid metabolism—little is known of the changes that may occur with "normal" aging (Kitani, 1978). As is the case with other multifunctional organs, not all functions age at the same pace. In this section, we shall consider some changes in morphology and function, particularly bile excretion. Changes in enzyme activity with aging and hepatotoxicity of various drugs, especially in the elderly, are considered in Chapters 6 and 24, respectively.

STRUCTURAL CHANGES

Atrophy and decreased weight of the liver are common in elderly individuals and are often independent of organ sclerosis and fibrosis. The reduced weight is due to a decrease in cell number rather than in cell size, in contrast to other instances, such as malnutrition, in which reduction of cell size is the cause of decreased liver weight. In fact, cell size is often increased. Cell loss begins in the 60s, slowly at first and then more rapidly in the 80s and thereafter.

Hepatic Cells. The liver is organized in lobules formed of hepatic cells, hepatocytes, lined up in rows irradiating from the center of the lobule to the periphery. The hepatic veins are situated in the center of the lobule, and the biliary ducts, the portal veins, and the hepatic arteries at the periphery. The specialized capillaries, the sinusoids, are lined with phagocytic cells (Kupffer's cells) that engulf bacteria or other foreign particles (see Chapter 8). The lobules are separated by a small amount of interlobular connective tissue in which are found the blood vessels and the beginnings of the biliary ducts and lymphatic vessels (Figure 21–6).

Binucleate cells appear with advancing age and, after 70 years, hypertrophy of the cells and polyploidization (increased nucleus size) (Tauchi and Sato, 1978). The enlarged cells are interspersed with "dark," degenerating cells, probably products of the usual cycle of cell degeneration/regeneration of the hepatic parenchyma. With aging, cell regeneration would be slowed down, perhaps owing to the absence or deficit of growth factors for cell replication or to the excess of growth inhibitory factors. Hence, cell hypertrophy may be interpreted as a compensatory reaction to cell loss. That this is the case and that aged hepatic cells are active is supported by the increased activity of some enzymes (e.g.,

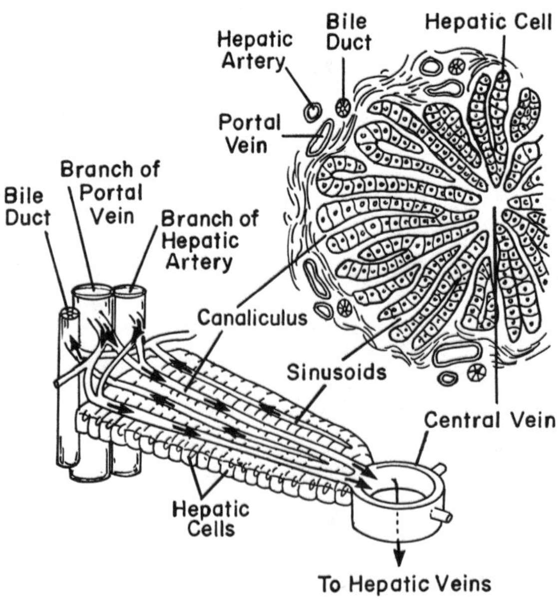

Figure 21–6. *Diagrammatic representation of the liver, which is organized in lobules formed of hepatic cells, hepatocytes, lined up in rows irradiating from the center of the lobule to the periphery, shown in sagittal plane, top, and a closer view, bottom.*

The hepatic veins are situated in the center of the lobule and the biliary ducts, the portal veins and hepatic arteries at the periphery. The specialized capillaries, the sinusoids, are lined with phagocytic cells (Kupffer's cells) that engulf bacteria or other foreign particles. The lobules are separated by a small amount of interlobular connective tissue in which are found the blood vessels and the beginnings of the biliary ducts and lymphatic vessels.

succinic dehydrogenase). The number of mitochondria is decreased whereas their size is increased, mitochondrial hypertrophy being a compensatory response to decreased number. The increased mitochondrial volume and the presence of "giant" mitochondria may be ascribed to the incompleteness of their division following synthesis of new mitochondrial material in the presence of hypertrophy. However, regeneration of liver after partial hepatectomy is slower in older rats, even after hormonal (cortisol, thyroxine) administration. Indeed, the very compensatory increase in volume when regenerative power is more limited would accelerate cell loss and thereby result in a vicious cycle of cell destruction and compensatory hypertrophy.

Smooth endoplasmic reticulum is decreased in the rat hepatocytes, a morphologic correlate underlining the age-related reduction in the hepatic capacity to metabolize drugs (Chapter 24). Other aspects of hepatic structure are not markedly altered in the old rat, and maintenance of normal morphology agrees with minimal or no alteration of hepatic metabolic functions such as protein synthesis (Schmucker, 1978). Some changes with aging of hepatic enzymes and their regulation by hormones and other factors have been discussed in Chapter 6.

Only a few studies have investigated whether collagen changes in the liver with aging; those conducted so far suggest a moderate increase (Barrows *et al.*, 1980) ascribed, perhaps, to hepatic injury (Popper, 1975).

FUNCTIONAL CHANGES

Alteration of hepatic structure and enzymatic functions with aging is moderate. In the healthy elderly, routine tests of liver function involving the metabolism and elimination of specific dyes (e.g., bromsulphalein) and radioisotopes and protein synthesis do not show significant differences between individuals ages 50 to 69 and 70 to 89 years (Koff *et al.*, 1973; Kampmann *et al.*, 1975) (Table 21–5). Similarly, tests of liver dysfunction, including cholestasis (blockage of bile flow), cell necrosis, inflammation, and impaired detoxification, are usually negative in the absence of specific liver damage and systemic disease.

Table 21–5. LIVER FUNCTION TESTS

FUNCTION	TEST
1. Hepatic clearance	Serum bilirubin levels
	Bromsulphalein and other dyes
	Radioisotope scans
2. Synthesis	Plasma albumin
	Prothrombin time
	Blood urea
3. Cell necrosis	Transaminases
	Lactic acid dehydrogenase
4. Cholestasis	Conjugated bilirubin levels
	Alkaline phosphatase
	5'-nucleotidase
	Gamma-glutamyltranspeptidase
5. Inflammation	Gamma-globulin level
6. Detoxification	Ammonia
	Mercaptans

In contrast to humans, studies in experimental animals (rats) show consistent reduced removal of many of the dyes used to measure hepatic function from the blood, storage, and transport maxima (van Bezooijen and Knook, 1978; Skaunic *et al.*, 1978). These changes have been ascribed to both circulatory alterations and increased collagen deposition (and hence impaired transport) in the liver.

BILE FORMATION

Bile production is a major function of the liver. Bile, considered as both a secretion and an excretion, is formed continuously by the hepatic cells. It is a greenish-yellow fluid composed of water, bile salts, bile pigments (bilirubin), cholesterol, and various inorganic salts.

The Biliary System. Bile formed by the hepatic cells is carried through several bile caniculi to the right and left hepatic ducts, which join to form, outside the liver, the common hepatic duct. This duct joins the cystic duct that drains in the gallbladder, the reservoir for bile located on the undersurface of the liver. The hepatic duct unites with the cystic duct to form the common bile duct, which enters the duodenum, usually united with the pancreatic duct, and pours the bile into the duodenum.

The bile, primarily through the action of its salts, has several important functions in the digestion by emulsifying lipids and activating the lipid enzymes, lipases. Bilirubin, the major pigment of the bile, results from the breakdown of hemoglobin, myoglobin, and respiratory enzymes in the

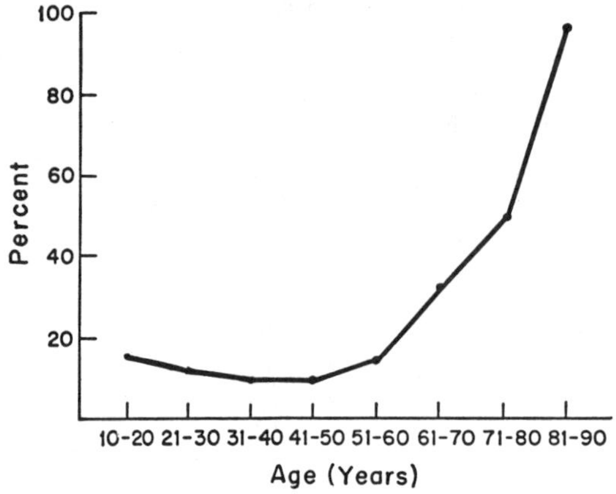

Figure 21–7. *Incidence of bile duct stones at cholecystectomy in relation to age.*

Note the sharp increase from 60 years on.

reticuloendothelial system of the liver and spleen. Unconjugated bilirubin thus formed is carried to the liver cell where it is conjugated and bound to proteins; this conjugated form is water-soluble. In the colon, conjugated bilirubin is hydrolyzed to urobilin and excreted.

Little is known of changes with aging in bilirubin metabolism. However, biliary disease is common and its incidence increases steadily with age (Figure 21–7). Biliary disease (gallstones), a common problem of most Western societies, affects 15 to 20 percent of adults of all ages and 30 to 50 percent of elderly persons by age 75 with a ratio of 2:1 for females to males (Hermann, 1983). As people live longer, the incidence of biliary disease has increased in the last 20 years. Forty to sixty percent of patients with gallstones show no symptoms, and it is possible that the condition starts this way in most individuals.

In the gallbladder, the bile is concentrated by absorption of water (water is 97 percent in the liver bile and 89 percent in the gallbladder bile). Stones (gallstones) form in the gallbladder or bile ducts when a substance that is not normally present appears in the bile or the composition of the bile changes so that a normal constituent precipitates. For example, cholesterol stones form when the proportion of cholesterol, lecithin, and bile salts in the bile is altered.

Several aspects of biliary disease are characteristic of the elderly. These include: a greater incidence of acute versus chronic cholicystitis (i.e., inflammation of the gallbladder); the presence of stones in the bile duct and other complications; the recurrence of the disease after a previous operation; and the greater severity of the disease and the higher mortality.

An increasing incidence of stones in bile ducts and gallbladder with aging has been well documented. With this increase, the incidence of related complications (e.g., jaundice, pancreatitis, cholecystitis, liver abscesses, and systemic sepsis) also rises. The treatment of choice is surgical and consists in the removal of the stone(s); it entails, in the elderly, more complicated operations to control or correct the disease.

Bilirubin is an Antioxidant. Bilirubin is generally regarded as a potentially cytotoxic, lipid-soluble waste product that needs to be excreted. However, bilirubin is also capable of efficiently scavenging peroxyl radicals (Stocker *et al.*, 1987). In this function, it would join other metabolic products such as uric acid (a product of purine metabolism) and taurine (a product of cysteine metabolism) with antioxidant properties. Thus, bilirubin would be "beneficial as a physiological, chain-breaking antioxidant." Therefore, the study of alterations in bilirubin metabolism with aging, hitherto little investigated, is clearly worth pursuing.

References

Allen, E. F.: Statistical study of primary causes of extractions. *J. Dent. Res.*, **23**:453–458, **1944.**

Amstad-Jossi, M., and Schroeder, H. E.: Age-related alterations of periodontal structures around the cemento-enamel junction of the gingival connective tissue composition in germ-free rats. *J. Peridont. Res.*, **13**:76–90, **1978.**

Barrows, G. H.; Schrodt, G. R.; Greenberg, R. A.; and Tamburro, C. H.: Changes in stainable collagen in the aging normal human liver. *Gastroenterology*, **79**:1099, **1980.**

Baum, B. J.: Characteristics of participants in the oral physiology component of the Baltimore longitudinal study of aging. *Commun. Dent. Oral. Epidemiol.*, **9**:128–134, **1981.**

Beaumont, D. M., and James, O. F. W.: Aspects of nutrition in the elderly. *Clin. Gastroenterol.*, **14**:811–827, **1985.**

Brocklehurst, J. C.: The problem of faecal incontinence. In Hellemans, J., and Vantrappen, G. (eds.): *Gastrointestinal Tract Disorders in the Elderly*, Churchill Livingstone, London, **1984.**

Fry, R. J. M.; Lesher, S.; and Kohn, H. I.: Influence of age on the transit time of cells of the mouse intestinal epithelium. III. Ileum. *Lab. Invest.*, **11**:289–293, **1962.**

Fuchs, E., and Hanukoglu, I.: Epidermal α-keratins:

structural diversity and changes during tissue differentiation. In Bereiter-Hahn, J.; Matoltsy, A. G.; and Richards, K. S. (eds.): *Biology of the Integument*, Springer-Verlag, Berlin, **1986.**

Garrett, J. R.: Some observations on human submandibular salivary glands. *Proc. R. Soc. Med.*, **55:**488–491, **1962.**

Grad, B.: Diurnal, age, and sex changes in the sodium and potassium concentrations of human saliva. *J. Gerontol.*, **9:**276–286, **1954.**

Hellemans, J.; Vantrappen, G.; and Pelemans, W.: Oesophageal problems. In Hellemans, J., and Vantrappen, G. (eds.): *Gastrointestinal Tract Disorders in the Elderly*, Churchill Livingstone, London, **1984.**

Hermann, R. E.: Biliary disease in the aging patient. In Texter, E. C. (ed.): *The Aging Gut*, Masson, New York, **1983.**

Hollis, J. B., and Castell, D. O.: Esophageal function in elderly men—A new look at "presbyesophagus." *Ann. Intern. Med.*, **80:**371–374, **1974.**

Holt, P. R.: Intestinal absorption and malabsorption. In Texter, E. C. (ed.): *The Aging Gut*, Masson, New York, **1983.**

Ireland, P., and Fordtran, J. S.: Effect of dietary calcium and age on jejunal calcium absorption in humans studied by intestinal perfusion. *J. Clin. Invest.*, **52:**2672–2681, **1973.**

Kampmann, J. P.; Sinding, J.; and Moller-Jorgensen, I.: Effect of age on liver function. *Geriatrics*, **30:**91–95, **1975.**

Kitani, K. (ed.): *Liver and Aging*, Elsevier/North Holland, Amsterdam, **1978.**

Kitani, K.; Kanai, S.; and Miura, R.: Hepatic metabolism of sulfobromophthalein (BSP) and indocyanine green (ICG) in aging rats. In Kitani, K. (ed.): *Liver and Aging*, Elsevier/North Holland, Amsterdam, **1978.**

Koff, R. S.; Garvey, A. J.; Burney, S. W.; and Bell, B.: Absence of an age effect on sulfobromophthalein retention in healthy men. *Gastroenterology*, **65:**300–302, **1973.**

Kumpuris, D.: Gastrointestinal bleeding in the older patient. In Texter, E. C. (ed.): *The Aging Gut*, Masson, New York, **1983.**

Laugier, R., and Sarles, H.: Pancreatic function and diseases. In Hellemans, J., and Vantrappen, G. (eds.): *Gastrointestinal Tract Disorders in the Elderly*, Churchill Livingstone, London, **1984.**

Magendie, F.: *A Elementary Compendium of Physiology: For Use of Students* (translated by E. Milligan), J. Webster, Philadelphia, **1824,** pp. 219–223.

Marks, I. N.: Peptic ulcer and its complications. In Hellemans, J., and Vantrappen, G. (eds.): *Gastrointestinal Tract Disorders in the Elderly*, Churchill Livingstone, London, **1984.**

McCay, C. M.; Crowell, M. F.; and Maynard, L. A.: The effect of retarded growth upon the length of life span and upon the ultimate body size. *J. Nutr.*, **10:**63–79, **1935.**

McEvoy, A., and James, O. F. W.: Malabsorption syndromes. In Hellemans, J., and Vantrappen, G. (eds.): *Gastrointestinal Tract Disorders in the Elderly*, Churchill Livingstone Press, Edinburgh, London, **1984.**

McGinty, D. P.; Bowles, M. H.; Patel, G. K.; and Texter, E. C.: Vascular ectasias of the gastrointestinal tract: A new problem in our aging population. In Texter, E. C. (ed.): *The Aging Gut*, Masson, New York, **1983.**

Meyer, J., and Necheles, H.: Studies in old age: IV. The clinical significance of salivary, gastric, and pancreatic secretion in the aged. *JAMA*, **115:**2050–2055, **1940.**

Morris, J. S., and Dew, M. J.: Age and gastrointestinal disease. In Pathy, M. S. J. (ed.): *Principles and Practice of Geriatric Medicine*, John Wiley & Sons, Chichester, UK, **1985.**

National Research Council, Food and Nutrition Board: *Recommended Dietary Allowances*, 9th ed., Washington, National Academy of Sciences, **1980.**

Nordin, B. E. C.; Wilkinson, R.; Marshall, D. H.; Gallagher, J. C.; Williams, A.; and Peacock, M.: Calcium absorption in the elderly. *Calc. Tis. Res.*, **21:**442–445, **1976.**

Patel, G. K.; Diner, W. C.; and Texter, E. C.: Swallowing and pharyngoesophageal function in the aging patient. In Texter, E. C. (ed.): *The Aging Gut*, Masson, New York, **1983.**

Pettersson, T.; Wegelius, O.; and Skrifvars, B.: Gastrointestinal disturbances in patients with severe rheumatoid arthritis. *Acta. Med. Scand.*, **188:**139–144, **1970.**

Popper, H. (ed.): *Collagen Metabolism in the Liver*, Stratton Intercontinental Book Corp., New York, **1975.**

Rosenberg, I. R.; Friedland, N.; Janowitz, H. D.; and Dreiling, D. A.: The effect of age and sex upon human pancreatic secretion of fluid and bicarbonate. *Gastroenterology*, **50:**191–194, **1966.**

Schmucker, D. L.: A quantitative morphological evaluation of hepatocytes in young, mature and senescent Fischer 344 male rates. In Kitani, K. (ed.): *Liver and Aging*, Elsevier/North Holland, Amsterdam, **1978.**

Segall, P. E., and Timiras, P. S.: Pathophysiologic findings after chronic tryptophan deficiency in rats: A model for delayed growth and aging. *Mech. Ageing Dev.*, **5:**109–124, **1976.**

Segall, P. E.; Ooka, H.; Rose, K.; and Timiras, P. S.: Neural and endocrine development after chronic tryptophan deficiency in rats: I. Brain monoamine and pituitary responses. *Mech. Ageing Dev.*, **7:**1–17, **1978.**

Segall, P. E.; Timiras, P. S.; and Walton, J. R.: Low tryptophan diets delay reproductive ageing. *Mech. Ageing Dev.*, **23:**245–351, **1983.**

Shannon, I. L.: A saliva substitute for dry mouth relief. In Toga, C. J.; Nandy, K.; and Chauncey, H. H. (eds.): *Geriatric Dentistry*, Lexington Books, Lexington, MA, **1979.**

Shklar, G.: Oral pathology in the aging individual. In Toga, C. J.; Nandy, K.; and Chauncey, H. H. (eds.): *Geriatric Dentistry*, Lexington Books, Lexington, MA, **1979.**

Skaunic, V.; Hulek, P.; and Martinkova, J.: Changes in kinetics of exogenous dyes in the ageing process. In Kitani, K. (ed.): *Liver and Aging*, Elsevier/North-Holland, Amsterdam, **1978.**

Skerrow, D.: Epidermal α-keratin: Structure and chemical composition. In Bereiter-Hahn, J.; Matoltsy, A. G.; and Richards, K. S. (eds.): *Biology of the Integument*, Springer-Verlag, Berlin, **1986.**

Soergel, K. H.; Zboralske, F. A.; and Amberg, J. R.: Presbyesophagus: Esophageal motility in nonagenarians. *J. Clin. Invest.*, **43:**1472–1479, **1964.**

Sonnenberg, A.; Schmid, P.; Muller-Lissner, S. A.; Vogel, E.; and Blum, A. L.: What makes duodenal ulcer heal and relapse. *Gastroenterology*, **78:**1266, **1980.**

Stewart, E. T., and Dodds, W. J.: Predictability of rectal incontinence on barium enema examination. *Am. J. Roentgenol.*, **132:**197–200, **1979.**

Stocker, R.; Yamamoto, Y.; McDonagh, A. F.; Glazer, A. N.; and Ames, B. N.: Bilirubin is an antioxidant of possible physiological importance. *Science*, **235:**1043–1046, **1987.**

Tauchi, H., and Sato, T.: Hepatic cells of the aged. In Kitani, K. (ed.): *Liver and Aging*, Elsevier/North-Holland, Amsterdam, **1978.**

Toga, C. J.; Nandy, K.; and Chauncey, H. H.: *Geriatric Dentistry*, Lexington Books, Lexington, MA, **1979.**

Tonna, E. A.: Explorations into the aging of skeletal-dental tissues: an ultrastructural study of aging cementum. In Toga, C. J.; Nandy, K.; and Chauncey, H. H. (eds.): *Geriatric Dentistry*, Lexington Books, Lexington, MA, **1979.**

Tune, J. M.; McGinty, D. P.; Navab, F.; Patel, G. K.; and Texter, E. C.: The spectrum of mesenteric vascular insufficiency. In Texter, E. C. (ed.): *The Aging Gut*, Masson, New York, **1983.**

Tytgat, G. N. J., and van Dongen, R. J. M.: Ischaemic disease of the small and large intestine. In Hellemans, J., and Vantrappen, G. (eds.): *Gastrointestinal Tract Disorders in the Elderly*, Churchill Livingstone, London, **1984.**

van Bezooijen, C. F. A., and Knook, D. L.: A comparison of age-related changes in bromsulfophthalein metabolism of the liver and isolated hepatocytes. In Kitani, K. (ed.): *Liver and Aging*, Elsevier/North-Holland, Amsterdam, **1978.**

Waldron, C. A., and Shafer, W. G.: Leukoplakia revisited. A clinicopathological study of 3,256 oral leukoplakia. *Cancer*, **36:**1386–1392, **1975.**

Walker, D. M.: Oral disease. In Pathy, M. S. J. (ed.): *Principles and Practice of Geriatric Medicine*, John Wiley & Sons, Chichester, UK, **1985.**

Warren, P. M.; Pepperman, M. A.; and Montgomery, R. D.: Age changes in small intestinal mucosa. *Lancet*, **2:**849–850, **1978.**

Webster, S. G. P.: Small bowel morphology and function. In Hellemans, J., and Vantrappen, G. (eds.): *Gastrointestinal Tract Disorders in the Elderly*, Churchill Livingstone, London, **1984.**

Webster, S. G. P.: Absorption of nutrients in old age. In Pathy, M. S. J. (ed.): *Principles and Practice of Geriatric Medicine*, John Wiley & Sons, Chichester, UK, **1985.**

Webster, S. G. P., and Leeming, J. T.: The appearance of the small bowel mucosa in old age. *Age Ageing*, **4:**168–174, **1975.**

Wienbeck, M., and Erckenbrecht, J.: Motor function of the large intestine. Constipation and diarrohea. In Hellemans, J., and Vantrappen, G. (eds.): *Gastrointestinal Tract Disorders in the Elderly*, Churchill Livingstone, London, **1984.**

CHAPTER

22 AGING OF THE SKELETON, JOINTS, AND MUSCLES

As with other systems of the body, the musculoskeletal system, including the skeleton, joints, and muscles, passes through phases of growth, maturation, and decline. The first two phases have been studied extensively because of their bearing on pediatric medicine. The postmature phase, characterized primarily by involutional processes, is less well understood. It is this latter phase that is addressed in the present chapter.

As indicated in Chapter 2, the various body systems in humans and other animals do not follow identical timetables of development and aging. Some systems move more smoothly and more rapidly than others in the phase of maximum efficiency, and some resist deterioration more stubbornly than others. Compared with other systems, the skeleton is rugged and durable; it usually carries on its tasks into advanced years, and normal and/or abnormal aging of the skeleton is seldom the cause of death. However, it is subject, as are other parts of the body, to various hazards, primarily trauma, deficient metabolism and nutrition, and multiple degenerative changes. The skeleton generally resists damage well and has an efficient self-repair capability.

While aging of the skeleton usually occurs without conscious awareness of the changes on the part of the individual, aging of the articulations (joints) induces considerable physical pain and causes severe disability. Arthritic diseases, some of the most common expressions of joint aging, are among the most frequent and debilitating diseases of old age. The functional impairment and pain resulting from normal or pathologic aging of the joints limit the movement of elderly individuals, thus hindering their ability to care for themselves, eroding their independence, and, by forcing them to varying degrees of immobility, contributing to the decline in competence of other systems (such as the circulatory system). Some pathology of the joints begins at a relatively young adult age (rheumatoid arthritis may begin in adolescence) but with increasing prevalence with advancing age. Thus, prevalence of rheumatoid arthritis is less than 1 percent before the age of 30 years and thereafter rises in each decade to 1 to 3 percent in the late 50s and 8 to 11 percent in the late 60s. Other manifestations of articular aging occur at later ages; osteoarthritis that affects 85 percent of persons 70 to 79 years of age is one of the major causes of invalidism confining the affected individuals to bed or to the wheelchair.

The aging process in skeletal muscle is greatly complicated by the fact that the muscle fibers do not constitute a homogeneous tissue and the state of the tissue at any time depends on the extent and nature of many influences (e.g., nutritional, neural, hormonal, exertional). The characteristic decline of muscular performance associated with advancing age is, therefore, variable and may be caused not only by primary aging changes in the muscle fibers, but also by aging of other body systems, nervous, vascular, and endocrine.

AGING OF THE SKELETON

The skeleton, the heaviest and most durable part of the body, provides the body framework and derives its properties from the unique characteristics of bone. In addition to this function of body support, the bone provides storage for calcium and other minerals thereby aiding in mineral homeostasis; it also contributes, in association with the lungs and kidneys, to the maintenance of acid-base balance by providing additional phosphate and carbonate for buffers.

Structure and Function of Bone. Bone is a hard form of connective tissue consisting of bone cells or osteocytes embedded in a collagenous protein matrix that has been impregnated with mineral salts, especially phosphates of calcium. The matrix occurs in two phases: an organic phase that consists of collagen, proteins, and glu-

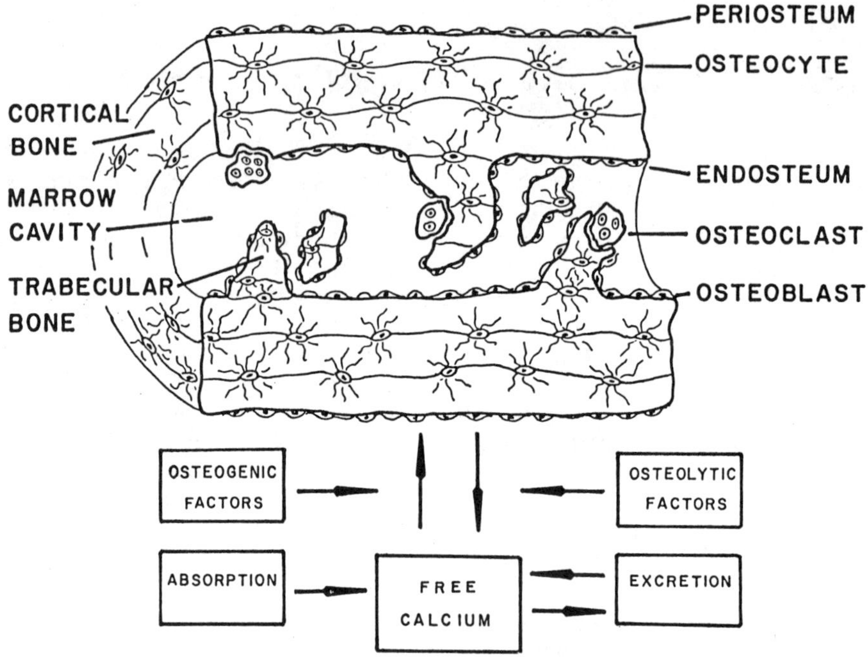

Figure 22–1. *Factors responsible for maintenance of bone structure.*

Calcium in bone is derived from circulating free calcium which depends on calcium absorption and excretion. Formation of new bone (osteogenesis) depends on osteoblasts and destruction of all bone (osteolysis) depends on osteoclasts. New bone is continuously formed in the periosteum and endosteum. Active bone is formed of osteocytes, which are part of the cortical and trabecular bone. Blood cells are continuously produced in the bone marrow. (Drawing by S. Oklund).

cosaminoglycans (see also Chapter 23) and an inorganic phase that consists mainly of hydroxyapatites (calcium phosphate) and minor amounts of other minerals. The collagen fibers provide resilience and the minerals hardness. Given individual variations, it can be stated that in childhood about two-thirds of the bone substance is composed of connective tissue, whereas in aged individuals about two-thirds consists of minerals. This transposition in content results in decreased flexibility and increased brittleness with advancing age.

Bone Histology. Bone is distinguished, histologically, as "compact bone" found in shafts of long bones and outer surfaces (periosteum) of flat bones; "cancellous bone" making up the trabecular space containing the bone marrow; and the "woven bone" an immature form of bone also involved in fracture repair. The cells in bone are primarily concerned with bone formation and resorption. Osteocytes, mainly in cancellous bone, maintain bone structure; osteoblasts in the periosteum and endosteum form the bone matrix; osteoclasts in the same regions as the osteoblasts resorb bone by phagocytosis and digestion in their cytoplasm. Bone is well vascularized and contains an abundant nervous network.

BONE REMODELING

Maintenance of bone structure and function is a dynamic process regulated by a number of factors, as illustrated in Figure 22–1. Calcium in bone is derived from circulating free calcium, which is dependent on adequate calcium absorption, mainly through the gastrointestinal tract. Circulating calcium also depends on its excretion, mainly through the kidneys. A number of osteogenic factors promote bone formation through stimulation of osteoblastic activity, or bone resorption through osteoclastic activity.

Bone is in a continuous state of flux. Although net bone mass does not change throughout much of adult life, bone is never metabolically at rest and constantly remodels and reappropriates its mineral stores along lines of mechanical stress. The major site of remodeling is the cancellous bone, lining the bone marrow cavities. Thus, bone maintenance includes formation of new bone by the osteoblasts, resorption of old bone by osteoclasts, and carrying out of mature bone functions by osteocytes (Enlow, 1963). The mechanisms responsible for the calcification of newly formed bone matrix are uncertain despite intensive investigation: precipitation of calcium phosphate may depend on some critical concentration (e.g., the solubility product) and is associated with the activity of certain enzymes (e.g., alkaline phosphatase) and specific proteins capable of binding calcium.

With aging, the balance between rates of bone formation and bone resorption is disturbed and the ensuing changes lead to a decrease in bone mass (Garn *et al.,* 1967; Garn, 1970; Tonna, 1981; Rogers, 1982; Exton-Smith, 1985). After age 40, formation rates remain constant while resorption rates increase. Over several decades, the skeletal mass may be reduced to half the value it had at 30 years. Progression of this loss may be measured by counting the number of Haversian canals or osteons. These are cylinders of bone containing a central blood vessel. With advancing age, the number of these osteons increases together with an increase in the bone shaft beginning at the ends of long bones (Kerley, 1970). Between the ages of 42 and 52 years this central (marrow or medullary) cavity extends to the neck of the femur; between 61 and 74 years it reaches the epiphyseal line close to the articular ends (Ubelaker, 1978). Similar changes occur in the humerus: after 61 years, the outer surface becomes rough and the cortex thinner; the medullary cavity reaches the epiphyseal line; after 75 years, there is little spongy tissue left and the cortex is very thin (Schranz, 1959). Articular surfaces become very thin and may collapse (Cobb, 1985).

The major factor in these age-related changes is a loss of bone matrix. However, this loss is confined primarily to the inner bone core. In the elderly, the periosteal tissue at the outer surface of the bones tends to remain constant or even increases in some bones (e.g., metacarpal bone of the hand) (Garn *et al.,* 1967), but the endosteal tissue at the interior of bones is increasingly resorbed (Roche, 1966).

Bone Strength

Bone strength is an important property that allows bones to withstand the forces applied in the various movements of daily life. Several tests of bone strength have been studied and the results show life cycle trends from youth through maturity into old age (Figure 22–2) and disclose a consistent decline of strength with aging (Smith *et al.,* 1981). Comparison of the timetable of aging of several musculoskeletal components reveals the fastest decrease in strength of the cartilage, followed by muscle, bone, and last tendon (Figure 22–3). Also, the comparison of bone with other tissues shows a much slower rate of decline for bone than for intestine and muscle but faster than for kidney (Figure 22–4) (Yamada, 1970).

Factors Affecting Bone Aging: Changes in Calcium Metabolism

While factors that affect bone remodeling are not completely known, adequate circulating calcium is vital in maintaining bone mass. Indeed, the body regulates few parameters with greater fidelity than the concentration of extracellular calcium. The constancy of these levels depends in part on its absorption in the intestinal mucosa and its excretion from the kidneys (Figure 22–5).

The human body contains 1100 g of calcium or 1.5 percent of body weight; 99 percent of this calcium is in the skeleton. The need for calcium increases with aging. For example, while for young adults the recommended daily allowance is 800 mg, for women over 50 years of age it is increased to over 1500 mg. This increased need for calcium may be explained by a progressively less efficient absorption from the upper intestinal tract (Francis *et al.,* 1983). Thus, in the elderly more dietary calcium is needed to maintain an adequate calcium balance.

Calcium Metabolism. Three hormones, parathyroid hormone, calcitonin (see Chapter 15), and calcitriol, are primarily concerned with calcium metabolism (Figure 22–6).

Parathyroid hormone acts directly on bone to increase its resorption and to mobilize calcium, thereby elevating plasma calcium. It also de-

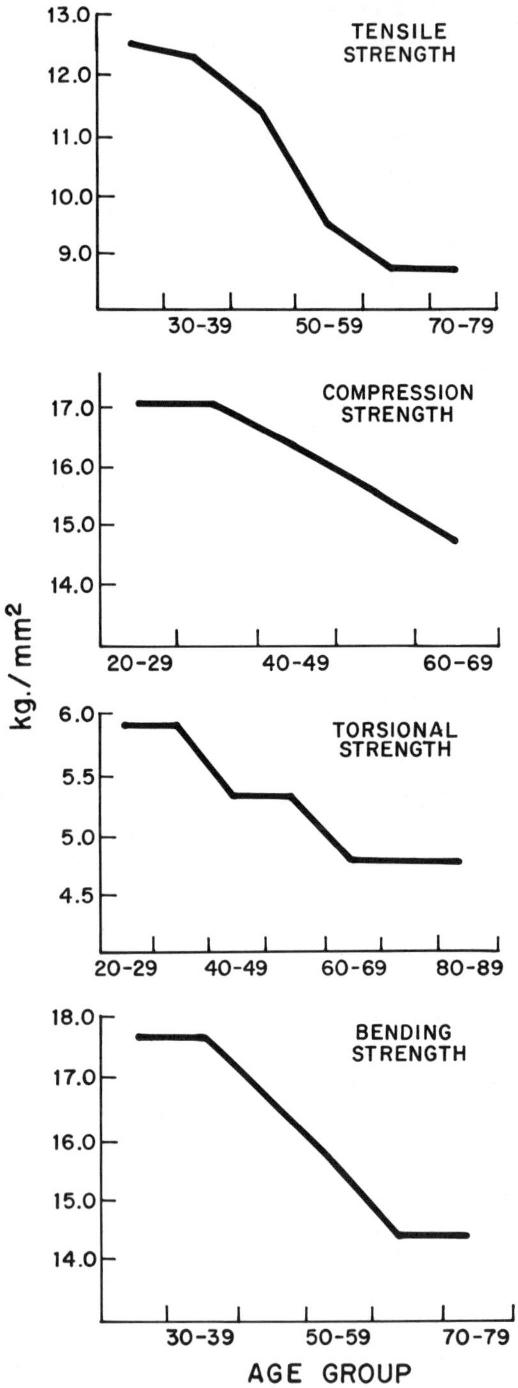

Figure 22–2. *Changes in bone strength with aging.**

Bone strength provides the ability of the bone to undergo force applied in (bottom to top) bending, twisting (torsional strength), compressing, and stretching (tensile strength).
*Data from Yamada, 1970.

presses plasma phosphate by increasing its urinary excretion.

Calcitonin lowers body calcium by inhibiting bone resorption.

Calcitriol (dehydroxycholecalciferol, vitamin D_3), a sterol derivative, increases calcium and phosphate absorption from the intestine and decreases their renal excretion; it also enhances bone resorption. Calcitriol derives through a series of steps either from the diet through absorption in the intestine, or through transformation of cholesterol in the skin by the action of sunlight. In the skin the first step is the formation of previtamin D_3, which is converted to vitamin D_3 or cholecalciferol. Vitamin D_3 from the skin and intestine is carried to the liver where it is hydroxylated to calcidiol, which, in turn, is carried to the kidney where it is again hydroxylated to form the active product calcitriol.

The regulation of the relationship between calcium in blood and in bone depends primarily on parathyroid hormone, but it also involves other factors acting on calcium in tissues and cells. Indeed, calcium has many functions and is known to be a "universal regulator" (Anghileri and Tuffet-Anghileri, 1982; Campbell, 1983). A summary of the many actions of calcium is presented in Table 22–1 where these actions are grouped into six categories: (1) cell movement; (2) cell excitability; (3) cell secretion; (4) phagocytosis; (5) intermediary metabolism and respiration; and (6) cell reproduction.

In each category, changes in intracellular calcium translate into specific actions Table 22-1. For example in (1) by promoting cell movement, calcium causes muscle contraction, ciliate and flagellate movement, and chemotaxis. In (2), the production of an action potential in appropriate cells causes muscle contraction or photoreceptor response. In (3), another pertinent example related to neural and endocrine functions is the role of calcium in cell secretion of neurotransmitters and hormones. In (4), calcium is involved in the uptake of particles by phagocytosis or uptake of soluble substances by vesiculation. (5) refers to the role of calcium in glucogenesis, lipolysis, and prostaglandin synthesis. And, finally, (6) intracellular calcium acts in the regulation of various phases of cell reproduction.

Despite the universal role of calcium in cell function and metabolism, few studies have inquired into the potential changes in calcium activity with aging. The most

	20-29	30-39	40-49	50-59	60-69	70-79
BONE	0	1	10	14	20	22
CARTILAGE	0	1	21	26	29	30
TENDON	0	1	1	1	6	18
SKELETAL MUSCLE	0	8	16	19	24	24

Age Group

Figure 22–3. *Aging rates for human locomoter tissues.**

Aging rates represent values on an arbitrary scale from 0 at 20–29 years of age to 30 at 70–79 years of age.
*Data from Yamada, 1970.

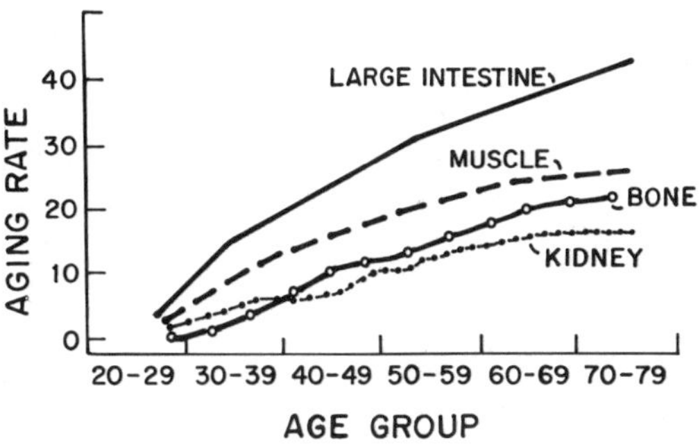

Figure 22–4. *Aging rates of several tissues.**

Aging rates represent values on an arbitrary scale from 0 at 20–29 years of age to 40 at 70–79 years of age.
*Data from Yamada, 1970.

prominent involvements of calcium related to aging (Table 22–2) appear to be: (1) triggering the intracellular production of oxygen radicals, which, as discussed in Chapter 7, would lead to the accumulation of potentially toxic substances (Hallett and Campbell, 1984); (2) a possible role of calcium in the pathogenesis of a number of diseases such as arthritis, obesity, diabetes, cystic fibrosis, etc.; (3) normal and abnormal bone metabolism; (4) calcification of injured and necrotic tissues such as occurs in atherosclerotic lesions (Chapter 17); (5) a possible role of calcium in age-related changes in cell excitability and in the action of several classes of drugs such as anesthetics, analgesics, and cardiovascular drugs (Godfraind *et al.*, 1985); (6) by its involvement on ion movement, calcium may affect neurotransmitter and hormone production and secretion; (7) its participation in phagocytosis may relate to aging of the immune system (Chapter 8). Considering the many actions of calcium in cell metabolism and function, it seems reasonable to hypothesize that alterations in metabolism and intracellular actions have an important bearing on the causes and course of the aging process. Research in this direction is lacking and should be pursued actively.

HORMONAL REGULATION OF BONE METABOLISM

Bone changes with aging apparently occur without marked alterations in the parathyroid gland or in the levels of parathyroid hormone (Chapter 15). However, in some women, parathyroid hormone levels increase with aging (Table 22–3). These higher levels have been interpreted as detrimental and probably contribute to bone loss. There seem to be some racial differences, with black and oriental postmenopausal women having lower levels of parathyroid hormone and higher levels of calcium well into advanced age than white women. There seems to be a sex difference as well, with men maintaining lower levels coincident with a lower incidence of osteoporosis than women (see also Chapters 13 and 14).

The increase in parathyroid hormone levels with aging may represent a compensatory response to reduced intestinal absorption of calcium, hence lower plasma calcium levels. Reduced exposure to sunlight in the immobile and housebound elderly will also impair vitamin D manufacture in the skin and accentuate any dietary

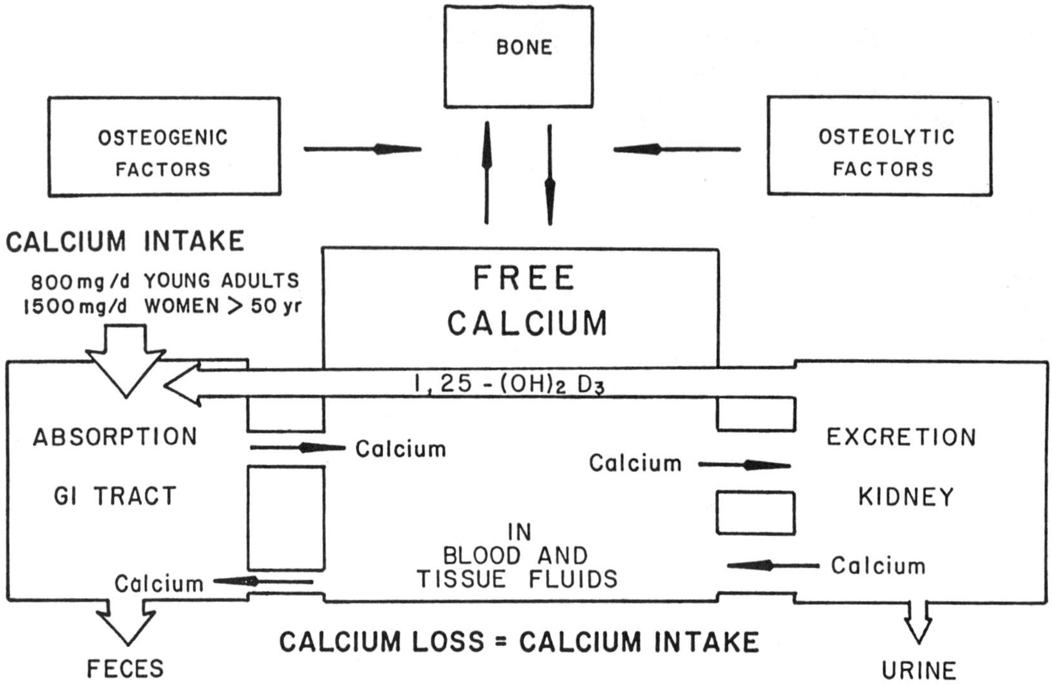

Figure 22–5. *Calcium metabolism.*

Note the different daily requirements of calcium with age: almost double in women after 50, as compared to young adults. (Drawing by S. Oklund)

deficiencies. Reduced renal degradation and excretion of parathyroid hormone may be another important factor; however, still controversial is whether such a reduction occurs and how serious it is.

Diseases of the Parathyroid Gland. Diseases of this gland are infrequent at all ages; however, they bear mentioning here for the symptoms associated with aging may mask parathyroid pathology. Indeed, if the disorder is recognized as a possible parathyroid dysfunction and is corrected, the symptoms described as aging changes may be ameliorated. Hyperparathyroidism presents with a variety of symptoms such as increased plasma calcium (hypercalcemia), renal calculi, peptic ulceration, and, in a few individuals, mental aberrations with psychotic components. The latter have been sometimes erroneously identified as senile dementia of the Alzheimer type (for a discussion of this condition see Chapter 9). In advanced stages, characteristic bone lesions are present. Hypoparathyroidism is quite rare at all ages and is easily recognizable for it generally follows ablation of the glands during thyroid gland surgery.

Regulation of bone metabolism depends on several hormones and in aging may depend on a number of endocrine changes. In women, the decrease in estrogen levels at menopause plays a key role in the induction of a common age-related degenerative bone disorder known as osteoporosis, already discussed in Chapter 13. Other hormones that influence bone metabolism include: glucocorticoids, which lower plasma calcium levels and over long periods of time may cause osteoporosis by decreasing bone formation (due to inhibition of cellular replication, protein synthesis, vitamin D absorption of calcium from the intestine and function of osteoblasts), and increasing bone resorption (due to stimulation of parathyroid hormone secretion). Growth hormone increases calcium excretion in urine, but it also increases intestinal absorption of calcium and this effect is greater than that on excretion and hence produces a positive calcium balance. Somatomedins, induced by growth hormone, stimulate protein synthesis in bone. Thyroid hormones may induce hypercalcemia and hypercalciuria and in some cases may also produce osteoporosis, but the mechanisms of these actions

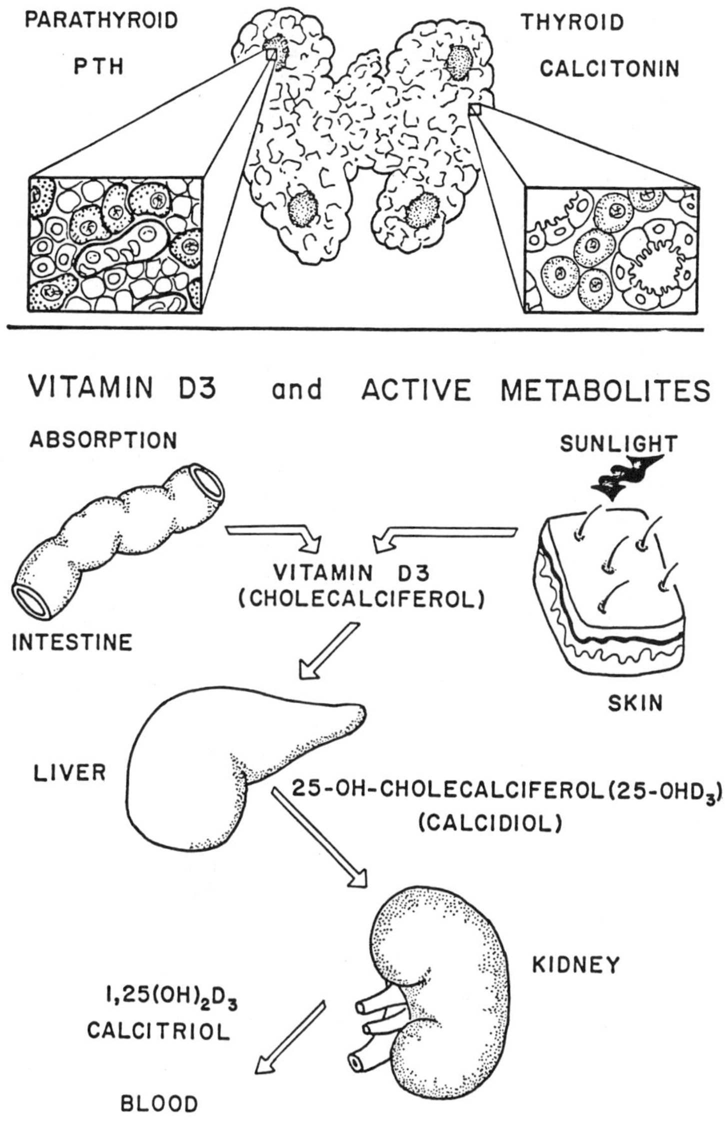

Figure 22–6. *Major hormones that regulate calcium metabolism.*

(At the top) The parathyroid gland secretes the parathyroid hormone (PTH) which acts directly on bone to increase its resorption and to mobilize calcium, thereby increasing plasma calcium. Calcitonin from the thyroid gland inhibits bone resorption and lowers serum calcium.

(At the lower part) Calcitriol, a sterol derivative, increases calcium absorption from the intestine and decreases renal excretion. It also enhances bone resorption. Vitamin D3 derives from dietary sources and is absorbed in the intestine or is formed in the skin under the influence of ultraviolet radiation. In the liver, vitamin D3 is converted to calcidiol which, in turn, is activated in the kidney to calcitriol, the most active form in calcium regulation. (Drawing by S. Oklund).

Table 22–1. INTRACELLULAR CALCIUM ACTIONS

ACTION	EXAMPLES OF CHANGE OF STATE
Cell movement	Muscle contraction Ciliate and flagellate movement Chemotaxis
Cell excitability	Muscle action potential Myocardial action potential Response of the eye and other photoreceptor types to light
Cell secretion	Neurotransmitter and hormone secretion Exocrine secretion gland
Cell phagocytosis	Vesiculation of particles or soluble substances
Intermediary metabolism and respiration	Glucose production Lipolysis Blood coagulation
Cell reproduction	Lymphocyte transformation Ovum fertilization and sperm capacitation Ovum maturation and meiosis

Table 22–2. INTRACELLULAR CALCIUM-DEPENDENT CHANGES RELATING TO AGING

ACTIONS	RELATION TO AGING
Intermediary metabolism and respiration	Activation of oxygen radicals Obesity and diabetes Arthritis and other diseases
Tissue calcification	Loss of bone calcium (osteoporosis) Abnormal deposition on normal and injured tissues (e.g., atherosclerotic lesions)
Cell excitability	Changes in cell potentials Changes in response to drugs
Cell secretion	Alterations in neurotransmitter and hormone production
Phagocytosis	Alterations in immune responses

Table 22–3. PARATHYROID HORMONE CHANGES WITH AGING

Increased Parathyroid Hormone Plasma Levels

Causes
- Decreased calcium intestinal absorption
- Decreased production of vitamin D (skin)
- Parathyroid tumors

Consequences
- Increased bone resorption (osteoporosis)
- Symptoms resembling SDAT
- Experimental progeria-like syndrome (rats)

Lesser Increase of Parathyroid Hormone Levels

Men
Black and Oriental women
- Lower incidence and severity of osteoporosis

are unclear. Estrogens prevent osteoporosis (Chapter 13), but the absence of estrogen receptors in bone leaves the mechanism of action unsettled. Insulin promotes bone formation and there is significant bone loss in diabetes.

Local factors also influence bone formation and resorption but their significance is uncertain, although it has been suggested that they may be involved in the continuing remodeling of bone, perhaps in response to stress. Most of these factors (e.g., epidermal growth factor, fibroblast growth factor, platelet-derived growth factor) promote bone growth. Prostaglandins E secreted by certain tumors increase plasma calcium levels. Osteoclast-activating factor, produced by the lymphocytes, induces bone loss in tumors of the bone marrow. It has been suggested, but not proven, that this factor may be involved in the formation of marrow cavities in normal bones. Physical activity also affects bone in several ways; it increases stress and strain on the skeleton due to muscular contraction and gravity; it improves blood flow to exercising muscles and, indirectly, increases venous return; and it stimulates bone mineral accretion. These effects are most marked in the young but are also effective, although to a lesser degree, in the old (Smith, 1981).

Age-Related Fractures. Fracture patterns in the elderly differ markedly from those in the younger adult. Whereas in the younger adult (20 to 50 years) considerable violence is required to break the bones, in the elderly fractures result from minimal or moderate trauma. This is due to the progressive loss of absolute bone volume, both compact and spongy bone, with aging. While bone loss has been shown to begin at 40 to 45 years of age in women and 50 to 60 years in men, it may in fact begin much earlier, at the end of the growth period.

In younger adults, fracture incidence is lower in females than in males; in the elderly, however, fracture incidence is much higher in females than in males, especially for fracture of the vertebral bodies, the lower end of the forearm, and the proximal femur. The relation between menopause and accelerated bone loss (osteoporosis) in females is discussed in Chapter 13.

Not only is the incidence of fractures higher in the elderly than the young, but the sites of fracture are often different. In the elderly, fractures occur through cancellous bone, usually next to a joint, rarely through the shaft of the bones, the most frequent site of fracture in the young.

In addition to osteoporosis, other age-related

bone disorders are associated with fractures. One of the most frequent is Paget's disease or osteitis deformans, characterized by pain, deformity, and fractures of the bones. It affects men more than women. The early lesions are localized osteolytic lesions and are followed by active remodeling leading to excessive and somewhat disorganized ("mosaic" or "woven" aspect) bone tissue balance. The resulting bone, although more dense than normal bone, has lost part of its elastic properties and is more susceptible to fractures (Courpron and Druguet, 1985). Complications include neoplastic transformation, neurologic signs due to compression of CNS structures, and heart failure. Management is based on symptomatic administration of aspirin for pain relief and of calcitonin and diphosphonates for decrease of bone resorption and bone formation.

AGING OF THE JOINTS*

The pattern and prevalence of joint changes in the elderly reflect (1) that certain disorders arise more frequently with increasing age and (2) that since many joint disorders are chronic, there is a steady cumulative effect with age (Gibson, 1985). By age 65, 80 percent of the population has some articular disorder (Harris, 1971; Kolodny and Klipper, 1976). Beyond the aging changes affecting the articulations themselves, the problems of added illness, frailty, diminished motivation, and social isolation affect the problems of management and outcome of the disorder (Gibson and Grahame, 1981).

Osteoarthritis and rheumatoid arthritis are examples of articular disorders occurring with increasing frequency from middle to old age. In fact, osteoarthritis is so common among the elderly that it is often assumed to be a normal accompaniment of aging rather than a disease. Radiologic signs of osteoarthritis are universal in the later decades of life, and in many cases, the changes are not associated with significant pain or disability. The dividing line between disease and normal aging is particularly difficult to draw with respect to degenerative changes of the cartilage (Gibson, 1985).

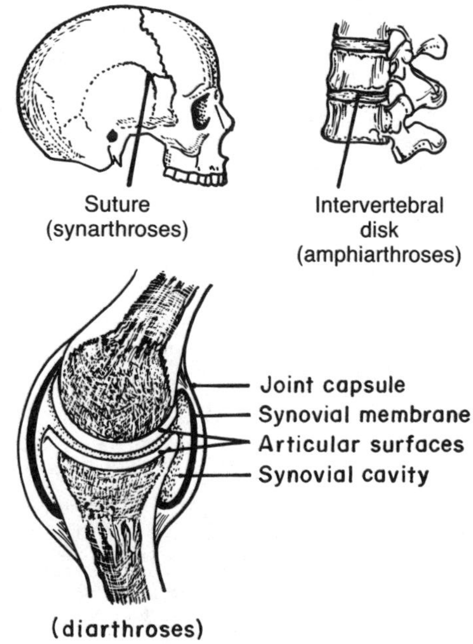

Figure 22–7. *The three major types of joints.*

Structure of the Joints. The articular system is comprised of simple and complex joints associated with the skeletal system and with their blood and nerve supplies. They represent junctions between two or more bones or cartilages (Figure 22–7). In the skull, the joints (synarthroses) are immovable and the connected bones are separated by a very thin layer of connective tissue. The articulations between the vertebrae (amphiarthroses) are a little more movable and the bones, in this case, are united by dense fibrous tissue and intervening cartilage. Most bones are freely movable (diarthroses), as the adjoining ends are coated with smooth cartilage separated by a short tube of strong fibrous tissue containing a fluid, synovial fluid. Joint cartilage is a special type of connective tissue with an extracellular matrix of proteoglycans and collagen, synthesized by the cartilage cells or chondrocytes.

AGE-RELATED CHANGES IN JOINTS

With aging, bony excrescences or osseous outgrowths (called osteophytes or bone spurs) occur on the heads of lone bones, for example, on the head of the femur in 33 percent of individuals beyond 50 years of age; they are not progressive and are viewed as a purely age-related phenomenon (Byers *et al.*, 1970). Areas where smooth cartilage has been replaced by a rough surface occur in all joints and are often seen as early as the second decade and spread to the periphery of the joint with age. The undulations and hollows that can

*This section (pp. 357–361) was contributed by M. L. Timiras.

be seen on the cartilage surface by electron microscopy increase both in depth and in diameter with increasing age and the outer surface irregularities become more common. Whether these consistent surface changes may be related to the development of osteoarthritis is not known. Osteoarthritis is associated with cartilage thinning. It is puzzling to note that in general, cartilage actually becomes thicker with increasing age (Armstrong and Gardner, 1977) with the exception of the patella (kneecap), which becomes thinner, especially in women (Meachim *et al.,* 1977). As cartilage ages, it loses some of its elasticity and becomes more easily stretched. Such changes lead to easier fatigability and higher susceptibility to osteoarthritis. There is a progressive pigmentation of the cartilage cells due to deposition of amino acid derivatives (probably from the protein of the matrix) and a gradual reduction in collagen, but no change in water content; the latter change is invariably associated with the early stages of osteoarthritis. The lack of changes or the presence of relatively minor biochemical changes with aging negates a generalized time-dependent deterioration of chondrocyte function in articular cartilage (Ball and Sharp, 1978).

PATHOLOGIC AND CLINICAL ASPECTS OF MUSCULOSKELETAL AGING

Normal and pathologic changes of the musculoskeletal system in the elderly are frequent and severely curtail the well-being of this population. They contribute significantly to Immobility, one of the dreaded Five I's of geriatrics (Chapter 3). It is difficult at best to encourage an elderly individual to maintain a program of physical fitness or activity if mobility is limited by joint pain. Chronic pain and disability of whatever cause or nature inflicts psychologic pain and dampens the morale of any individual, especially the elderly already prone to depression. The loss of the ability to participate in certain physical activities can be quite devastating to an elderly individual who may be suffering from other concomitant losses.

The list of musculoskeletal disorders of the elderly is quite long and an all-inclusive description of these disorders is beyond the scope of this text. A few of the more common entities will be described briefly in this section as a comparison and elucidation of "normal" aging changes. Musculoskeletal disorders can essentially be divided into two major types: those that affect joints without involvement of other organ systems, and those that affect the musculoskeletal system as a manifestation of systemic disease involving several organ systems (Table 22–4). Most of the systemic disorders mentioned in this section are often referred to as "collagen-vascular" as they are frequently manifested by changes in connective and/or vascular tissues. Several of these disorders are also referred to as "autoimmune" because they are associated with the presence of antibodies that attack and damage the host's own tissue (see Chapter 8; also Kay *et al.,* 1980).

OSTEOARTHRITIS AND GOUT

As already indicated, the most common articular disorder of the elderly is *osteoarthritis* or degenerative joint disease (Howell, 1980; Hamerman, 1983). The former term is preferable because it carries less negative connotation of decay and degeneration. Although it affects over three-quarters of the elderly, only 30 percent have any

Table 22–4. TYPES OF MUSCULOSKELETAL DISORDERS

	NONSYSTEMIC	SYSTEMIC
Noninflammatory	Osteoarthritis	
Inflammatory	Gout	Nonautoimmune Polymyalgia rheumatica Giant cell arteritis Autoimmune Rheumatoid arthritis Systemic lupus erythematosus

symptoms thereof and only 10 percent suffer significant disability therefrom. In a large proportion of the elderly, osteoarthritic lesions are discovered incidentally (for example on a chest x-ray). Risk factors include heredity as well as a history of trauma or injury to a certain body part or bone. Little is known of the pathogenesis of osteoarthritis. Why the process occurs at an accelerated pace in some individuals and why it affects certain joints and not others remain a mystery.

The early changes occur in the articular cartilage that lines the joint surfaces of the bones and are due to a loss of proteoglycans (Hamerman and Klagsbrun, 1985). Eventually the joint space narrows. The bone underlying the articular cartilage is itself undergoing aging changes and becomes more susceptible to damage and microfractures. In the attempt to repair the damage, cysts and osteophytes form in addition to sclerosis.

Osteoarthritis is not a systemic disease; it affects only individual joints. Susceptible locations include the hands, hips, knees, feet, and spine. Symptoms usually begin with aches and pain in the involved joints. Initially pain occurs with motion or weight bearing. In later stages, pain can occur at rest. Hand involvement occurs more frequently in women than in men and usually affects the distal interphalangeal joints. Small paired dorsal cysts of these affected joints are called Heberden's nodes. The first carpometacarpal joint at the base of the thumb is also commonly affected and gives the thumbs a squared-off appearance. Hip involvement occurs more frequently in men and can present with knee or groin pain.

Diagnosis and Treatment of Osteoarthritis. Diagnosis is made from clinical presentation and x-rays. It is important to differentiate the disease from other much more serious and life-threatening illnesses. For example, an elderly person with back pain should be carefully evaluated to ensure that no serious pathology, such as metastatic malignancy, exists before attributing the symptoms to osteoarthritis.

There is no cure for osteoarthritis. There are no measures known that prevent or reverse the progressive joint damage. Therefore, management revolves around symptomatic relief of pain (Table 22–5). In view of the lack of inflammatory activity in the infected joints, some argue that acetaminophen (Tylenol) is a good first-line medication particularly in those susceptible to the gastrointestinal effects of aspirin, which is just as effective. The nonsteroidal antiinflammatory agents (such as ibuprofen) are more potent but potentially have more side effects.

Table 22–5. MANAGEMENT OF OSTEOARTHRITIS

PHYSICAL INTERVENTIONS	MEDICAL TREATMENT
Weight loss	Acetaminophen (Tylenol)
Cane	Aspirin
Exercise to increase muscle strength	Nonsteroidal antiinflammatory drugs
Orthotics	Intraarticular steroid injection
Intraarticular lavage	
Arthroplasty (joint replacement)	

Avoidance of heavy weight bearing can be helpful especially in osteoarthritis of the knee. Weight loss, use of a cane, and orthotic (for the feet) can aid in diminishing some of the weight bearing. Muscle strengthening is also to be encouraged especially in knee osteoarthritis. Intraarticular steroid injection and lavage have been used with temporary amelioration of the symptoms. For osteoarthritis of the hip and knee, joint replacement or arthroplasty is available to individuals who present low operative risk and to whom continued activity is important (Wilcock, 1978).

Another localized joint disorder is *gout*. Unlike osteoarthritis, however, gout induces, in the articulation involved, an inflammatory response that is manifested by joint swelling (due to fluid accumulation), warmth, and the presence of white blood cells in the joint fluid. Urate crystals in the fluid are diagnostic of gout. This disease can occur in persons younger than 60 years of age who have a metabolic defect in the breakdown of uric acid, a product of protein metabolism formed from the breakdown of purines and synthesized from glutamine. Gout occurs commonly in the elderly because of decreased urate excretion by the kidney. This diminished urinary excretion can be further exacerbated by the use of diuretics (for reducing hypertension), which further decrease urate excretion (Chapters 20 and 24). The most frequently affected joint is the great toe (podagra), but other joints such as ankle, knee, elbow, and wrist can also be involved. An articular alteration similar to gout is pseudogout, or chondrocalcinosis, or calcium pyrophosphate deposition disease. This condition is distinguished from gout by the presence in the joint fluid or in the calcifications in joint cartilage of calcium pyrophosphate crystals. In both conditions, management involves the use of nonsteroidal antiinflammatory drugs (e.g., aspirin, indomethacin). The routine use of substances that either decrease production of uric acid (naproxen, colchicine) or increase its excretion (probenecid, sulfinpyrazone) is recommended only when serum uric acid levels are moderately increased and gouty attacks occur frequently.

AUTOIMMUNE ARTHRITIDES

Cartilage is an avascular tissue that is usually protected from immune recognition and, in this sense, is truly an immunologically privileged structure (Herman, 1980). However, both proteoglycans of the cartilage matrix and chondrocytes manifest antigenic properties, which are usually sequestered in the intact tissue. It is possible to envision that alteration of the integrity of cartilage, irrespective of the cause, may facilitate a leaching out into the circulation or may promote exposure of antigenic molecules of the tissue. An ensuing humoral or cell-mediated immune response would induce not only inflammation, but also cartilage degradation. Furthermore, because of the antigenic cross-reactivity between matrix constituents and tissues elsewhere in the body, sensitization initiated at one particular articulation may be responsible for the genesis of autoimmunicity throughout the body, thereby creating a systemic autoimmune disease. This is the case of *rheumatoid arthritis,* which is a systemic disease involving several organ systems in addition to the musculoskeleton (Vaughan, 1980). It occurs in all age groups but is more frequent in the elderly. Seventy-five percent of the elderly undergo a clinical course similar to that of young patients (e.g., weight loss, malaise, vasomotor disturbances, symmetric joint swelling with stiffness, redness, warmth, and pain, subcutaneous nodules, and sometimes enlarged spleen and lymph nodes). One-fourth, however, can exhibit atypical symptoms such as more severe proximal muscle weakness, more marked morning stiffness, higher fever, more severe weight loss, and malaise, while the inflammatory involvement of the joints may be less evident.

Pathogenesis of Rheumatoid Arthritis. Although rheumatoid arthritis is considered an autoimmune disease, multiple factors may contribute to its pathogenesis, including genetic predisposition and neural involvement, besides impaired immunologic control of virus infection and autoantibody formation. Involvement of the nervous system is suggested by the release at the sensory nerve endings to the joint tissues of the neuropeptide, substance P, involved in the transmission of pain signals (Lotz *et al.,* 1987). Substance P would stimulate the release of prostaglandin and activate the enzyme collagenase from the synovial cells (synoviocytes). In addition, substance P would stimulate proliferation of these cells. The symmetric distribution of the joints affected and the role of psychologic trauma in the onset and exacerbation of the disease are clinical observations that support a role for the nervous system in the disease. These observations point to a pathway by which the nervous system might be directly involved in diseases of the joints.

Differentiation from osteoarthritis is based on the different preferential localization of the joint lesions and the presence in rheumatoid arthritis of some markers such as rheumatoid factor, increased antinuclear antibodies, elevation of erythrocyte sedimentation rate, and gamma globulins. The management of rheumatoid arthritis is complex and includes both steroidal (corticosteroids) and nonsteroidal antiinflammatory drugs. Gold injections and, more recently, oral gold and agents used in chemotherapy are also effective.

Another autoimmune disease involving also the articulations is *systemic lupus erythemathosus*. The disease can occur in all age groups; however, it is less common and generally exhibits a clinically milder course in the elderly than in younger individuals.

Polymyalgia rheumatica (PMR) is a clinical syndrome that rarely occurs in persons less than 50 years of age. The average annual incidence in a studied population increased from about 20 per 100,000 persons aged 50 to 59 years to 112 per 100,000 persons aged 70 to 79 years (Chuang *et al.,* 1982). It occurs in females more than in males and virtually never occurs in blacks or Orientals. PMR is characterized by pain and stiffness in pelvic and shoulder girdles, which is worse in the morning (making it difficult to get out of bed) and after periods of inactivity. This reflects the inflammatory involvement of the synovial membranes of these joints (Chou and Schumacher, 1984). This is a systemic disease, and in some elderly individuals, there may be only general symptoms such as weight loss, fever, anorexia, malaise, and apathy. Anemia is commonly a complication. An elevated erythrocyte sedimentation rate is one of the nonspecific diagnostic findings. A prompt response to moderate doses of corticosteroids is also characteristic of this disorder.

Giant cell arteritis (GCA) or temporal arteritis often overlaps with PMR, 60 percent of patients with GCA having PMR as well. This disorder involves an inflammatory response in medium-sized arteries incorporating giant cells; hence the diagnosis is made by biopsy of arteries. The temporal arteries are most commonly affected (hence the name) and are more readily accessible for biopsy. Headache is the most common symptom; however, painful chewing caused by inflammation of the facial artery, transient double vision due to ischemia of the extraocular muscles, and sudden unilateral blindness due to occlusion of the terminal branches of the ophthalmic artery can also occur. This illness can lead to very serious problems stemming from the ischemia that results when an artery is affected. High doses of corticosteroids are required, and patients may have to remain on lower doses to prevent relapse (Goodman, 1979). It is important to exclude the possibility of GCA complications in patients with PMR, although obtaining temporal artery biopsies in all PMR patients is controversial.

PATTERN AND MANAGEMENT OF JOINT DISORDERS IN THE ELDERLY

Most of the disorders involving the articulations and described here become manifest for the first time beyond the age of 60 years. They represent a disease process that begins at a much younger age, is often generalized to the entire organism, and at the level of the articulations may be superimposed on normal aging processes. Establishing the diagnosis of an arthritis, especially when it is acute, tends to be more problematic in the elderly, but in view of the high incidence of these disorders in the aged population, it is important that the diagnosis be carefully conducted in order that the appropriate treatment may be rendered. The goal of such treatment is rarely the cure of the disease, still unavailable at present; rather, the present goal is to keep the symptoms under sufficient control to maintain mobility and independence of living as long as possible (see also Chapter 26).

AGING OF SKELETAL AND CARDIAC MUSCLE

It is well known that muscle strength declines with increasing age irrespective of the muscle group considered. Peak of muscle strength occurs between 20 and 30 years of age, and the decline is continuous thereafter, accelerating progressively with aging, although the rate of aging may vary depending on the muscle groups studied and the type of test used for measurement of muscle function (Figure 22–8). For example, the diaphragm remains active throughout life and undergoes little change with aging (see also Chapter 19). In contrast, the soleus muscle of the leg may be relatively inactive in the less mobile elderly and shows decreased strength with aging (Pearson *et al.*, 1985). Many of the age-related changes identified in muscle are similar to those of other tissues, but those occurring in muscle are particularly prominent because of the proportionally high distribution of muscle throughout the body and its relationship to lean body mass (body mass minus bone, mineral, fat, and water) (Kaldor and DiBattista, 1978; Seals *et al.*, 1984; Cunningham *et al.*, 1987). However, physical training, even in the elderly, can increase muscle power (Aniansson *et al.*, 1980).

Skeletal Muscle Structure and Function. The major function of muscle is to contract with utilization of energy and production of work and heat. Muscle is formed of individual muscle fibers containing fibrils that are divisible in filaments made up of contractile proteins, myosin, actin, tropomyosin, and troponin. Myosin forms the thick muscle filaments, and the three other proteins form the thin filaments. Cross-linkages are formed between myosin and actin molecules. During contraction, by breaking and reforming of cross-linkages between myosin and actin, the thin filaments slide over the thick filaments thereby shortening muscle length and utilizing ATP for energy.

Muscle fibrils are surrounded by the sarcotubular system formed of vesicles and tubules distinguished into a T system and a sarcoplasmic re-

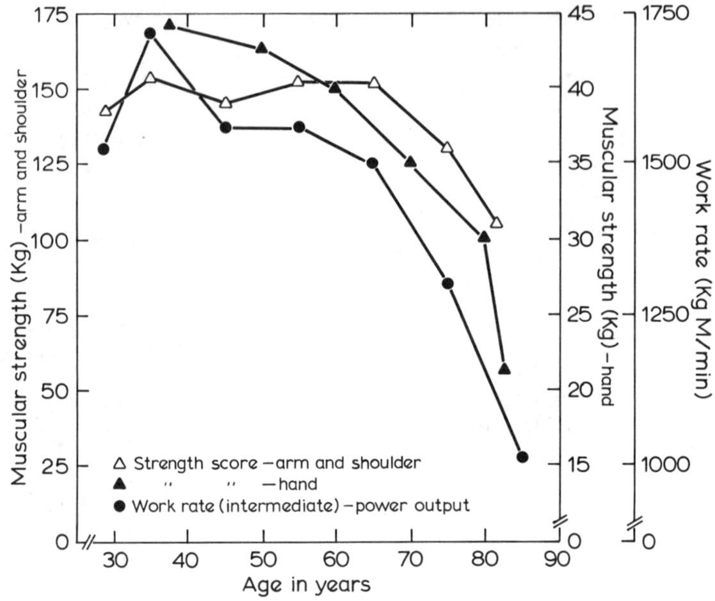

Figure 22–8. *Changes with age in muscular strength and maximum work rate.*

The test, used to assess changes in the strength of the arms and shoulders with age, is carried out in a subject who is seated and asked to pull, with maximum effort, different levers that are arranged to demand exertion of these muscles. Composite strength scores are calculated by summating the highest values recorded (in kilograms) for each of the pulls. Muscular strength did not change significantly from age 20 to age 65 and, even in the 70- and 80-year-old subjects, the reduction in muscle strength (although significant) was less marked when allowance was made for the lower body weight of this age group. Conversely, however, muscular strength as measured in the muscle of the hand with the Smedley dynamometer appears to undergo a progressive decline already significant at 50 years of age. Thus, the decline in strength varies with the muscular group considered.

Maximum work rate is assessed by having the subject, recumbent in bed, crank a drive spocket wheel with maximum effort, over 10- to 15-sec periods at four different "load" settings. Since the duration of the cranking exercise is short, the involvement of cardiovascular and pulmonary responses is minimal. Work rate is measured in terms of power output expressed in KgM/min; only values for intermediate loads are presented here. With all load rates, power output is seen to decline at 40 years of age and to progressively decrease thereafter, even when the values are corrected for the lower body weights in the 70- and 80-year-old subjects. Reduced coordination, involving both muscular and nervous function, is the most likely cause for the decline in power output with age.

ticulum. The function of the T system is rapid transmission of the action potential from the cell membrane to all myofibrils. The sarcoplasmic reticulum regulates calcium movement and muscle metabolism.

Muscle contraction is initiated by calcium release through depolarization at the neuromuscular junction; the action potential is transmitted to all fibrils via the T system and triggers the release of calcium from the sarcoplasmic reticulum. This process is called excitation-contraction coupling.

AGING-RELATED CHANGES IN SKELETAL MUSCLE

As muscles age they become smaller in size (i.e., become atrophic) and lose the usual red-brown color of normal muscle due to the myoglobin pigment. Instead they become yellow owing to the deposition of lipofuscin pigment and increased fat cells or gray owing to increased amounts of connective (fibrous) tissue (Larsson, 1982). Microscopically, muscle fibers are decreased in number and usually increase in size variability. Whether or not this is the most striking feature of the aging muscle or whether the proliferation of the T system and sarcoplasmic reticulum or the decrease in the synthesis of contractile protein or the reduction in the number of mitochondria are the primary phenomena remains controversial (Gutmann *et al.*, 1977; Florini, 1978; Fitts, 1981; Shafiq *et al.*, 1978, 1984).

Together with the muscular changes, the capability of the neuromuscular junction to sustain transmission of the nerve impulse from the neuronal axon to the muscle fiber decreases, the amount of acetylcholine (ACh), the neurotransmitter at the neuromuscular junction, declines, and the balance between nerve terminal growth and degeneration becomes less stable. These changes, which are characterized by their high variability (i.e., some neuromuscular junctions remain unaffected), are associated with altered membrane structure. Membrane alterations are manifested in reduced membrane potentials, lowered uptake of choline (the ACh precursor), and less uniform distribution of ACh receptors (Smith and Rosesheimer, 1984).

Motor nerve conduction velocity is reduced in old age while muscle and nerve fibers show increased refractoriness (Delbeke *et al.*, 1978). Thus senile muscle atrophy may be due to intrinsic muscle changes, to alterations of the neuromuscular junctions, and/or to mental impairment, as observed in demented individuals (Mortimer *et al.*, 1982; Denham, 1985).

AGING-RELATED CHANGES IN CARDIAC MUSCLE

The major function of the heart is to pump blood through the systemic and pulmonary circulations and thereby transport respiratory gases, nutrients, and metabolic products to and from tissues. It is not surprising, therefore, that any alteration in cardiac function will have life-endangering consequences (Weisfeldt, 1980). Indeed, heart disease, associated with advancing age and atherosclerosis, remains the most important single cause of death worldwide in old age in both sexes (Chapter 17). In individuals over the age of 65, heart disease accounts for approximately 70 percent or more of all cardiovascular deaths in many countries, including the United States. Usually, pathologic changes in the heart are superimposed on physiologic changes, which may be relatively minor but which, with the consistent and marked vascular atherosclerotic lesions, predispose the heart to a variety of pathologic conditions, most of them lethal.

Physiologic changes may be primary to the heart or they may be secondary to vascular lesions or to pulmonary disease. They may be so severe as to be present at rest, or they be manifest only under conditions of increased demand, such as physical exercise. They involve, in varying degrees, all cardiac elements, muscle, connective tissue, conduction tissue, endocardium, valves, and cardiac vasculature. When present, aging changes usually result in a general decline of all aspects of organ and integrated functions. This decline, associated with concomitant atherosclerosis of the coronary arteries, the major arteries of the heart, leads to severe pathology such as coronary heart disease, the major cause of cardiovascular disease in the elderly (Chapter 17). Another consequence of age-related changes in heart and vasculature is hypertension, which today is amenable to successful treatment (Chapters 17 and 24).

Structural changes with aging involve all components of the heart, including the myocardium, the cardiac muscle (closely resembling the skeletal muscle with the difference that myocardial fibers act as a syncytium), the cardiac conduction system (the specialized pacemaker tissue that can initiate repetitive action potentials), and the endocardium (the endothelial layer lining the internal surface of the cardiac cavities) (Figure 22–9).

Cardiac size and weight remain essentially unchanged with aging although some studies suggest enlargement, perhaps due to adipose tissue deposition, or atrophy, due to loss of muscle mass. The most constant change in cardiac muscle cells is the accumulation of lipofuscin (see also Chapters 4 and 5) often associated with accumulation of basophilic material, perhaps a possible byproduct of glycogen metabolism. Connective tissue represents 20 to 35 percent of cardiac mass, and this proportion either remains unchanged or increases slightly with aging.

Adipose tissue accumulates as fat deposits both in the ventricles and in the interatrial septum. In the latter, such deposits may displace conduction tissue in the sinoatrial node and lead to disturbances of conduction in some severe cases. Other extracellular deposits include some degree of fibrosis and amyloidosis. Fibrosis such as occurs in myocardial infarction (Chapter 17) reduces the contractile efficiency of cardiac muscle; amyloid degeneration and accumulation is also found in some alterations of the aged brain, such as neuritic plaques and congophilic deposits around cerebral vessels in SDAT (Chapter 9).

Specialized conducting cells (forming the si-

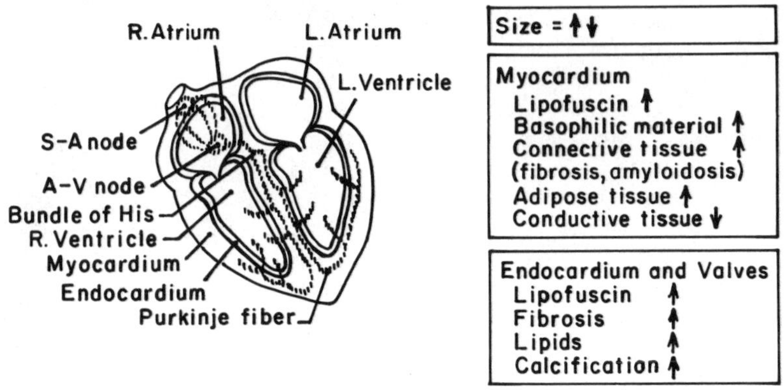

Figure 22–9. *Some age-related changes in the heart.* (Drawing by S. Oklund).

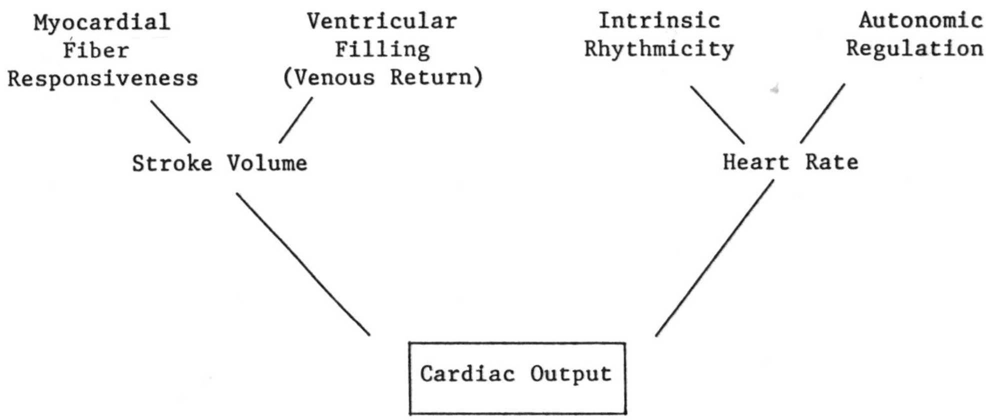

Figure 22–10. *Factors regulating cardiac output.*

noatrial and atrioventricular nodes and the intraventricular bundle of His) may be lost with aging, although this loss is usually moderate and may be associated with an increase in connective tissue elements, particularly collagen and elastin. It is not clear, however, whether and to what extent these changes interfere with conduction.

Endocardial changes—lipofuscin deposition and varying degrees of fibrosis—are probably influenced by mechanical factors such as blood flow. These mechanical factors may also be responsible for thickening of the atria and valves, which also show lipid deposition and calcification. The timetable of these valvular lesions varies with each valve.

One of the most consistent age-related changes in the human heart is a decrease in cardiac output, a significant functional change reflecting alterations in both cardiac stroke volume and cardiac rate (Figure 22–10). The reduction in stroke volume, the amount of blood ejected with each cardiac contraction, results from decreased muscle contractility and reduced stimulatory action of catecholamines (the sympathetic neurotransmitters). Reduced contractility leads to less forceful blood ejection in systole (the period of ventricular contraction) and reduced ventricular filling at diastole (the period of ventricular relaxation). As both systolic and diastolic efficiency decline with aging, cardiac output decreases correspondingly at a rate of approximately 1 percent per year over the age range of 20 to 80 years, so that by the age of 80, cardiac output is 2.5 l/minute, approximately half that at age 25.

Table 22–6. EFFECTS OF AGING ON VENOUS RETURN

Venous competence depends on:
- Venous diameter
- Intrathoracic pressure
- Total blood volume

With aging:
- Altered venous smooth muscle and elastin (Varicose veins, hemorrhoids)
- Thrombophlebitis
- Orthostatic hypotension (Sympathetic tone, baroreceptor activity, polypharmacy)

Role of Venous Return in Decreased Cardiac Output. Cardiac output depends, in addition to the factors previously discussed, on the amount of blood returning to the heart, the so-called venous return. This depends on the competence of the veins. For example, constriction of the peripheral veins reduces the size of the venous pools and reservoirs and, thus, increases venous return. Likewise, an increase in the normal negative intrathoracic pressure increases blood flow to the heart.

With aging, the venous compartment is altered, probably owing to changes in the elastic and smooth muscle components (Table 22–6). One example is represented by the varicose veins, tortuous and enlarged veins, most frequently found in the lower limbs; another example are hemorrhoids, enlargement of the rectal veins. Both of these occur at all ages, but are more frequent at older ages. Another condition related to the aging of the venous tree is thrombophlebitis, an inflammation of the veins due to the presence of a thrombus induced by slow blood flow in the unusually dilated veins.

Postural hypotension is common in the elderly and its incidence increases with age. This condition, characterized by a fall in blood pressure rising from the supine to the standing position, has been ascribed to autonomic, particularly sympathetic, insufficiency, to low circulating levels of epinephrine, or to decreased activity of the baroreceptors that sense blood pressure.

CARDIAC OUTPUT DURING PHYSICAL EXERCISE

The decreasing cardiac output with age may not have significant impact on the circulation at rest, but severely curtails the ability of the heart to respond to increased demand such as with physical exercise. This potential cardiac insufficiency is particularly reflected in the cardiac rate, which remains essentially unchanged at rest but cannot adjust efficiently to physical exercise. During exercise, the expected rise in cardiac rate necessary to increase cardiac output in order to provide for the increased oxygen consumption by the exercising muscles is much lower in the elderly than in the young. The maximum achievable heart rate with exercise decreases linearly with age and may be calculated empirically taking 220 beats/minute as the maximum in the adult. The age changes can be calculated by subtracting the age of the individual from the 220 value (Figure 22–11). Thus, in an 80-year-old the maximal heart rate that can be achieved while exercising is 220 − 80 = 140 beats/minute. Although the decline is progressive, the change is more precipitous after 50 years of age.

During exercise in the young adult cardiac output is also increased by increasing stroke volume. Here, the most important factor is the vasodilation in exercising muscles; vasodilation leads to a fall in vascular resistance, thereby augmenting venous return to the heart and increasing stroke volume. With aging, vascular resistance is increased owing to atherosclerosis and cannot be overcome by the strength of cardiac contraction inasmuch as muscle mass decreases with aging.

Cardiac Changes with Disuse. Decreased cardiac output similar to that described for the elderly is also found in young individuals after as little as a few weeks of muscle disuse, as found with bed rest, or in individuals exposed to low gravity, as astronauts (Chapter 3). Typical in the older individual after retirement is reduced physical activity; therefore, the reduced physical capacity of the elderly may be ascribed to aging *per se* and may have superimposed thereon the consequences of disuse. If, truly, a part of the reduced physical capacity of the elderly is the consequence of disuse, then, indeed, exercise may be of benefit in conditioning and rehabilitating cardiac function, in particular, and in the overall functional competence of the elderly.

NEURAL CONTROL OF CARDIAC FUNCTION

With aging, the regulatory competence of both the intrinsic (cardiac conduction system) and extrinsic (autonomic nervous system) cardiac innervations undergoes a progressive decline, particularly evident when the heart is required to respond to increased demand, as during physical exercise. The major factors involved in the regulation of cardiac contraction and likely to be altered with aging include loss of myocardial tis-

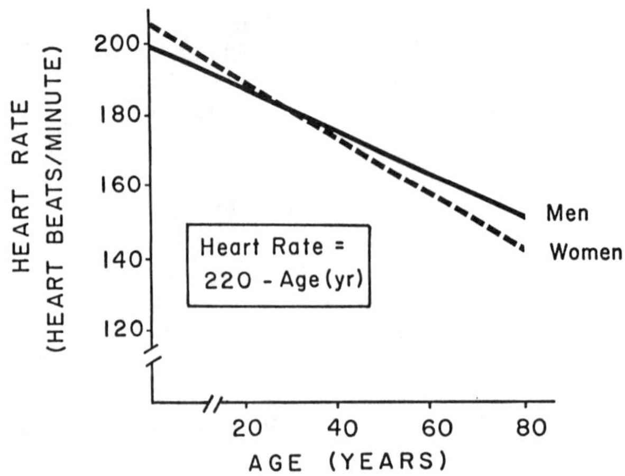

Figure 22–11. *Changes in cardiac rate with age.*

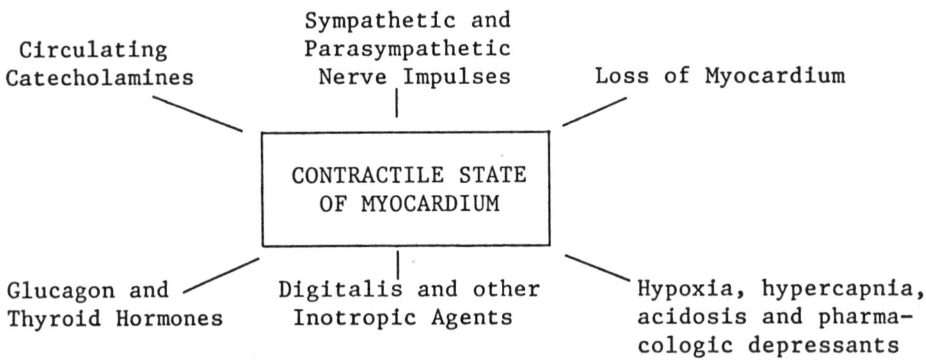

Figure 22–12. *Factors that influence the contractile state of the myocardium.*

sue, alterations in autonomic nervous control particularly with respect to levels of catecholamines, effects of hormones and selected drugs, and alterations in blood oxygen, electrolytes, and pH (Figure 22–12).

Cardiac Innervation and Some Disorders with Aging. Intrinsic conduction tissue is characterized by an unstable potential related to an unstable permeability to potassium. With aging, intracellular accumulation of lipofuscin, extracellular amyloidosis, loss of conduction cells, and fatty and fibrotic infiltrates lead to a decline in function and an increase in instability. Thus, cardiac dysrhythmias or arrhythmias (alterations of cardiac rhythmic contractions) are frequent in elderly subjects, whose hearts are more vulnerable to such biochemical insults as hypoxia (decreased oxygen), hypercapnia (increased carbon dioxide), acidosis (decreased pH), and hypokalemia (decreased blood potassium). All these conditions increase cardiac irritability, particularly of the atria. This, coupled with reduced cardiac output and coronary blood flow, leads, in the elderly more than in young adults, to cardiac failure and death.

Another conduction defect in the elderly is the interruption or block of conduction, most often between atria and ventricles. Cardiac blocks reflect potential cardiac disorders but are themselves usually asymptomatic and non-life-threatening.

The extrinsic innervation of the heart involves the two branches of the autonomic nervous system: the parasympathetic vagal innervation slows heart rate, the sympathetic increases cardiac rate and strength of contraction (Table 22–7). Both undergo changes with aging. Some constant findings are decreased inotropic (force of cardiac contraction) responses to catecholamines (primarily, epinephrine and norepinephrine) and decreased sensitivity to a variety of drugs (e.g., sympathetic agonists or antagonists) or hormones (e.g., thyroid hormones). Decreased sympathetic responses may be due to loss of neural cells resulting in reduced catecholamine content. In the rat, for example, cardiac norepinephrine is halved between the age of 1 month (young) and 28 months (old). Another contributing factor may be the reduction in number and/or affinity of beta recep-

Table 22–7. AUTONOMIC CARDIAC REGULATION

Parasympathetic stimulation
↓ Heart rate
↓ Conduction
↑ Refractory period
Sympathetic stimulation
↑ Heart rate
↑ Strength of contraction

tors. Although little is known in man, in experimental animals the number of receptors appears to be markedly decreased.

Hormonal and Chemical Influences on the Aging Heart. Some hormones, such as glucagon and thyroid hormones, influence myocardial contractility (Figure 22–11). Glucagon (see Chapter 16) increases the formation of cAMP through its binding to receptors other than beta receptors. Its inotropic action therefore can be beneficial to individuals suffering from toxicity due to the administration of beta-adrenergic blockers. Thyroid hormones increase the number of beta-adrenergic receptors in the heart, and their effects resemble those of sympathetic stimulation.

Various drugs also affect myocardial contractility. Xanthines, such as caffeine, exert their inotropic effect by inhibiting the breakdown of cAMP. The inotropic effect of digitalis and related drugs is due to their inhibitory effects on $Na^{+}K^{+}$-ATPase; this inhibition increases intracellular sodium, which, in turn, increases calcium availability to the cell and initiates contraction. Depressants such as barbiturates depress myocardial contractility.

To what extent age-related changes in myocardial function will influence and be influenced by hormones and drugs in elderly individuals is still not certain. Responses to inotropic agents are altered in the aged under some conditions. Evaluation of these data should take into consideration that cardiac responses depend in large measure on the condition of the vascular tree and that the agents considered exert both cardiac and extracardiac effects and the latter may, indirectly, influence the myocardium.

EXCITATION-CONTRACTION COUPLING IN THE AGING HEART

In skeletal muscle, the nerve impulse triggers the release of calcium from its stores in the sarcoplasmic reticulum and initiates contraction. Calcium binds to troponin C and, in so doing, uncovers several myosin-binding sites on actin. These molecular changes result in a decrease in the number of cross-linkages that bind myosin to actin and facilitate the sliding of the actin and myosin filaments along each other and induce shortening of the muscle during contraction. In cardiac muscle during the action potential, calcium ions diffuse into the myofibrils from stores in the sarcoplasmic reticulum and also from the T system. Cardiac T tubules are much larger and contain many times more calcium than those in skeletal muscle. This extra supply of calcium from the T tubules is at least one factor responsible for prolonging the cardiac muscle action potential for as long as one-third of a second, 10 times longer than in skeletal muscle. Once calcium concentration is lowered, chemical interaction between myosin and actin ceases and the muscle relaxes. ATP provides the energy necessary for the active transport of calcium.

With aging, the excitation-contraction coupling in the heart appears altered. In experimental animals or using isolated heart models, excitation appears insufficient—or less sufficient than in the young—to trigger the release of calcium from its stores; the calcium stores themselves would be reduced and the accumulation of calcium in the sarcoplasmic reticulum would be slowed. Likewise, the active transport of calcium appears inhibited and the duration of contraction and relaxation is prolonged (Lakatta *et al.*, 1975). Alterations with aging in calcium stores and movements are also reflected in diminished cardiac responses to inotropic agents such as catecholamines. These agents exert their stimulatory action on cardiac contraction by loading calcium stores and by facilitating calcium transport in the cells. With aging, both calcium storage and movements would be altered, hence the reduced effectiveness of the inotropic factors to activate cardiac contraction.

MUSCLE ENERGY SOURCES AND METABOLISM

Muscle activity requires energy; the muscle has been called a machine for converting chemical energy to mechanical. In the case of the heart, the requirement is for continued sustained work with limited resting time when compared to skeletal muscle activity. Activity in skeletal muscle is on demand with intervening periods of contractile inactivity. To provide for the energy requirements of cardiac muscle, the heart has an abundant blood supply, numerous mitochondria, and a high content of myoglobin.

Myoglobin is an iron-containing pigment, resembling hemoglobin. It serves as an oxygen supply during contractions that cut off blood flow and also facilitates the diffusion of oxygen to mitochondria where the oxidative reactions occur.

Normally, less than 1 percent of the energy liberated in cardiac tissue is due to anaerobic metabolism; the heart is highly dependent on aerobic processes. Under basal (at rest) conditions, 35 percent of the caloric needs of the heart are provided by carbohydrates, 5 percent by ketones and amino acids, and 60 percent by fat. The proportion of these substrates varies with the nutritional state. Oxygen consumption of the heart is primarily dependent on the heart rate and the contractile state of the myocardium, among other factors. Increasing the heart rate increases oxygen consumption, at least temporarily until the appropriate compensatory adjustments enter into effect, and so, too, does increased peripheral resistance, which causes the heart to work harder. This explains why in angina pectoris (described in Chapter 17) there is a relative deficiency of oxygen due to the greater oxygen demand to expel blood against increased peripheral pressure.

PHYSICAL ACTIVITY PROGRAMS FOR THE AGED

Physical activity programming for the older adult requires more individualized care and more knowledge of the musculoskeletal system than with any other age group. Several factors must be recognized and critically evaluated before establishing a useful program, one that provides the most benefits without endangering the individual. These factors include: (1) the wide spectrum of physical abilities displayed by the older individuals and the considerable variability among individuals; (2) the difficulty of detecting and assessing these abilities by medical examination, including electrocardiogram under exercise (e.g., treadmill) (stress ECG) and forestalling any potential dangers to safety; (3) the need to distinguish between the "young" old (still preserving some lifelong activity habits) and the "old" old (with mental and physical disorders restricting activity) (Morse and Smith, 1981; Serfass, 1981; Shephard, 1981; Sidney, 1981). While many older individuals are limited in their ability to pursue regular physical activity, the need for a minimum level of daily exercise to prevent cardiovascular and musculoskeletal complications and further age-related deterioration is well established (Morse and Smith, 1981). A number of exercise programs are being tested and implemented to improve mechanical functioning, including amelioration of performance of skeletal muscle and cardiovascular function (Moritani, 1981; Sidney, 1981), joints (Munns, 1981), and bone (Smith, 1981).

In addition, enhancement of body image through physical exercise and improved fitness is another important reason for encouraging further exploration and implementation of physical fitness programs in the elderly population (see also Chapter 26).

References

Anghileri, L. J., and Tuffet-Anghileri, A. M.: *The Role of Calcium in Biological Systems,* CRC Press, Boca Raton, FL, **1982.**

Aniansson, A.; Grimby, G.; Rungren, A.; Svanborg, A.; and Olander, J.: Physical training in old men. *Age Ageing,* **9:**186–187, **1980.**

Armstrong, G. G., and Gardner, D. L.: The thickness and distribution of human femoral head articular cartilage changes with age. *Ann. Rheum. Dis.,* **36:**407–412, **1977.**

Ball, J., and Sharp, J.: Osteoarthrosis. In Scott, J. T. (ed.): *Copeman's Textbook of the Rheumatic Diseases,* 5th ed., Churchill Livingstone, London, New York, **1978.**

Byers, P. D.; Contempomi, C. A.; and Farkas, T. A.: A post mortem study of the hip joint including the prevalence of the features of the right side. *Ann. Rheum. Dis.,* **29:**15–31, **1970.**

Campbell, A. K.: *Intracellular Calcium,* John Wiley & Sons, London, UK, **1983.**

Chen, J. C.; Warshaw, J. B.; and Sanadi, D. R.: Regulation of mitochondrial respiration in senescence. *J. Cell. Physiol.,* **80:**141–148, **1972.**

Chou, C- T., and Schumacher, H. R., Jr.: Clinical and pathologic studies of synovitis in polymyalgia rheumatica. *Arthritis Rheum.,* **27:**1107–1117, **1984.**

Chuang, T- Y.; Hunder, G. G.; Ilstrup, D. M.; and Kurland, L. T.: Polymyalgia rheumatica. A 10-year epidemiologic and clinical study. *Ann. Intern. Med.,* **97:**672–680, **1982.**

Cobb, W. M.: Skeleton. In Lansing, A. I. (ed.): *Cowdry's Problems of Ageing: Biological and Medical Aspects,* 3rd ed., Williams & Wilkins, Baltimore, **1952.**

Courpron, P., and Druguet, M.: Bone disorders. In Pathy, M. S. J. (ed.): *Principles and Practice of Geri-*

atric Medicine, John Wiley & Sons, Chichester, UK, **1985.**

Cunningham, D. A.; Rechnitzer, P. A.; Howard, J. H.; and Donner, A. P.: Exercise training of men at retirement: A clinical trial. *J. Gerontol.,* **42:**17–23, **1987.**

Delbeke, J.; Kopec, J.; and McComas, A. J.: Effect of age, temperature and disease on the refractoriness of human nerve muscle. *J. Neurol. Neurosurg. Psychiatry,* **41:**65–71, **1978.**

Denham, M.: Diseases of muscle and connective tissues. In Pathy, M. S. J. (ed.): *Principles and Practice of Geriatric Medicine,* John Wiley & Sons, Chichester, UK, **1985.**

Enlow, D. H.: *Principles of Bone Remodeling: An Account of Postnatal Growth and Remodeling Processes in Long Bones and the Mandible,* Charles C Thomas, Springfield, IL, **1963.**

Exton-Smith, A. N.: Mineral metabolism. In Finch, C. E., and Schneider, E. L. (eds.): *Handbook of the Biology of Aging,* Van Nostrand Reinhold, New York, **1985.**

Fitts, R. H.: Aging and skeletal muscle. In Smith, E. L., and Serfass, R. C. (eds.): *Exercise and Aging: The Scientific Basis,* Enslow Publishers, Hillside, NJ, **1981.**

Florini, J. R.: Biosynthesis of contractile proteins in normal and aged muscles. In Kaldor, G., and DiBattista, W. J. (eds.): *Aging in Muscle,* Raven Press, New York, **1978.**

Francis, R. M.; Peacock, M.; Storer, J. H.; Davies, A. E. J.; Brown, W. B.; and Nordin, B. E. C.: Calcium malabsorption in the elderly: The effect of treatment with oral 25-hydroxyvitamin-D3. *Eur. J. Clin. Invest,* **13:**391–396, **1983.**

Garn, S. M.: *The Earlier Gain and the Later Loss of Cortical Bone,* Charles C Thomas, Springfield, IL, **1970.**

Garn, S. M.; Rohmann, C.; Wagner, B.; and Ascoli, W.: Continuing bone growth throughout life: A general phenomenon. *Am. J. Phys. Anthropol.,* **26:**313–317, **1967.**

Gibson, T.: Disease of joints. In Pathy, M. S. J. (ed.): *Principles and Practice of Geriatric Medicine,* John Wiley & Sons, Chichester, UK, **1985.**

Gibson, T., and Grahame, R.: Rehabilitation of the elderly arthritic patient. *Clinics Rheum. Dis.,* **7:**485–495, **1981.**

Godfraind, T.; Vanhoutte, P. M.; Govoni, S.; and Paoletti, R.: *Calcium Entry Blockers and Tissue Protection,* Raven Press, New York, **1985.**

Goodman, B. W.: Temporal arteritis. *Am. J. Med.,* **67:**839–852, **1979.**

Gutman, E.: Muscle. In Finch, C. E., and Hayflick, L. (eds.): *Handbook of Biology of Ageing,* Van Nostrand Reinhold, New York, **1977,** pp. 445–469.

Hallett, M. B., and Campbell, A. K.: Is intracellular Ca^{++} the trigger for oxygen radical production by polymorphonuclear leucocytes? *Cell Calcium,* **5:**1–19, **1984.**

Hamerman, D.: Current leads in research on the osteoarthritic joint. *J. Am. Geriatr. Soc.,* **31:**299–304, **1983.**

Hamerman, D., and Klagsbrun, M.: Osteoarthritis. Emerging evidence for cell interactions in the breakdown and remodeling of cartilage. *Am. J. Med.,* **78:**495–499, **1985.**

Harris, A. I.: *Handicapped and Impaired in Great Britain,* Part 1, Social Survey Division, Office of Population Censuses and Surveys, HMSO, London, **1971.**

Herman, J. H.: Cartilage as an immune stimulator and target tissue in rheumatoid diseases. In Kay, M. M. B.; Galpin, J.; and Makinodan, T. (eds.): *Aging, Immunity, and Arthritic Disease,* Raven Press, New York, **1980.**

Howell, D. S.: Aging in osteoarthritis (Osteoarthrosis or degenerative joint disease). In Kay, M. M. B.; Galpin, J.; and Makinodan, T. (eds.): *Aging, Immunity, and Arthritic Disease,* Raven Press, New York, **1980.**

Kaldor, G., and DiBattista, W. J. (eds.): *Aging in Muscle,* Raven Press, New York, **1978.**

Kay, M. M. B.; Galpin, J.; and Makinodan, T. (eds.): *Aging, Immunity, and Arthritic Disease,* Raven Press, New York, **1980.**

Kerley, E. R.: Estimation of skeletal age: After about age 30. In Stewart, T. D. (ed.): *Personal Identification in Mass Disasters,* National Museum of Natural History, Smithsonian Institute, Washington, **1970.**

Kolodny, A. L., and Klipper, A. R.: Bone and joint diseases in the elderly. *Hosp. Pract.,* **11:**91–101, **1976.**

Lakatta, E. G.; Gerstenblith, G.; Angell, C. S.; Shock, N. W.; and Weisfeldt, M. L.: Prolonged contraction duration in aged myocardium. *J. Clin. Invest.,* **55:**61–68, **1975.**

Larsson, L.: Aging in mammalian skeletal muscle. In Mortimer, J. A.; Pirozzolo, F. J.; and Maletta, G. J. (eds.): *The Aging Motor System,* Praeger, New York, **1982.**

Lotz, M.; Carson, D. A.; and Vaughan, J. H.: Substance P activation of rheumatoid synoviocytes: Neural pathway in pathogenesis of arthritis. *Science,* **235:**893–895, **1987.**

Meachim, G.; Bentley, G.; and Baker, R.: Effect of age on thickness of adult patellar articular cartilage. *Ann. Rheum. Dis.,* **36:**563–568, **1977.**

Moritani, T.: Training adaptations in the muscles of older men. In Smith, E. L., and Serfass, R. C. (eds.): *Exercise and Aging: The Scientific Basis,* Enslow Publishers, Hillside, NJ, **1981.**

Morse, C. E., and Smith, E. L.: Physical activity programming for the aged. In Smith, E. L., and Serfass, R. C. (eds.): *Exercise and Aging: The Scientific Basis,* Enslow Publishers, Hillside, NJ, **1981.**

Mortimer, J. A.; Pirozzolo, F. J.; and Maletta, G. J. (eds.): *The Aging Motor System,* Praeger, New York, **1982.**

Munns, K.: Effects of exercise on the range of joint motion in elderly subjects. In Smith, E. L., and Serfass, R. C. (eds.): *Exercise and Aging: The Scientific Basis,* Enslow Publishers, Hillside, NJ, **1981.**

Pearson, M. B.; Bassey, E. J.; and Bendall, M. J.: Muscle strength and anthropometric indices in elderly men and women. *Age Ageing,* **14:**49–54, **1985.**

Roche, A. F.: Aging in the human skeleton. *Med. J. Aust.,* **2:**943–946, **1966.**

Rogers, S. L.: *The Aging Skeleton—Aspects of Human Bone Involution,* Charles C Thomas, Springfield, IL, **1982.**

Schranz, D.: Age determinations from the internal structure of the humerus. *Am. J. Physiol. Anthropol.,* **17** (4):273–277, **1959.**

Seals, D. R.; Hagberg, J. M.; Hurley, B. F.; Ehsani, A. A.; and Holloszy, J. O.: Endurance training in older men and women. I. Cardiovascular responses to exercise. *J. Appl. Physiol.,* **57:**1024–1029, **1984.**

Serfass, R. C.: Exercise for the elderly: What are the benefits and how do we get started? In Smith, E. L., and Serfass, R. C. (eds.): *Exercise and Aging: The Scientific Basis,* Enslow Publishers, Hillside, NJ, **1981.**

Shafiq, S. A.; Lewis, S. G.; Dimino, L. C.; and Schutta, H. S.: Electron microscopic study of skeletal muscles in elderly subjects. In Kaldor, G., and DiBattista, W. J. (eds.): *Aging in Muscles,* Raven Press, New York, **1978.**

Shafiq, S. A.; Lewis, S.; Leung, B.; and Schutta, H. S.: Fine structure of aging skeletal muscle. In Johnson, J. E., Jr. (ed.): *Aging and Cell Structure,* vol. 1,

Plenum Press, New York, **1984.**

Shephard, R. J.: Cardiovascular limitations in the aged. In Smith, E. L., and Serfass, R. C. (eds.): *Exercise and Aging: The Scientific Basis,* Enslow Publishers, Hillside, NJ, **1981.**

Sidney, K. H.: Cardiovascular benefits of physical activity. In Smith, E. L., and Serfass, R. C. (eds.): *Exercise and Aging: The Scientific Basis,* Enslow Publishers, Hillside, NJ, **1981.**

Smith, E. L.: Bone changes in the exercising older adult. In Smith, E. L., and Serfass, R. C. (eds.): *Exercise and Aging: The Scientific Basis,* Enslow Publishers, Hillside, NJ, **1981.**

Smith, E. L.; Sempos, C. T.; and Purvis, R. W.: Bone mass and strength decline with age. In Smith, E. L., and Serfass, R. C. (eds.): *Exercise and Aging: The Scientific Basis,* Enslow Publishers, Hillside, NJ, **1981.**

Smith, D. O., and Rosenheimer, J. L.: Aging at the neuromuscular junction. In Johnson, J. E. (ed.): *Aging and Cell Structure,* Plenum Press, New York, **1984.**

Tonna, E. A.: Electron microscopy of skeletal aging. In Johnson, J. E., Jr. (ed.): *Aging and Cell Structure,* vol. 1, Plenum Press, New York, **1981.**

Ubelaker, D. H.: *Human Skeletal Remains: Excavation, Analysis, Interpretation,* Aldine Publishing Company, Chicago, **1978.**

Vaughan, J. H.: Aging, immunity and rheumatoid arthritis. In Kay, M. M. B.; Galpin, J.; and Makinodan, T. (eds.): *Aging, Immunity, and Arthritic Disease,* Raven Press, New York, **1980.**

Weisfeldt, M. L.: *The Aging Heart. Its Function and Response to Stress,* Raven Press, New York, **1980.**

Wilcock, G. K.: Benefits of total hip replacement to older patients and the community. *Br. Med. J.,* **2**:37–39, **1978.**

Yamada, H.: *Strength of Biological Materials,* Williams & Wilkins, Baltimore, **1970.**

CHAPTER

23 AGING OF THE SKIN AND CONNECTIVE TISSUE

Mary L. Timiras

INTRODUCTION

Perhaps no aspect of aging is as dramatic or readily obvious as that which occurs in the skin and its appendages. The development of either gray hair or facial wrinkles is irrefutable evidence of the passage of time and the aging process. Many descriptions of aging skin fail to distinguish between intrinsic aging changes and changes caused by environmental insults that accumulate with exposure time. For example, chronic solar damage changes are far more prevalent in the elderly since they result from cumulative exposure over time (Forbes *et al.*, 1979). Intrinsic changes in the structure and function of skin that occur with aging also make the skin more vulnerable to external insults. It is not surprising, then, that dermatologic problems are common in the elderly. Several studies describe how almost one-half of persons over 65 years of age have at least one dermatologic disease requiring medical attention (Johnson and Roberts, 1977; Gilchrest, 1982). About one-third of these have more than one skin problem. Multiple skin conditions are characteristic of the very old, and the common ones are different from those affecting the young (Kligman *et al.*, 1985; Marks, 1985).

A connective tissue component particularly involved in skin changes with aging is collagen. Because it is ubiquitous throughout the body and undergoes identifiable changes with age, collagen has been intensively studied as a possible primary source for the onset of aging processes. It has been proposed, for example, that the striking changes that take place with age in the structure and chemistry of collagen fibers and the surrounding extracellular matrix (previously designated as ground substance) may derive from metabolic alterations in tissues—as manifested by the occurrence of cross-linkages—and, thus, represent a fundamental mechanism by which overall functional impairment is induced in the aged (Verzar, 1968). In order to provide an understanding of the nature and origin of age-related changes in the skin and of how these changes lead to dermatologic problems in the aged, this chapter will review some of the anatomic and physiologic changes that occur in the skin and collagen with normal senescence. Pressure sores will be discussed as a clinical example of skin dysfunction in the elderly.

AGE-RELATED CHANGES IN THE SKIN

The skin is one of the largest organs of the body and accounts for approximately 16 percent of the total body weight. It is part of the integument, a covering of the entire body, which, in addition to the skin, includes the nails, hair, and various types of glands, all accessory organs derived from the skin. The following are the major functions of the skin: (1) it provides a barrier to exclude harmful substances and prevents desiccation; (2) it plays a role in the control of body temperature; (3) it readily repairs itself; (4) it receives sensory stimuli: touch, pressure, temperature, and pain; (5) it excretes waste products through sweat glands and secretes special products such as milk from mammary glands. The skin consists of an epithelium, the epidermis, and the dermis considered as part of the connective tissue.

Epidermis and Dermis. The main layers of the skin consist of the surface layer, known as the epidermis, and a deeper connective tissue layer, known as the dermis. The interface between the epidermis and dermis is normally uneven and forms wavy interdigitations. The projections of the dermis into the epidermal layer are called dermal papillae.

The epidermal cells produce keratin, a fibrous protein essential for protection, and form the dead superficial layers of the skin (stratum corneum). The superficial keratinized cells are continuously exfoliated and are replaced by cells that arise from the basal layer of the epidermis. The sequence of changes of an epidermal cell from the basal layer of the epidermis to keratinization and exfoliation normally takes from 15 to 30 days, depending on the region of the body.

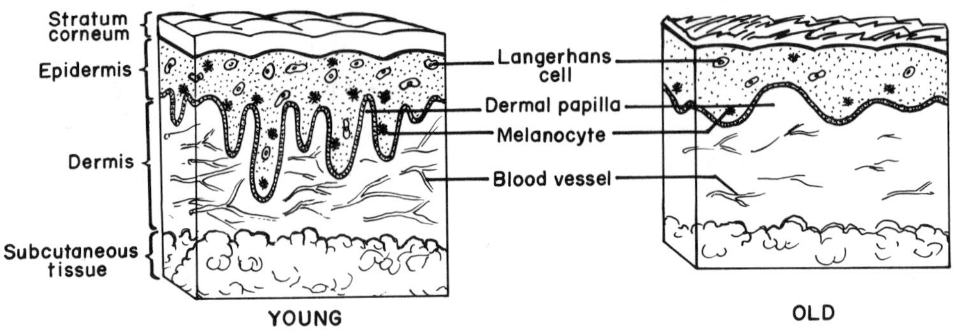

Figure 23–1. *Histologic changes in normal aging skin.*

Changes from top to bottom include (1) rougher stratum corneum, (2) fewer melanocytes and Langerhans cells, (3) flattening of the dermo-epidermal junction, (4) fewer blood vessels in the dermis and, (5) less subcutaneous tissue.

The epidermis is locally specialized to form various skin appendages such as the hair, nails, sweat glands, and oil or sebaceous glands. Other types of cells that are found in the epidermis include melanocytes, which produce the pigment melanin that protects against ultraviolet irradiation, and Langerhans cells which are believed to be responsible for recognition of foreign antigens.

Since the epidermis has no blood vessels, the dermis, which has abundant blood vessels, plays an important role in supplying the epidermis with nutrients. Although the epidermis does contain nerve endings, there are more in the dermis because it also contains the nerves that lead to the sensory nerve endings. In addition, epidermal appendages such as the hair follicles and sebaceous and sweat glands extend down into the dermis. Below the dermis is looser connective tissue, which usually consists of subcutaneous adipose tissue that plays a role in fat metabolism.

EPIDERMAL CHANGES

Dryness and/or roughness of the aging skin is one of the most readily appreciated changes that occur. This could be due either to a decrease in the moisture content of the stratum corneum or to a decrease in vertical height and increase in overall surface area of epidermal cells. The increased dryness results in a surface likened to "shingles on an old roof" (Fenske and Lober, 1986) (Figure 23–1). The exact pathogenesis of the drying process is still unclear but probably represents a combination of several contributing factors.

Another well-recognized change that occurs with aging is the increased incidence of both benign and malignant epidermal neoplasms. Although there is no question that chronic ultraviolet-light exposure contributes to this problem, some intrinsic cellular alterations of basal cells may also contribute to the increased incidence of skin cancer in the elderly.

One of the histologic changes that occurs most consistently in the elderly is flattening of the dermoepidermal interface and effacement of the dermal papillae. This reduces the total area of dermoepidermal junction per area of external body surface area. This change predisposes older persons to blister formation and shear-type injuries and easy abrasions. Another observation is an age-associated decrease in epidermal turnover rate of about 50 percent between the third and seventh decades of life. This means fewer basal cells are replaced and it takes longer for a basal cell to reach the stratum corneum and be exfoliated. The slower movement prolongs the exposure of epidermal cells to potential carcinogens and contributes to an increased incidence of skin cancer; in addition, it is responsible for the slowing of wound healing.

The number of melanocytes decreases with age by approximately 8 to 20 percent per decade after the age of 30 in both exposed and unexposed areas (Quevedo *et al.*, 1969). This reduction leads to irregular pigmentation, especially in sun-exposed areas (hence the "age spots" frequently seen on the back of the hands), and to the inability to tan as deeply as when younger. However, other studies seem to negate or at least to minimize this reduction in melanocytes (Kligman *et al.*, 1985). The number of Langerhans cells decreases as well. This change is expected to contribute to a decline in the skin's cell-mediated immune response (see Chapter 8). The reduction of melanin and its protective action, the reduced inflammatory warning signs, and the reduced immune capacity combine to increase the risk for tumorigenesis. In fact, elderly patients require longer ultraviolet exposure to develop erythema and edema (sunburn) than younger patients. Thus, the body's warning system as well as its defense system in relation to skin cancer become blunted with age. In addition, ultraviolet light further reduces the quantity of Langerhans cells. These changes together with the increase in cumulative irradiation exposure may explain why nonmelanomatous skin cancers are prone to occur on sun-exposed skin.

DERMAL CHANGES

The dermis in elderly individuals has a decreased density and fewer cells and blood vessels. The total amount of collagen decreases 1 percent per year in adulthood; therefore, skin thickness decreases linearly with age after 20. Collagen itself becomes thicker, less soluble, and more resistant to digestion by collagenase with age. Changes in the number and type of cohesive bonds make collagen stronger and more stable. Collagen alteration predisposes the dermis to tear-type injury since there is less "give" in the tissue. Architectural rearrangements of fibers may also be responsible for changes in dermal tissue properties.

The total amount of hyaluronic acid and dermatan sulfate, components of the extracellular matrix, decreases in the dermis with aging, affecting the viscosity of the dermis, which, in turn, may alter the rate of dermal clearance of substances. Changes in the elastic fibers of the dermis also result in loss of stretch and resilience. A consequence is skin sagging and wrinkling and predisposition to injury of the underlying tissues following trauma. While even the very old (beyond 85 years) can effectively repair extensive wounds, elderly individuals, in general, lag behind younger controls at every stage of wound healing (Grove, 1982; Grove and Kligman, 1983).

Pale skin results from the decrease in dermal blood vessels. Skin surface temperature is also decreased owing to the diminished vascularity. These changes, together with a decrease in the thickness of the subcutaneous tissue, make thermoregulation more difficult in the elderly. The vascular changes described above also result in a decrease in dermal clearance of foreign materials, which can prolong or exacerbate cases of contact dermatitis.

AGE-RELATED CHANGES IN SKIN APPENDAGES

Older individuals produce less sweat because sweat glands decrease in either number or functional efficiency, a decrease that interferes further with thermoregulation. Although the number of sebaceous glands remains constant with age, their size increases, while the sebum output as well as wax production decline with age. The diminished sweat and oil production no doubt contribute to skin dryness and roughness in the elderly.

The rate of linear nail growth decreases with aging. Nail plates usually become thinner, more brittle, and fragile.

Hair graying occurs because of a progressive loss of functional melanocytes from hair bulbs. By the age of 50, it is said that in 50 percent or more of the population at least 50 percent of the body hair is gray regardless of sex or hair color. Heredity plays an important role in hair graying as well. A decrease in the number of hair follicles in the scalp and consequent increased balding have also been described (Selmanowitz *et al.*, 1977).

Although no changes in the free nerve endings in aged skin have been found, the number of Pacinian and Meissner's corpuscles (end-organs responsible for the sensation of pressure and light touch) decrease with age. This results in decreased sensation, which predisposes the elderly to injury. It also decreases the ability to perform fine maneuvers with the hands. A summary of structural and functional changes with aging in the main skin components, epider-

Table 23–1. CHANGES IN NORMAL AGED SKIN

Epidermis	*Dermis*
↑ Dryness and roughness	↓ Density
Flattening of dermoepidermal junction	↓ Cells
↓ Epidermal turnover rate	↓ Blood vessels
↓ Number of melanocytes	Stiffer collagen
↓ Langerhans cells	Stiffer elastic fibers
Appendages	↓ Clearance of foreign substances
↓ Sweat production	
↓ Sebaceous glands	
↓ Hair follicles	
Gray hair	
↓ Rate of nail growth	
Thinner nails	
↓ Sensory end-organs	

Table 23–2. FUNCTIONAL CHANGES IN AGING SKIN

↓ Wound healing capability	↑ Blister formation
↓ Cell-mediated immune response	↑ Incidence of infection
↓ Thermoregulation	↑ Incidence of cancer
↓ Clearance of foreign substances	↑ Dryness
↓ Tanning	↑ Roughness
↓ Elasticity	↑ Fragility
↓ Sweat and oil production	↑ Sensory deprivation
↓ Thickness	

mis, dermis, and appendages, is presented in Tables 23–1 and 23–2, respectively.

Projecting the Image. Upon a first encounter, the older individual, like any other, is judged by the image he projects. The skin is a major signpost of time. We estimate age, personality, status, race, and health merely by looking. A psychologic study shows that aged persons who are physically attractive are more optimistic and have better personality and health than the unattractive (Graham, 1983). One must always have a proper regard for the skin and bear in mind that a number of the skin lesions affecting the elderly are preventable. As noted previously, some of the lesions are due to the passage of time, but most are due to cumulative environmental insults and should, and can, be avoided.

Pressure Sores. The pathophysiology of pressure sores illustrates several principles in geriatric management (Agate, 1985). Although not the most commonly seen dermatologic diagnosis in the elderly (skin cancer is), the problem of pressure sores is frequent enough and produces serious enough consequences to deserve discussion. Pressure sores were formerly seen more often in younger patients with chronic diseases or spinal cord injuries (Reuler and Cooney, 1981). Now they are becoming more of a problem in the elderly. The prevalence of pressure ulcerations increases with age such that patients over 70 years of age account for 70 percent of those affected. In this age group, 70 percent of patients develop pressure sores within 2 weeks of hospital admission (Cooney and Reuler, 1984). As with urinary incontinence, the presence of pressure ulcers and their status frequently play a prominent role in the decisions made regarding the ultimate management of a patient.

Pressure sores represent a dreaded complication of one of the five "I's" of geriatrics: immobility (see Chapter 3). The role of pressure is the most critical in the development of the pressure ulcer. The average period of time necessary to produce pressure-associated changes varies but averages about 2 hours. Hence a patient who does not move him/herself every 2 hours, for whatever reason, is at risk for developing sores. Other factors include shearing forces that are produced by an improper position, friction that occurs with improper handling of the patients, and moisture due to perspiration or urinary and fecal incontinence. Due to all these factors, the skin changes previously described increase the risk of developing pressure sores.

The most common and serious complication of a pressure sore is infection. The elderly are more at risk of infection because of their altered immune system, decreased vascularity, and decreased epithelialization. There is no cure for a pressure sore once it develops. Even if an ulcer heals, there is always a significant chance that it will recur (Constantian and Jackson, 1980). Therefore, prevention of the development of pressure sores, as with many other geriatric problems, is the most important aspect of management. Once patients at risk are identified, specific measures need to be taken to avoid the causative factors mentioned earlier. Relief from pressure is the most important factor in preventing pressure sores. In patients at risk, this may necessitate turning the patient in bed every 2 hours. Although such a maneuver is seemingly burdensome on the nursing staff, the nursing care of pressure sores, and the physical and emotional pain that accompany them, are far more burdensome to the patient as well as the caregivers.

AGING OF COLLAGEN

Collagen, with elastin and ground substance, is one of the components of connective tissue, generally found around the structural elements that constitute organs and tissues but ubiquitous throughout the body. Connective tissue itself, formed of cells, fibers, and extracellular matrix, functions in a number of important ways—serving as mechanical support, means of exchange of metabolites between blood and tissues, storage of fuel in its adipose cells, protection against infection, and repair of injury. Collagenous fibers are present in all types of connective tissue but vary greatly in their abundance as well as in the importance of their function and the range of aging effects (Hall, 1976). Collagen undergoes continuous changes with age. It forms a large portion (30 to 40 percent) of all proteins of the body. It is easily available and its structure and chemistry are fairly well known. Therefore, it offers a valuable model for gerontologic tissue studies. Indeed, the demonstration that cross-linkages do occur biologically and that highly cross-linked collagen structures increase proportionally during the course of natural aging has been largely responsible for the cross-linking theory of aging (see Chapters 4 and 7).

Structure and Chemistry of Collagen. Collagens are a family of macromolecules deposited in the form of fibers. They occur almost chemically pure in the tendons, as a convolute of fibers in an extracellular matrix in the skin, as the substance of bones on which calcium is deposited, or as the interstitial fibrous tissue between muscle fibers, in membrane of articulations, in the arterial wall, and so on. The central feature of all collagen molecules is their stiff, triple-stranded helical structure. Three collagen polypeptide chains, called α chains, are wound around each other in a regular helix to generate a ropelike collagen molecule conventionally referred to as tropocollagen, about 300 mm long and 1.5 mm in diameter. In unstained preparations of loose connective tissue, the collagen fibers appear as colorless strands. When collagen fibers are treated with a special stain and viewed at high magnification, several transversal bands can be resolved at intervals of 649 Å. The explanation of this striation has been based on the generally accepted view that tropocollagen molecules (see below) come together in a parallel arrangement and overlap each other by about one-quarter of their length to produce a staggered array resulting in cross-striations (Figure 23–2).

Although flexible, collagen fibers offer great resistance to a pulling force. For example, the breaking point of human collagenous fibers (as in tendon) is only reached with a force of several hundred kilograms per square centimeter and their elongation at this point is only a few percentage points. In this respect, the flexibility and stability of the collagen fiber have been related to that of a cable that ties a ship to shore; it is sufficiently flexible to be curled when not in use and, yet, does not allow movement of the ship at anchor. Similarly, blood vessels, skin, and tendon are capable of transmitting tension and compression as they are simultaneously restrained from deformation by their collagen (and elastin) fibers (Verzar, 1968).

Of the amino acids comprising the polypeptide chains, two, hydroxyproline and hydroxylysine, do not occur in significant amounts in other animal proteins, and their content in a tissue, therefore, can be taken as an index of its collagen content. Collagen molecules are held together by electrostatic bonds, and the different amino acid chains are connected by intermolecular cross-links to form fibrils; the strength of these bonds increasing progressively with age. From the moment the collagen is formed, the completed fiber does not take part in metabolism and is regarded as a metabolically inert component of the extracellular space.

Tropocollagen fibers are usually embedded in a matrix of amorphous ground substance, a very viscous solution formed mainly of proteoglycans. Originally, the polysaccharides are modified hexose polymers usually bound to proteins: some contain a sulfate group (chondroitin-6-sulfate) whereas others carry a large number of negatively charged ions (hyaluronate) and are therefore described as polyanions. Ground substance also contains interstitial fluid filtered from the capillaries, and water is loosely absorbed to the ground substance components as water of hydration. Plasma proteins may also penetrate the ground substance and be bound to the polysaccharides. Both water and proteins are returned to the circulation—in the case of water, through the lymphatic system, and in the case of proteins, either directly (for the free proteins) or after release from the polysaccharides by the action of proteases (for the bound proteins). Thus, ground substance may serve not only as a lubricant (to facilitate the movement of the joints), as a barrier to the spread of bacteria (that have gained access to the tissues), and as a "plasticizer" (to diminish friction and wear between collagen fibers), but also as a storage site for water, ions, and proteins (Sobel, 1967).

Collagen is produced by fibrocytes, the cellular elements of the connective tissue, from amino acids that are extruded into the ground substance where they then undergo maturational changes leading to the typical structure of the adult tropocollagen (Figure 23–3). The collagen chains are originally formed from larger precursors, which

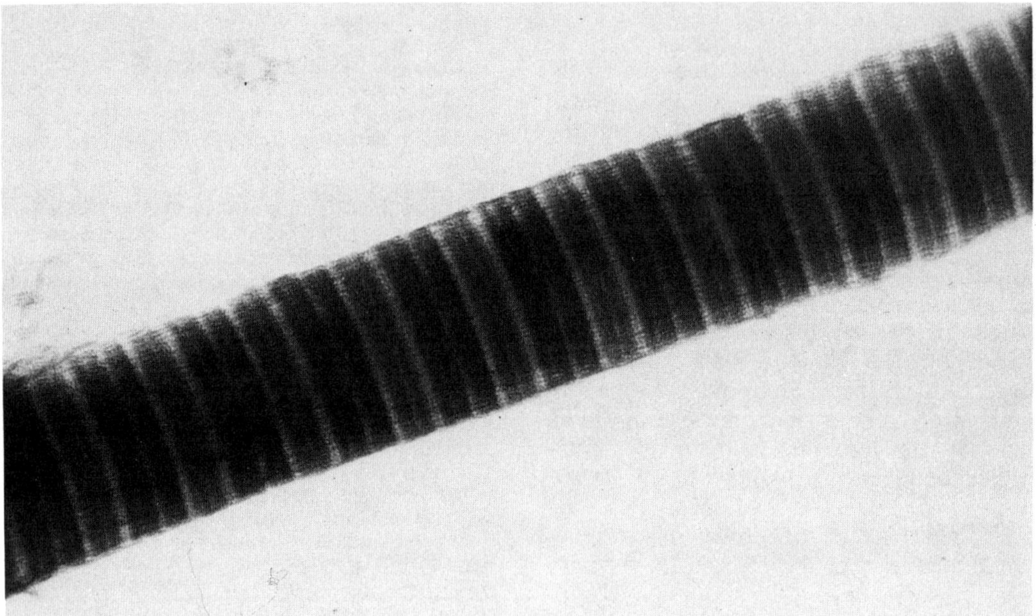

Figure 23–2. *Electron micrograph of a negatively stained microfibril of collagen isolated from rat tendon.*

One dark and one light segment represent a period produced by the arrangement of tropocollagen molecules. Magnification 128,722×. (Courtesy of Dr. N. B. Gilula).

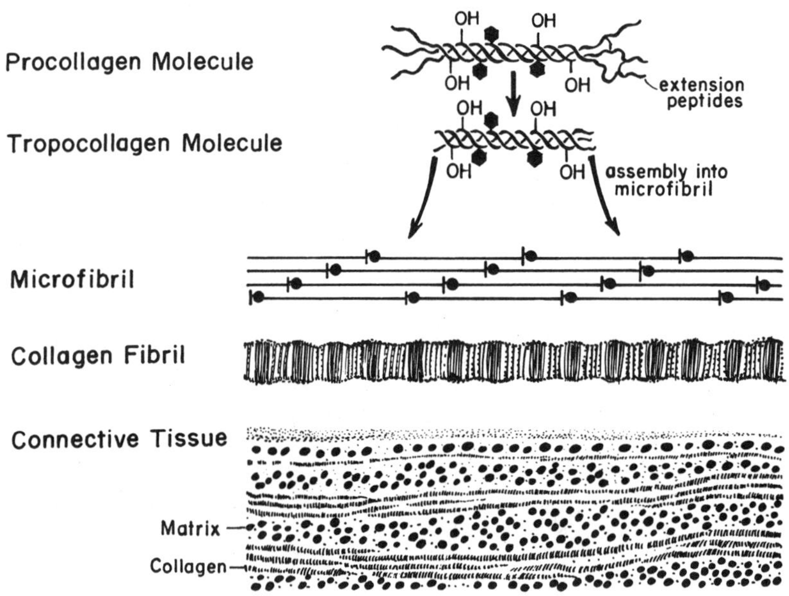

Figure 23–3. *Schematic representation of the composition of a collagen fibril and the distribution of tropocollagen molecules in the connective tissue.*

Tropocollagen molecules, 2800 Å in length, are aligned in a staggering fashion, overlapping by one quarter of their length (640 Å).

contain both the amino acids that give rise to collagen and some extra amino acids, called extension peptides, that do not form collagen. These extension peptides have at least two important functions: (1) they guide the intracellular formation of the triple-stranded collagen molecule and (2) they prevent the intracellular formation of large collagen fibrils, which would be catastrophic for the cell. With aging, either of these functions could be altered as well as the proteolysis of this material.

GROWTH AND AGING OF COLLAGEN

Growth of the collagen fibers after their birth proceeds in two phases: the tropocollagen fibers aggregate in the axial direction and continue to grow in thickness by apposition, i.e., by accretion of more soluble particles. Extracellular matrix is also produced by fibrocytes, and when newly formed, it appears under the electron microscope as vacuolated, consisting of a water-rich phase (the vacuoles) and a less water-rich phase (the walls of the vacuoles). Some time after secretion of the ground substance, the tropocollagen begins the end-to-end alignment process, with the fibrils orienting themselves parallel to each other in the denser (less water-rich) areas of the ground substance (Bondareff, 1957). The formation and maturation of tropocollagen and extracellular matrix are closely interrelated: for example, proteoglycans from the ground substance seem to regulate fibril formation, as shown by the observation of a decrease in the quantity of these proteins in tendons when the tropocollagen fibers have grown to their ultimate size.

With the passage of time, both tropocollagen and extracellular matrix undergo molecular changes leading to structural, biochemical, and functional alterations, including: decreased chemical extractability, decreased effectiveness of enzymatic degradation, increased cross-linkage, increased hydrophobicity. As a result of these changes, the collagen becomes tougher, more crystalline, and more difficult to dissolve; its tensile strength is reduced; and its plasticizing function is impaired or lost. In the case of the extracellular matrix, age-related changes in its physicochemical composition and a decrease in turnover of some of its constituents induce an increase in density and aggregation, thereby rendering the ground substance less permeable to the flow of substances moving through it; as a consequence, cellular nutrition becomes altered.

Collagen solubility decreases with age and this decrease has been related to increased cross-linking (Houck *et al.*, 1967). The appearance of cross-links between collagen fibers is well documented and is generally regarded as a normal index of maturational change. With increasing age, however, as the collagen becomes less degradable, the number of cross-linkages and especially of intra- and inter-molecular ester bonds increases (Seifter *et al.*, 1961).

Other properties of collagen, such as its extractability and solubility, are also affected by age. In young rats, for example, the chemically insoluble fraction of collagen can be effectively degraded when treated with cortisol or other hormones of the adrenal cortex, whereas in older animals hormonal treatment does not restore the reduced capacity of the animal to degrade collagen (Houck *et al.*, 1967). The greater resistance of older collagen to enzymatic degradation may be ascribed to either or both of two factors: the decrease in amount and activity of collagenase or the increased resistance of the more tightly held cross-linked fibers to collagenase activity. In relation to the first factor, cortisol is capable of stimulating collagenase activity in young but not in old animals. In this regard, it should be recalled that glucocorticoids secreted by the adrenal cortex have a gluconeogenic activity; that is, they are capable of converting amino acids to glucose. Some of the amino acid components of collagen are strongly gluconeogenic, and it has been suggested that in case of stress, the increased levels of glucocorticoids would be capable of stimulating activity, thereby releasing the amino acids from collagen converting them to glucose, thus producing the energy necessary to withstand the stressful situation. In older animals, however, such an energy conversion is prevented because of the metabolic inertia of senile collagen with the result that resistance to stress is decreased in advancing age (Houck *et al.*, 1967).

Heating of collagen (e.g., tendon fibers from the rat tail) to approximately 60°C induces shrinkage of the fibers to about one-fourth their original length. Shrinkage is greater and the contraction and subsequent relaxation periods are more prolonged in older than in younger animals. These differences in thermal responses are accompanied by chemical differences. For example, hyroxyproline, the amino acid characteristic of collagen, is liberated during contraction: in the young animal, the contracting tendon fibers release hydroxyproline quickly and in large quantities, whereas in the old animal, hydroxyproline is released more slowly and to a much smaller extent. Progressive changes in mechanical tension and chemical composition occur throughout life. The liberation of hydroxyproline complexes from collagen during thermal contraction is quantitatively related to the age of the animal. This observation has facilitated the study of aging of collagen in such tissues as skin, skeletal muscles, and arterial walls, in which mechanical shortening of the fibers cannot be measured. Regardless of the index chosen, however, the quantity of labile collagen was shown to decrease with age in all tissues studied (see Verzar, 1968).

Aging of Collagen and Body Temperature. Besides its sensitivity to relatively high temperatures, collagen appears also to be influenced by comparatively low temperatures, such as those of the internal and external environment. The hypothesis that aging of collagen *in vivo* is caused by body temperature is based on brownian molecular movement (i.e., the movement of particles suspended in a liquid), which brings the molecules together and thus permits the formation of intermolecular bonds (Sinex, 1957). Extrapolating from 58°C, the temperature at which thermal contraction takes place, to body temperature of 38°C, the aging of elastin, and probably also collagen fibers, can be attributed to thermal denaturation. This interpretation raises the question of whether the shrinkage temperature of collagen varies between organisms that live in hot or cold environments; for example, a certain difference in the collagen reactivity of the skin and degree of extractability of collagen has been reported between Eskimos and the individuals living in warmer climates, but the evidence is not conclusive. Such relationships between thermal denaturation and aging may also be challenged on the basis that animals with the same body temperatures vary widely in lifespan and presumably, their respective rates of aging, e.g., 2 to 3 years in rats, 12 to 14 years in cattle, and 50 to 70 years in humans.

OTHER CHANGES—CONNECTIVE TISSUE ELEMENTS

It is difficult to envision that changes in collagen would occur independently from alterations in the other components of the connective tissue. Changes with age in elastin structure and function have been thoroughly investigated (Sinex, 1964). A marked reduction in the volume of the extracellular matrix or in relation to the collagen content of a tissue is also a typical consequence of aging and is often accompanied by a decrease in interstitial water content. Indeed, a progressive reduction in the relative tissue content of water is consistently observed throughout the lifespan in many organs and species. The decrease in extracellular matrix has been explained by its faster turnover as compared to that of collagen, for extracellular matrix must be renewed within days or weeks, whereas the more inert collagen persists for a considerably longer period of time. Changes in the composition of the extracellular matrix with age have also been described and appear to differ from tissue to tissue with a progressively increasing occurrence of cross-links.

Connective Tissue, a "Poor" Substitute for Specialized Tissues. Unique to connective tissue is its ability to intervene in the repair of tissue at all sites and after all types of damage. The fibrocytes, the cellular elements of the connective tissue, are generally stimulated by cell injury and death; thus, proliferation of fibrocytes replaces the loss of more specific cells, an event that, in itself, represents a functional decrement: fibrocytes lay down more collagen and extracellular matrix to fill up the areas vacated by the dead cells and, in this manner, contribute to functional loss. The response of the organism to injury is to attempt to replace the loss. Many tissues cannot regenerate and, instead, connective tissue proliferates. In the aged, even such proliferation is slowed. Under the best of conditions, the connective tissue replacement always lacks the functional competence of the original elements.

Pathogenicity of the Aging Collagen. Aging of the connective tissue has been implicated in the etiopathology of a number of diseases often associated with old age (Hall, 1976; Denham, 1985). Only a few examples will be mentioned here; others are discussed in the context of aging of specific organs and systems. Alterations with age in collagen and matrix in bone, cartilage, and articulation are responsible for several diseases of the skeleton (osteoporosis) and joints (osteoarthritis) (see Chapter 22). Changes in the composition of the extracellular matrix and increased cross-linking in collagen and elastin fibers with advancing age may reduce lung flexibility to such a degree that pulmonary vital capacity is impaired, as occurs dramatically with emphysema (see Chapter 19). As previously discussed, in the skin, the oxidation of elastin fibers with age results in their degeneration and replacement by less flexible collagen fibers, which age, in turn, and become progressively less resilient. Profound changes also occur in elastin and collagen fibers of the arterial walls, and such alteration is viewed by some as one of the primary causes of arteriosclerosis (see Chapter 17). Total collagen content of the heart increases with age, as does that of the cardiac valves, which, as a consequence, become rigid. As a result of changes in the extracellular matrix, alterations occur in the basement membrane of the capillaries, reducing their permeability and slowing down transport processes and metabolic exchanges between blood and tissues. When such a decrease in permeability involves the capillaries of the kidney, the glomerular filtration rate is decreased; thus, so is the efficiency of renal excretory function (Chapter 20). When the permeability of cellular membrane is affected, the transport of substances in and out of the cell may be retarded; indeed, diabetes in older persons has been attributed to a decreased sensitivity of the cell membrane to insulin, thereby deterring the transport of glucose (Chapter 16).

References

Agate, J. N.: Pressure sores. In Pathy, M. S. J. (ed.): *Principles and Practice of Geriatric Medicine,* John Wiley & Sons, Chichester, UK, **1985.**

Bondareff, W.: Submicroscopic morphology of connective tissue ground substance with particular regard to fibriollogenesis and aging. *Gerontologia,* **1:**222–233, **1957.**

Cooney, T. G., and Reuler, J. B.: Pressure sores. *West J. Med.,* **140:**622–624, **1984.**

Constantian, M. B., and Jackson, H. S.: Biology and care of the pressure ulcer wound. In Constantian, M. B. (ed.): *Pressure Ulcers. Principles and Techniques of Management,* Little, Brown, Boston, **1980.**

Denham, M.: Diseases of muscle and connective tissue. In Pathy, M. S. J. (ed.): *Principles and Practice of Geriatric Medicine,* John Wiley & Sons, Chichester, UK, **1985.**

Fenske, N. A., and Lober, C. W.: Structural and functional changes of normal aging skin. *J. Am. Acad. Dermatol.,* **15:**571–585, **1986.**

Forbes, P. D.; Davies, R. E.; and Urbach, F.: Aging, environmental influences, and photocarcinogenesis. *J. Invest. Dermatol.,* **73:**131–134, **1979.**

Gilchrest, B. A.: Age-associated changes in the skin. *J. Am. Geriatr. Soc.,* **30:**139–143, **1982.**

Graham, J. A.: The psychotherapeutic value of cosmetics. *Cosmetic Technol.,* **5:**25–26, **1983.**

Grove, G. L.: Age-related differences in healing of superficial skin wounds in humans. *Arch. Dermatol. Res.,* **272:**381–385, **1982.**

Grove, G. L., and Kligman, A. M.: Age-associated changes in human epidermal cell renewal. *J. Gerontol.,* **38:**137–142, **1983.**

Hall, D. A.: *The Ageing of Connective Tissue,* Academic Press, London, **1976.**

Houck, J. C.; DeHesse, C.; and Jacob, R.: The effect of aging upon collagen catabolism. *Symp. Soc. Exp. Biol.,* **21:**403–425, **1967.**

Johnson, M. L. T., and Roberts, J.: Prevalence of dermatologic disease among persons 1–74 years of age, *Advance Data.* US Department of Health, Education and Welfare, Washington, DC, **1977.**

Kligman, A. M.; Grove, G. L.; and Balin, A. K.: Aging of human skin. In Finch, C. E., and Schneider, E. L. (eds.): *Handbook of the Biology of Aging,* 2nd ed., Van Nostrand Reinhold, New York, **1985.**

Marks, R.: Skin disorders. In Pathy, M. S. J. (ed.): *Principles and Practice of Geriatric Medicine,* John Wiley & Sons, Chichester, UK, **1985.**

Quevedo, W. C.; Szabo, G.; and Vicks, J.: Influence of age and ultraviolet on the populations of dopa-positive melanocytes in human skin. *J. Infect. Dis.,* **52:**287–290, **1969.**

Reuler, J. B., and Cooney, T. G.: The pressure sore: Pathophysiology and principles of management. *Ann. Intern. Med.,* **94:**661–666, **1981.**

Seifter, S.; Gallop, P. M.; and Franzblau, C.: Some aspects of collagenolytic action. *Trans. NY Acad. Sci.,* **23:**540–547, **1961.**

Selmanowitz, V. J.; Rizer, R. L.; and Orentreich, N.: Aging of the skin and its appendages. In Finch, C. E., and Hayflick, L. (eds.): *Handbook of the Biology of Aging,* Van Nostrand Reinhold, New York, **1977.**

Sinex, F. M.: Aging and the lability of irreplaceable molecules. *J. Gerontol.,* **12:**190–198, **1957.**

Sinex, F.: Cross-linkage and aging. In Strehler, B. L. (ed.): *Advances in Gerontological Research,* Vol. 1, Academic Press, New York, **1964.**

Sobel, H.: Aging of ground substance in connective tissue. In Strehler, B. L. (ed.): *Advances in Gerontological Research,* Vol. 2, Academic Press, New York, **1967.**

Verzar, F.: Intrinsic and extrinsic factors of molecular aging. *Exp. Gerontol.,* **3:**69–75, **1968.**

PART

IV

Prevention and Rehabilitation

CHAPTER

24 PHARMACOKINETICS AND DRUG MANAGEMENT IN THE ELDERLY

Doherty B. Hudson

As the age of the population increases, so does the incidence of medical complaints. Some of these complaints are the consequence of age-induced physical changes; others are due to disease. In all, the older individuals have a greater number of illnesses and a greater number of prescriptions written for them. Although the elderly currently account for 11 percent of the U.S. population, the cost of their medications is 25 to 30 percent of this nation's expenditures for medications. The percentage of the population taking prescription medications increases with age as does the number of prescriptions per person (Figure 24–1), and as a consequence of this increase in the number of drugs taken, the incidence of adverse drug reactions rises. In fact, in hospitalized patients, those over 65 years of age have adverse drug reactions three times more frequently than those under 50 years of age.

With the passage of time, stature as well as lean body mass and body water decrease, renal function declines, and the liver loses some of its detoxifying capacity and protein-synthesizing ability. Insults to the body in the form of abuse and disease accumulate over the years. The abuses to the body include recreational drugs (including alcohol), smoking, and possibly dangerous dietary habits. When the foregoing factors are combined with some type of disease and many medications, some of them very potent, the incidence of adverse drug reactions rises. Of course, some adverse reactions are also due to noncompliance (Table 24–1).

Noncompliance, the failure of a patient to follow instructions regarding medications, occurs with 30 to 40 percent of the elderly. Half of these are noncompliant because they fail to take the medication owing to forgetfulness, lack of funds, or not having the prescription filled. Other forms of noncompliance are taking the medications at the wrong time, taking too much ("more is better"), discontinuing the drug too soon—as with antibiotics—or taking interfering prescribed or nonprescribed medications (Table 24–2).

PHARMACOKINETICS

Basically, pharmacology is concerned with the effects of chemical agents on living matter—our immediate concern is with drugs in humans (Gilman *et al.,* 1985). Two aspects must be considered, the drug and the human body. The potential actions of the drug are independent of aging; however, the aging-induced physiologic changes in the body can alter the pharmacokinetics, the absorption, metabolism, storage, and excretion of the drug (Bergener and von Hahn, 1981; Vestal and Dawson, 1985; O'Malley *et al.,* 1985).

The drug is a chemical agent, possibly even a hormone, that can be altered or me-

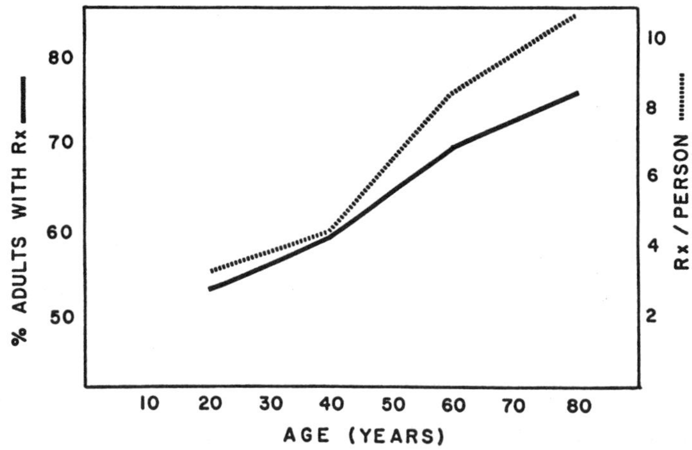

Figure 24–1. *Increase with age in the percentage of adults receiving prescriptions (———) and in the number of medication prescribed per person (··········).*

Table 24–1. FACTORS ASSOCIATED WITH INCREASED INCIDENCE OF ADVERSE DRUG REACTIONS

1. Reduced (small) stature
2. Reduced renal and hepatic function
3. Cumulative insults to body
   - Disease
   - Faulty diet
   - Drug abuse
4. Medications, multiple and potent
5. Altered pharmacokinetics
6. Noncompliance

Table 24–2. CAUSES OF NONCOMPLIANCE

1. Failure to take medication
2. Incorrect dosage of medication
   - Prescribed
   - Self-administered
3. Premature discontinuance
4. Interactions with other medications

tabolized in specific ways. In the body many different enzymes act to metabolize drugs, but the manner in which a drug can be altered is limited and is generally known as a pathway. Such a pathway for the amino acid tyrosine is tyrosine—dihydroxyphenylalanine (DOPA)—dopamine—norepinephrine—epinephrine. A specific enzyme is necessary at every step and the presence or absence of that particular enzyme in a cell determines the end-product. Dopamine is the active substance released by certain cells of the caudate nucleus of the brain (Chapter 9) because these cells do not contain dopamine hydroxylase, the enzyme necessary for the progression on to norepinephrine. However, postganglionic cells of the superior cervical ganglion contain this enzyme and produce norepinephrine. To carry this one step further, cells of the adrenal medulla also contain PNMT (phenylethanolamine-*N*-methyltransferase), and consequently norepinephrine can be converted to epinephrine at this site (Chapter 12). These three agents are effective neurotransmitters whose actions must be terminated. The metabolic process continues and the agent may be inactivated or combined with another substance and is eventually eliminated from the body.

What does the drug do? Over the ages man has concocted and brewed beverages, elixers, and so forth to counteract his pain and suffering. Some of these proved to be effective drugs that were identified because they produced immediate and unmistakable results. The only effect a drug can produce is to alter a function or process that maintains the living organism. All drugs act by producing changes in some known physiologic function or process; they may increase or decrease a normal function, but they cannot initiate a new function. Their effects are quantitative, not qualitative. The particular effect of a drug is expressed in relative terms—relative to the physiologic condition that exists at the time of drug administration, such as reduction of tem-

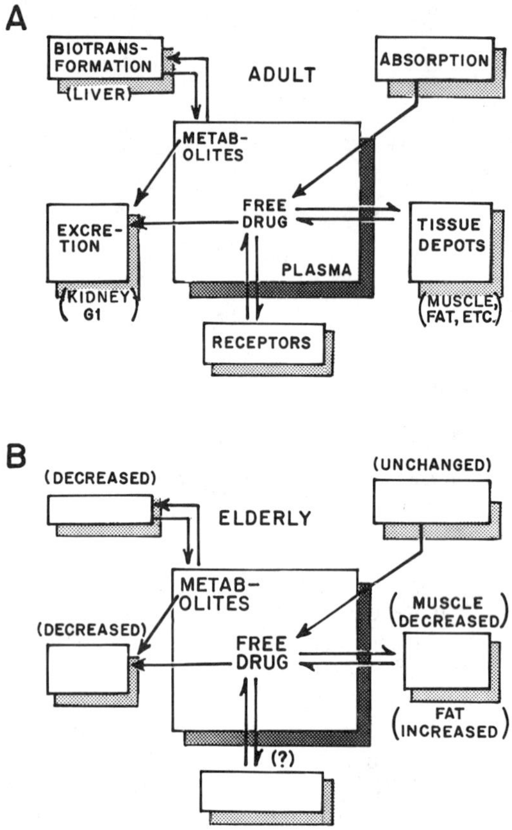

Figure 24–2. *Drug Kinetics in Adults and Elderly.*

A. In the adult, active free drug depends upon absorption, metabolism and excretion. It also depends on type of tissue for deposition and duration of time in body. The cellular action is dependent on receptor binding. B. In the elderly, persistance and elevated active free drug due to decreased metabolism, excretion. Tissue depots change and the net result is prolonged duration of action. Receptor changes are as yet unknown. (Drawing by S. Oklund.)

perature, reduction of pain, lowering of blood pressure.

The effect of a drug on the body may readily be measured, yet how this effect was produced is a fundamental question. What is the action of the drug? The actions are characterized in terms of what is known of physiologic functions and processes. The action of a drug is formulated on understanding the physiologic or biochemical process with which the drug interacts. The drug may act extracellularly, as does heparin by combining with and removing proteins from the blood to reduce clotting; at the cell membrane to bind with a receptor, as does curare at the neuromuscular junction to block the acetylcholine receptor and cause paralysis; or intracellularly to alter a biochemical reaction, as do the nitrates (nitroglycerin) by activating guanylate cyclase and setting in motion the intracellular events that relax vascular smooth muscle in angina pectoris.

What is the fate of a drug in the body? The drug must first be absorbed and then enter the bloodstream in order that it may be distributed throughout the body and reach its potential site of action. Most drugs are metabolized in the body, transformed into a form that is more readily excreted from the body, and then eliminated (Figure 24–2A).

Some orally administered drugs remain in the gastrointestinal tract and never enter the circulation, but most therapeutic agents are absorbed across the intestinal mucosa and enter the circulation. However, the presence of food in the stomach or the pH of a particular region of the gut may reduce the solubility of the drug or bind it so that it cannot readily pass into the circulation. In the elderly, who are often prone to using antacids, stool softeners, and laxatives, drug absorption may be reduced and this interferes with the amount of drug entering the blood.

Drug distribution may be altered because of changes in body size and composition (Chapter 20). Body fat increases while total body water and lean body mass decline, causing the concentration of a drug in tissues and blood to be elevated, and so, too, the effects of the drug. Fat-soluble drugs may have a longer retention time because more drug can be sequestered in the increased amount of body fat and, as a consequence, the duration of action of such a drug is prolonged as it is slowly returned to the blood. Serum albumin decreases as the rate of protein synthesis declines with aging and, consequently, bound drug in the circulation decreases. Thus, more free (unbound) drug is available for distribution to the body's tissues and the chance of an adverse drug reaction increases.

Whether or not the elderly have a decreased capacity to metabolize certain drugs is questionable. The most recent studies indicate that the induction of liver enzyme synthesis by drugs is not impaired (Pearson and Roberts, 1984), but other hepatic enzymes are also unchanged or reduced (Kiechel, 1982). Hepatic blood flow decreases 40 to 50 percent between 25 and 65 years of age along with a smaller hepatic mass, and this may, indeed, lower the rate of drug detoxification. The excretion of drugs relies to a great extent on renal function. Renal excretion is altered by changes in renal blood flow (1 percent per year decrease), glomerular filtration rate, and tubular reabsorption or excretion (Chapter 20). The system least changed by the passage of time is the gastrointestinal tract, for drug absorption is essentially unchanged although gastric emptying may be somewhat slowed, as may intestinal motility and blood flow (Figure 24–2B).

In the aging population, the incidence of certain disorders increases, and pharmacologic agents are employed to ameliorate or alleviate the symptoms. The current therapeutic regimens are predicated on overcoming the symptoms of the disease and returning the individual to as near-normal a condition as is possible. It must be borne in mind that a drug acts to alter the rate of a normal process and such process may occur in tissues other than those with apparent dysfunction, giving rise to side effects of the drug. Often a second drug may be necessary to control the side effects of the first drug—thus contributing to or initiating polypharmacy.

DRUG MANAGEMENT

POLYPHARMACY

Multisystem disease and nonspecific presentation of disease are more prevalent in the older population. Since compensatory mechanisms and functional reserves are impaired, the response of the elderly to illness can vary. Awareness of such altered responses to illness in the elderly is important in diagnosis as well as in treatment.

The multiple pathology of aging individuals leads to the prescription of a greater number of drugs to this group. Over the last 25 years the development of new and more potent drugs has been striking. The "multiple" pathologies lead to "multiple" drugs to treat "multiple" symptoms and side effects of these "multiple" drugs—initiating polypharmacy (Table 24–3). Polypharmacy, originally meaning many drugs, has acquired a derogatory connotation of excessive and unnecessary use of medication. Features of this practice include: (1) Medications for which there is no indication. For example, digoxin, a digitalis agonist effective in normalizing heart rate and contractility but with quite narrowly defined limits for use, may be given to patients with heart problems without assessment or reassessment for its use. (2) The use of duplicate medications—for example, two different sedatives with the same pharmacologic effect and, therefore, possible toxic effects. (3) The concurrent use of interacting medications, such as digoxin and kaopectate, an antidiarrheal that decreases the absorption of digoxin by binding and retaining it in the

Table 24–3. FEATURES OF POLYPHARMACY

1. Medication not indicated
2. Duplicate medications
3. Concurrent interacting medications
4. Contraindicated medications
5. Inappropriate dosage
6. Drug treatment of adverse drug reaction
7. Improvement following discontinuance

gastrointestinal tract. (4) The use of contraindicated medications, because of failure to consider the total health problems of the individual—for example, to treat hypertension using a beta-blocker (see below), which decreases cardiac contractility, in a patient who is also suffering from heart failure. (5) The use of inappropriate dosage; administration of a drug may be too frequent, the unit dosage too high, deviation from the prescribed dose or noncompliance. (6) Treating an adverse drug reaction with a drug that may have side effects of its own. (7) Improvement of an individual's condition following discontinuation of medications.

While the problem of polypharmacy with prescription drugs exists, it may be compounded with over-the-counter medications that the elderly are prone to self-prescribe. Another consideration is the altered presentation of disease in the elderly (Chapter 3) and a misdiagnosis of the problem, which can lead to iatrogenic (physician-induced) disease. Therefore, a precise diagnosis is needed before initiating treatment and a complete assessment of the physiologic and pathologic profile of the individual is prerequisite to initiating treatment (Chapter 2). Such treatment may, indeed, require multiple medications, which can be most efficacious when properly programmed.

EXAMPLES OF PHARMACOLOGIC MANAGEMENT OF SOME COMMON DISEASES OF THE ELDERLY

Rather than listing a series of drugs and the altered responses thereto with aging, it was elected to consider the regimens employed to treat specific disorders. We chose, specifically, multidrug regimens as these are most commonly utilized in the elderly. The diseases most frequent in the elderly and most likely to lead to death are diseases of the cardiovascular system such as coronary heart disease and hypertension (see Chapter 17).

Management of coronary heart disease may be medical or surgical or both (Mock *et al.*, 1985; Gersh *et al.*, 1985). Medical treatment, on which we focus, includes changes in the life style as well as pharmacologic therapy (Table 24–4).

Table 24–4. MAJOR TYPES OF CORONARY HEART DISEASE TREATMENT

Medical treatment
Diet
Exercise
No smoking
Pharmacologic agents
Surgical treatment
Aortocoronary bypass graft
Percutaneous transluminal coronary angioplasty with streptokinase anticoagulant therapy

Table 24–5. PHARMACOLOGIC THERAPY OF CORONARY HEART DISEASE

Angina pectoris
Nitroglycerine and nitrates
Beta-adrenergic blockers
Calcium channel blockers
Myocardial infarction
Anticoagulants
Antithrombotics
Thrombolytics

Surgical treatment consists primarily of two types of interventions, which will be mentioned only briefly here. One intervention, aortocoronary bypass graft, is based on the detection of discrete areas of coronary narrowing by angiography and bypass of these areas by implantation of a graft. This procedure often produces marked and sustained relief, but it is unsettled whether it protects against myocardial infarction or produces significant prolongation of life when compared to medical treatment.

Another promising technique is percutaneous transluminal coronary angioplasty, which consists of dilation of constricted areas by a balloon inserted in the coronary vessel under fluoroscopic control.

Both interventions may be combined with medical treatment, particularly with the injection of streptokinase to dissolve the clot and anticoagulant therapy.

Medical treatment consists of amelioration of the diet (see Chapters 18 and 25), appropriate exercise and no smoking (see Chapter 26), and pharmacologic agents (Stamler, 1985). The pharmacologic therapies of coronary heart disease have the goal of reestablishing blood flow to the heart before the cardiac muscle has incurred irreversible damage. This goal has been approached in different ways (Table 24–5). In angina pectoris, the major goal is to reduce the work of the heart. This is achieved by vasodilation produced by agents such as nitroglycerine and other nitrates and antihypertensive drugs such as beta-adrenergic and calcium channel blockers. In myocardial infarction, there are three major goals: to prevent blood from clotting, to prevent thrombus formation, and to dissolve a thrombus that has already formed. Representatives of each type are: heparin, as an anticoagulant; aspirin, as an antithrombotic agent; and streptokinase, as a thrombolytic.

The strategy involved in the pharmacologic treatment of angina pectoris is to improve the balance between myocardial oxygen supply and demand. This means increasing blood flow to the heart or decreasing its work load. The vasodilator nitroglycerin has been known to be effective in relieving and preventing anginal attacks for more than 100 years. More recently, the beta-adrenergic antagonists and the calcium channel blockers, to be discussed later, have been added for long-term prophylaxis of angina (Needleman, Corr, and Johnson, 1985).

Anginal attacks can be relieved by the sublingual administration of nitroglycerin in tablet form. It is rapid acting, in 1 or 2 minutes, but the effects fall off rapidly and are undetectable within 1 hour. Nitroglycerin in various forms can be used prophylactically before undertaking a strenuous task. Nitrates (Table 24–6) do not increase *total* coronary blood flow in patients with typical angina due to atherosclerosis; they do, however, cause redistribution of blood flow in the heart when there is partial occlusion of the coronary circulation. They also reduce the oxygen requirements of the myocardium by decreasing resistance in the systemic circulation.

High doses of nitrates given orally can cause a small decrease in blood pressure, preferably avoided in the elderly already prone to orthostatic hypotension (Chapter 17). They may also cause other troublesome side effects such as headache and induce tolerance (increased dose to obtain the same effect). These substances are available in various forms, some particularly useful for the elderly because they do not require frequent administration. This is the case of a cutaneous nitroglycerin disk bonded into an adhesive bandage, which permits gradual absorption over 24 hours.

Table 24–6. CLINICALLY USED ORGANIC NITRATES

NITRATE	FORM
Nitroglycerin	Sublingual tablet Sustained-release tablet Buccal tablet Oral tablet Ointment Transdermal disk Intravenous
Isosorbide dinitrate	Sublingual tablet Chewable tablet Oral tablet Sustained-release tablet
Erythrityl tetranitrate	Sublingual tablet Chewable tablet
Pentaerythritol tetranitrate	Oral tablet Sustained-release tablet

Table 24–7. PHARMACOLOGIC INTERVENTIONS IN MYOCARDIAL INFARCTION

Anticoagulant	Heparin
Antithrombotic	Aspirin
Thrombolytic	Streptokinase Tissue-type plasminogen activator

The pharmacology of myocardial infarction includes, as we have already indicated, a three-pronged approach (Table 24–7). Anticoagulant therapy has been used for many years in the hope of reducing the incidence of thromboembolism.

Clotting Mechanisms. A clot follows transection or damage to blood vessels. It functions to seal off the vessel and prevent blood loss. It consists of a plug of platelets (one type of blood cell) (Zucker, 1980) embedded in a net of fibrin and is formed by a cascading reaction. The first step is the conversion of the plasma protein fibrin into an insoluble fibrin catalyzed by the enzyme thrombin. Fibrin consolidates further under the influence of calcium. Each of these reactions is activated by a number of factors, which are indispensable and whose absence leads to various diseases of blood clotting. The knowledge of these factors has led to the discovery of agents that enhance or prevent blood clotting. In our discussion we are concerned with the anticoagulants of which heparin, capable of inhibiting the actions of thrombin, is a common example. Clotting can also be prevented by the removal of calcium, either by precipitation or by binding.

Fibrin thrombi occur primarily in the venous system. Anticoagulants such as heparin are used to prevent blood clotting by interfering with the formation of clotting factors necessary for the production of fibrin and the coagulation of blood. Oral anticoagulants are widely used in attempts to reduce the risk of emboli forming and causing recurrent myocardial infarctions. However, their effectiveness is far from proven and, in addition, they may induce unwanted effects in the elderly, such as increased risk of hemorrhagic complications.

Among the antithrombotic drugs, aspirin is effective, easy to administer, and inexpensive; it has potent and long-lasting effects in inhibiting platelet aggregation, and a single, adult (325 mg) tablet, daily, may be prescribed for patients with angina or those who have recovered from a myocardial infarct. Aspirin interferes with a particular enzyme, cyclooxygenase, active in the platelet aggregation process. Platelets cannot synthesize this enzyme and, therefore, when the enzyme is destroyed, aggregation is inhibited.

If the embolus that is occluding a coronary artery and causing infarction can be dissolved, blood flow will resume. If this is accomplished soon enough after infarction (within hours) and revascularization is complete, the chances of 1-year survival are greater than 90 percent.

Streptokinase is a protein with demonstrated efficacy in treating acute thromboembolic disease. Streptokinase stimulates a proteolytic enzyme that hydrolyzes fibrin and promotes dissolution of the thrombus. By injecting the drug directly into the occluded coronary artery, systemic side effects, such as bleeding, may be avoided (Kennedy *et al.,* 1985; Koren *et al.,* 1985).

The most recent addition to the thrombolytic armamentarium is the tissue-type plasminogen activator (TPA). This activator preferentially initiates and confines fibrinolysis to a thrombus in a particular tissue type and avoids systemic effects. The plasminogen activator can be prepared by recombinant DNA technology. The intravenous administration of tissue-type plasminogen activator to patients with acute myocardial infarction results in a recanalization of the occluded coronary artery in about half the cases—a value significantly higher than achieved with intravenous streptokinase (TIMI Study Group, 1985; Zivin *et al.,* 1985).

The benefit of multipronged approach to a disease such as cardiac ischemia, which has widespread consequences on the total organism, is well illustrated by the foregoing discussion of angina and myocardial infarction. Although we have emphasized the pharmacologic interventions, medical treatment also includes diet and exercise. Medical treatment with its components, pharmacology, diet, and exercise, is effective not only in the overt disease but also in its prevention or eventually in rehabilitation. If this combined medical treatment proves to be unsatisfactory, surgery is performed.

Similarly, myocardial infarction is initially treated medically with either streptokinase or tissue plasminogen activator and/or nitrates, calcium channel blockers, and beta blockers as with angina. Narcotics and tranquilizers are also used to control pain and keep the patient sedated. If this fails, then the patient undergoes cardiac catheterization and, if a bypassable blockage is found, undergoes bypass surgery.

The exercise treadmill is a simple test that involves monitoring the patient's electrocardiogram while he/she exercises and provides an intermediate diagnostic step for patients in whom there is question about the diagnosis of coronary artery disease. Patients who have had an uncomplicated course after their myocardial infarction may use the treadmill to determine whether or not ischemia consequent to coronary disease persists and the degree of rehabilitation. The performance under exercise also provides guidelines for a safe physical fitness program to improve exercise tolerance and counteract unnecessary invalidism and depressive symptoms that usually occur in elderly patients with coronary artery disease.

Management of hypertension is presented in Table 24–8 as a stepped flowchart, starting with health measures at the top and progressing through various steps of pharmacologic treatment using one, two, three, and more drug combinations.

Once the diagnosis of hypertension has been made, the first attempt at treatment is to prescribe weight reduction, exercise, and

Table 24–8. STEPWISE APPROACH TO ANTIHYPERTENSIVE THERAPY

Nonpharmacologic Approach	
Weight reduction	
Exercise	
Sodium restriction	
Pharmacological Approach	
Step I	Administration of a single drug: Thiazide-diuretic *or* beta-adrenergic blocker
Step II	Administration of two drugs: Thiazide-diuretic *and* beta-adrenergic blocker
Step III	Administration of three drugs: Vasodilator added to the two drugs above
Step IV	Administration of a fourth drug: e.g., inhibitor of renin-angiotensin system

dietary sodium restriction. Modest results may be seen, but most patients with hypertension require treatment with drugs. The aim of the therapy is to achieve and maintain blood pressure at an acceptable level, particular a diastolic pressure below 90 mm Hg (O'Malley and O'Brien, 1980; Franklin, 1983; Gavra and Gavra, 1983; Williams, 1985).

In a stepped-care pharmacologic approach, treatment is initiated with small doses of a single agent, a thiazide diuretic or a beta-adrenergic blocker. The dose chosen is increased gradually until the desired blood pressure is attained, side effects interfere, or the maximum recommended dose has been reached. If the desired reduction of blood pressure has not been attained, then on to step 2 and the gradual addition of a second drug. Table 24–8 shows the results of combined therapy in patients of different ages and demonstrates the changes necessary to maintain a diastolic pressure of 90 mm Hg.

The most common antihypertensive drug combination is a thiazide-diuretic plus a beta-blocker. This approach allows flexibility and use of the complementary interaction of the different agents as well as minimizing the dose of each drug and its possible adverse side effects (Tables 24–9 and 24–10).

Antihypertensive Diuretics. The first choice to initiate pharmacologic therapy is, especially in the elderly, the thiazide diuretic (Table 24–9). Although the term diuretic (capable of increasing urine excretion) is used, the major hypotensive effect with chronic administration appears to be due to vasodilatation and not to sodium or water loss, which could, however, contribute to the antihypertensive action.

Table 24–9. ANTIHYPERTENSIVE EFFECTS OF THIAZIDES

Effects	Reduction of blood pressure Diuresis Synergism with other antihypertensives
Mechanism of action	Vasodilation Loss of interstitial fluid
Side effects	Potassium loss Reduced glucose tolerance Increased serum uric acid

Table 24–10. ANTIHYPERTENSIVE EFFECTS OF BETA-BLOCKERS

Effects	Reduction of blood pressure Reduction of cardiac output Inhibition of renin secretion
Mechanism of action	Blocks $beta_1$ and $beta_2$ adrenergic receptors Hypotensive action unknown
Side effects	Bronchospasm Cardiac failure Cold extremities Insulin blocked response (caution in diabetes)

There is no way to predict the hypotensive responses to thiazide from the duration or severity of hypertension in a given patient. Patients generally respond to thiazide within 2 to 4 weeks. The antihypertensive effect lasts longer and occurs at lower doses than does the diuretic effect. The timing of the drug for the elderly should be such that sleep is not unduly interrupted. Susceptible patients with problems of mobility may develop nocturia and urinary incontinence.

Potassium supplements are often necessary as the elderly are more sensitive to the potassium-losing effect of the thiazide, their dietary potassium intake may be reduced, and their capacity for renal conservation may be impaired. Potassium-retaining diuretics are available and are used in combination with other diuretics to prevent or correct potassium loss.

Postural hypotension should not be a problem with small doses. Side effects include a tendency to reduced glucose tolerance and a rise in serum uric acid; therefore, thiazide may not be advisable in individuals with diabetes or gout.

Adrenergic Beta-Blockers. Among drugs with peripheral sympatholytic action are the beta-adrenergic antagonists or blockers (Table 24–10). These agents are effective for treatment of hypertension and are usually well tolerated. In whites, the two types of drugs, thiazides and beta-blockers, are about equally effective for initial treatment. However, the response to beta-blockers is reduced in the elderly patient in whom the autonomic nervous system is less active (Buhler *et al.*, 1972; Roberts and Steinberg, 1986).

Beta-adrenergic blockers competitively inhibit the action of circulating catecholamines, epinephrine and norepinephrine, on beta-receptors, but the blockers' actual hypotensive mechanism is not yet established. They do reduce cardiac output and inhibit renin secretion. All beta-blockers appear to be equally effective for the treatment of hypertension, and any one can be used alone as initial therapy; however, they are more effective in combination with other antihypertensive drugs such as thiazide.

All beta-blockers can aggravate congestive heart failure; they cannot be used to treat hypertensive patients with asthma or obstructive pulmonary disease. Heart rate and contractility as well as relaxation of the pulmonary bronchioles are under beta-sympathetic control. Blocking these receptors reduces the rate and strength of the heartbeat and allows constriction of the bronchioles. Side effects are usually minor, but the dosage should be lowered in case of bronchospasm, vivid dreams, cardiac failure, or cold extremities.

Should the two-drug antihypertensive treatment combination not be adequate, a third drug is introduced; one with vasodilating properties, such as hydralazine, is most likely to be effective (Table 24–11). Following the same rationale, as a fourth step, other agents can be added—many of these are newer agents such as the atrial natriuretic hormone and the calcium blockers.

Hydralazine acts to produce arteriolar dilation (Table 24–11). Hydralazine causes direct relaxation of arteriolar smooth muscle, not through sympatholytic actions. Used alone, compensatory reactions to the vasodilatation such as increased heart rate and contractility, increased plasma renin activity, and fluid retention would occur and would counteract the antihypertensive effect to some degree. However, used in combination with a beta-blocker, which counteracts the effects on the heart and renin secretion, and the thiazide, which reduces fluid retention, it is most effective. The preferential dilatation of arterioles rather than veins reduces the incidence of orthostatic hypotension, more frequent in the elderly (see Chapter 17).

The total daily dose should be kept below 200 mg. This drug fell into disfavor years ago when administered in high doses and given alone as it produced a lupuslike syndrome. This is not seen with the currently approved doses. Headache may occur as an undesirable side effect and necessitates cessation of administration.

In the elderly, hydralazine may be a successful adjunct to the stepped-care approach in the treatment of hypertension because it does not produce drowsiness or postural hypotension, side effects of a number of other agents.

Table 24–11. ANTIHYPERTENSIVE EFFECTS OF THE VASODILATOR HYDRALAZINE

Effects	Reduction of blood pressure
Mechanism of action	Direct relaxation of arteriolar smooth muscle
Side effects	Alone:
	Increased heart rate and contractility
	Increased renin release
	Fluid retention
	Lupuslike syndrome (high dose)
	In combination with thiazide and beta-blocker:
	None, except headache

Table 24–12. ANTIHYPERTENSIVE EFFECTS OF MISCELLANEOUS DRUGS

Captopril	Angiotensin-converting enzyme inhibitor
	Reduces circulating angiotensin II
Calcium-channel blockers	Inhibit calcium movement
	Relax arterial smooth muscle
Atrial natriuretic hormone	Reduces circulating renin

The rationale in the stepped-care approach of hypertension is the use of drugs that are capable of lowering blood pressure by different mechanisms: so thiazides reduce extracellular fluid, beta-blockers reduce cardiac output and renin activity, hydralazine dilates arterioles—all of them lower blood pressure.

Patient compliance is, of course, basic to the establishment and maintenance of such a program. If a drug can be administered once a day, it is less likely to be forgotten; also, the fewer the number of pills, the less chance of being overlooked. As technology improves, other methods of administration besides oral are being introduced, such as transdermal administration with an adhesive patch, which acts for several days and is impervious to showering and daily activities.

There are other drugs available that have still other mechanisms of action (Table 24–12). Among these, one of the most effective or promising is an inhibitor of the angiotensin-converting enzyme (Doyle and Bearn, 1984). The representative substance captopril slows the formation of angiotensin II, the most powerful vasoconstrictor. The consequent fall in blood pressure results from reduced total peripheral resistance, and captopril increases the compliance of large arteries, which contributes to the reduction of systolic pressure. Low doses of captopril may be effective with a low incidence of adverse effects in patients with mild to moderate hypertension and without diabetes. Captopril is more effective with thiazide than alone.

Other effective antihypertensive drugs are calcium channel blockers. These agents are particularly effective in manipulating the function of smooth and cardiac muscle. As a group they are potent arterial vasodilators. Again, combination with a thiazide is beneficial. Still other antihypertensive drugs are the lipoprotein lowering drugs (see Chapter 18) as well as the atrial natriuretic hormone.

Calcium Channel Blockers. Even such a short consideration of calcium metabolism as presented here cannot overlook a new group of substances that act to control calcium movement. We are referring to the calcium channel blockers. Calcium channels are proteins of specific molecular weight that promote the entry of calcium across the plasma membrane into the cell cytosol. They are prevalent in excitable tissues such as nerve and muscle; they contain pores of specific sizes and, on their surface, many charged groups, which shift when the channel moves from the closed to the open position. Opening of the channel is also known as channel activation and depends on depolarization of the cell membrane. Calcium blockers inhibit the entry of calcium into cells or its mobilization from intracellular stores. The two major types are:

- heavy metals, which irreversibly block the channels and have general toxic effects on the organism and are, therefore, not used clinically, and
- inorganic blockers, which modify "gating" patterns, that is opening and closing patterns, and have proven useful in a number of cardiovascular disorders and, therefore, they have been ascribed as having an indirect antiaging affect.

The major actions of these blockers are relaxation of arterial smooth muscle, slowing of atrioventricular conduction, reduction of cardiac muscle contraction, decrease of coronary vascular resistance, and increase of coronary blood flow. The major untoward effects include excessive vasodilation, bradycardia, and sinoatrial block. Drug modifications and additional applications with regard to disorders of old age can be anticipated (Needleman *et al.*, 1985; Draper and Robison, 1986).

Atrial Natriuretic Hormone. The heart, in addition to being a pump, also has endocrine functions represented by the secretion of a hormone called atrial natriuretic hormone (ANH). In humans undergoing cardiac catheterization, stretching of atrial cells signals the release of ANH; likewise, an increase in blood volume will cause release of ANH. Experimental animals with hypertension or with congestive heart failure show a depletion of ANH within the atria. There appear to be specific binding sites on the cell of the responsive organs. This hormone relaxes smooth muscle cells throughout the vascular system. It is hypothesized that ANH affects either the entry of calcium into the cells or its relocation within the cell, through activation of intracellular cyclic AMP and GTP (adenylate and guanylate cyclases). The hypotensive actions have been ascribed to inhibition of renin, aldosterone, and vasopressin secretions, thus involving blood vessels, adrenals, and kidneys. The powerful vasorelaxant effects of this hormone are being studied as new and alternate means to control and treat hypertension and congestive heart failure (de Bold, 1985; Laragh, 1985; Sonnenberg and Maack, 1986; Blaine, 1986).

Hypertension in the elderly is a pathologic process leading to severe life-threatening diseases. Although precise parameters for treatment of hypertension remain controversial and each case must be considered on an individual basis, some general guidelines, once the diagnosis of hypertension has been made, include the following (Table 24–13):

1. One should try, first, nonpharmacologic treatment such as weight loss, salt reduction, and exercise, when appropriate;
2. If the nonpharmacologic treatment fails or is not appropriate, do not hesitate to use pharmacologic therapy. Keep in mind, however, that drugs are handled differently in the elderly and need to be tailored according to their special needs (Figure 24–2A). Therapy usually follows a stepped approach. Diuretics are used first with monitoring of blood potassium levels. A combination of two or three

Table 24–13. GENERAL GUIDELINES FOR TREATMENT OF HYPERTENSION IN THE ELDERLY

Use nonpharmacologic maneuvers when possible
Use pharmacologic therapy cautiously
Avoid sudden changes in blood pressure
Watch for orthostatic hypotension

drugs can be utilized if needed and with careful monitoring of possible side effects.

3. One should strive to maintain a blood pressure ranging from 140/80 to 160/95 without causing any sudden drops in blood pressure as elderly patients do not tolerate quick changes in pressure.
4. One must not forget to check for postural or orthostatic hypotension as the elderly are prone to this problem. In view of the relative ease of diagnosis, the high prevalence in the elderly population, and the severe consequences that result from neglect of hypertension, vigorous screening for this condition and reliable follow-up treatment are essential components of the health care of any elderly individual.

PHARMACOLOGY AND WELL-BEING IN THE ELDERLY

Pharmacology has emerged as a discipline over the last century and a quarter, and it is within the last 50 years that the greatest advances have been made. Over this same time period we have seen a prolongation of the lifespan, with a higher percentage of the population over 60 years of age, and pharmacology has had a great hand in this. Pharmacology is concerned with therapeutics, with how to correct or ameliorate dysfunction. However, assessment of drugs is primarily done in the healthy adult and we now realize that age and physical condition can alter the response to a drug. Our awareness was aroused by observation of the unique response of children to some medications—a substance that would sedate an adult would stimulate a child. Consequently, pediatric pharmacology has developed. Only now, as the older population is increasing, are we becoming aware that these older individuals also respond uniquely to some medications and have special needs. Thus, a geriatric pharmacology must also be established to benefit this sector of the population.

Studying pharmacology in the elderly embraces two concepts: (1) How and to what extent does aging influence the effect of drugs? (2) How and to what extent do drugs affect the elderly? Drug treatment of the elderly involves the use as well as the misuse of medication. In this group, self-medication and nonmedical influences, morbidity patterns, and socioeconomic parameters are also operative.

A strategy of treatment must be defined for the individual and should include the following: (1) Establish the most accurate diagnosis possible. (2) Define a therapeutic goal. (3) Rank the medications required for treatment. (4) Establish appropriate communication regarding the treatment. (5) Monitor serum levels of medication for proper dosage and compliance.

The elderly cover a considerable span of ages, generally have concomitant disease, are smokers and nonsmokers, engage in different physical activities, and subsist at different nutritional levels. Therefore, wide variations exist within the group. General facts that can be summarized are that old human beings often have diminished organ and body clearances of drugs and are thereby endangered to develop higher-than-expected plasma and tissue levels of a drug.

This older group also bears the consequences of current and past diseases and is physiologically less able to reestablish homeostasis. The group as a whole is at risk of being the victims of polypharmacy due to the increased pattern of disease occurring in the aged.

A judicious therapeutic regimen should be established and its implementation determined by screening the serum levels of active agents to verify they are in the therapeutic, not toxic, range or that the patient has, indeed, been taking the medication(s).

Although a vast armamentarium of therapeutic products exists, their pharmacodynamic actions must be adapted to the particular pharmacokinetic situation of old human beings. It is probable that we need new drugs and increased understanding for the great number of conditions encountered particularly in old age.

References

Bergener, M. K., and von Hahn, H. P. B. (eds.): Satellite Symposium XII Internatl Cong. Geront July 10–11, 1981 Kerger, Basal Influence of old age on the effect of drugs. *Gerontology*, **28** (Suppl. 1):**1981.**

Blaine, E. H. (Chrmn.): Atrial natriuretic factor, *Fed. Proc., FASEB Bull.*, **45**:2360–2391, **1986.**

de Bold, A. J.: Atrial natriuretic factor: A hormone produced by the heart. *Science,* **230**:767–770, **1985.**

Buhler, F. R.; Laragh, J. H.; Baer, L.; Vaughn, D. E.; and Brunner, H. R.: Propranolol inhibition of renin secretion. *N. Engl. J. Med.,* **287**:1209–1214, **1972.**

Doyle, A. E., and Bearn, A. G. (eds.): *Hypertension and the Angiotensin System: Therapeutic Approaches,* Raven Press, New York, **1984.**

Draper, H. H., and Robison, G. A. (Chrmn.): Controversy in pharmacology: Calcium and hypertension, *Fed. Proc., FASEB Bull.,* **45**:2732–2762, **1986.**

Franklin, S. S.: Geriatric hypertension. *Med. Clin. North Am.,* **67**:395–417, **1983.**

Gavra, H., and Gavra, I.: *Hypertension in the Elderly,* John Wright PSG, Boston, **1983.**

Gersh, B. J.; Kronmal, R. A.; Schaff, H. V.; Frye, R. L.; Ryan, T. J.; Mock, M. B.; Myers, W. O.; Athearn, M. W.; Gosselin, A. J.; and Kaiser, G. C.: Comparison of coronary artery bypass surgery and medical therapy in patients 65 years of age or older. A nonrandomized study from the Coronary Artery Surgery Study (CASS) registry. *N. Engl. J. Med.,* **313**:217–224, **1985.**

Gilman, A. G.; Goodman, L. S.; Rall, T. W.; and Murad, F. (eds.): *Goodman and Gilman's The Pharmacological Basis of Therapeutics,* 7th ed., Macmillan Pub. Co., New York, **1985.**

Kennedy, J. W.; Ritchie, J. L.; Davis, K. B.; Stadius, M. L.; Maynard, C.; and Fritz, J. K.: The Western Washington randomized trial of intracoronary streptokinase in acute myocardial infarction. *N. Engl. J. Med.,* **312**:1073–1078, **1985.**

Kiechel, J. R.: Biotransformation of drugs during aging. *Gerontology,* **28** (Suppl. 1):101–112, **1982.**

Koren, G.; Weiss, A. T.; Hasin, Y.; *et al.*: Prevention of myocardial damage in acute myocardial ischemia by early treatment with intravenous streptokinase. *N. Engl. J. Med.,* **313**:1384–1389, **1985.**

Laragh, J. H.: Atrial natriuretic hormone, the renin-aldosterone axis, and blood pressure—electrolyte homeostasis. *N. Engl. J. Med.,* **313**:1330–1340, **1985.**

Mock, M. B.; Schaff, H. B.; Holmes, D. R.; Vlietstra, R. E.; Smith, H. C.; and Gersh, B. J.: Comparison of coronary bypass surgery and medical therapy in patients 65 years of age or older. *N. Engl. J. Med.,* **312**:916–919, **1985.**

Needleman, P.; Corr, P. B.; and Johnson, E. M., Jr.: Drugs used for the treatment of angina: Organic nitrates, calcium channel blockers and beta-adrenergic antagonists. In Gilman, A. G.; Goodman, L. S.; Rall, T. W.; and Murad, F. (eds.): *Goodman and Gilman's The Pharmacological Basis of Therapeutics,* 7th ed., Macmillan Pub. Co., New York, **1985.**

O'Malley, K.; Meagher, F.; and O'Callaghan, W.: The pharmacology of aging. In Pathy, M. S. J. (ed.): *Principles and Practice of Geriatric Medicine,* John Wiley & Sons, Chichester, UK, **1985.**

O'Malley, K., and O'Brien, E.: Management of hypertension in the elderly. *N. Engl. J. Med.,* **302**:1397–1404, **1980.**

Pearson, M. W., and Roberts, C. J. C.: Drug induction of hepatic enzymes in the elderly. *Age Ageing,* **13**:313–316, **1984.**

Roberts, J., and Steinberg, G. M. (ed.): Effects of aging on adrenergic receptors. *Fed. Proc.,* **45**:40–64, **1986.**

Sonnenberg, H., and Maack, T. (Chrmn.): Atrial natriuretic factors I and II, *Fed. Proc., FASEB Bull.,* **45**:2079–2132, **1986.**

Stamler, J.: Coronary heart disease: Doing the "right things." *N. Engl. J. Med.,* **312**:*1053–1055,* **1985.**

TIMI Study Group: The thrombolysis in myocardial infarction (TIMI) trial. *N. Engl. J. Med.,* **312**:932–936, **1985.**

Vestal, R. E., and Dawson, G. W.: Pharmacology and aging. In Finch, C. E., and Schneider, E. L. (eds.): *Handbook of the Biology of Aging,* Van Nostrand Reinhold, New York, **1985.**

Williams, B. H. O.: The cardiovascular system. In Pathy, M. S. J. (ed.): *Principles and Practice of Geriatric Medicine,* Wiley & Sons, New York, **1985.**

Zivin, J. A.; Fisher, M.; DeGirolami, U.; Hemenway, C. C.; and Stashak, J. A.: Tissue plasminogen activator reduces neurological damage after cerebral embolism. *Science,* **230**:1289–1292, **1985.**

Zucker, M. B.: The functioning of blood platelets. *Sci. Am.,* **242**:86–103, **1980.**

CHAPTER

25 EFFECTS OF DIET ON AGING

Brian J. Merry and Anne M. Holehan

STUDIES IN LABORATORY ANIMALS

In seeking to gain insight into the biochemical mechanisms that underlie aging, particularly in mammals, it has to be recognized that merely cataloguing physiologic changes with age will give little understanding of such a complex process. Aging is both multifaceted and hierarchic in its expression, with subtle changes occurring simultaneously with time at the molecular, cellular, tissue, and organ levels. Further complexity arises at each of these levels as metabolic and homeostatic compensations are made in an attempt to accommodate these age-induced changes in the normal functioning of the animal. To distinguish "cause" and "effect" in the assessment of the biologic mechanisms of aging is therefore extremely difficult, a problem frequently exacerbated by the existence of underlying chronic pathology.

Recognizing these difficulties, attempts have been made to develop experimental models in which the rate of aging can be manipulated in a predictable manner, thus facilitating the distinction between "cause" and "effect." Of the many experimental approaches that have been attempted to achieve this end, the most successful strategies have incorporated some form of dietary restriction.

THE DIETARY RESTRICTION MODEL

The observation that restricted feeding had a beneficial effect on survival in a laboratory rodent population has been known for many years (Osborne and Mendel 1915; McCay *et al.,* 1939; Ross, 1966, 1969). The effect was both reproducible and observed in spite of widely differing experimental designs, dietary composition, and severity of restricted feeding. One of the simplest but most effective methods of extending lifespan, and therefore, by implication, slowing the rate of aging, has been to limit access to the normal diet in rodents so that the body weight of experimental animals is maintained at about 50 percent that of age-matched, fully fed control animals. This is approximately equivalent to maintaining age-matched animals on half-rations throughout postweaning life. This allows for a continuous slow rate of growth to occur throughout life and results in a 36 to 42 percent extension in mean and maximum lifespan (see Figure 25–1). Such survival data may be transformed into linear form by the Gompertz equation (Gompertz, 1825):

$$R_m = R_0 e\alpha^t = \frac{-1}{n} \times \frac{dn}{dt}$$

where n = number of survivors at time t, and α (the slope constant) and R_0 (the hypothetical mortality at time 0) are constants. The time to double the rate of mortality for a population can be represented by $T_d = 0.693/\alpha$. Calculation from survival data of the time required to double the rate of mortality in fully fed control rats gives a period of about 100 days, while in animals dietary-restricted throughout postweaning life the figure is approximately 200 days.

Composition of the Diet

Numerous studies have been reported that attempt to elucidate the component in the diet responsible for the effect on the rate of aging. Most of the studies have concentrated on the protein and carbohydrate content of the diet, and conflicting conclusions have been reported. In one detailed investigation into whether the beneficial effects of underfeeding were derived mainly from either protein or caloric restriction, 1600 male rats were divided into five di-

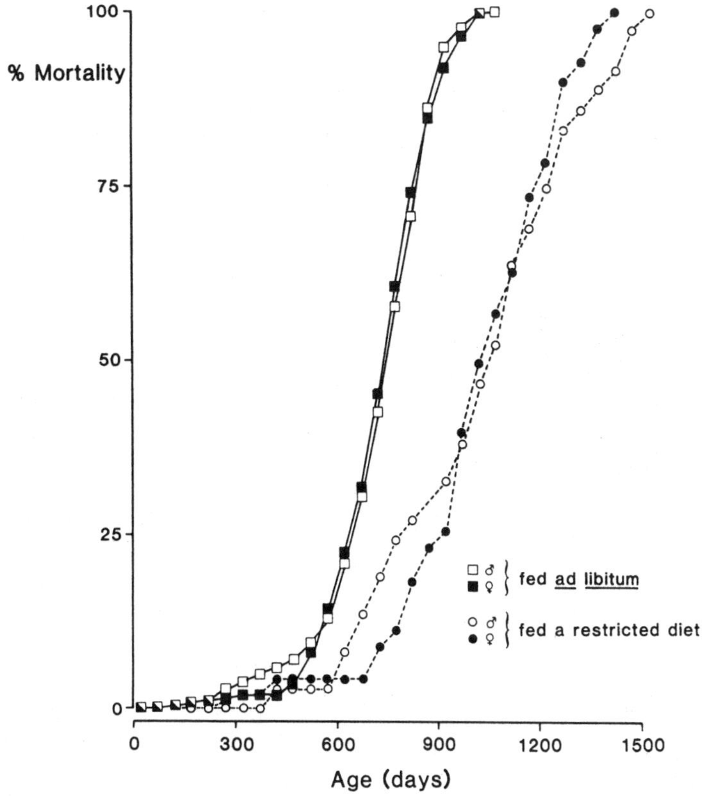

Figure 25–1. *Mortality profiles of CFY Sprague Dawley rats fed* ad libitum *(■ ♀ □ ♂) or a restricted diet (● ♀ ○ ♂) such that body weight was maintained at 50 percent that of the fully fed animals.*

Group numbers: *ad libitum* = 200♀, 397♂; dietary restricted = 100♀, 100♂. Reprinted with permission from (Merry, B.J. and Phillips, J.G.; Basic Gerontology, In: Green, M.: (ed.): *Clinics in Endocrinology and Metabolism,* vol. 10, no. 1). Copyright (1981) W.B. Saunders Company Ltd.)

etary groups (Ross, 1959). One group was fed a commercial diet *ad libitum* and the other four were fed restricted diets designated low protein–low carbohydrate, low protein–high carbohydrate, high protein–low carbohydrate, and high protein–high carbohydrate. The results from this study were again equivocal in their interpretation with the exception that all four dietary-restricted groups had a greater life expectancy than those fed *ad libitum*. Animals fed high-protein diets had markedly superior survival in the first half of life, but feeding high carbohydrate either with high or low protein intake resulted in a steep late mortality. The low-protein–low-carbohydrate diet yielded a high early mortality resulting from cecal impaction but showed the best late-life survival. It was further concluded that the caloric intake of these five dietary groups was linearly related to the lifespan with a slope of approximately −3.9 days kcal/day.

Subsequent attempts to resolve this confused aspect of the model have utilized experimental designs that provide restricted rats with the same amount of protein as *ad libitum* controls but with varying amounts of carbohydrate (Davis *et al.*, 1983). It was concluded that rats fed calorically restricted diets survive longer than those fed *ad libitum* even when both groups have a similar protein intake. Low levels of dietary protein in both calorie-restricted and *ad li-*

bitum–fed animals were associated with a decrease in survival rates and caloric intake appeared to have a greater effect on survival than protein intake. It is, however, difficult to separate the effects of calorie versus protein restriction on subsequent survival because of the metabolic compensations that occur when energy intake in the diet is a limiting factor. As the severity of energy restriction is increased, more protein is utilized for energy purposes and thus dietary-restriction regimes invariably result in a complex interaction of energy and protein restriction.

INITIATION OF DIETARY RESTRICTION: EFFECT OF AGE

It had been concluded in earlier studies using rats, mice, and hamsters that dietary restriction for 1 year followed by a return to full feeding was the most effective nutritional regimen for delaying aging in these species (Stuchlikova *et al.*, 1975). These conclusions, however, were based, not on maximum lifespans or the survival of the last decile (last 10 percent of the population), but on mean lifespan data. Changes in the shape of the survival curve will radically alter the average survival age without affecting maximum lifespan and the rate of aging. In the three dietary regimes in which dietary restriction was imposed for (1) the total postweaning lifespan, (2) the first year of life, or (3) the second year of life, little variation in maximum lifespan occurred. It is now accepted that the greatest effect of dietary restriction regimes on subsequent survival is recorded for animals underfed throughout the postweaning period of life. The question therefore arises as to whether there are periods in the life of an animal that are more susceptible to the effects of undernutrition in extending lifespan. Early dietary restriction followed by *ad libitum* feeding has been found not to extend maximum lifespan (Nolen, 1972; Holehan and Merry, 1986), but restricted feeding for only 7 weeks after weaning has been claimed to delay tumor onset and reduce subsequent mortality risk by 20% (Ross, 1972).

Successful food restriction of adult rodents appears dependent on the gradual adaptation of the animals to the reduced rations (Weindruch and Walford, 1982). Adult mice from two long-lived strains were food-restricted at 12 months by restricting food intake for the first month of underfeeding to 72 percent and then in the second month to 56 percent that of *ad libitum* intake. An increase in maximum and mean lifespan of 10 to 20 percent was achieved by this procedure (see Figure 25–2).

While the greatest effect on slowing the rate of aging is achieved by dietary-restricting animals throughout postweaning life, the immediate postweaning period is clearly not the only phase of the lifespan sensitive to the effects of underfeeding. Observations from a number of groups indicate that either refeeding previously dietary-restricted animals or underfeeding rodents during the preweaning period is detrimental to subsequent survival.

EFFECT ON AGE-RELATED PATHOLOGY

It has been recognized from many studies on nutrition and aging that age-related pathologies in laboratory rodents are exquisitely sensitive to the dietary history of the individual animal. A beneficial effect of undernutrition on reducing the incidence of chronic glomerulonephritis, myocardial fibrosis, peribranchial lymphocytosis, periarteritis, prostatitis, and endocrine hyperplasias in rats has been recorded (see Figures 25–3 and 24–4) (Ross, 1959, 1964; Berg, 1960).

TUMOR INCIDENCE

The majority of studies on chronic underfeeding and pathology have concentrated on the incidence of neoplastic lesions, which is a linearly increasing function of caloric intake or body weight and the protein component of the diet (Ross and Bras, 1965; 1973; Payne, 1979). The protein content of the diet has a complex action, with some types of tumor being commonest at high-protein intake and others at low-protein intake. Dietary restriction has been observed to reduce the frequency of tumors of the pituitary gland, lung, and pancreatic islet cells, while in tumors of soft tissue origin and those of the thyroid gland and the bladder the frequency of appearance was

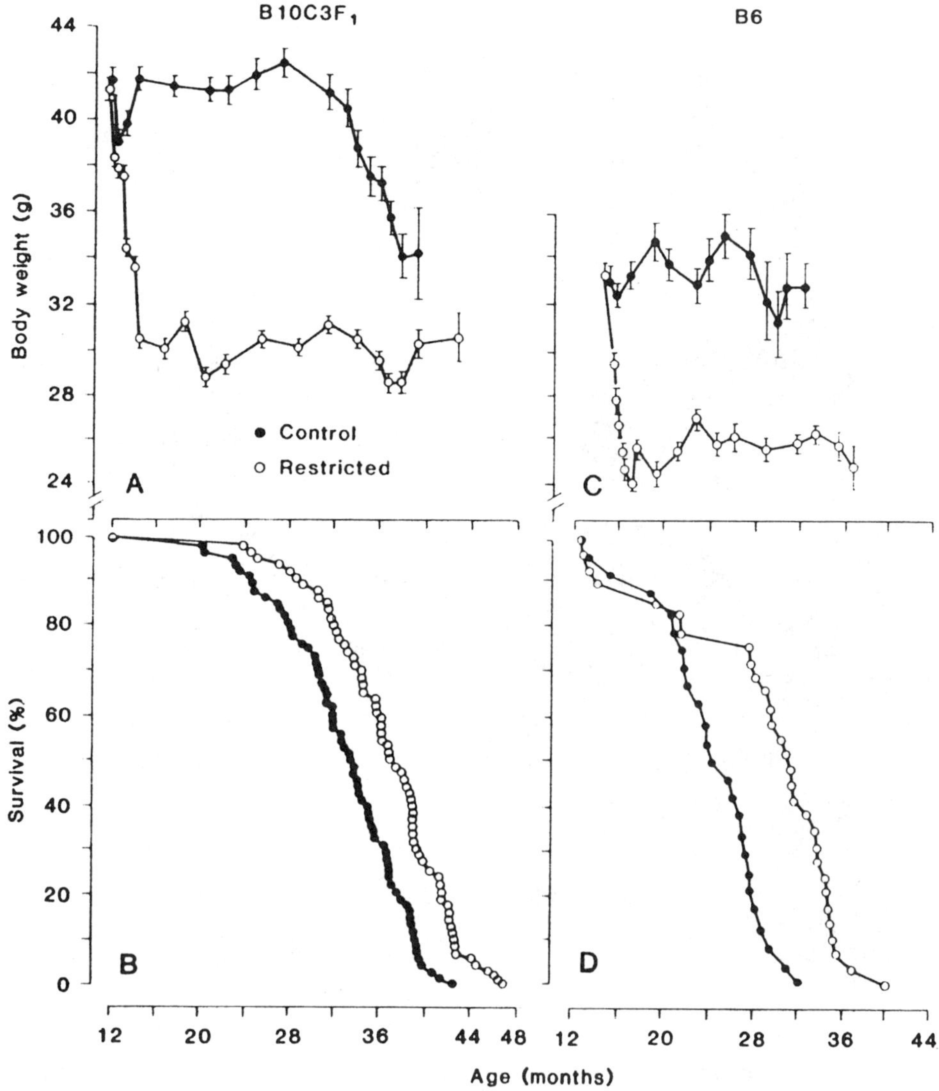

Figure 25–2. *Body weights and survival of B10C3F$_1$ mice (A and B) and B6 mice (C and D) fed on control and restricted diets.*

Weights are plotted as means ± standard error for all mice alive at the indicated ages. Each point in the survival curves represents one mouse. Reprinted with permission from (Weindruch, R. and Walford, R.L.: Dietary restriction in mice beginning at 1 year of age: Effect on life-span and spontaneous cancer incidence. *Science,* 215:1415–1418). Copyright (1982) by the AAAS.

unaffected although a delay in onset was observed. Conversely, malignant epithelial tumors, adrenal, parathyroid gland tumors, and reticulum cell sarcomas of the lymphoid glands were significantly increased (Ross and Bras, 1971). These observations have been confirmed in mice and rats where a reduction of only 20 percent of the normal food intake resulted in a significant reduction of the most common tumor for each species (mice—liver; rats—pituitary, mammary gland, skin) (Tucker, 1979) (see Figure 25–5). The formation of spontaneous lymphoma is inhibited in mice underfed from 12 months of age, but no effect of diet on hepatoma incidence was observed

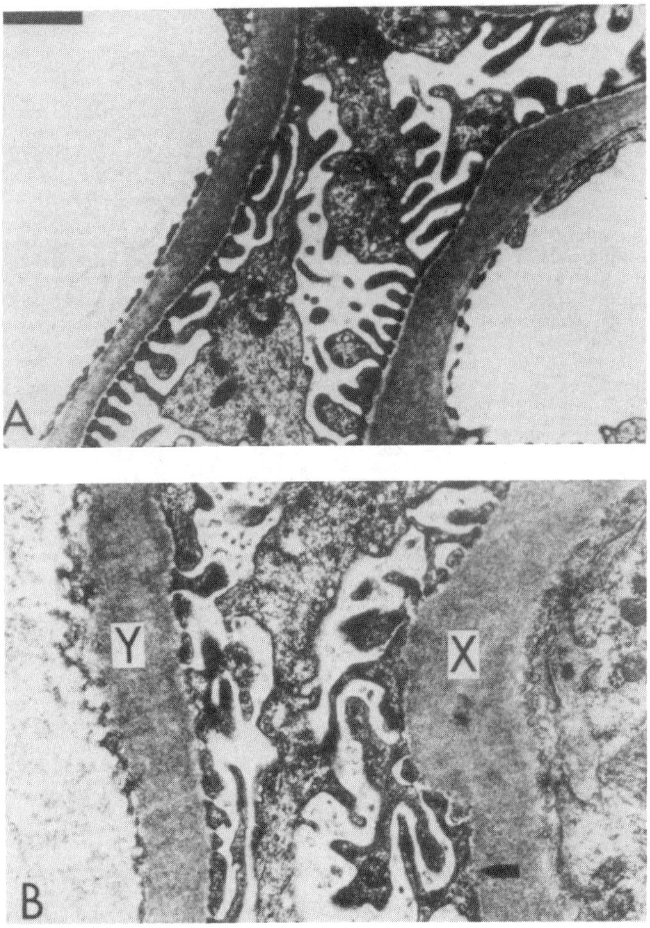

Figure 25–3. **(A)** Section showing the peripheral edges of the adjacent capillary loops in a normal glomerulus taken from an old, isolated, dietary restricted rat (1302 days). The basement membrane shows only slight thickening and the foot processes are well formed and discrete. **(B)** Comparable area from an abnormal glomerulus taken from an old isolated *ad libitum* fed rat (1010 days). The basement membrane is markedly thickened, showing a scallop in the area indicated at *X*. Thickening at *Y* is partly due to oblique sectioning of the membrane at that point. The spreading out of the foot processes along the membrane is clearly illustrated (arrow). (Magnification × 7332; scale bar is 2.11 μm). Reproduced with permission (*Arch. Gerontol. Geriatr.*, 2, Wyndham, J.R., *et al.*, Effects of isolation and food restriction begun at 50 days on the development of age-associated renal disease in the male Wistar rat). Copyright (1983) Elsevier Science Publishers B.V. (Biomedical Division) Amsterdam.

(Weindruch and Walford, 1982). Thus, a selective effect of diet on the inhibition of tumor formation is again evident.

Response to Carcinogens. Chronic dietary restriction confers a degree of protection against the highly mutagenic action of exogenous carcinogens. The polycyclic hydrocarbon carcinogen dimethylbenz(a)anthracene, which binds covalently to DNA after conversion to a reactive epoxide, demonstrates significantly reduced binding to skin DNA from mice maintained on 60 percent of *ad libitum* food intake (Pashko and Schwartz, 1983). It is suggested that a reduction in the binding of the carcinogen to DNA would retard the initiation of tumor formation. Similarly, specific protection against the initiation of intestinal tumors by methylazoxymethanol (MAM) in the highly susceptible Lobund Sprague-Dawley (SD) rat has been demonstrated when such animals are maintained on restricted feeding (Pollard *et al.*, 1984). Fully fed male Lobund (SD) rats produce a high percentage of visible tumors in the colon and small intestine 20 weeks after a single subcutaneous injection of MAM. When rats were fed 75 percent the *ad libitum* food intake 10 days after exposure to MAM, significantly fewer intestinal tumors were observed 20 weeks after injection of the carcinogen (see Table 25–1). The moderate degree of dietary restriction utilized in this experiment appeared to be acting in a suppressive rather than a chemopreventive mode in which the timing of initiation of restricted feeding was critical. Delayed onset of un-

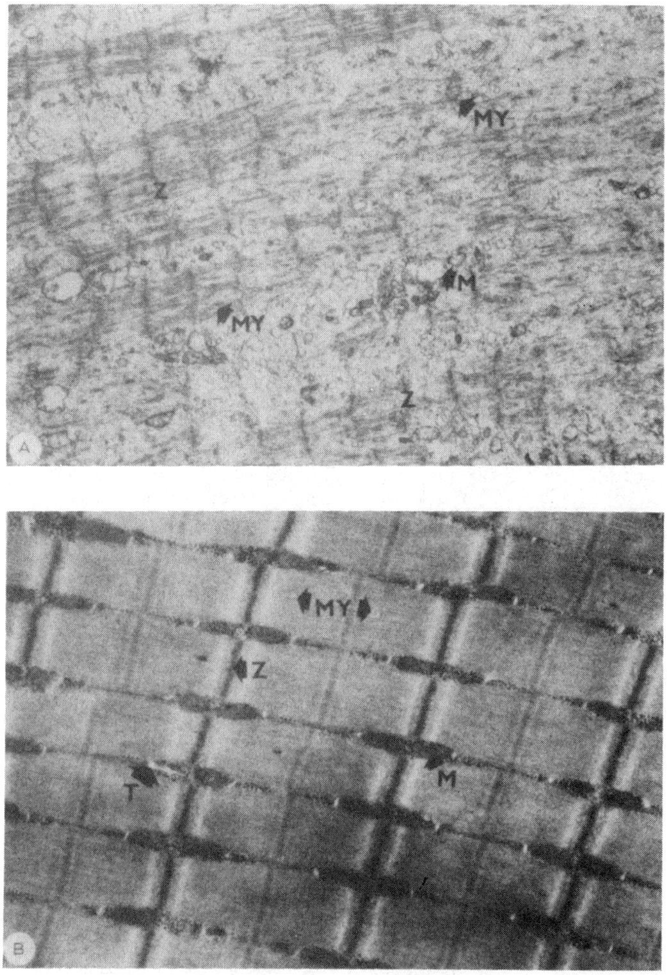

Figure 25–4. (**A**) Longitudinal section through the gastrocnemius muscle of a control male Wistar rat aged 1010 days. Myofibrillar breakdown is significant with only thin diffuse Z-bands (arrowed) remaining to support the sparse, degenerated myofibrils. The sarcoplasm contains few mitochrondria, vesicles, and fine filamentous remnants. (**B**) Electron micrograph of a longitudinal section through the gastrocnemius muscle of a food restricted male Wistar rat aged 1284 days. There is no evidence of myofibrillar breakdown or structural abnormalities in mitochondria or t-tubules. Abnormal amounts of lipid were not detected. Magnification × 10,290, Z = Z band, M = mitochondrion, MY = myofilaments, T = tubule. Reproduced with permission from (*Arch. Gerontol. Geriatr.*, 4, Everitt, A.V., *et al.*, Skeletal muscle aging in the hind limb of the old male Wistar rat: inhibitory effect of hypophysectomy and food restriction). Copyright (1985) Elsevier Science Publishers B.V. (Biomedical Division) Amsterdam.

derfeeding until 63 days after the injection of MAM was ineffective in preventing tumor development. The moderate degree of dietary restriction imposed on the rats did not induce a depressed metabolic state, and paradoxically, alternate days of fasting and full feeding (an alternative strategy of restricted feeding frequently used to extend maximum lifespan in rodents) was ineffective in preventing MAM-induced tumors. This diversity in tumor formation under the alternative restricted feeding regimes remains an intriguing but unexplained observation.

HYPERTENSION

The major causes of death in an aging human population are pathologies associated with the cardiovascular system in which hypertension has been a major risk factor. Consequently, animal models have been developed to facilitate a detailed study of the genetic and environmental components of this pathology. Hypertension for which no recognizable cause can be found is called essential or idiopathic. The spontaneously hypertensive rat (SHR), selectively bred from a strain of Wistar rats, has been claimed to be a good model for the study of essential hypertension in humans since the condition is spontaneous, increases in severity with age, is more severe in males, and is often associated with complications of several organs, including heart, brain, and kidneys, similar to those found in human hypertension. The development of hypertension occurs prematurity followed by

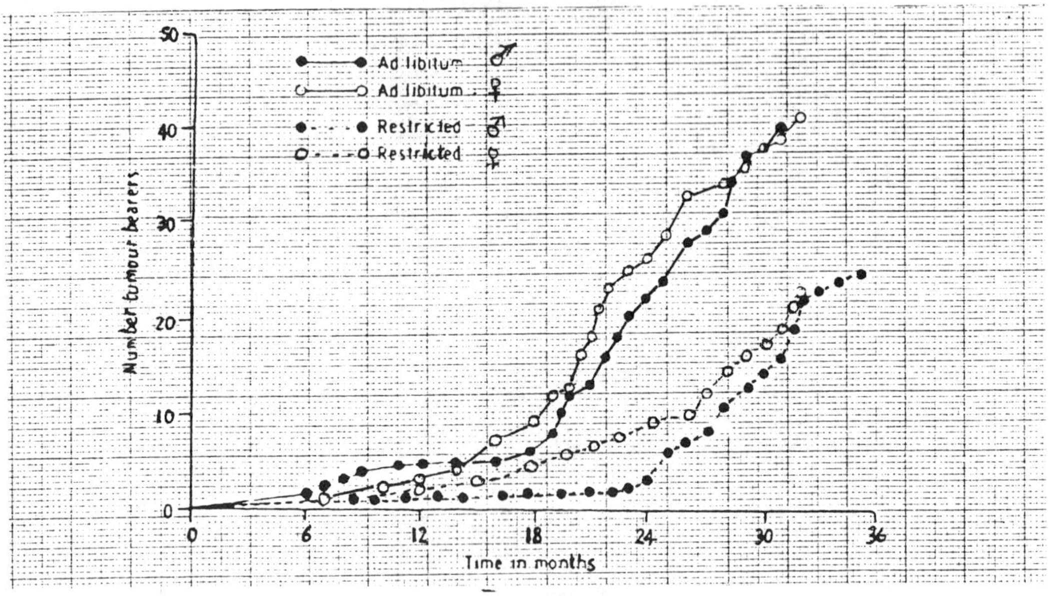

Figure 25–5. *Cumulative totals of tumor bearing specific-pathogen-free Swiss albino mice of the Alderley Park strain.*

Control animals were fed *ad libitum* (from 5g/mouse/day) whereas dietary restricted animals were fed 4g/mouse/day. Each experimental group consisted of 50 animals. Reprinted with permission from (Tucker, M.J.: The effect of long-term food restriction on tumors in rodents. *Int. J. Cancer,* 23, 803–807), Copyright (1979) International Journal of Cancer.

a secondary slower increase in blood pressure throughout life with death resulting at about 18 months compared to 24 months in the normotensive WKY control rats (see Figure 25–6). The early death is attributed to six specific lesions: interstitial fibrosis of the kidney, myocardial edema, fatty infiltration of the myocardium, atrial thrombosis, congestion, and vacuolization in the adrenal. Restriction of the normal rat diet to 40 percent *ad libitum* intake extended mean and maximum lifespan in both normotensive and hypertensive animals (Lloyd and Boyd, 1981; Lloyd, 1984). Mean lifespan in normotensive animals was increased by 8 months (from 24 to 32 months) while mean lifespan in underfed SH rats was increased by over 12 months (from 18 to over 30 months) (see Figure 25–7). The extension in lifespan in the SH rat was accompanied by a decrease in the specific lesions associated with the hypertensive state to a frequency not significantly different from the dietary-restricted normotensive WKY controls. Paradoxically, the development of the hypertension was not affected by the restricted diet, but conversely underfeeding appears to convey protection against end-organ damage and subsequent pathology resulting from the elevated blood pressure.

Immunologic Response to Dietary Restriction

The delayed appearance and enhanced resistance to many pathologies associated with aging in chronically underfed rodents has inevitably resulted in a detailed evaluation of the immune system in these animals. Most of the studies have been conducted with dietary-restricted mice in which the genetics of individual strains are clearly defined. A general response common to mice, rats, and guinea pigs exposed to moderate chronic protein restriction is a depression in antibody production but, conversely, enhanced cell-mediated immunity (Walford *et al.*, 1974) (see Figure 25–8). Although dietary restriction will modify longevity in all strains of mice evaluated, the

Table 25–1. EFFECTS OF DIETARY RESTRICTIONS ON MAM-INDUCED INTESTINAL TUMORS[a]

GROUP	NO. OF RATS	L-485 DIET	INTERVAL (DAYS) TO RESTRICTION	INTERVAL (DAYS) TO AUTOPSY	AVERAGE BODY WEIGHT (G)	NO. OF RATS WITH TUMORS/ NO. OF RATS AT RISK	TOTAL NO. OF TUMORS	AVERAGE NO. OF TUMORS/ RAT	P VALUE[b]
A	11	*Ad libitum*	10	140	460	10/11	30	2.72	<0.0001
	10	12 g/day		140	320	3/10	4	0.4	
B	8	*Ad libitum*	63	140	382	6/7	11	1.57	NS
	7	12 g/day		140	308	7/7	16	2.2	
C	10	*Ad libitum*	8	140	431	6/10	14	1.4	NS
	10	*Ad libitum*/alternate days		140	341	6/10	11	1.1	
D	10	*Ad libitum*	31	140	418	9/10	20	2.0	NS
	10	*Ad libitum*/alternate days		140	385	6/9	18	2.0	

[a]Weanling male S–D rats were inoculated sc once with MAM (30 mg/kg of body weight). Thereafter, groups were fed either *ad libitum* or restricted diet until day 140, when they were killed and examined.

[b]NS = not significant.

Reprinted with permission from Pollard, M., *et al.:* Inhibition of intestinal tumorigenesis in methylazoxymethanol-treated rats by dietary restriction. *Cancer Treat. Rep., 68:*405–408, 1984.

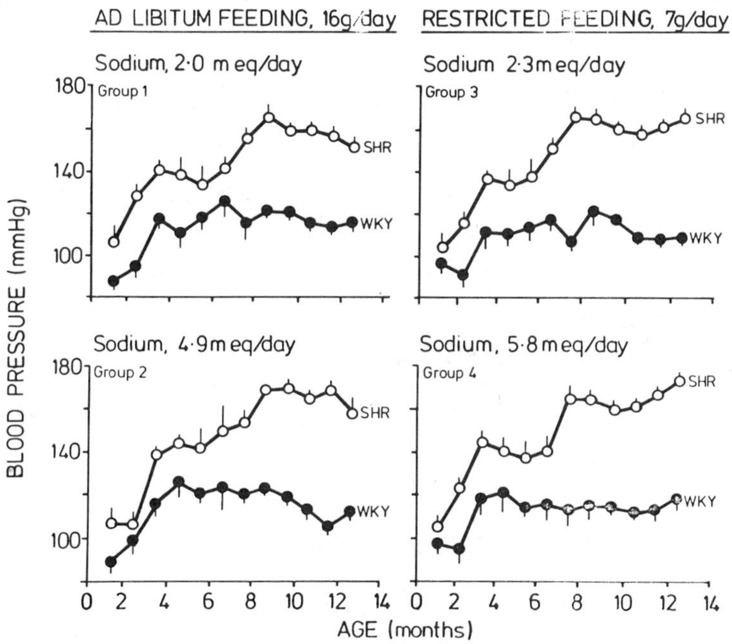

Figure 25–6. *The effects of restricted feeding and dietary sodium intake on the development and maintenance of hypertension in the spontaneously hypertensive rat (SHR) compared to the normotensive Wistar Kyoto (CWKY) substrain.*

Reprinted with permission from (Lloyd, T. and Boyd, B.; Development and regulation of hypertension in the spontaneously hypertensive rat; enzymatic and nutritional studies. In Usdin, E.; Weiner, N.; Youdin M.B.H.: (eds): *Function and regulation of monoamine enzymes: Basic and clinical aspects*). Copyright (1981) Macmillan Publishing Co., London.

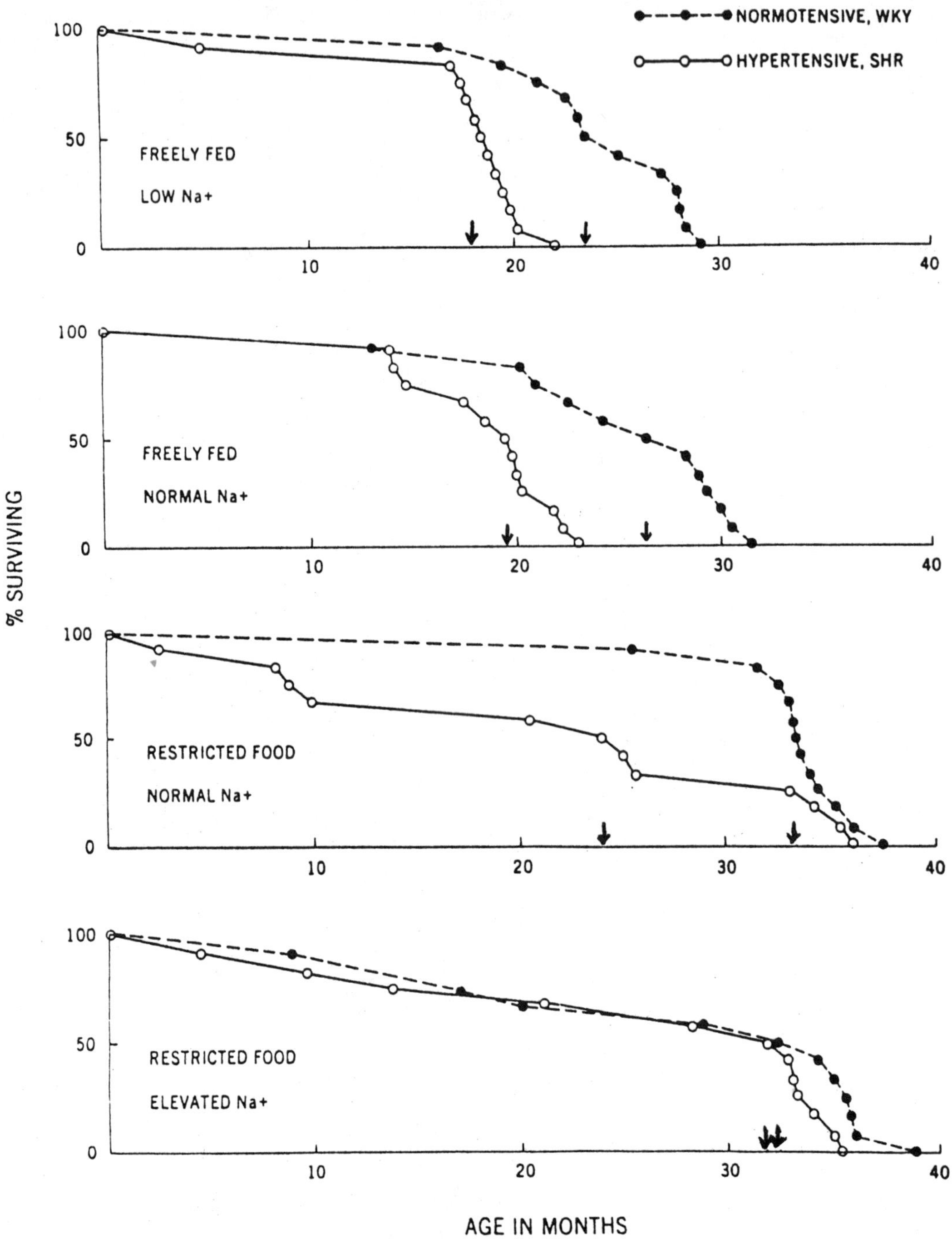

Figure 25–7. *Survival curves of* ad libitum *fed and dietary restricted spontaneously hypertensive rats (SHR) and normotensive controls (WKY).*

The arrows indicate the mean life time for each strain under the differing dietary conditions. Reprinted with permission from (*Life Sciences,* 34, Lloyd, T., Food restriction increases lifespan of hypertensive animals.) Copyright (1984), Pergamon Press).

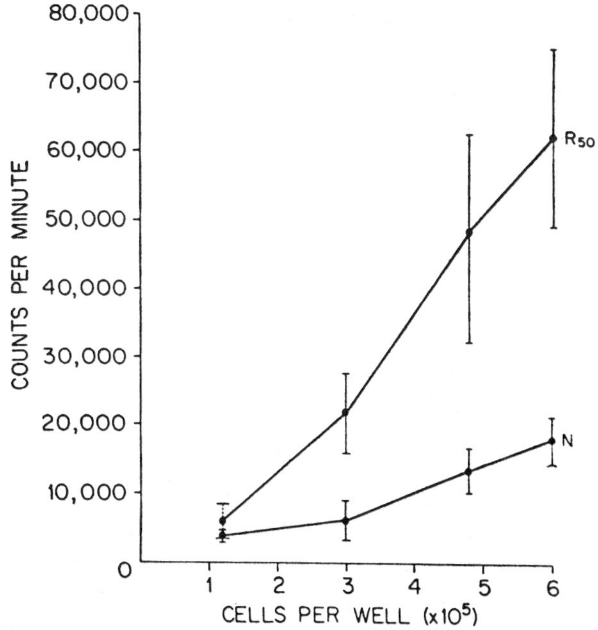

Figure 25–8. *Cell dosage study of spleen cell phytohemagglutinin reactivity in 13–14.5 month old* ad libitum *fed and dietary restricted mice.*

Animals on restricted feeding were fed alternate days 50 Kcal/week. Values plotted are the mean ± standard error for ^{3}H-thymidine uptake for individual mice with background counts per minute subtracted. Reprinted with permission from (*Exp. Gerontol.*, 17, Weindruch, R.H., Kristie, J.A., Naeim, F., Mullen, B.G. and Walford, R.L.: Influence of weaning-initiated dietary restriction on responses to T cell mitogens and on splenic T cell levels in a long-lived F_1-hybrid mouse strain). Copyright (1982), Pergamon Journals Ltd.

early immunologic effects of underfeeding seem to be strain dependent. In assays of T-cell function, restricted female $B_{10}C_3F_1$ mice outperformed fully fed controls, but when young C_{57}BL/6J mice were assessed, control mice outperformed dietary-restricted animals. While dietary influences on the immune system have been shown to be profound, the effects are clearly modified by genetic factors and the associated predisposition to develop particular pathologies, rendering the strain short-lived. This effect can be illustrated by the two short-lived mouse strains DBA/2f and (NZB × NZW)F_1 (B/W). Caloric restriction in B/W mice prolonged lifespan more than protein restriction, whereas DBA/2f mice showed enhanced survival only when the diet was restricted for protein (Fernandes *et al.,* 1976). The diversity of response of these two strains to caloric and protein restriction in terms of subsequent survival appears to result from the influence of diet on the rapidly progressive, highly destructive, autoimmune renal disease that occurs in B/W mice.

Autoimmune Disease. In an earlier section (see Response to Carcinogens), attention was directed to the protective effect of dietary restriction against tumor formation even when implemented 10 days after exposure to the carcinogen MAM. A somewhat similar effect has been reported in mice susceptible to autoimmune disease. It is a characteristic of the MRL/1 mouse strain that both males and females develop lymphoproliferative diseases, autoimmunity, and a rapidly progressive renal disease. Consequently MRL/1 mice live approximately 6 months when fed *ad libitum* but survival can be doubled to over 1 year if mice are underfed even if the restricted feeding regimen is not implemented until after the onset of the disease. Such delayed

Table 25–2. EFFECT OF DIETARY RESTRICTION ON LYMPHOCYTE FUNCTION AND PROTEIN SYNTHESIS

	PROLIFERATION (CPM/5 × 10^6 CELLS)	IL-2 PRODUCTION (CPM/2 × 10^4 CELLS)	PROTEIN SYNTHESIS (CPM/10^7 CELLS)
Ad libitum	30,176 ± 516	4011 ± 237	11,209 ± 1,305
Restricted	58,762 ± 462	6051 ± 589	15,758 ± 785

Male Fischer F344 rats were fed *ad libitum* or a 40 percent caloric-restricted diet beginning at 6 weeks of age. Phytohemagglutinin-induced proliferation, concanavalin A-induced IL-2 production, and protein synthesis by spleen lymphocytes isolated from 19-month-old male Fischer F344 rats fed *ad libitum* or the restricted diet were determined. Each value is the mean ± SD of data obtained from two animals. Reprinted with permission from Richardson, A., and Cheung, H.T.: I. The relationship between age-related changes in gene expression, protein turnover, and the responsiveness of an organism to stimuli. *Life Sci.*, 31. Copyright (1982) Pergamon Press, Ltd.

dietary restriction very dramatically influenced the appearance of renal pathology and the autoimmune reaction (Kubo *et al.*, 1984). The mechanism of this protective action of underfeeding is again not understood, for neither the formation of anti-DNA nor antigen-antibody complexes are reduced by dietary restriction, a paradox similar to that noted for the protective effect of underfeeding in the SH rat (see Hypertension). It was observed, however, that dietary-restricted MRL/1 mice were no longer deficient in interleukin-2 production, particularly in the lymph nodes. This finding is in agreement with the report that in rats maintained on chronic dietary restriction regimes mitogen-induced lymphocyte proliferation, interleukin-2 induction, and protein synthesis were increased in spleen lymphocytes (see Table 25–2) (Richardson and Cheung, 1982). Autoimmune-prone mice strains characteristically have very deficient production of interleukin-2 (Altman *et al.*, 1981).

METABOLIC RESPONSE TO DIETARY RESTRICTION

The early studies that attempted to measure the basal metabolic rate of dietary-restricted rats reported it as lying between normal young and normal old animals (Horst *et al.*, 1934). More precisely, when measured at 850 days it was reported to be lower than in control animals if expressed as heat production per unit surface area or, alternatively, higher if expressed against body weight (Will and McCay, 1943). Indirect support for the idea that the metabolic rate was depressed was presented by Sacher (Sacher, 1977), when he reviewed the data from the earlier study of Ross (Ross, 1969), in which five dietary regimes were used to observe the effect of calorie intake on survival. It appeared from the calculations that total calorie intake during the lifespan per gram of body weight was the same for each of the five dietary groups, being approximately 102 kcal/g body weight. This conclusion was interpreted as support for the rate-of-living theory of aging (Rubner, 1908). Two subsequent studies have failed to substantiate this conclusion. Male Fischer 344 rats fed 60 percent of the *ad libitum* in take from 6 weeks consumed a greater number of calories per gram of body weight during their lifetime than did rats fed *ad libitum* (Masoro *et al.*, 1982). This observation was confirmed in female CFY strain Sprague-Dawley rats (Holehan, 1984).

Direct measurement of basal metabolic rate utilizing modern technology has confirmed that it is not depressed in chronically dietary-restricted rats. Male and female rats adapted over an 8-week period from weaning to a 50 percent restriction of energy intake at two levels of protein intake (20 percent and 10 percent) showed no change in basal metabolic rate (Mohan and Narasinga Rao, 1983). The growing rats adapted to low energy intake by reducing tissue deposition and increasing the efficiency of energy utilization for tissue maintenance. This observation was confirmed in male Fischer 344 rats maintained at 60 percent of *ad libitum* food intake. A comparison of oxygen consumption for fully fed and restricted animals at 6 months of age showed no difference in metabolic rate when expressed per kg lean body mass. If

Table 25–3. METABOLIC RATE OF RATS FED *AD LIBITUM* AND FOOD RESTRICTED

				METABOLIC RATE			
GROUP	*N*	BW,G	LBM,G	KCAL.KG $BW^{-1} \cdot DAY^{-1}$	KCAL.KG $LBM^{-1} \cdot DAY^{-1}$	KCAL.KG $BW^{-0.67} \cdot DAY^{-1}$	KCAL.KG $BW^{-0.75} \cdot DAY^{-1}$
1	6	378 ±19	313 ±16	112.8 ±4.8	136.4 ±6.8	82.1 ±1.9	88.1 ±2.9
2	6	234 ±5	208 ±6	124.3 ±1.8	142.5 ±2.9	77.7 ±1.1	87.4 ±1.1
P		<0.05	<0.05	<0.05	NS	NS	NS

Values are means ± SE. Group 1, rats fed *ad libitum*; group 2, food-restricted rats; BW, body weight; LBM, lean body mass; NS, no significant difference between mean values of groups 1 and 2. $BW^{-0.67}$ and $BW^{-0.75}$ represent body weights to the two-third and three-fourth powers, common modes of expressing metabolic rate.

Reprinted with permission from McCarter, R., *et al.*: Does food restriction retard aging by reducing the metabolic rate? *Am. J. Physiol.*, 248:E488–E490. *Endocrinol. Metab.*, 11.) Copyright (1985) the American Physiological Society.

the data were normalized to kg body weight, then the metabolic rate was higher in restricted animals, but not when normalized to $kg^{0.67}$ body weight (McCarter *et al.*, 1985) (see Table 25–3).

CORE BODY TEMPERATURE

The measurement of metabolic rate and body temperature in female C56BL/6J mice fed *ad libitum* either a 26 percent protein intake or a 4 percent protein intake revealed higher oxygen consumption but significantly lower rectal temperature in animals maintained on the 4 percent protein intake (Leto *et al.*, 1976b). A significantly lower body temperature in mice exposed to early-onset dietary restriction has been confirmed, but late-onset underfeeding (1 year) did not induce a fall in core temperature when compared to age-matched *ad libitum* fed controls (Weindruch *et al.*, 1979).

Conflicting results have, however, been reported for the effect of chronic dietary restriction on core body temperature in rats. It was observed that in Sprague-Dawley rats (Crl:CD[SD]BR strain) the circadian variation of body temperature was similar in restricted and control animals (Volicer *et al.*, 1984). Technical difficulties, particularly relating to the stress of handling, elevated the core temperature, especially in the younger age groups. It was therefore concluded that the effect of chronic underfeeding on body temperature was different in the two species. Reexamination of core body temperature using rectal probes in Sprague-Dawley rats (CFY strain) has revealed a complex response of body temperature to dietary restriction, which may explain in part the conflicting observations previously reported (Holehan and Merry, 1986). Male rats maintained at 50 percent the body weight of age-matched controls showed a fall in core temperature of up to 2°C prior to feeding. Immediately after meal feeding, core temperature rose to control values, but after 9 hours at 70 and 120 days, the temperature was again significantly lower in the restricted group. It was noted that with increasing age a subtle adaptation in the body temperature was observed. At 1 year the rhythm in core temperature was similar to that observed in the young animals, with the exception that core temperature after feeding was now significantly higher than in fully fed animals. This significant elevation in core temperature after feeding was again observed in 525-day-old animals, but at this age no significant depression in core temperature prior to feeding could be observed. It was concluded that the response of core temperature in rodents to chronic postweaning dietary restriction involves two components. The metabolic response to the timing and periodicity of feeding are superimposed on the changes in core temperatures that occur with age in both experimental and control animals (Holehan and Merry, 1986) (see Figure 25–9).

MITOCHONDRIAL RECOVERY

This was assessed in mice dietary restricted from weaning (Weindruch *et al.*, 1980). Increased state 3 rates but not state 4 rates for respiration supported by gluta-

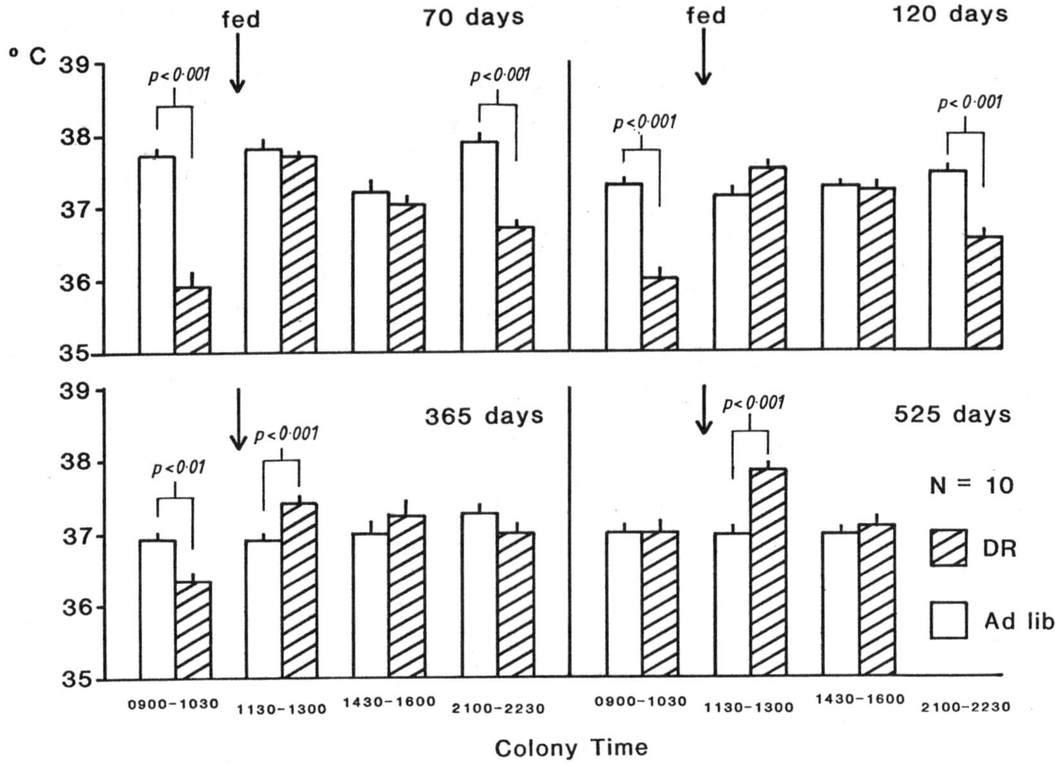

Figure 25–9. *Rectal temperature of* ad libitum *fed and dietary restricted male rats from 70 to 525 days.*

Temperatures were recorded during four time periods each day which span the period of meal feeding for the restricted animals. Dietary restricted (DR) animals were fed the same diet as control rats but in a limited amount so as to restrict their body weight to 50 percent that of *ad libitum* fed age-matched rats. Reprinted with permission from *Biol. Reviews, 61*:329–368, 1986, Holehan, A.M. and Merry, B.J.: The experimental manipulation of ageing by diet). Copyright (1986), Cambridge University Press.

mate or pyruvate plus malate were observed for liver mitochondria. Dinitrophenol-uncoupled rates were also increased by restricted feeding. The interpretation of these data was that the more efficient uncoupling of mitochondria observed in tissue from dietary-restricted mice would result in a reduction of free-radical generation in the intact animal and thus retard age-induced mitochondrial damage.

Enzyme Activities in Response to Dietary Restriction

Studies of the response of specific enzyme activity in tissues from dietary-restricted animals have yielded conflicting results. A delay in the maximum activity of liver ATPase, from 200 to 600 days, was observed in rats (Ross, 1959); however no effect of restricted feeding on kidney catalase activity could be detected (Stoltzner, 1977). Animals maintained on a low-protein diet (4 percent protein) showed a decrease in the activity of kidney and liver cholinesterase, lactic and malic dehydrogenase, and succinoxidase while heart alkaline phosphatase and cathepsin were unaffected (Barrows and Kokkonen, 1982). In a detailed study of the hepatic metabolic response to early- and late-onset dietary restriction five experimental groups were utilized (Yu *et al.*, 1984). Male Fischer 344 rats were divided at 6 weeks of age into:

Group 1. *Ad libitum* fed.
Group 2. Restricted to 60 percent food intake of group 1.
Group 3. Restricted to 60 percent food intake of group 1 until 6 months and then fed *ad libitum*.
Group 4. Fed *ad libitum* until 6 months and then restricted to 60 percent food intake of group 1.
Group 5. Fed the same caloric intake as group 1 but 60 percent of the protein intake.

Hepatic cholesterol concentration increased with age only in group 1 animals fed *ad libitum*. In groups 2 and 4, which had the longest periods of restricted feeding, postabsorptive hepatic glycogen concentrations were significantly higher, and enhanced microsomal activity, as indicated by microsomal 3-hydroxy-3-methyl-glutaryl-coenzyme A reductase, was enhanced.

The response of the activity levels of many enzymes is dependent on the type (protein and/or caloric), degree, and duration of the restricted feeding. As the degree of restriction of a 20 percent protein diet (fed over a period of 6 weeks) increased (75, 50, and 25 percent of *ad libitum* intake), the activity of liver tryptophan oxygenase activity increased, while conversely quinolinate phosphoribosyl-transferase activity decreased (Satyanarayana and Narasinga Rao, 1977). This trend was reversed for quinolinate phosphoribosyl-transferase activity when the degree of restriction exceeded 50 percent of *ad libitum* intake. A similar observation has been recorded for the specific activities of liver lysosomal enzymes: acid phosphatase, β-galactosidase, arylsulfatase B, and cathepsin D in rats fed 90, 70, and 50 percent of *ad libitum* intake from weaning (Solomon *et al.*, 1984). It was noted that in the early phase of restricted feeding (3 weeks) increased activity of acid phosphatase was observed only in the 50 percent restricted group while arylsulfatase B activity increased in all restricted groups, with the greatest effects being recorded in the animals restricted to 50 percent food intake. These biochemical changes were associated with ultrastructural modification of the hepatocytes and with the appearance of increased number of autophagic vacuoles and residual bodies. Both the ultrastructural and biochemical changes were interpreted to be a catabolic adaptation to the nutritional stress, and by 7 weeks of restricted feeding the specific activity of acid phosphatase and hepatocyte ultrastructure were similar to those in fully fed animals. The activity of arylsulfatase B remained significantly higher in the dietary-restricted groups for the duration of the experiment, 24 weeks of restricted feeding. It appears from the available data that there is no consistent age-related pattern of enzyme activity in either control (Finch, 1972) or restricted animals. The lack of consistency in the reports on the effects of chronic dietary restriction on enzyme levels would be expected in view of the differing experimental designs and the complex metabolic adaptations that would be induced.

LIPID PEROXIDATION

The activity of the free radical scavenger superoxide dismutase has been shown to be inversely related to the protein level of the diet, while lipid peroxidation activity in liver homogenates is positively correlated with the dietary intake of protein (De *et al.*, 1983). Thus in both hepatocytes and alveolar macrophages (Watson *et al.*, 1976) enhanced superoxide dismutase activity is associated with a reduced capacity for lipid peroxidation in animals fed a low-protein diet. The classical cellular biomarker of aging, lipofuscin, is a fluorescent pigment thought to be derived from lysosomal enzyme-induced lipid peroxidation, which accumulates with time in neurons, heart, testis, adrenals, and other tissues of many mammalian species. It has been confirmed in the heart and brain of male Swiss albino mice examined during the first 12 months of the lifespan that lower levels of such fluorescence age pigments are present when these animals are maintained on a diet containing 4 percent protein (see Figure 25–10) (Enesco and Kruk, 1981).

PROTEIN SYNTHESIS

The activity levels of individual enzymes represent a balance between the synthesis and degradation rates; therefore, it is pos-

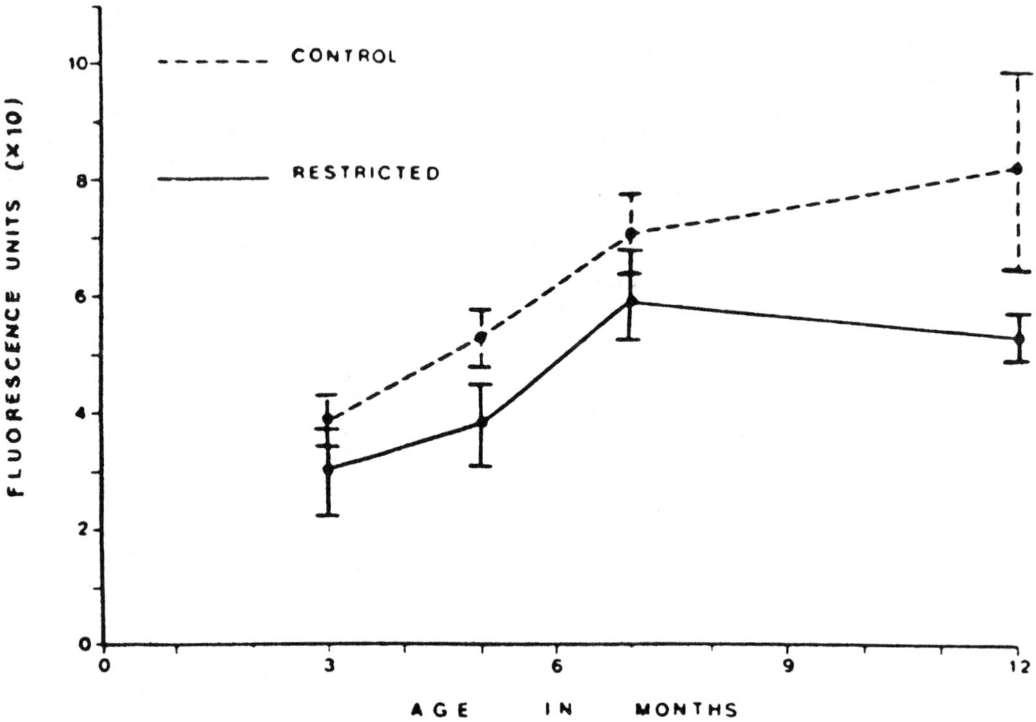

Figure 25–10. *Brain levels of lipid peroxidation fluorescent products expressed as fluorescence units per 0.2 g of tissue with age.*

The level is consistently lower in the brains of mice on the restricted diet of 4 percent protein as compared to the brains of mice on the control, 26 percent protein diet. Reprinted with permission (*Exp. Gerontol.*, 16, Enesco, H.E. and Kruk, P.: Dietary restriction reduces fluorescent age pigment accumulation in mice). Copyright (1981) Pergamon Journals Ltd.

sible that much of the conflicting conclusions derived from studies on specific activity levels may be resolved by observations on protein renewal. *In vitro* protein synthesis and turnover has been studied in a number of tissues from dietary-restricted rats (Richardson and Cheung, 1982; Richardson and Birchenall-Sparks, 1983; Richardson *et al.*, 1984; Richardson, 1985; Birchenall-Sparks *et al.*, 1985). A significantly higher rate of protein synthesis was recorded in suspensions of freshly isolated kidney cells and cell-free homogenates prepared from testis and spleen lymphocytes from dietary-restricted animals (60 percent of *ad libitum* intake) than from fully fed control animals. In the second year of life in Fischer 344 rats a significant decline in testicular protein synthesis can be shown *in vitro*, but when rats have been maintained on a restricted diet, no age-related decrease in protein synthesis is observed over the same period. Similarly protein synthesis in isolated hepatocytes from *ad libitum*-fed rats declined 55 percent between 2.5 and 19 months of age, whereas only a slight decrease with age in protein synthesis was observed in hepatocytes isolated from dietary-restricted rats. This had the consequence that at advanced age hepatocytes from dietary-restricted animals had a significantly higher rate of protein synthesis than hepatocytes from age-matched, fully fed controls. The general effect of restricted feeding, as determined by studies *in vitro*, was to retard the normal age-related decline of protein synthesis and, by implication, protein degradation.

This observation was confirmed *in vivo* for whole-body protein turnover in Sprague

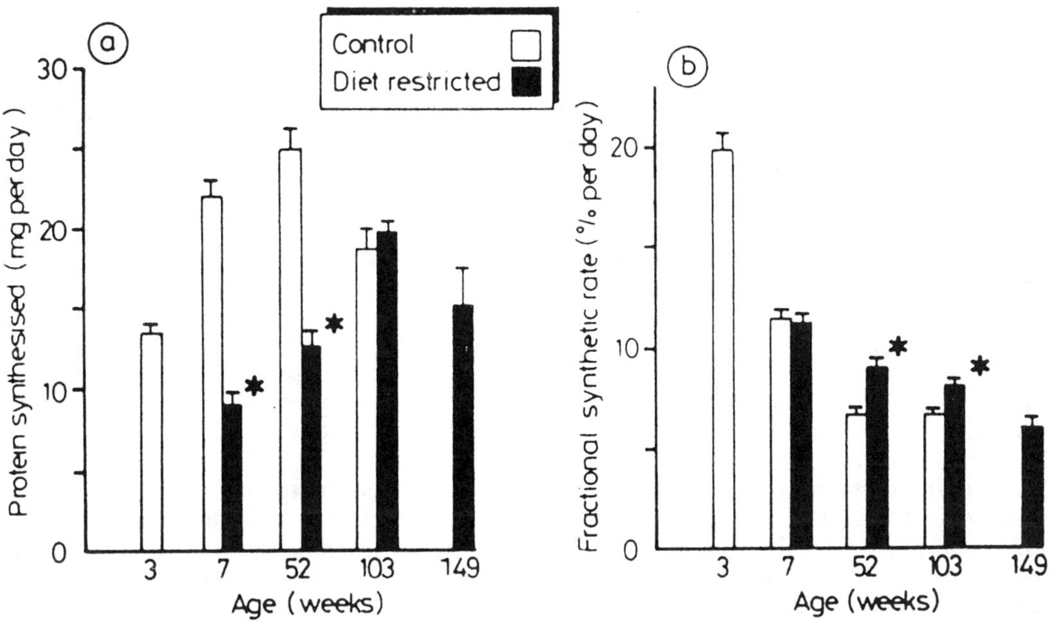

Figure 25–11. *Rates of ventricular protein synthesis during postnatal development and long term dietary restriction.*

Values are mean ± SEM of a minimum of 5 tissues expressed either as the total amount of protein synthesized per day (a) or the fractional rate (k = , the percentage of protein mass synthesized per day) (b), $*p < 0.01$. Dietary restricted male rats were fed limited amounts of the normal diet so as to maintain body weight at 50 percent that of *ad libitum* fed age-matched controls. Reprinted with permission from (*Cardiovascular Research,* 20, Goldspink, D.F., Lewis, S.E.M., and Merry, B.J.: Effects of aging and long term dietary intervention on protein turnover and growth of ventricular muscle in the rat heart). Copyright (1986) Cardiovascular Research, British Medical Association, London.

Dawley rats (Lewis *et al.,* 1985). Dietary restriction (50 percent *ad libitum* intake) retarded the developmental decline in protein turnover, resulting in significantly higher fractional synthetic rates (proportion of total protein renewed every 24 hours) and degradation rates for restricted animals from 1 year of age. While the data from the whole-animal protein turnover studies confirmed the *in vitro* observations, when the same dietary-restricted model was utilized to observe the effect on discrete tissues, the response was found to be more complex. Protein turnover in the ventricular muscle of the heart (see Figure 25–11) and the small intestine closely followed the response observed for the whole animal, but the general effect on skeletal muscle and lung was a lowering of the rate of protein turnover (Goldspink *et al.,* 1986, 1987; El Haj *et al.,* 1986). The general effect on skeletal muscle of chronic dietary restriction was to slow down cellular proliferation and to delay the normal age-related morphologic changes.

Protein synthesis in the liver of dietary-restricted rats was depressed when measured *in vivo* in contrast to the findings of the *in vitro* studies with isolated hepatocytes. It was not possible to calculate breakdown and turnover rates for hepatic proteins in this *in vivo* study because of the unknown proportion of the total protein synthesized that was exported from the liver of rats fed a restricted diet. While *in vitro* studies provide for a greater control of experimental conditions, they do have the disadvantage of removing the tissue from the metabolic and endocrine constraints pertaining in the experimental animal.

That the rate of hepatic protein synthesis is directly dependent on the level of circulating thyroid hormones has been clearly demonstrated in surgically thyroidectomized rats (Mathews *et al.*, 1973). The hormonally sensitive aspect of the translation mechanism is the rate of peptide elongation, and it appears to be independent of any metabolic effect on mitochondrial activity. Surgically thyroidectomized rats that are thyroxine and triiodothyronine deficient have a significantly slower *in vivo* rate of peptide elongation during protein synthesis. Elongation rates can be returned to or above normal by subcutaneous injections of triiodothyronine. It has been established for a number of years that underfeeding in mammals results in a depression of serum levels of thyroxine and triiodothyronine, an observation confirmed in the long-lived dietary-restricted rat (Merry and Holehan, 1985). It was therefore plausible that the depressed rates of hepatic protein synthesis may be explained, at least in part, by changes in the rate of elongation of the nascent polypeptides.

Chronic underfeeding has been found to have two effects on the average transit time for polypeptide synthesis in liver. The initial response observed shortly after the imposition of restricted feeding at weaning was to significantly increase the time required to assemble the average polypeptide from 76.4 to 177.3 seconds. With increasing age the transit time in fully fed male rats increased to 96.9 seconds at 2 years whereas in the underfed animals a decrease in transit time was recorded as the animals recovered from the initial acute response to restricted feeding. By 2 years of age the dietary-restricted animals had an average ribosomal transit time significantly faster than that of age-matched controls. Ribosomal transit times and hepatic protein synthesis in young dietary-restricted rats could be returned almost to normal values after 3 days of subcutaneous injections of the hormone triiodothyronine. Administration of this hormone was more effective in restoring transit time values to control levels than was refeeding although the rate of hepatic protein synthesis rapidly increased on return to refeeding. A period of about 1 month of *ad libitum* feeding was required before ribosome transit times were returned to control values whereas circulating thyroxine levels returned to control values within a few days (Holehan and Merry, 1986). One possible explanation for these observations is a persistent impaired peripheral conversion of thyroxine to triiodothyronine in refed dietary-restricted rats. Most of the hormonal potency of thyroxine is derived from its conversion to triiodothyronine at peripheral conversion sites, a process impaired during caloric deprivation (van Doorn *et al.*, 1984). It is this peripheral conversion of thyroxine to the more active derivative that appears central to the effect on ribosome transit time and, in particular, the delayed recovery observed on return to full feeding.

A decrease in protein synthesis is a characteristic of many organisms with aging, and it has been suggested from observations recorded in brain, kidney, liver, and skeletal muscle of mice that such a decrease results mainly from an increase in ribosome transit time, i.e., decreased rates of peptide elongation (Blazejowski and Webster, 1984). The increase in the ribosomal transit time for protein synthesis appears to result from a lowered activity of elongation factor 1, the translatable mRNA for which disappears with the decline in activity. It has been proposed that the loss of activity of elongation factor 1 with age results from a decline in its synthesis rather than from posttranslational inactivation of normally synthesized molecules (Webster and Webster, 1985). That the decline in protein synthesis with age in cells results primarily from increased ribosomal transit times is still a point of contention, but based on available data the stages of protein synthesis most affected by aging are the ribosomal aggregation to mRNA and the elongation step. Data has been published that suggest that the rate of protein initiation may also be decreased with aging, and further studies are required to resolve this issue.

Response of Collagen to Dietary Restriction

The rate of cross-linkage (the formation of stable covalent bonds) between the fibers of the structural protein collagen has been used for many years as a biomarker for the rate of aging. Dietary restriction has

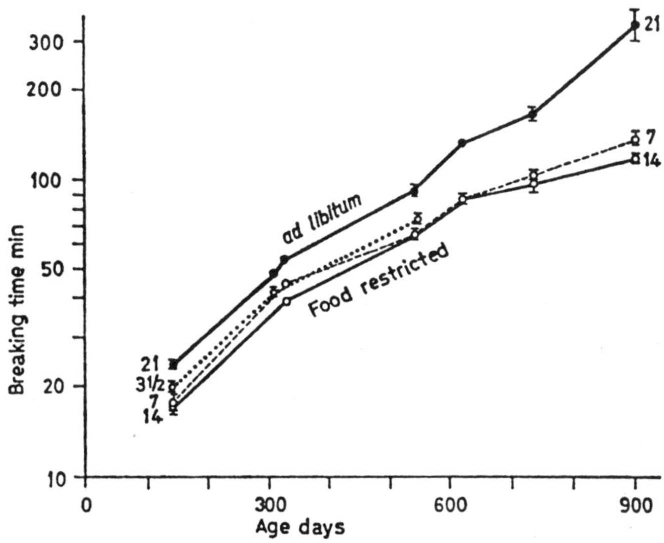

Figure 25–12. *The effect of increasing the food intake from 3.5 to 21 g/day, on the aging of tail tendon collagen fibers in the male rat.*

Collagen age was measured in individual fibers by determining the breaking time in mins in 7M urea at 40°C under a load of 2 g. Reprinted with permission from (*Gerontologia,* 17, Everitt, A.V., Food intake, growth and the ageing of collagen in rat tail tendon). Copyright (1971) S. Karger AG, Basel.

been shown in a number of studies to retard the aging of collagen and the deposition of collagen in the kidneys, lung, and liver (see Figure 25–12) (Chvapil and Hruza, 1959; Giles and Everitt, 1967; Deyl *et al.,* 1971). No effect of diet was found on age-related changes in collagen for the skin (Leto *et al.,* 1976a). Early studies had reported an increase in the level of calcification for the aorta and kidney in the dietary-restricted rat, but this observation may reflect the relatively high mineral content of the early diets rather than a real response to long-term dietary restriction.

The mammalian eye lens has provided over recent years a model system in which to observe age-related posttranslational changes in structural proteins and enzymes (Bloemendal, 1981). A consistent finding with age in both rodents and humans is a significant decrease in the amount of soluble gamma crystallin, an observation often associated with cataract development. In a study of a long-lived mouse strain fed either 85 kcal/week (controls) or 50 kcal/week (dietary restricted), the high-performance liquid chromatography profiles of the soluble lens proteins of restricted and control mice showed no differences at 2 months, but at 11 months of age significantly different profiles were apparent (Leveille *et al.,* 1984). The amounts of gamma crystallin in lenses from middle-aged mice maintained on the restricted diet were significantly greater than in lenses from age-matched control mice. This difference was confirmed by sodium dodecylsulfate polyacrylamide gel electrophoresis and persisted in a comparison of 30-month-old animals (see Figure 25–13).

Physiologic measurements on vascular smooth muscle have shown that restricted feeding prevented the normal age-related loss in tension observed in late life for *ad libitum*-fed rats (Herlihy and Yu, 1980). Individual muscles respond in different ways to chronic underfeeding. In the gastrocnemius muscle a delay in the age-related decline in mass and associated accumulation of collagen was reported (Yu *et al.,* 1982). Examination of the lateral omohyoideus, a fast twitch muscle, at 6 months of age in underfed rats revealed no effect on the mechanical properties, resting metabolism, ul-

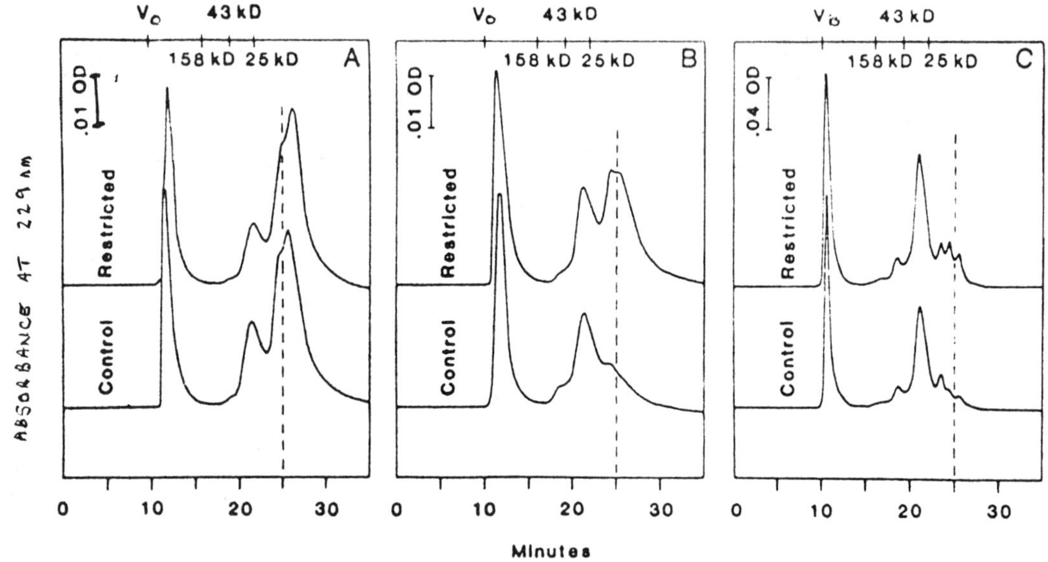

Figure 25–13. *High Performance Liquid Chrometography (HPLC) elution profiles of soluble proteins from lenses of diet-restricted and control mice aged (A) 2 months, (B) 11 months, (C) 30 months.*

The proteins were monitored at 229 nm and each profile is a representative of an individual lens (N = 4, by age and by diet). Within each age and diet group the chromatograms were highly reproducible and superimposable under identical conditions. It was consistently found that the third peak, gamma crystallins (identified by the dotted line), was significantly greater in 11 and 30 month old mice on the restricted diet. Mice were fed a semipurified diet providing either 85kcal per week (controls) or 50kcal per week (restricted). Abbreviations are V_0, void volume and OD, optical density. Reprinted with permission from (*Science*, 224, 1247–1249, Leveille, P.J., *et al.*, Dietary restriction retards age-related loss of gamma crystallins in the mouse lens). Copyright (1984) by the AAAS.

trastructure, or number of muscle fibers although muscle mass and fiber diameter were decreased (McCarter *et al.*, 1978).

THE PHYSIOLOGIC RESPONSE TO CHRONIC UNDERFEEDING

Reproduction

The original work utilized such a severe degree of restricted feeding that rats were maintained for prolonged periods (up to 900 days) in a prepubertal condition (McCay *et al.*, 1939). This gave rise to the idea that arrested development and enhanced survival were inextricably linked. Refeeding such animals resulted in rapid sexual maturation, which was followed by a much foreshortened adult phase of the lifespan although total survival was increased. It has subsequently been shown for the rat that increased longevity can be achieved with less severe dietary restriction, which does not inhibit sexual maturation or result in the loss of fertility (Merry and Holehan, 1979; Holehan, 1984). In male Sprague-Dawley rats maintained at 50 percent the body weight of age-matched *ad libitum*-fed animals, puberty was delayed by approximately 20 days, as shown by breeding trials and the circulating levels of the hormones, luteinizing hormone, follicle-stimulating hormone, testosterone, and its peripheral metabolite 5α-dihydrotestosterone (Merry and Holehan, 1981). The decline with age in fertility for male rats was similar in both fully fed and dietary-restricted animals, decreasing to 30 to 50 percent by 2 years. The most notable endocrine disturbance resulting from underfeeding initiated at weaning was a premature fall in serum follicle-stimulating hormone following the initial prepubertal rise, and this may explain the slight delay in the timing of puberty for these animals.

In contrast puberty in similarly restricted

female Sprague-Dawley rats was delayed until 63 to 189 days (range in fully fed rats 34 to 39 days). The delay in the onset of puberty was again associated with decreased circulating levels of follicle-stimulating hormone. Serum progesterone values were significantly depressed in the prepubertal dietary-restricted rats while estradiol-17β levels were significantly elevated (Holehan and Merry, 1985a). The decrease in serum progesterone appears to result from a failure to release pituitary gonadotropins for there was no significant difference in the elevation of circulating progesterone in response to exogenous gonadotropin stimulation of the ovarian follicles. After sexual maturation more than 70 percent of dietary-restricted female rats demonstrate a normal 5-day cycle characteristic of the CFY strain.

With increasing age the estrous cycle length in fully fed females increases in length and is associated with characteristic irregularities. The most common perturbations of the normal cycle with age are an extension of the period of cornification (persistent estrus) or an increase in the frequency of recurrent pseudopregnancy. Cycle length extension in fully fed female rats is observed as early as 148 to 168 days while persistent estrus or recurrent pseudopregnancy is typical of the second year of life. Chronic underfeeding abolishes the age-related increase in cycle length and results in a much later appearance of the cycle irregularities. The age-related irregularities of the estrous cycle in fully fed rats are dependent on changes in ovarian endocrine secretion and in the threshold sensitivity of the hypothalamic-pituitary system (Lu, 1983). Comparison of the serum profiles for luteinizing hormone, follicle-stimulating hormone, progesterone, and estradiol-17β at 3-hour intervals across the 5-day cycle in fully fed and dietary-restricted rats of 180 to 200 days supports the contention of retarded endocrine aging in underfed animals. At this age fully fed females are beginning to show the first age-dependent changes in the normal estrous cycle and clear differences are evident in the temporal relationships of the individual hormones when a comparison is made with dietary-restricted animals. The preovulatory peak of luteinizing hormone was reduced in height by underfeeding but occurred approximately 6.6 hours earlier in the cycle whereas a delay of 6 hours was observed in the rise of serum estradiol-17β. Significantly greater amounts of follicle-stimulating hormone were released over the cycle of dietary-restricted rats but the total amounts of estradiol-17β and progesterone were reduced (Holehan and Merry, 1985b).

A series of *in vitro* studies have been undertaken to gain greater insight into the effect of age and diet on the steroid pathways within individual follicles. The follicular content and the release over 4 hours of estradiol-17β, progesterone, testosterone, androstenedione, and 20α-dihydroprogesterone were measured during unstimulated steroid synthesis and after luteinizing hormone- or testosterone-stimulated synthesis (Merry and Holehan, 1986). It was observed that with increasing age in control follicles there was increased release of progesterone after luteinizing hormone stimulation and enhanced aromatization of available androgen, resulting in a greater activity of the delta-4 pathway to estradiol-17β and reduced activity of the pathway of progesterone metabolism. These age changes were retarded by chronic underfeeding and correlated with the observations on serum hormone levels. A comparison of follicular steroid synthesis in dietary-restricted animals of 1 year with that from fully fed animals of 3 months showed no differences. When, in contrast, follicular steroid synthesis was compared in 3-month-old and 1-year-old fully fed animals, a significant age effect was seen. Estradiol-17β synthesis in response to luteinizing hormone or testosterone (a precursor of estradiol-17β) in the incubation media was increased over all stages of the cycle while the release from the follicle of testosterone and 20α-dihydroprogesterone was reduced.

Extended fertility has been reported in a number of studies where previously dietary-restricted animals have been returned to full feeding before being allowed to breed. Female rats dietary restricted from 45 days and then returned to *ad libitum* feeding at 6 to 17 months all successfully produced three to six litters when bred at 16 to 23 months, an age when control fe-

Table 25–4. MAXIMUM AGE OF MOTHER AT BIRTH OF LITTER AND BREEDING PERIOD (DAYS)

	GROUP HOUSED[a] CONTINUOUSLY BRED		GROUP HOUSED[b] INTERMITTENTLY BRED		INDIVIDUALLY[c] HOUSED	
AGE AT ONSET OF BREEDING (DAYS)	MAXIMUM AGE (DAYS)	BREEDING PERIOD (DAYS)	MAXIMUM AGE (DAYS)	BREEDING PERIOD (DAYS)	MAXIMUM AGE (DAYS)	BREEDING PERIOD (DAYS)
28	507	479	599	571	—	—
Puberty	532	492	585	545	613	573
100	598	498	552	452	610	510
175	630	455	647	472	677	502
250	565	315	583	333	675	425
325	587	262	537	212	603	278
400	472	72	720	320	537	137

	DIETARY RESTRICTED[d]		DIETARY RESTRICTED–*AD LIBITUM*[e]	
	MAXIMUM AGE (DAYS)	BREEDING PERIOD (DAYS)	MAXIMUM AGE (DAYS)	BREEDING PERIOD (DAYS)
259	737	478	—	—
350	769	419	520	170
530	871	341	724	194
760	937	177	952	192

[a]Females allowed *postpartum* mating and caged in groups of four. *ad libitum* feeding.
[b]Females caged in groups of four and mated 21 days after last litter weaned.
[c]Females caged individually and mated 21 days after last litter weaned. *ad libitum* feeding.
[d]Restricted to 50 percent *ad libitum* food intake, caged individually, and mated 21 days after last litter weaned.
[e]As group 4 but returned to *ad libitum* feeding 75 days prior to first mating.

males were infertile (Osborne and Mendel, 1915). Maintaining A strain mice on a calorie-deficient diet induced a state of near sterility but a return to *ad libitum* feeding at 240 days allowed animals to produce 13 times as many litters after 240 days as their fully fed controls (Ball *et al.,* 1947). This finding was confirmed in a later study using A strain mice but it was observed that although fertility was enhanced on a return to full feeding, the animals were unable to successfully wean their litters (Visscher *et al.,* 1952). Growth in Long-Evans rats can be suspended or retarded by feeding a diet deficient to varying degrees in the amino acid tryptophan. If growth is reinitiated or accelerated at 17 to 33 months by a return to a complete diet, such animals are then able to reproduce at an age when all control animals are infertile (Segall and Timiras, 1975; Segall *et al.,* 1983). Female Sprague-Dawley rats (CFY strain) dietary-restricted from weaning at 21 days are fertile, but overall fertility and litter size are reduced compared to control animals. These females do, however, retain their fertility to an age far exceeding that of the fully fed group (as late as 937 days compared to approximately 550 days) (Merry and Holehan, 1979; Holehan, 1984). In these studies the animals were fertile while retained on the restricted diet and were not returned to full feeding prior to the breeding trial (see Table 25–4).

NONREPRODUCTIVE ENDOCRINOLOGY

In view of the early studies on the dietary-restricted rat in which animals were sexually immature, and the findings that hypophysectomy linked with hormone replacement therapy could mimic many of the aspects of the restricted feeding model (Everitt, 1976, 1982), the endocrine response of the long-lived rat is of importance and has been reviewed in some detail elsewhere (Merry and Holehan, 1985).

The release of growth hormone in rats in which the growth rate is retarded by dietary means is very dependent on the duration and degree of underfeeding. Starvation of adult animals for 2 to 5 days will elevate circulating growth hormone, but chronic, less severe underfeeding results in a depression of both circulating and pituitary growth hormone (Sorrentino *et al.*, 1971). Growth hormone release and plasma values in the rat are characterized by an episodic rhythm of approximately 3.3 hours (Tannenbaum *et al.*, 1978). In 4-month-old male dietary-restricted rats fitted with indwelling cannulae and maintained at 50 percent the normal growth rate, the frequency of release and the plasma concentrations of growth hormone were unaffected although a restriction in peak duration was observed. That such animals are not growth hormone deficient has been confirmed by the administration of exogenous ovine growth hormone injected subcutaneously each day over a 3-week period. In fully fed rats daily injection of ovine growth hormone significantly accelerated the growth rate when compared with saline-injected fully fed controls. No difference in growth rate was evident between growth-hormone- or saline-injected dietary-restricted rats (Merry and Holehan, 1985). The action of growth hormone on growth promotion is postulated to occur through a family of peptides, the somatomedins, which are depressed in undernutrition. It has been suggested that the somatomedins play a role in the maintenance of body weight and nutritional homeostasis at the level of the central nervous system. Whether specific changes in the somatomedins are important in the dietary-restricted long-lived rat has yet to be determined.

It has been shown that maintaining rats on 60 percent of the average food intake of *ad libitum*-fed animals will increase mean lifespan by 50 percent and this is associated with delayed skeletal maturation. In such animals the peak of immunoreactive serum parathyroid hormone observed at advanced age in the fully fed animals is not seen in the dietary-restricted rats (Kalu *et al.*, 1984). This age-related hyperparathyroidism in control rats was linked to enhanced bone resorption and bone loss, a process markedly attenuated in the dietary-restricted animals. The detailed mechanism by which food restriction prevents age-induced hyperparathyroidism is not understood, but a concomitant decrease in the incidence of renal lesions has been reported (Kalu *et al.*, 1984). Utilizing the same degree of restricted feeding, it has been shown that the normal age-associated increase in circulating and thyroidal calcitonin is significantly retarded (Kalu *et al.*, 1983).

A depression in the circulating levels of thyroxine and triiodothyronine is observed within 3 to 7 days of the initiation of restricted feeding, but thyroxine levels could be returned to or above age-matched control values by a return to *ad libitum* feeding for 7 days. The peaks of plasma thyroxine and triiodothyronine associated with the onset of puberty were delayed by approximately 20 days in the timing of their appearance in dietary-restricted rats, which is in agreement with the observations for plasma testosterone (Merry and Holehan, 1981, 1985). The greater effect of underfeeding was recorded for plasma triiodothyronine, the peripheral conversion product of thyroxine. During caloric restriction in the rat, total-body thyroxine-to-triiodothyronine conversion is significantly reduced (van Doorn *et al.*, 1984). Thus moderate restricted feeding sufficient to prolong lifespan has a greater effect on the peripheral conversion of the thyroid hormones than on their central neuroendocrine control through the release of thyroid-stimulating hormone.

In contrast to the thyroid hormones but in agreement with the effect on progesterone synthesis and release, the changes in plasma glucocorticoids in underfed rats originate primarily through changes in hypothalamic-pituitary control. Elevation in the corticotropin-releasing-factor content of the median eminence, plasma adrenocorticotropic hormone, plasma corticosterone levels, and adrenal hypertrophy have been reported as the initial response to dietary restriction in rats (Chowers *et al.*, 1969; Bouille and Assenmacher, 1970; Everitt, 1976). Prolonged underfeeding is associated with depressed adrenocortical function while calorie restriction is acknowledged to desynchronize the circadian corticoid rhythm between individual animals (Bouille and Assenmacher, 1970; Gallo and Weinberg, 1981). It has been shown that 14 days of dietary restriction commenced at weaning (21 days) was sufficient to eliminate the rise in plasma corticosterone normally observed in response to an environmental stress in rats (Merry and Holehan, 1985). The stress response was gradually recovered throughout the first year of life and at 1 year of age had returned to that of fully fed animals. In agreement with the observations on thyroxine, 7 days of full feeding were sufficient to return the stress elevation of plasma corticosterone to normal. This inability to elevate the plasma corticosterone to a perceived stress appears to originate at the hypothalamic-pituitary level, for the adrenal cortex in young dietary-restricted rats will respond with an elevation in plasma corticosterone to exogenous adrenocorticotropic hormone when administered to conscious animals through indwelling cannulae.

It is recognized that there is a synergistic induction of growth hormone messenger ribonucleic acid biosynthesis by glucocorticoid and thyroid hormones. These hormones can modify the rate of transcription of the growth hormone gene in the normal rat (Rosenfeld *et al.,* 1983). Such an interplay of two hormones to influence the synthesis of a third has not been studied in the dietary-restricted animal.

The morphologic appearance of islet cells in the pancreas of underfed rats is characteristic of those of a chronologically younger animal, and in agreement with the observations for calcitonin and parathyroid hormone, the age-related increase observed in fully fed animals for serum insulin is eliminated by restricted feeding. Serum glucose concentration is not generally depressed by restricted feeding, and in an *in vitro* evaluation of the responsiveness of isolated pancreatic cells to glucose stimulation, the decline in insulin secretion with age and the loss of glucose responsiveness were unaffected by dietary restriction (Reaven and Reaven, 1981). It has been suggested that this apparent contradiction with the histologic findings in islet cells from underfed rats reflects a reduced functional demand thereby delaying morphologic deterioration in comparison to *ad libitum*-fed rats. The age-dependent loss in glucagon-promoted lipolysis in adipocytes is prevented by restricted feeding, and a study of fat cell metabolism with age in response to insulin and epinephrine has shown a reduction in basal glyceride synthesis (Bertrand *et al.,* 1980; DiGirolamo *et al.,* 1984). Underfeeding preserved the response to insulin and completely prevented the age-related decline in the lipolytic response; however, in both control and restricted rats the basal conversion of glucose to fatty acids declined rapidly with age. In an *in vitro* culture of vascular smooth muscle cells that retained the age-dependent decrease in β-adrenergic responsiveness characteristic of whole blood vessels, dietary restriction retarded the loss of this response (Volicer *et al.,* 1983).

NEUROLOGY

In a study on the formation of lipid peroxidation fluorescence products (age pigments) in the brain and heart of mice that had been maintained on a low-protein diet, significantly lower fluorescence was recorded in the brain by 3 months and in the heart by 12 months of age. Chronic dietary restriction delayed age-related loss of pineal cells in CD rats and resulted in the retention of a more juvenile type of pineal gland. The loss of striatal dopamine receptors that play an integral role in the altered dopaminergic control of physiologic and behavioral functions in the old fully fed rat was delayed by dietary restriction (by feeding every other day) (Levin *et al.,* 1983) (see Figure 25–14). This type of restricted feeding increased mean survival by 40 percent, and further studies have established that the sparing effect on striatal dopamine receptors is a chronic effect rather than an acute response to restricted food intake (Roth *et al.,* 1984). These biochemical responses to underfeeding are reflected in the retention of behavioral stereotypes more characteristic of younger control animals when 2-year-old dietary-restricted rats are challenged with dopaminergic agonists (Joseph *et al.,* 1982). A selective effect has so far been seen for the effect of chronic underfeeding on brain aging in rodents. Choline acetyl transferase activity was increased in the striatum, hippocampus, and cerebellum of dietary-restricted 2-year-old rats, but little effect was observed in the same brain regions for the activity of glu-

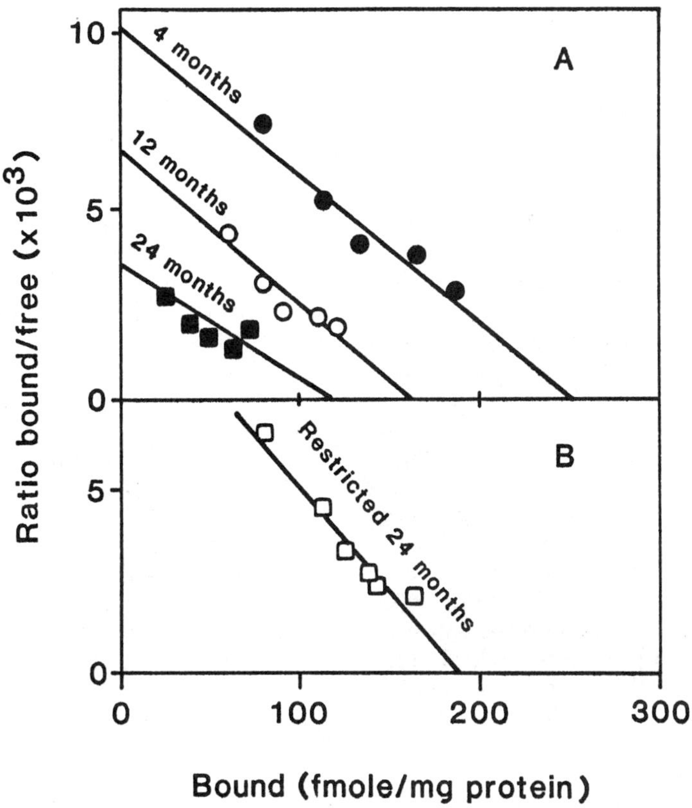

Figure 25–14. *Scatchard analyses of the binding of ³H-labeled amino-6,7-dihydroxy-1,2,3,4-tetrahydronaphthalene (ADTN) to rat striatal membranes.*

Rat striatal dopamine receptors were measured by the specific binding of 3.5nM to 17nM ^{3}H-labeled ADTN with unlabeled 10^{-5} M (+)-butaclamol being used as competitor. Wistar control rats were allowed free access to NIH or Laboratory Chow: the rats on the restricted diet had access to the same food but only on alternate days from weaning. (A) Typical Scatchard analysis of control animals aged 4,12 and 24 months. (B) Typical Scatchard analysis of 24 month old rats maintained on the restricted diet. Loss of striatal dopamine receptors in the brain was substantially reduced by restricted feeding. Striata from three rats were pooled for each individual analysis. Reprinted with permission from (*Science,* 214, 561–562, Levin, P., *et al.,* Dietary restriction retards the age-associated loss of rat striatal dopaminergic receptors). Copyright (1981) by the AAAS.

tamic acid decarboxylase, the synthetic enzyme for the neurotransmitter γ-amino butyric acid (London *et al.,* 1983).

PROPOSED MECHANISMS OF ACTION OF RESTRICTED FEEDING

Although in recent years studies have proliferated detailing the effect of restricted feeding on the physiology and pathology of aging, the molecular mechanism by which these effects can be satisfactorily explained has remained elusive.

METABOLIC

Attempts have been made to explain aging and, more recently, the effects of restricted feeding on the basis of a limited total lifetime energy expenditure. An inverse correlation can be demonstrated within the Mammalia between lifespan and lifetime energy expenditure (approximately

200 kcal/g) in animals ranging in lifespan from 2 years (mouse) to 70 years (elephant). Although most mammalian species have about the same lifespan energy expenditure, in primates it is higher (an average expenditure of 488 kcal/g), and data based on 77 mammalian species indicate that there are three major classes of lifespan energy expenditure (Cutler, 1983). Attempts have been made to calculate the total lifespan energy expenditure for varying degrees of restricted feeding in rats (Sacher, 1977). Two subsequent studies have not substantiated the idea that total energy expenditure per gram of tissue was similar in fully fed and dietary-restricted rats. Direct measurement of the metabolic rate has confirmed that total lifetime energy expenditure per gram of tissue in dietary-restricted rats is significantly greater than for *ad libitum*-fed controls (Masoro *et al.,* 1982; Holehan, 1984; McCarter *et al.,* 1985). Such observations, taken together with protein turnover in underfed rats, suggest that a simple metabolic explanation is extremely unlikely.

PROTEIN TURNOVER

It has been proposed that the rate of aging could be retarded if the rate of synthesis of specific ribonucleic acids and proteins that control the occurrence of programmed events during the lifespan could be decreased and delayed in their synthesis (Barrows and Kokkonen, 1982). Thus, as an organism ages new genetic information is transcribed and translated at different ages, and dietary restriction operates by modifying the rate of occurrence of such programmed events. The delayed appearance of the age-related enzymatic activity profile reported by some groups working with the dietary-restricted rat has been interpreted as support for this hypothesis (Ross, 1959). It is difficult to adapt such an hypothesis to explain the extension of lifespan observed with underfeeding in the adult rat, and no direct experimental data have been presented to support this idea. On the contrary, prolonged dietary protein deficiency has been shown to result in increased transcription and turnover of ribosomal RNA and ribosomes (Kawada *et al.,* 1977; Conde and Franze-Fernandez, 1980). Accelerated degradation rates for RNA are reported in response to restricted dietary protein, which is reversed by amino acid absorption from the gut. Lower RNA:DNA ratios in the liver are seen in dietary-restricted rats (50 percent *ad libitum* intake) because of the rapid degradation of newly synthesized RNA the consequence of which is an increase in the free nucleotide content of the plasma (Srivastava *et al.,* 1978; Merry and Holehan, 1985). It appears from the limited data available relating to RNA metabolism and chronic underfeeding that it is the transfer RNA and the insoluble RNA (with a sedimentation coefficient of 4 to 18 Svedberg units) that are most sensitive to the dietary manipulations (Srivastava *et al.,* 1972).

It is a general observation that the rate of protein synthesis in many organisms and cells declines with age, and this appears to be associated with a similar decrease in the rate of protein degradation (Makrides, 1983; Richardson, 1985). It can therefore be predicted that with age an increase in the half-life of proteins will occur with a decrease in the rate of protein turnover. This can be illustrated by consideration of the two liver enzymes ornithine decarboxylase and aldolase, the turnover for which declines significantly with age in C57BL/6J mice (Jacobus and Gershon, 1980; Reznick *et al.,* 1981). Further support for a decrease in protein turnover with age has been published, and it is suggested that this increase in protein half-life is an important contributory factor in the appearance of altered proteins in the tissues of older organisms (Adelman and Dekker, 1985). While providing for a mechanism for the removal of defective proteins, turnover is an important component in enzyme regulation endowing the cell with the versatility to respond to metabolic change.

As previously stated, in rodents maintained on chronic dietary restriction for all their postweaning life, whole-body protein turnover at advanced chronologic age is enhanced while individual tissue response *in vivo* and *in vitro* is more variable. It has been proposed that the decrease in protein turnover with age is the molecular basis for many of the physiologic changes associated with aging, and a retention of a higher rate of protein turnover into advanced chronologic age in underfed rats would be predicted. Comparison of the labile component of glucose-6-phosphate dehydrogenase in young and old fully fed and dietary-restricted mice revealed a 50 percent decrease in the proportion of labile enzyme in tissue from underfed animals (Wulf and Cutler, 1975). The control of protein degradation rates is little understood and the molecular details whereby diet can modify the rate of protein turnover are still to be elucidated.

NEUROENDOCRINE

Retention of the immature state for prolonged periods of time, the length of which was shown to be directly correlated with the extension in lifespan but inversely correlated with the length of the adult period of life remaining after refeeding, has led to the repeated suggestion that restricted feeding operates through a neuroendocrine mechanism. Early studies had shown, particularly when adult animals were used, that severe prolonged undernutrition can induce a pseudohypophysectomized state (Mulinos and Pomerantz, 1940). Further support for this idea has come from the studies utilizing early hypophysectomy linked to cortisone replacement therapy (Everitt *et al.*, 1980). Such treatment, begun at 70 days, greatly retards growth and aging of tail collagen and prevents the development of proteinuria and subsequent renal disease. Tumor incidence is significantly decreased and survival in dietary restricted and hypophysectomized rats is similarly increased compared to *ad libitum*-fed control animals. Maximum lifespans for *ad libitum*-fed, dietary-restricted, and hypophysectomized (with hormone replacement) rats were 1120, 1282, and 1342 days, respectively. The relationship between the antiaging actions of hypophysectomy and underfeeding still need to be resolved since it is clear from the data cited earlier that the induction of a pseudohypophysectomized state is not obligatory for lifespan extension. Moderate degrees of restricted feeding have produced a far greater effect on survival in terms of maximum lifespan achieved (up to 1800 days) in the rat than have been reported for hypophysectomized animals. It is postulated that growth hormone secretion in the adult phase of the lifespan may have an aging-promotion effect, but although hypophysectomy eliminates this hormone, growth hormone release continues in the dietary-restricted animal.

The suggestion has been made that hypophysectomy linked with appropriate hormonal maintenance will induce a reversal of age-related pathology and a physiologic rejuvenation in rats. This conclusion is based on specific physiologic changes known to occur with age, designated biomarkers of aging, but not on survival data. It is known that under certain experimental conditions changes in such biomarkers may be retarded without a true retardation of aging in the whole animal. Indeed it has been reported that hypophysectomized mice had increased motor activity and presented a more youthful appearance even though they were shorter lived than control animals (Harrison *et al.*, 1982). It is therefore possible that surgical hypophysectomy is an alternative means of inducing chronic underfeeding and that the endocrine changes resulting from such a procedure are secondary to the primary response induced by underfeeding.

Over a number of years a specialized form of restricted feeding has been developed and studied in which rats are maintained on a diet deficient only in one amino acid, tryptophan (Segall and Timiras, 1976; Segall *et al.*, 1983). Such a regime severely retards growth and development and delays the onset of reproductive senescence and tumorigenesis in a manner somewhat similar to severe dietary restriction. The hypothesis has been advanced that this form of restricted feeding may operate through a complex neuroendocrine adjustment involving the neurotransmitter serotonin. It is well established that dietary tryptophan is the sole source of serotonin in the rat and that brain serotonin levels decrease in rats maintained on a diet low in tryptophan (Fernstrom and Wurtman, 1971). Brain serotonin concentrations are subject not only to the plasma levels of unbound tryptophan, but also to the concentration of several other large neutral amino acids that share the same transport system at the blood-brain barrier. Since serotonin stimulates growth hormone release while dopamine exerts an inhibitory effect, the possibility exists that diet can modify the monoaminergic innervation of the hypothalamus directly and so disturb the endocrine status of the animal. The synthesis of the neurotransmitter acetylcholine and the synthesis and release of dopamine and norepinephrine can be similarly manipulated by altering the dietary levels of their precursor molecules, choline and tyrosine. Thus it is plausible that dietary restriction can act through a complex neuroendocrine response, which modifies specific gene expression. Since the neuroendocrine system is central to other ontogenetic processes, such as the timing and onset of puberty, it is feasible that the timing and process of senescence may be under similar controls (Segall, 1979). Thus dietary restriction could be seen to operate through such a pathway to modify the coordination and timing of ontogenesis.

Tryptophan, however, while being an important precursor for neurotransmitter synthesis, is equally important as a key amino acid in the regulation of polysome profile in protein synthesis since it is often the amino acid of lowest concentration in the diet. The interrelationship of endocrine status and protein synthesis and degradation is extremely complex, with at least seven hormones or groups of hormones being known to affect the rate of protein synthesis or protein degradation: insulin, growth hormone, somatomedins, glucagon, thyroid hormones, corticosteroids, and prostaglandins. Modification of the endocrine status of the animal through diet will inevitably have consequences for enzyme induction and protein half-lives, and it is plausible that this effect is the molecular expression of the neuroendocrine response to dietary restriction.

IMMUNOLOGIC

It has been argued that much of observed aging can be explained on the basis of increased autoimmunity and decreased heteroimmunity (Walford, 1972). Data on the immune function in the long-lived dietary-restricted rodent support this general contention for a delay in thymic involution, and enhanced T-cell function compared to aged matched controls has clearly been established. The age-related decline in heteroimmunity is retarded in such animals and autoimmune pathologies are suppressed even in strains of mice genetically predisposed to such pathology. Enhanced survival in underfed rodents results in part from the retention of a competent immune system to a greater age than observed in fully fed animals, but conversely, it is difficult to see how in young dietary-restricted rats the immune system can offer enhanced surveillance against tumor induction by administered carcinogens, particularly when the imposition of restricted feeding is delayed until some weeks after exposure to the carcinogen.

Some data suggest that involution and atrophy of the thymus are important in the control of aging in the immune system, and several mechanisms have been advanced to explain this observation (Pierpaoli and Sorkin, 1967; Everitt, 1976). It has been suggested that thymic involution and atrophy are a result of clonal exhaustion, the possibility existing that a genetically programmed clock mechanism induces cell death after undergoing a fixed number of cell divisions similar to the fixed *in vitro* cell-doubling potential observed for somatic cells in culture (Burnet, 1974). In dietary-restricted rats mitogen-induced lymphocyte proliferation, interlukin-2 induction, and protein synthesis in spleen and lymph node lymphocytes are characteristic of physiologically younger animals, supporting the idea of delayed clonal exhaustion for such animals. The primary control of immune aging may lie within the endocrine system, a decline in trophic factors with age resulting in a decline in T-cell maturation or an increase in suppressor cell activity. The relationship of enhanced immunologic function to altered hormonal control of the immune system in dietary-restricted rats has not been studied in detail. The retention of enhanced immunologic surveillance to a greater age in dietary-restricted animals clearly facilitates survival by delaying the appearance of and reducing the intensity of age-related pathology. It is far from certain, however, whether this is the primary action of underfeeding since it may well represent another aspect of molecular adaptation common to many cells and tissues.

The molecular mechanism whereby diet can so modify age-related pathology, the response to external carcinogens, and the genetic predisposition to hypertension-related disease while retarding physiologic aging is far from understood. Progress in understanding the mechanism of action of diet on the aging process has been disappointingly slow primarily because of the complexity of the homeostatic response of mammals to the dietary stress. We have attempted to bring together some of the disparate ideas that have been proposed to explain the underlying mechanism of action of restricted feeding (see Figure 25–15). Central to this integrated hypothesis is the idea that enhanced protein turnover with age, amplified through homeostatic adjustments in the endocrine system, reduces the cellular load of defective proteins while facilitating metabolic regulation and immunologic surveillance, (Richardson and Cheung, 1982; Rothstein, 1981). Further experimental work is required to determine whether the enhanced rates of protein turnover observed in some tissues from dietary-restricted animals are central to the mechanism of action.

THE EFFECTS OF DIET ON AGING IN THE HUMAN

The use of chronic underfeeding to extend lifespan has so far been restricted to short-lived rodent species. We are unaware of any data relating the effect of chronic underfeeding to survival in longer-lived animals, particularly primate species. This lack of data in nonrodent species is to be expected, for research projects of 10 to 20 years' duration are prohibitive both in financial terms and in the experimental commitment required. Whether it is possible to modify the rate of aging in nonrodent species by dietary means is as yet unresolved, but this fact should not, however, detract from the advantages that the rodent model offers to probe the biochemistry of aging.

With respect to human aging, comparatively little is known of the nutritional requirements of the elderly or the effect of the dietary history on the predisposition to age-related pathology. The data presented earlier demonstrate in rodents a clear effect of diet on both the timing and intensity of cardiovascular disease, cancer, and brain aging. It is acknowledged that such pathologies in the human account for two-thirds of all deaths in the United States. Nutritional requirements are governed by many factors, including body size and composition, rate of growth, physical activity, metabolic rate, and, importantly, age, for the optimum diet in the elderly has been shown to be quite different from that for the young adult (Weg, 1979). In the human many diseases associated with aging are susceptible to dietary intervention, and the proposal has been made that nutrition will become a major strategy in reducing the incidence of the major causes of death (Weg, 1979).

SENILE DEMENTIA OF ALZHEIMER'S TYPE

As the proportion of elderly persons in Western society has risen sharply in the last century, so concomitantly have the number of individuals who will show symptoms of cognitive impairment or senile dementia. Senile dementia of the Alzheimer's type (SDAT) is usually characterized by a progressive loss of mental faculties associated with memory, learning, and concentration. Such a progressive impairment of mental function has been formulated into specific stages and is associated with characteristic histologic changes in the cortex at autopsy (neurofibrillary tangles and neuritic plaques composed of amyloid) (Sinex and Myers, 1982). In SDAT there is a significant and selective loss of cholinergic neurons and the activity of the choline acetyltransferase (CAT) enzyme responsible for the conversion of choline to the neurotransmitter, acetylcholine. This dramatic loss of CAT activity appears specific to SDAT and is not a noticeable feature in patients with multiinfarct dementia (dementia induced by vascular disease) or in normal age-matched controls. A significant correlation has been demonstrated between CAT levels from brain biopsy data and the degree of cognitive impairment (Perry *et al.*, 1978; Spillane *et al.*, 1977). It has been shown in both an-

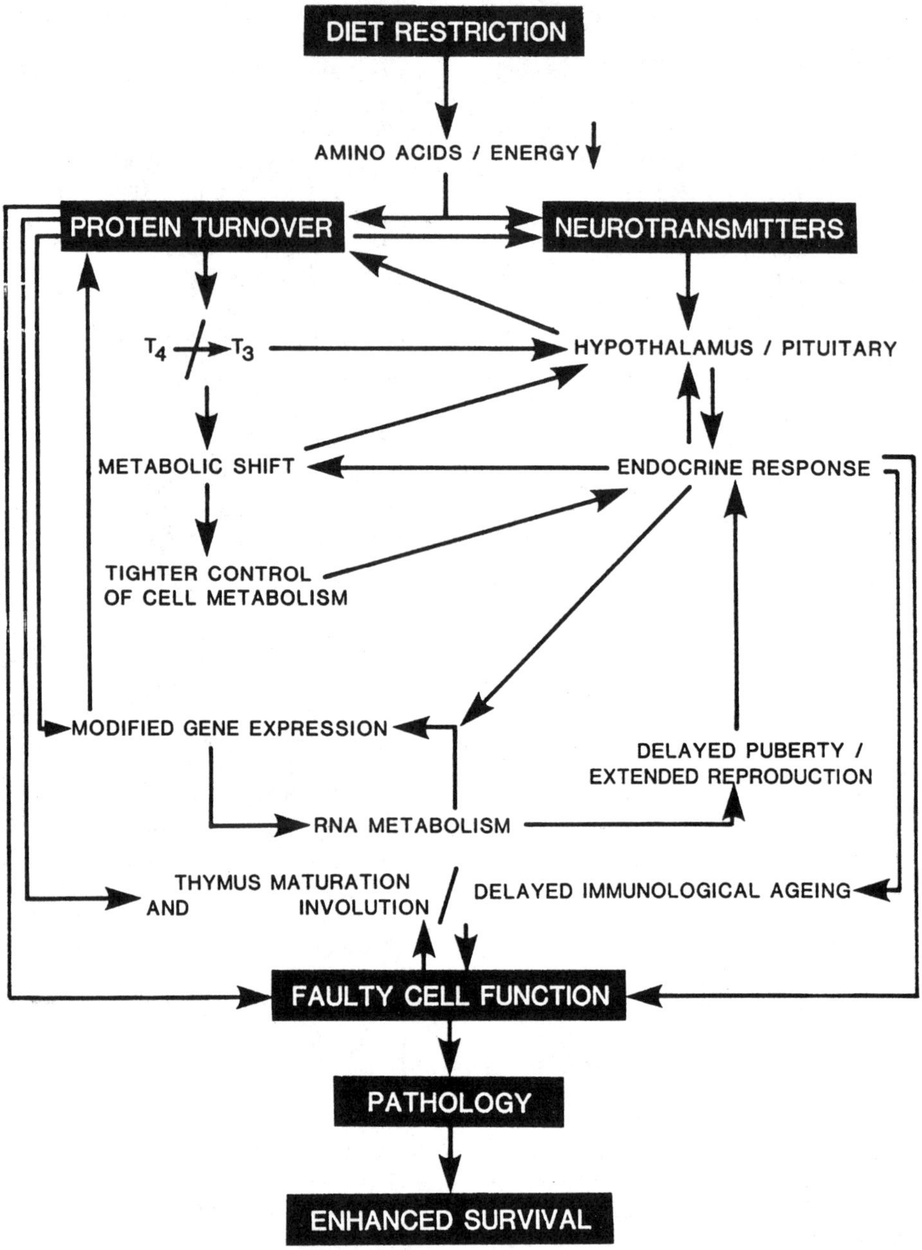

Figure 25–15. *Retarded aging is envisaged to result from two major effects of underfeeding.*

The primary mechanism of action would be an increased rate of turnover for those proteins central to the regulation of cell function. A secondary complex neuroendocrine adjustment to limited neurotransmitter precursor availability, further modified by a reduction in the half life of regualtory enzymes in neural tissue, would amplify the initial effects on cell and tissue homeostasis. Such a dual strategy would decrease with age the cellular load of labile and defective proteins while retaining immunological surveillance. Reprinted with permission from (*Biol. Reviews, 61*:329–368, 1986. Holehan, A.M. and Merry, B.J., The experimental manipulation of ageing by diet). Copyright (1986) Cambridge University Press.

imal and human studies utilizing anticholinergic compounds such as scopolamine that the cholinergic neurotransmitter system is directly involved in memory processes (Dismukes and Rake, 1972; Drachman and Leavitt, 1974; Drachman, 1977). The provision of acetylcholine precursors, choline chloride and lecithin, in the diet of rats elevates brain acetylcholine levels (Cohen and Wurtman, 1975; Hirsch and Wurtman, 1978). When the precursor is dietary choline, then an increase in the activity of tyrosine hydroxylase in the nuclei of dopaminergic neurons of rats is also observed, associated with increased activity of nicotinic acetylcholine receptors. Addition of choline to the diet will also reduce the cholinergic blocking action of atropine. It is suggested that dietary levels of choline have the potential to affect synaptic activity as well as acetylcholine levels. In the human, addition of choline or lecithin to the diet will increase the plasma concentration of these precursors, but a direct effect on brain acetylcholine has not been demonstrated.

Based on this background attempts have been made in a series of studies to improve human memory through dietary manipulation of acetylcholine precursors. The results of such trials are equivocal with respect to the dietary administration of choline salts (Reisberg *et al.,* 1984). This may reflect in part the metabolism of choline salts by intestinal bacteria to di- and trimethylamines. Diets high in lecithin content have been shown to be more effective in elevating serum choline levels. Clinical trials that have studied the effects of enhanced dietary lecithin on cognitive performance in patients with senile dementia have been very limited. Preliminary data suggest that it is possible to elevate plasma choline concentrations by such an approach but that only a proportion of patients at an early stage of Alzheimer's disease showed improved learning ability, which persisted only as long as oral lecithin was administered (Etienne *et al.,* 1978).

CARBOHYDRATE METABOLISM

During aging in humans fasting blood glucose significantly increases, and this is associated with glucose intolerance, an abnormality in carbohydrate metabolism identifiable in a large proportion of the elderly population. Concomitantly after the age of 50 there is an increased incidence of non-insulin-dependent diabetes mellitus, a condition of unknown etiology. Obesity is a very common observation in type II (non-insulin-dependent) diabetes and is associated with tissue insensitivity to insulin, which is reversible with weight loss. Modest loss of weight can result in a marked reduction of plasma glucose, and hypocaloric diets have previously been recommended as part of the therapeutic regimen for diabetics. Unfortunately, diets low in carbohydrates are often high in fats as an alternative source of calories and as such may be atherogenic; accelerated atherosclerosis is the major cause of death in type II diabetes. Reduction of body weight in overweight type II diabetics is still the primary objective not only because of the strong association between adiposity and diabetes, but also because of the benefits of a reduction in hyperlipidemia and hypertension. There is some evidence to indicate that weight loss results in an increase in the number of insulin receptors on the cell membrane. While total caloric restriction is the most effective dietary approach to control type II diabetes in overweight patients, it has been observed that feeding high-carbohydrate diets to such diabetics does not cause a deterioration in the condition. Conversely, increasing the proportion of carbohydrate in the diet enhances the sensitivity of tissues to insulin and results in improved glucose tolerance (Podolsky and El-Beheri, 1984).

Substantial epidemiologic data now exist to suggest that a lack of dietary fiber in the diet may in part be responsible for higher incidences of diverticular disease of the colon and rectum, diabetes mellitus, and ischemic heart disease (Burkitt and Trowell, 1975). Several studies have shown that high-fiber diets have a beneficial effect on the control of hyperglycemia in diabetes mellitus. The most likely mechanism for the attenuation of postprandial hyperglycemia is a delay in the absorption of nutrients from the small intestine. The short-term use of a high-carbohydrate, high-fiber diet has been shown to result in lowering of plasma insulin in nonobese diabetics while still maintaining glucose control. The exact role of dietary fiber in glucose control in diabetes mellitus is still very controversial, and the favorable effects reported for high-fiber diets may reflect simultaneous changes in the proportion of dietary carbohydrate and fat rather than being a direct effect of the plant fiber.

NUTRITION AND CANCER

Nutrition is important in the etiology of human cancers, and certain kinds of nutritional manipulations may be important in the treatment of specific types of cancer. A number of studies have related dietary and nutrient changes to the development of cancers in the esophagus, stomach, colon, pancreas, liver, and breast (Marks, 1977). Indeed it has been suggested that over 50 percent of all female cancer deaths and 30 percent of male cancer deaths may be related to nutritional factors. Epidemiologic studies on the distribution of cancers between racial groups before and after migration to the United States give strong support to a role for nutrition in cancer incidence. Cancer of the stomach is much more common in Japan than in the United States but cancer of the large intestine, breast, and prostate is less so. On migration to the United States a partial reversal of the Japanese incidence pattern to that of the United States is observed, a trend that is continued through the first generation of sons born to Japanese immigrants. Somewhat similar observations have been reported for Jewish populations that have migrated to Israel from Europe or the United States. Initially the immigrant population reflects the cancer incidence of the country of origin but over time, particularly in the first generation who adopt the cultural and dietary habits of the new country, the cancer incidence concomitantly changes.

Studies on rats and mice have indicated that a high-fat diet favors the development of mammary tumors, and epidemiologic data show a significant correlation between dietary saturated animal fat intake and mortality from breast cancer in humans (Carroll, 1975). In animals dietary fat appears to act as a cocarcinogen to promote tumor formation after the preneoplastic stage. In the hormonally dependent mammary tumors of rodents dietary fat promotes tumor growth by increasing the ratio of circulating prolactin to estrogen (Chan and Cohen, 1975). Whether a similar mechanism exists in the human female is as yet uncertain. Alternative mechanisms by which dietary fat can effect mammary tumorigenesis have been postulated, e.g., modification of membrane structure and function, DNA repair, and immunocompetence (Hopkins and West, 1976). Significant correlations have been demonstrated between dietary fat intake and mortality from intestinal cancer, leukemia, and ovarian, skin, and pancreatic cancer.

The role of dietary fiber in protecting against colon cancer is still a matter for debate. It has been postulated that fiber shortens intestinal transit time of food and, hence, shortens the exposure time to potential carcinogens derived from bacterial action. The water retention properties of many fiber types increase fecal mass and aid peristaltic action.

NUTRITION AND CARDIOVASCULAR DISEASE

Coronary heart disease and cerebrovascular disease as a group of pathologies are the major causes of death in Western societies. In the United Kingdom they account for 40 percent of deaths in men and 38 percent of deaths in women. Most deaths from cardiovascular disease occur in old age, the median age of death being 74 years for coronary heart disease and 79 years for stroke in the United Kingdom, although nearly 30,000 deaths occur annually in men under the age of 65. Many countries have recently experienced dramatic declines in mortality from coronary heart disease, with the United Kingdom being a notable exception (Department of Health and Social Security, 1984).

Epidemiologic data show a significant positive correlation between the proportion of dietary energy derived from saturated fatty acids and mortality from coronary heart disease. A negative correlation has been demonstrated between mortality from coronary heart disease and both dietary intake and blood and adipocyte lipid contents of linoleic acid (a polyunsaturated fatty acid). Diets high in saturated fatty acids are associated with increased plasma total cholesterol, which is known to be positively related to the incidence of coronary heart disease, while conversely dietary polyunsaturated fatty acids decrease plasma total cholesterol. A combination of diet or diet and cholesterol-lowering drugs to lower plasma cholesterol in patients with high total plasma cholesterol has been shown to be associated with a reduced incidence of coronary heart disease. Such a lowering of plasma cholesterol may also be reflected in a slower progression of atherosclerotic arterial lesions.

High intake of dietary fiber or complex carbohydrates has been shown to be associated with a reduced incidence of coronary heart disease, and certain types of fiber reduce blood concentrations of cholesterol and glucose. Since complex carbohydrate and dietary fiber are usually present together in high-fiber diets, it is uncertain as to the exact effect of fiber on coronary heart disease.

In the last 40 years for the United Kingdom an increase in weight for height has been observed, leading to an increase in the proportion of men and women who are overweight. Obesity has been defined as weight that is 20 percent above the upper level of the standard for height and build. Overweight is associated not only with an increased risk of coronary heart disease, but also with hypertension, increased plasma cholesterol, and diabetes mellitus (Royal College of Physicians, 1983).

Hypertension and the intake of salt (sodium chloride) in the diet have frequently been linked. Epidemiologic studies have shown statistical associations between the average blood pressure of populations and their dietary salt intake. Reduction of the salt intake of normotensive and hypertensive individuals has resulted in small reductions of blood pressure, with the hypertensive individuals showing the greatest effect. The effect is complicated by the existence of subpopulations of salt-sensitive individuals and the possibility that the chloride component of salt may induce changes in blood pressure through changes in renin and aldosterone secretion (WHO Report, 1983).

References

Adelman, R. C., and Dekker, E. E.: *Modifications of Proteins During Aging*. Modern Aging Research, Vol. 7, Alan R. Liss, New York, **1985.**

Altman, A.; Theofilopoulos, A. N.; Weiner, R.; Katz, D. H.; and Dixon, F. J.: Analysis of T cell function in autoimmune murine strains. *J. Exp. Med.*, **154:**791–808, **1981.**

Ball, Z. B.; Barnes, R. H.; and Visscher, M. B.: The effects of dietary caloric restriction on maturity and senescence with particular reference to fertility and longevity. *Am. J. Physiol.*, **150:**511–519, **1947.**

Barrows, C. H., and Kokkonen, G. C.: Dietary restriction and life extension—Biological mechanisms. In Moment, G. B. (ed.): *Nutritional Approaches to Aging Research*, CRC Press, Boca Raton, FL, **1982.**

Berg, B. N.: Nutrition and longevity in the rat. I. Longevity and onset of disease with different levels of food intake. *J. Nutr.*, **71:**255–263, **1960.**

Bertrand, H. A.; Lynd, F. T.; Masoro, E. J.; and Yu, B. P.: Changes in adipose mass and cellularity through the adult life of rats fed *ad libitum* or a life-prolonging restricted diet. *J. Gerontol.*, **35:**827–835, **1980.**

Birchenall-Sparks, M. C.; Roberts, M. S.; Staecker, J.; Hardwick, J. P.; and Richardson, A.: Effect of dietary restriction on liver protein synthesis. *J. Nutr.*, **115:**110–116, **1985.**

Blazejowski, C. A., and Webster, G. C.: Effect of age on peptide chain initiation and elongation in preparations from brain, liver, kidney and skeletal muscle of the C57BL/6J mouse. *Mech. Ageing Dev.*, **25:**323–333, **1984.**

Bloemendal, H.: *Molecular and Cellular Biology of the Eye Lens*, John Wiley & Sons, New York, **1981.**

Bouille, C., and Assenmacher, I.: Effects of starvation on adrenal cortical function in the rabbit. *Endocrinology*, **87:**1390–1394, **1970.**

Burkitt, D. P., and Trowell, H. C.: *Refined Carbohydrate Foods and Disease*, Academic Press, London, **1975.**

Burnet, F. M.: *Intrinsic Mutagenesis: A Genetic Approach to Aging*, MTP: Medical and Technical Publishing Co., John Wiley & Sons, New York, **1974.**

Carroll, K. K.: *Progress in Biochemical Pharmacology*, Vol. 10, Lipids and Tumors, Karger, Basel, **1975.**

Chan, P. C., and Cohen, L. A.: Dietary fat and growth of rat mammary tumors. *Cancer Res.*, **35:**3384–3386, **1975.**

Chowers, I.; Einat, R.; and Feldman, S.: Effects of starvation on levels of corticotrophin releasing factor, corticotrophin and plasma corticosterone in rats. *Acta Endocrinol. (Copenhagen)*, **61:**687–694, **1969.**

Chvapil, M., and Hruza, Z.: The influence of aging and undernutrition on chemical contractility and relaxation of collagen fibres in rats. *Gerontologia*, **3:**241–252, **1959.**

Cohen, E. L., and Wurtman, R. J.: Brain acetylcholine: Increase after systemic choline administration. *Life Sci.*, **16:**1095–1102, **1975.**

Conde, R. D., and Franze-Fernandez, M. T.: Increased transcription and decreased degradation control the recovery of liver ribosomes after a period of protein starvation. *Biochem. J.*, **192:**935–940, **1980.**

Cutler, R. G.: Superoxide dismutase, longevity and specific metabolic rate. *Gerontology*, **29:**113–120, **1983.**

Davis, T. A.; Bales, C. W.; and Beauchene, R. E.: Differential effects of dietary caloric and protein restriction in the aging rat. *Exp. Gerontol.*, **18:**427–435, **1983.**

De, A. K.; Chipalkatti, S.; and Aiyar, A. S.: Some biochemical parameters of ageing in relation to dietary protein. *Mech. Ageing Dev.*, **21**:37–48, **1983.**

Department of Health and Social Security. *Diet and Cardiovascular Disease,* Report on Health and Social Subjects, number 28, HMSO, London, **1984.**

Deyl, Z.; Juricova, M.; Rosmus, J.; and Adam, M.: The effect of food deprivation of collagen accumulation. *Exp. Gerontol.*, **6**:383–390, **1971.**

DiGirolamo, M.; Crandall, D.; Fried, S. K.; Nickel, M.; and Hill, J. O.: Effects of chronic food restriction (CFR) and aging on rat adipocyte metabolic activities and hormonal responsiveness. *Proceedings of the 7th International Congress of Endocrinology,* Abstract number 573, Excerpta Medica, International Congress Series 652, Elsevier, Amsterdam, **1984.**

Dismukes, R. K., and Rake, A. V.: Involvement of biogenic amines in memory formation. *Psychopharmacologia,* **23**:17–25, **1972.**

Drachman, D. A.: Memory and cognitive functions in man: Does the cholinergic system have a specific role? *Neurology (NY),* **27**:783–790, **1977.**

Drachman, D. A., and Leavitt, J.: Human memory and the cholinergic system. *Arch. Neurol.*, **30**:113–121, **1974.**

El Haj, A. J.; Lewis, S. E. M.; Goldspink, D. F.; Merry, B. J.; and Holehan, A. M.: The effect of chronic and acute dietary restriction on the growth and protein turnover of fast and slow types of rat skeletal muscle. *Comp. Biochem. Physiol.*, **85A**:281–287, **1986.**

Enesco, H. E., and Kruk, P.: Dietary restriction reduces fluorescent age pigment accumulation in mice. *Exp. Gerontol.*, **16**:357–361, **1981.**

Etienne, P.; Gauthier, S.; Johnson, G.; Collier, B.; Mendis, T.; Dastoor, D.; Cole, M.; and Muller, H. F.: Clinical effects of choline in Alzheimer's disease. *Lancet,* **1**:508–509, **1978.**

Everitt, A. V.: The nature and measurement of aging. In Everitt, A. V., and Burgess, J. A. (eds.): *Hypothalamus, Pituitary and Aging,* Charles C Thomas, Springfield, IL, **1976.**

Everitt, A. V.: The genetic clock-hormone theory of aging. In International Union for the Scientific Study of Population: *Biological and Social Aspects of Mortality and the Length of Life,* Ordina Editions, Liege, **1982.**

Everitt, A. V.; Seedsman, N. J.; and Jones, F.: The effects of hypophysectomy and continuous food restriction, begun at ages 70 and 400 days, on collagen aging, proteinuria, incidence of pathology and longevity in the male rat. *Mech. Ageing Dev.*, **12**:161–172, **1980.**

Fernandes, G.; Yunis, E. J.; and Good, R. A.: Influence of diet on the survival of mice. *Proc. Natl. Acad. Sci. USA,* **73**:1279–1283, **1976.**

Fernstrom, J. D., and Wurtman, R. J.: Effect of chronic corn consumption on serotonin content of rat brain. *Nature,* **234**:62–64, **1971.**

Finch, C. E.: Enzyme activities, gene function and ageing in mammals. *Exp. Gerontol.*, **7**:53–67, **1972.**

Gallo, P. V., and Weinberg, J.: Corticosterone rhythmicity in the rat: Interactive effects of dietary restriction and schedule of feeding. *J. Nutr.*, **111**:208–218, **1981.**

Giles, J. S., and Everitt, A. V.: The role of the thyroid and of food intake in the aging of collagen fibres. *Gerontologia,* **13**:65–74, **1967.**

Goldspink, D. F.; Lewis, S. E. M.; and Merry, B. J.: The effects of ageing and chronic dietary intervention on protein turnover and the growth of ventricular muscle in the rat heart. *Cardiovasc. Res.*, **20**:672–678, **1986.**

Goldspink, D. F.; El Haj, A. J.; Lewis, S. E. M.; Merry, B. J.; and Holehan, A. M.: The influence of chronic dietary intervention on protein turnover and growth of the diaphragm and extensor digitarum longus muscles of the rat. *Exp. Gerontol.*, *22*:67–78, **1987.**

Gompertz, B.: On the nature of the function expressive of the law of human mortality and on a new mode of determining life contingencies. *Philos. Trans. R. Soc. Lond. (Biol.),* 513–585, **1825.**

Harrison, D. E.; Archer, J. R.; and Astle, C. M.: The effect of hypophysectomy on thymic aging in mice. *J. Immunol.*, **129**:2673–2677, **1982.**

Herlihy, J., and Yu, B. P.: Dietary manipulation of age-related decline in vascular smooth muscle function. *Am. J. Physiol.*, **238**:H652–H655, **1980.**

Hirsch, M. J., and Wurtmann, R. J.: Lecithin consumption increases acetylcholine concentrations in rat brain and adrenal gland. *Science,* **202**:223–225, **1978.**

Holehan, A. M.: *The effect of ageing and dietary restriction upon reproduction in the female CFY Sprague-Dawley rat,* Ph.D. thesis, University of Hull, England, **1984.**

Holehan, A. M., and Merry, B. J.: The control of puberty in the dietary restricted female rat. *Mech. Ageing Dev.*, **32**:179–191, **1985a.**

Holehan, A. M., and Merry, B. J.: Modification of the oestrous cycle hormonal profile by dietary restriction. *Mech. Ageing Dev.*, **32**:63–76, **1985b.**

Holehan, A. M., and Merry, B. J.: The experimental manipulation of ageing by diet. *Biol. Rev.*, *61*:329–368, **1986.**

Hopkins, G. J., and West, C. E.: Minireview: Possible roles of dietary fats in carcinogenesis. *Life Sci.*, **19**:1103–1116, **1976.**

Horst, K.; Mendel, L. B.; and Benedict, F. G.: The influence of previous diet, growth and age upon the basal metabolism of the rat. *J. Nutr.*, **8**:139–162, **1934.**

Jacobus, S., and Gershon, D.: Age-related changes in inducible mouse liver enzymes: ornithine decarboxylase and tyrosine aminotransferase. *Mech. Ageing Dev.*, **12**:311–322, **1980.**

Joseph, J. A.; Whitaker, J.; Ingram, D. K.; and Roth, G. S.: Dietary restriction retards age-related decrements in stereotypy following intrastriatal injection of DA-active agents. *Soc. Neurosci. Abstr.*, **9**:840, **1982.**

Kalu, D. N.; Cockerham, R.; Yu, B. P.; and Roos, B. A.: Lifelong dietary modulation of calcitonin levels in rats. *Endocrinology,* **113**:2010–2016, **1983.**

Kalu, D. N.; Hardin, R. R.; Cockerham, R.; Yu, B. P.; Norling, B. K.; and Egan, J. W.: Lifelong food restriction prevents senile osteopenia and hyperparathyroidism in F344 rats. *Mech. Ageing Dev.*, **26**:103–112, **1984.**

Kawada, T.; Fujisawa, T.; Imai, K.; and Ogata, K.: Effects of protein deficiency on the biosynthesis and degradation of ribosomal RNA in rat liver. *J. Biochem.*, **81**:143–152, **1977.**

Kubo, C.; Day, N. K.; and Good, R. A.: Influence of early or late dietary restriction on lifespan and immunological parameters in MRL/Mp-Ipr/Ipr mice. *Proc. Natl. Acad. Sci. USA,* **81**:5831–5835, **1984.**

Leto, S.; Kokkonen, G. C.; and Barrows, C. H.: Dietary protein, life-span and biochemical variables in female mice. *J. Gerontol.*, **31**:144–148, **1976a.**

Leto, S.; Kokkonen, G. C.; and Barrows, C. H.: Dietary protein, life-span and physiological variables in female mice. *J. Gerontol.*, **32**:149–154, **1976b.**

Leveille, P. J.; Weindruch, R.; Walford, R. L.; Bok, D.; and Horwitz, J.: Dietary restriction retards age-related loss of gamma crystallins in the mouse lens. *Science,* **224**:1247–1249, **1984.**

Levin, P.; Haji, M.; Joseph, J. A.; and Roth, G. S.: Effect of aging on prolactin regulation of rat striatal dopamine receptor concentrations. *Life Sci.*, **32**:1743–1749, **1983.**

Lewis, S. E. M.; Goldspink, D. F.; Phillips, J. G.; Merry, B. J.; and Holehan, A. M.: The effects of ageing and chronic dietary restriction on whole body growth and protein turnover in the rat. *Exp. Gerontol.*, **20**:253–263, **1985.**

Lloyd, T.: Food restriction increases lifespan of hypertensive animals. *Life Sci.*, **34**:401–407, **1984.**

Lloyd, T., and Boyd, B.: Development and regulation of hypertension in the spontaneously hypertensive rat: enzymatic and nutritional studies. In Usolin, E.; Weiner, N.; and Youdin, M. B. H. (eds.): *Function and Regulation of Monoamine Enzymes: Basic and Clinical Aspects,* Macmillan, London, **1981.**

London, E. D.; Ingram, D. K.; and Waller, S. B.: Effects of dietary restriction on neurotransmitter synthetic enzymes and binding in aging rat brain. *Soc. Neurosci. Abstr.*, **9**:98, **1983.**

Lu, J. K. H.: Changes in ovarian function and gonadotropin and prolactin secretion in aging female rats. In Meites, J. (ed.): *Neuroendocrinology of Aging,* Plenum Press, New York, **1983.**

Makrides, S. C.: Protein synthesis and degradation during aging and senescence. *Biol. Rev.*, **58**:343–422, **1983.**

Marks, P. A.: Nutrition and the cancer problem—An overview. In Winick, M. (ed.): *Nutrition and Cancer,* John Wiley & Sons, New York, **1977.**

Masoro, E. J.; Yu, B. P.; and Bertrand, H. A.: Action of food restriction in delaying the aging process. *Proc. Natl. Acad. Sci. USA*, **79**:4239–4241, **1982.**

Mathews, R. W.; Oronsky, A.; and Haschemeyer A. E. V.: Effect of thyroid hormone on polypeptide chain assembly kinetics in liver protein synthesis *in vivo*. *J. Biol. Chem.*, **248**:1329–1333, **1973.**

McCarter, R.; Masoro, E. J.; and Yu, B. P.: Does food restriction retard aging by reducing the metabolic rate? *Am. J. Physiol.*, **248**:E488–E490, **1985.**

McCarter, R.; Yu, B. P.; and Radicke, D.: Effects of caloric restriction on contraction of skeletal muscle. *Nutr. Rep. Int.*, **17**:339–342, **1978.**

McCay, C. M.; Maynard, L. A.; Sperling, G.; and Barnes, L. L.: Retarded growth, lifespan, ultimate body size and age changes in the albino rat after feeding diets restricted in calories. *J. Nutr.*, **18**:1–13, **1939.**

Merry, B. J., and Holehan, A. M.: Onset of puberty and duration of fertility in rats fed a restricted diet. *J. Reprod. Fertil.*, **57**:253–259, **1979.**

Merry, B. J., and Holehan, A. M.: Serum profiles of LH, FSH, testosterone and 5α-DHT from 21 to 1000 days of age in *ad libitum* fed and dietary restricted rats. *Exp. Gerontol.*, **16**:431–444, **1981.**

Merry, B. J., and Holehan, A. M.: The endocrine response to dietary restriction in the rat. In Woodhead, A. D.; Blackett, A. D.; and Hollaender, A. (eds.): *The Molecular Biology of Aging,* Vol. 35, Basic Life Sciences, Plenum Press, New York, **1985.**

Mohan, P. F., and Narasinga Rao, B. S.: Adaptation to underfeeding in growing rats. Effects of energy restriction at two dietary protein levels on growth, feed efficiency, basal metabolism and body composition. *J. Nutr.*, **113**:79–85, **1983.**

Mulinos, M. G., and Pomerantz, L.: Pseudo-hypophysectomy, a condition resembling hypophysectomy produced by malnutrition. *J. Nutr.*, **19**:493–504, **1940.**

Nolen, G. A.: Effects of various restricted dietary regimes on the growth, health and longevity of albino rats. *J. Nutr.*, **102**:1477–1494, **1972.**

Osborne, T. B., and Mendel, L. B.: The resumption of growth after long continued failure to grow. *J. Biol. Chem.*, **23**:439–454, **1915.**

Pashko, L. L., and Schwartz, A. G.: Effects of food restriction, dehydroepiandrosterone, or obesity on the binding of ^{3}H-7, 12-dimethylbenz(a)anthracene to mouse skin. *J. Gerontol.*, **38**:8–12, **1983.**

Payne, P.: Ageing and nutrition. In Crooks, J., and Stevenson, I. H. (eds.): *Drugs and the Elderly,* Macmillan, London, **1979.**

Perry, E. K.; Tomlinson, B. E.; Blessed, G.; Bergmann, K.; Gibson, P. H.; and Perry, R. H.: Correlation of cholinergic abnormalities with senile plaques and mental test score in senile dementia. *Br. Med. J.*, **2**:1457–1459, **1978.**

Pierpaoli, W., and Sorkin, E.: Relationship between thymus and hypophysis. *Nature,* **215**:834–837, **1967.**

Podolsky, S., and El-Beheri, B.: Nutrition and the elderly diabetic. In Ordy, J. M.; Harman, D.; and Alfin-Slater, R. (eds.): *Nutrition in Gerontology,* Raven Press, New York, **1984.**

Pollard, M.; Luckert, P. H.; and Pan, G-Y.: Inhibition of intestinal tumorigenesis in Methylazoxymethanol-treated rats by dietary restriction. *Cancer Treatment Rep.*, **68**:405–408, **1984.**

Reaven, E., and Reaven, G. M.: Structure and function changes in the endocrine pancreas of aging rats with reference to the modulating effects of exercise and caloric restriction. *J. Clin. Invest.*, **68**:75–84, **1981.**

Reisberg, B.; Ferris, S. H.; and Gershon, S.: Dietary treatment of Alzheimer's type senile dementia. In Ordy, J. M.; Harman, D.; and Alfin-Slater, R. (eds.): *Nutrition in Gerontology,* Raven Press, New York, **1984.**

Reznick, A. Z.; Lavie, L.; Gershon, H. E.; and Gershon, D.: Age-associated accumulation of altered FDP aldolase B in mice. Conditions of detection and determination of aldolase half life in young and old animals. *FEBS Lett.*, **128**:221–224, **1981.**

Richardson, A.: The effect of age and nutrition on protein synthesis by cells and tissues from mammals. In Watson, R. R. (ed.): *Handbook of Nutrition in the Aged,* CRC Press, Boca Raton, FL, **1985.**

Richardson, A., and Birchenall-Sparks, M. C.: Age-related changes in protein synthesis. In Rothstein, M. (ed.): *Review of Biological Research in Aging,* Vol. 1, Alan R. Liss, New York, **1983.**

Richardson, A., and Cheung, H. T.: The relationship between age-related changes in gene expression, protein turnover, and the responsiveness of an organism to stimuli. *Life Sci.*, **31**:605–613, **1982.**

Richardson, A.; Roberts, M. S.; and Birchenall-Sparks, M. C.: *The Possible Role of Protein Synthesis in the Aging Process,* Vol. 4, Modern Aging Research, Alan R. Liss, New York, **1984.**

Rosenfeld, M. G.; Amora, S. G.; Birnberg, N. G.; Mermod, J-J.; Murdoch, G. H.; and Evans, R. M.: Calcitonin, prolactin and growth hormone gene expression as model systems for the characterization of neuroendocrine regulation. *Recent Prog. Horm. Res.*, **39**:305–351, **1983.**

Ross, M. H.: Protein, calories and life expectancy. *Fed. Proc.*, **18**:1190–1207, **1959.**

Ross, M. H.: Nutrition, disease and length of life. In Wolstenholme, G. E. W., and O'Connor, M. (eds.): *Diet and Bodily Constitution,* Ciba Foundation Study Group, number 17, **1964.**

Ross, M. H.: Life expectancy modification by change in dietary regimen of the mature rat. *Proc. 7th Int. Congr. Nutr.*, **5**:35–38, **1966.**

Ross, M. H.: Aging, nutrition and hepatic enzyme activity patterns in the rat. *J. Nutr.* **97** (Suppl. 1):563–602, **1969.**

Ross, M. H.: Length of life and caloric intake. *Am. J. Clin. Nutr.*, **25**:834–838, **1972.**

Ross, M. H., and Bras, G.: Tumor incidence patterns and nutrition in the rat. *J. Nutr.*, **87**:245–260, **1965.**

Ross, M. H., and Bras, G.: Lasting influence of early caloric restriction on prevalence of neoplasms. *J. Natl. Cancer Inst.*, **47**:1095–1113, **1971.**

Ross, M. H., and Bras, G.: Influence of protein under and over nutrition on spontaneous tumor prevalence in the rat. *J. Nutr.*, **103**:944–963, **1973.**

Roth, G. S.; Ingram, D. K.; and Joseph J. A.: Delayed

loss of striatal dopamine receptors during aging of dietarily restricted rats. *Brain Res.*, **300**:27–32, **1984.**

Rothstein, M.: Posttranslational alteration of proteins. In Florini, J. R. (ed.): *CRC Handbook of Biochemistry in Aging*, CRC Press, Boca Raton, FL, **1981.**

Royal College of Physicians of London: Obesity report. *J. R. Coll. Physicians Lond.*, **17**:5–65, **1983.**

Rubner, M.: *Das Problem der Lebensdauer und seine Beziehungen zu Wachstum und Ernahrung*, R. Oldenbourg, Munchen, **1908.**

Sacher, G. A.: Life table modification and life prolongation. In Finch, C. E., and Hayflick, L. (eds.): *Handbook of the Biology of Aging*, Van Nostrand Reinhold, New York, **1977.**

Satyanarayana, U., and Narasinga Rao, B. P.: Effect of diet restriction on some key enzymes of tryptophan-NAD pathway in rats. *J. Nutr.*, **107**:2213–2218, **1977.**

Segall, P. E.: Interrelations of dietary and hormonal effects in aging. *Mech. Ageing Dev.*, **9**:515–525, **1979.**

Segall, P. E., and Timiras, P. S.: Age-related changes in thermoregulatory capacity of tryptophan deficient rats. *Fed. Proc.*, **34**:83–85, **1975.**

Segall, P. E., and Timiras, P. S.: Pathophysiologic findings after chronic tryptophan deficiency in rats: A model for delayed growth and aging. *Mech. Ageing Dev.*, **5**:109–114, **1976.**

Segall, P. E.; Timiras, P. S.; and Walton, J. R.: Low tryptophan diets delay reproductive aging. *Mech. Ageing Dev.*, **23**:245–252, **1983.**

Sinex, F. M., and Myers, R. H.: Alzheimer's disease, Down's syndrome and aging: The genetic approach. *Ann. NY Acad. Sci.*, **396**:3–13, **1982.**

Solomon, C.; Tuchweber, B.; Srivastava, U.; and Nadeau, M.: Liver lysosomal enzymes in rats during long-term dietary restriction. I. Changes during the developmental period of life. *Mech. Ageing Dev.*, **24**:9–27, **1984.**

Sorrentino, S.; Reitner, R. J.; and Schalch, D. S.: Interactions of the pineal gland, blinding and underfeeding on reproductive organ size and radioimmunoassayable growth hormone. *Neuroendocrinology*, **7**:105–115, **1971.**

Spillane, J. A.; White, P.; Goodhardt, M. J.; Flack, R. H. A.; Bowen, D. M.; and Davison, A. N.: Selective vulnerability of neurons in organic dementia. *Nature*, **266**:558–559, **1977.**

Srivastava, U.; Ganguli, P. K.; Brasseur, R.; and Gyenes, L.: The metabolism of liver RNA in adult rats subjected to prolonged dietary restriction during the period of growth and development. *Nutr. Rep. Int.*, **17**:367–375, **1978.**

Srivastava, U.; Vu, M. L.; Bhargava, S.; and Goswani, T.: Metabolism of nucleic acids and protein in the liver, brain and kidney of female rats subjected to dietary restriction during the period of gestation as well as the period of growth, gestation and lactation. *Can. J. Physiol. Pharmacol.*, **50**:832–839, **1972.**

Stoltzner, G.: Effects of life-long dietary protein restriction on mortality, growth, organ weights, blood counts, liver aldolase and kidney catalase in BALB/c mice. *Growth*, **41**:337–348, **1977.**

Stuchlikova, E.; Juricova-Horakova, M.; and Deyl, Z.: New aspects of the dietary effect of life prolongation in rodents. What is the role of obesity in ageing? *Exp. Gerontol.*, **10**:141–144, **1975.**

Tannenbaum, G. S.; Epelbaum, J.; Colle, E.; Brazeau, P.; and Martin, J. B.: Antiserum to somatostatin reverses starvation induced inhibition of growth hormone but not insulin secretion. *Endocrinology*, **102**:1909–1914, **1978.**

Tucker, M. J.: The effect of long-term food restriction on tumours in rodents. *Int. J. Cancer*, **23**:803–807, **1979.**

van Doorn, J.; Van der Heide, D.; and Roelfsema, F.: The influence of partial food deprivation on the quantity and source of triiodothyronine in several tissues of athyreotic thyroxine-maintained rats. *Endocrinology*, **115**:705–711, **1984.**

Visscher, M. B.; King, J. T.; and Lee, Y. C. P.: Further studies on influence of age and diet upon reproductive senescence in strain A female mice. *Am. J. Physiol.*, **170**:72–76, **1952.**

Volicer, L.; West, C. D.; Chase, A. R.; and Greene, L.: Beta-adrenergic receptor sensitivity in cultured vascular smooth muscle cells: Effect of age and of dietary restriction. *Mech. Ageing Dev.*, **21**:283–293, **1983.**

Volicer, L.; West, C.; and Greene, L.: Effect of dietary restriction and stress on body temperature in rats. *J. Gerontol.*, **39**:178–182, **1984.**

Walford, R. L.: Introduction to special issue. Immunology and aging. *Gerontologia*, **18**:243–246, **1972.**

Walford, R. L.; Liu, R. K.; Gerbase-Delima, M.; Mathies, M.; and Smith, G. S.: Long-term dietary restriction and immune function in mice. *Mech. Ageing Dev.*, **2**:447–454, **1974.**

Watson, R. R.; Rister, M.; and Baehner, R. L.: Superoxide dismutase activity in polymorphonuclear leucocytes and alveolar macrophages of protein malnourished rats and guinea pigs. *J. Nutr.*, **106**:1801–1808, **1976.**

Webster, S. L., and Webster, G. C.: Effect of age on the synthesis of individual cellular proteins. *Proc. XIIIth Int. Congr. Gerontol.*, New York, **1985,** pp. 354–346.

Weg, R. B.: *Nutrition and the Later Years*. University of Southern California Press, Los Angeles, **1979.**

Weindruch, R. L.; Cheung, M. K.; Verity, M. A.; and Walford, R. L.: Modification of mitochondrial respiration by aging and dietary restriction. *Mech. Ageing Dev.*, **12**:375–392, **1980.**

Weindruch, R. H.; Kristie, J. A.; Cheney, K. E.; and Walford, R. L.: Influence of controlled dietary restriction on immunologic function and aging. *Fed. Proc.*, **38**:2007–2016, **1979.**

Weindruch, R. H., and Walford, R. L.: Dietary restriction in mice beginning at 1 year of age: Effect on lifespan and spontaneous cancer incidence. *Science*, **215**:1415–1418, **1982.**

World Health Organisation: Primary prevention of essential hypertension. *W.H.O. Technical Report Series No. 686*, WHO, Geneva, **1983.**

Will, L. C., and McCay, C. M.: Ageing, basal metabolism and retarded growth. *Arch. Biochem.*, **2**:481–485, **1943.**

Wulf, J. H., and Cutler, R. G.: Altered protein hypothesis of mammalian aging process. I. Thermal stability of glucose-6-phosphate dehydrogenase in C57BL/6J mouse tissue. *Exp. Gerontol.*, **10**:101–117, **1975.**

Yu, B. P.; Masoro, E. J.; Murata, I.; Bertrand, H. A.; and Lynd, F. T.: Life span study of SPF Fischer 344 male rats fed *ad libitum* or restricted diets: Longevity, growth, lean body mass and disease. *J. Gerontol.*, **37**:130–141, **1982.**

Yu, B. P.; Wong, G.; Lee, H-C.; Bertrand, H. A.; and Masoro, E. J.: Age changes in hepatic metabolic characteristics and their modulation by dietary manipulation. *Mech. Ageing Dev.*, **24**:67–81, **1984.**

CHAPTER

26 PHYSIOLOGIC APPROACH TO REHABILITATION MEDICINE

Chang-Zern Hong
and Jerome S. Tobis

PHILOSOPHY OF REHABILITATION MEDICINE

Rehabilitation medicine for the geriatric patient is usually concerned with the care of the severely disabled and chronically ill who often have multiple-system disease with medical, psychologic, and social problems. The evaluation of such patients often requires a multidisciplinary approach with the participation of several disciplines, when feasible. This group forms a therapeutic team. Insofar as rehabilitation medicine is concerned with the functional status of a patient, it is the clinical application of a physiologic approach to the care of the disabled.

Historical Background: Development in Physical and Rehabilitation Medicine. The application of physical agents in the care of the sick was one of the few effective measures in ancient medicine. Of the many therapeutic agents used, heat and exercise were more extensively employed than others up until the very present. In the nineteenth century, the three main physical agents used were exercise (with massage), water (with heat), and electricity. The three principal divisions of physical therapy were exercise/massage, balneology, and electrotherapy. At the turn of the century, these three groups combined to be called *PHYSIOTHERAPY*, then *PHYSICAL THERAPY* and, in 1931, *PHYSICAL MEDICINE* (in England, but not until 1946 in the United States) (Gullickson and Licht, 1968).

The word "rehabilitation" was probably first mentioned in the mid-nineteenth century (Licht, 1984). The American Medical Association (AMA) endorsed the concept of specialty boards beginning in 1916. Among the 19 authorized boards, only one has in its title the word "rehabilitation." That board is called Physical Medicine and Rehabilitation. In 1947 the word "physiatrist" (physician who specializes in physical medicine and rehabilitation; *physikos* = physical, *iatros* = physician) was adopted by American specialists. The definition of rehabilitation medicine is: The medical management of the disabled, or the treatment and training of the patient to the end that he may attain his maximal potential for normal living physically, psychologically, socially, and vocationally (Gullickson and Licht, 1968).

Team Approach. The traditional REHABILITATION TEAM includes a physiatrist, rehabilitation nurse, physical therapist, occupational therapist, speech pathologist, orthotist/prosthetist, psychologist, social worker, and vocational counselor. Other disciplines may be included, such as the primary-care or family physician. Key participants should include the patient and the patient's family. Obviously not all frail, disabled elderly will require participation of all the above listed disciplines. The role and participation of each team member will change from case to case, and from time to time for the same case. The patient should be the center of the team, and the physiatrist is usually the team coordinator and case manager. Figure 26–1 shows the important concept of the rehabilitation team approach.

FUNCTIONAL ASSESSMENT

The traditional "medical model" is limited to identification of the characteristics of disease: etiology-pathology-manifestations (disease-oriented). Rehabilitation medicine extends its concerns to the person-oriented level (Granger, 1984). Its goal is restoring and/or maintaining independence. Basically rehabilitation medicine deals with disability as a consequence of functional limitations (Figure 26–2). Functional assessment is a method for describing abilities and activities in order to measure an individual's skills in performing the tasks necessary for daily living, vocational pursuits, social interactions, leisure activities, and other required behaviors (Chapter 2). The rehabilitation process can be made more effective through the use of a functional assessment. Table 26–1 shows the functional evaluation done by a physiatrist.

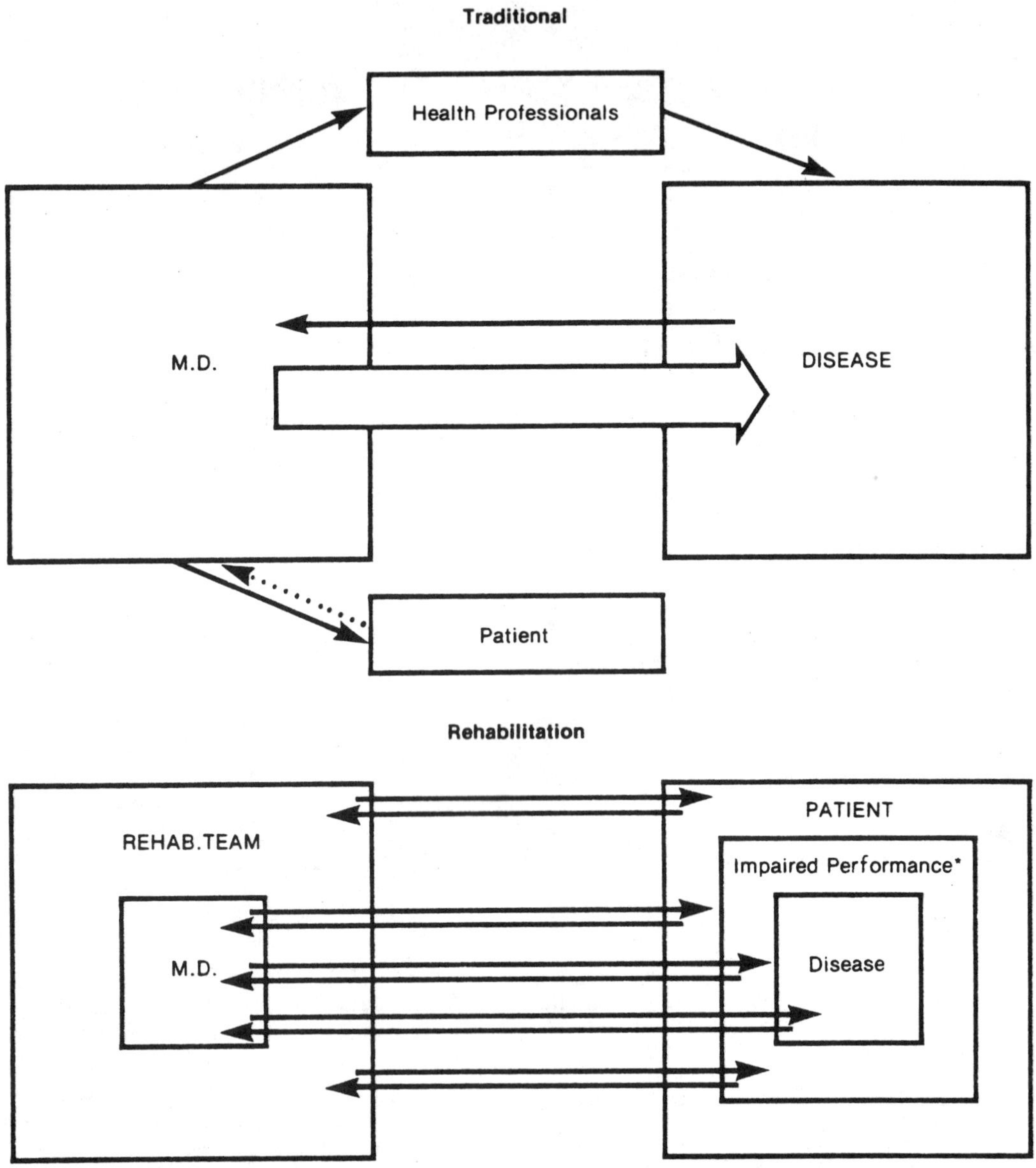

Figure 26–1. *Relationships: Traditional compared to the rehabilitation approach.*

(From Anderson, T.P.: Rehabilitation management and the rehabilitation team. In Basmajian, J. V., and Kirby, R. L. (eds.): *Medical Rehabilitation,* copyright 1984 by Williams and Wilkins. Used with permission.)

GOALS AND MANAGEMENT

Since rehabilitation medicine is problem-(functional limitation) oriented, the *specific goals* are essential guides toward a successful outcome. These goals are usually established by the team with the participation of the patient. The patient's functional level should be assessed periodically to reevaluate the goals and modify the therapeutic program (Figure 26–3). The rehabilitation process is an ongoing *dynamic process* as long as the patient has the potential for further functional improvement, that is, optimal adaptation in all aspects.

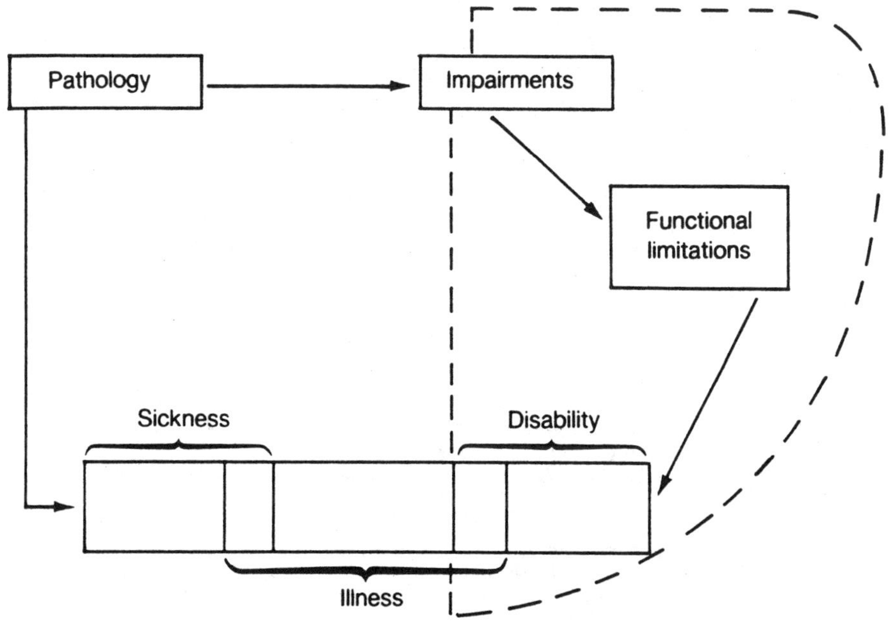

Figure 26–2. *The territory of rehabilitation medicine (area enclosed by the broken line).*

(From Duckworth, D.: Terminology and Classification. In Granger, C. U., and Gresham, G. E. (eds.): *Function Assessment in Rehabilitation Medicine,* copyright 1984 by Williams and Wilkins. Used with permission.)

Table 26–1. PHYSIATRIST EVALUATION

1. History
2. Physical examination
3. Functional assessment
   a. Musculoskeletal function
      • strength
      • endurance
      • coordination
      • balance
      • skills
      • posture
      • gait
   b. Activities of daily living (ADL)
      • self-care activities
      • homemaking activities
   c. Speech and language function
   d. Bladder and bowel function
   e. Cardiopulmonary fitness
4. Electrodiagnosis
5. Evaluation for orthosis and prothesis and other assistive devices/equipment
6. Psychologic assessment and psychosocial diagnosis
7. Vocational or recreational (for elderly) assessment

In the stage of acute illness, the program (early rehabilitative management) may facilitate functional improvement and/or prevent complications. For example, a stroke patient may be able to move his paralytic limbs in a few days through neuromuscular facilitation technique and thus shorten the period of being bedridden.

Elderly patients with multiple medical problems may have a short life expectancy and, ethically, intervention at this time may be questioned. However, through the rehabilitation program they have a better quality of life, although rehabilitation itself may not prolong life.

The expense of health care may be reduced dramatically if an appropriate rehabilitation program is provided. The decreased expense of attendant care, due to reduction of dependency or the reduced incidence of medical complications through rehabilitation, is cost effective.

The elderly active patient is more prone to accident than is his inactive counterpart. Physical activities as part of the rehabilitation programs may subject a geriatric patient to the risk of trauma or significant stress, so the elderly patient must be closely supervised to avoid undue risk (Tobis, 1979).

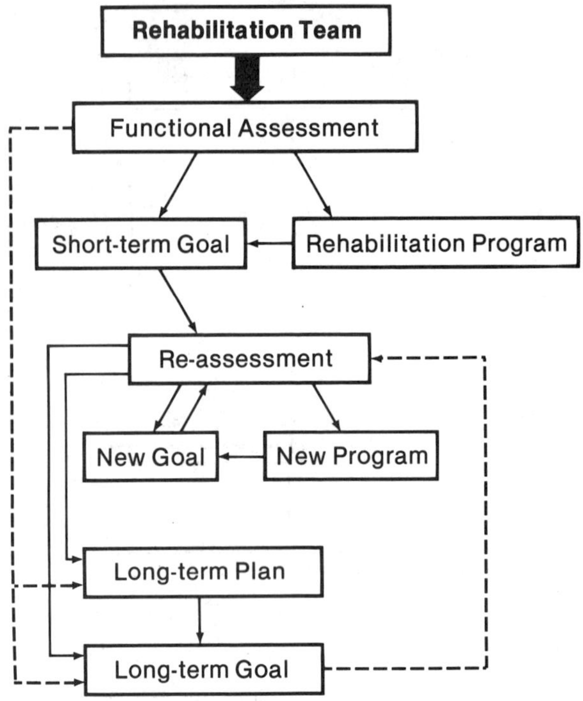

Figure 26–3. *Dynamic rehabilitation program—adjustment of goal as required to reach the new goal.*

CONCEPTS OF GERIATRIC REHABILITATION

As repeatedly emphasized throughout this book, aging is not a disease. New data suggest that the older person need not show decrements of function in many parameters until the "final drop." Much of what has been termed the "changes of aging" may represent unrecognized disease processes that are so often more widespread in the elderly. The physician may tell an older patient that his right knee pain is due to his age. However, this patient may ask the doctor, "What about my left knee? It is just the same age as my right one, but it never bothers me."

The principles of rehabilitation medicine apply to the care of the elderly as for any age group (Figure 26–4). However, because of the limited residual capacities that are often associated with the frail, chronically ill elderly, the goal and therapeutic program must take these limitations into account. Thus, a graduated exercise program to enable an 85-year-old hemiplegic to jog would be foolhardy, if not dangerous, because of cardiopulmonary and neuromuscular limitations.

LEVELS OF REHABILITATION

The different levels of rehabilitation care are summarized in Table 26–2. In the acute stage the patient should receive bedside rehabilitation care to prevent complications and to facilitate functional recovery. A comprehensive rehabilitation program can be carried out during the acute or subacute stage in the acute care hospital immediately after the patient's condition has become stabilized. The team may be involved in enabling the patient to reach his or her highest feasible functional level. The patient may participate in an intensive rehabilitation program, such as after an acute myocardial infarct, provided the acute care services are immediately available.

The care of the patient after the acute stage can be carried out in a rehabilitation

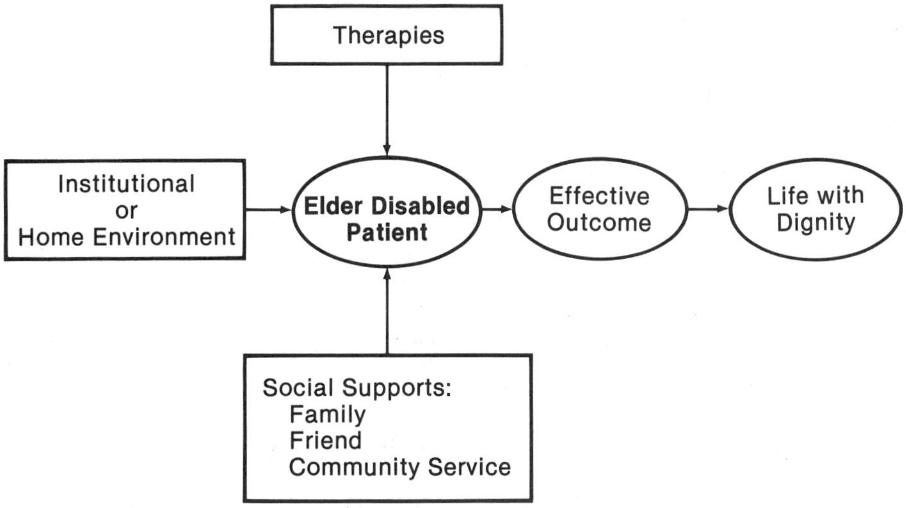

Figure 26–4. *Concept of geriatric rehabilitation—to improve quality of life.*

Table 26–2. LEVELS OF REHABILITATION CARE

		SUBACUTE		CHRONIC	
STAGE	ACUTE I	II	III	IV	V
Programs	Bedside care	Comprehensive rehab.	Comprehensive rehab.	Long-term rehab.	Maintenance rehab.
Site	Acute general hospital—acute ward	Acute general hospital—rehab ward	Acute general hospital—rehab ward or rehab center	Rehab center or ambulatory care or extended-care facilities	Nursing home or ambulatory care
Emergency services	Available	Available	Not immediately available	Not immediately available	Not immediately available
Rehab. staff involved	Limited	All	All	All	Very limited
Therapy time	Limited	As needed	As needed	Limited	Very limited
Criteria					
1. Rehab. potential	Uncertain	Good	Good	Fair	Poor
2. Function improved	Uncertain	Significant	Significant	Some	No
Cost	Moderate	High	High	Moderate	Low
Outcome	Uncertain	Good	Good	Fair	Poor

service of an acute care hospital or a rehabilitation center. More long-term care with rehabilitation services may be provided in a different setting, such as a lower-level-of-care rehabilitation center, a skilled-nursing home, an extended-care facility, home care, or outpatient care. It is important that the patient be placed in the appropriate setting at the right time in his or her progressive recovery from disability.

For patients receiving custodial care, minimum rehabilitation programs (maintenance rehabilitation programs) should be available to prevent medical complications and to reduce dependency. Without this minimum care, patients may deteriorate rapidly. This program can also be done at home if the family is supportive. A list of different places for rehabilitation care is shown in Figure 26–5.

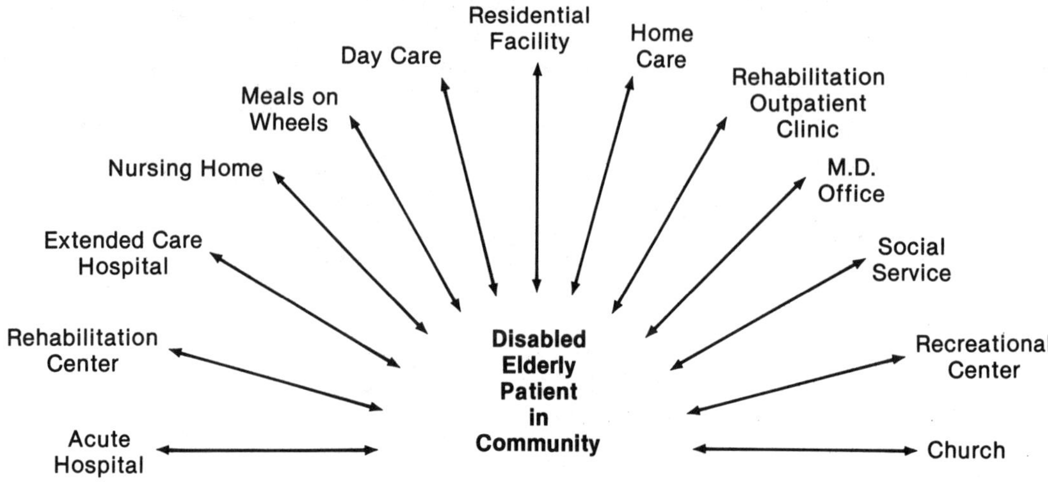

Figure 26–5. *Care for the disabled elderly from various resources.*

THERAPEUTIC REHABILITATION MODALITIES

THERAPEUTIC EXERCISE

Physiological Effects of Exercise Training. Table 26–3 provides an overview of the changes in organ systems that result from exercise training.

Skeletal Muscle. The functional changes of skeletal muscle that result from exercise training include increase of strength, endurance, speed, and flexibility. Exercise with high resistance and high rate is usually required to improve muscle strength and speed. This type of activity may stimulate certain morphologic changes (increase of myofibrils and surrounding connective tissue—hypertrophy) (Astrand and Rodahl, 1977; Taylor and Wilkinson, 1986), biochemical changes (increase of adenosine triphosphate and creatine phosphate, contractile proteins, glycolytic enzymes, phosphorylase, and myosin ATPase) (Astrand and Rodahl, 1977), and possible fiber-type changes (increase of type II fibers) (Herbison and Gordon, 1973; Saltin *et al.,* 1977). On the other hand, low resistance, low rate, and long duration of activities are required for the improvement of muscle endurance, as endurance exercise can cause other patterns of morphologic changes (increase of number of mitochondria), and biochemical changes (increase of oxidative enzymes, myoglobin content, muscle glycogen, sarcoplasmic protein, and intracellular fat) (Holloszy *et al.,* 1977).

In rehabilitation programs, both types of activities should be emphasized to improve muscle function to its optimal state. The maintenance of muscle flexibility is also very important in rehabilitation programs. A contracted muscle cannot work efficiently even with normal strength, speed and endurance.

Nervous System. Motor skill and coordination may be improved by practice, such as repetitive patterns of motor activities. Neuromuscular facilitation techniques have been well developed to facilitate motor recovery in upper-motor-neuron lesions such as cerebral infarction or multiple sclerosis (Harris, 1984). These techniques are based on neurophysiologic knowledge, including spinal reflex patterns, brain stem reflex phenomena, or higher-center reflex circuits, sensory feedback, and cortical integration.

Classical and Modern Training Methods, including Bobath technique (neurodevelopmental approach), Brunnstrom technique (central facilitation with initiating, facilitating, and shaping abnormal synergic pattern), Knott and Voss technique (proprioceptive neuromuscular facilitation, PNF), and Rood's approach (application of cutaneous stimuli), are still valuable if they are combined, coordinated, and modified depending on the individual problem.

The modern biofeedback training technique based on "central EMG (electromyogram)" has

Table 26–3. PHYSIOLOGIC EFFECTS OF EXERCISE TRAINING

ORGAN SYSTEM	STRUCTURAL CHANGES	BIOCHEMICAL CHANGES	FUNCTIONAL CHANGES
Skeletal muscle	Number of myofibrils ↑ Connective tissue thickening Capillarization ↑	Contractile protein ATP and CP ↑ Glycolytic enzyme ↑ Myoglobin ↑ Glycogen store ↑	Strength ↑ Endurance ↑
	Number of mitochondria ↑	Oxidative enzyme ↑ Myosin ATPase ↑	Speed ↑
Central nervous system		Serum endorphins ↑	Coordination ↑ Motor skills ↑ Neurologic recovery ↑ Pain tolerance ↑
Skeletal system	Bone density ↑	Mineral content ↑	Strength to stress ↑
Heart	Hypertrophy (athletic heart) Vascularity ↑ Size of coronary artery ↑	Myocardial enzyme ↑	At rest: Bradycardia stroke volume ↑ During exercise: Less tachycardia Higher stroke volume
Vascular system			At rest: Diastolic BP ↓ During exercise: Less BP ↑ Cardiac output ↑ Peripheral resistance ↓ Coronary blood flow ↑
Pulmonary			Pulmonary ventilation ↑ Diffusion capacity ↑

been proven to be effective (Basmajian, 1984). The plasticity of the central nervous system (CNS) has been well studied, and has clinical implication for recovery after CNS injury (Jen Yu, 1980, 1982a,b). The increase in serum concentrations of endorphins during exercise creates a new field of pain management (Sutton, 1985).

The lower motor neuron and its peripheral nerve may be influenced by exercise. The action potential of the motor neuron is followed by a prolonged after-hyperpolarization (AHP) that is the key factor in the control of maximum cell firing rates. The longer the AHP, the slower motoneurons tend to fire. Immobilizing muscles at shortened lengths may cause a decrease in the duration of AHP. This change can be prevented by muscle contraction from electric stimulation. These observations suggest that metabolic changes in muscle may have a retrograde trophic influence on motor nerve (Booth, 1982).

Skeletal System. Physical activity is an important factor in bone metabolism (Stillman *et al.*, 1986; Aloia, 1981). Immobilization leads to excessive loss of mineral content of the skeleton (Chapters 3 and 22). The density of bone is positively related to physical activity, with significantly higher bone mineral content in women who maintain an active lifestyle, particularly during their premenopausal years (Stillman *et al.*, 1986).

Cardiovascular System. Physiologic effects on cardiovascular function have been well studied and represent one of the most significant aspects of exercise physiology (Astrand and Rodahl, 1977; Clausen, 1977; Hammond and Froelicher, 1985; Leon, 1985; Scheuer and Tipton, 1977).

Structural Changes of Myocardium. Long-term heavy exercise may cause cardiac hypertrophy, and is known as "athletic heart" (Morganroth and Marion, 1977). Athletes participating primarily in isotonic exercise (e.g., walking, swimming, weight training, calisthenics, etc.) have an increase in left ventricular end-diastolic volume with little or no increase in left ventricular wall thickness, whereas athletes participating primarily in isometric exercise (e.g., gripping tennis ball, pressing against wall) have an increase in left ventricular wall thickness associated with normal left ventricular end-diastolic volume.

Therefore, endurance conditioning produces eccentric hypertrophy (increase in ventricular end-diastolic volume) as a result of chronic volume overloading. Strength conditioning produces concentric hypertrophy (increase in ventricular mass) as a result of chronic pressure overloading. Whether this is pathologic or physiologic is still controversial. In the ordinary rehabilitation setting such change usually does not occur. However, a patient with impending heart failure may develop cardiac hypertrophy earlier than might be expected, even though the amount of exercise is lower than that associated with "athletic heart."

In animal studies, some changes of myocardial ultrastructure have been observed. Small shifts in intracellular volume fractions as well as dilatation of transverse tubules and sarcoplasmic reticulum follow an acute bout of exercise to the point of exhaustion (Thomas, 1985). After repeated strenuous dynamic exercise for an extended period of time, the effects seem to be principally on the vasculature of the heart, with no alterations in composition of the myocardial cells. The size of the major coronary arteries increases with a corresponding change in the number of capillaries (Thomas, 1985). Thus, exercise appears to play both a preventive and rehabilitative role with respect to coronary heart disease.

Biochemical Changes of Myocardium. The activities of some myocardial enzymes, including glycogen synthetase, some oxidative and glycolytic enzymes, and myosin ATPase, were increased after exercise in animal studies (Baldwin, 1985; Scheuer and Tipton, 1977). These changes may partly explain the improvement in myocardial function from exercise training.

Hemodynamic Changes. Trained athletes have a lower heart rate and higher stroke volume at rest and during submaximal exercise than normal sedentary people owing to improvement of myocardial contractility (Clausen, 1977; Astrand and Rodahl, 1977; Hammond and Froelicher, 1985). Decrease of total peripheral resistance with increase of muscle blood flow during exercise causes less elevation of blood pressure from exercise. There is evidence that long-term exercise training might reduce blood pressure in hypertensive subjects, but not in normotensive individuals (Tipton, 1984).

Pulmonary Function and Oxygen Transport. Exercise training increases maximal oxygen uptake (aerobic capacity) and oxygen debt (anerobic capacity) (Astrand and Rodahl, 1977; Hammond and Froelicher, 1985). The improvement of aerobic capacity is due to many factors, including pulmonary function, oxygen transport, and tissue oxygen utilization. Changes of pulmonary function due to exercise training are usually not as remarkable as those of cardiovascular function. The maximal pulmonary ventilation and pulmonary diffusion capacity may be increased by training. Biochemical changes in skeletal muscle fibers cause improvement in tissue oxygen utilization. On the other hand, hemoglobin concentration is not significantly altered by exercise training (Martin *et al.*, 1977). Enhanced anaerobic capacity is probably due to an increased physiologic tolerance for lactic acid with its side effects such as tachypnea, tachycardia, etc., or a greater psychic ability to exert oneself (Astrand and Rodahl, 1977).

Metabolic Function. Physical training may increase the ability to utilize fat as an energy source for exercise. Long-term heavy exercise can decrease serum levels of triglyceride low-density lipoprotein and total cholesterol (Astrand and Rodahl, 1977; Hong and Lien, 1984; Haskell, 1984). However, no significant change in serum protein, liver enzymes, serum electrolytes, or serum creatinine have been found.

TYPE OF EXERCISE

Passive exercise is prescribed for maintenance of range of motion or to stretch tight muscles or soft tissue contractures. Active nonresistive exercise is the choice for severely weakened muscles, poor cardiopulmonary fitness, or difficulty in mobility due to pain (such as postoperative). Active resistive exercise can be static (isometric), or dynamic (isotonic or isokinetic). Static exercise is usually not recommended for the hypertensive or cardiac patient because of its high pressure load on the cardiovascular system. Static exercise may cause significant elevation of mean blood

Table 26–4. **PHYSIOLOGIC BASIS OF THERAPEUTIC HEAT**

ORGAN SYSTEM	PHYSIOLOGIC EFFECTS	CLINICAL APPLICATION
Connective tissue	Extensibility of collagen tissue ↑	Relief of joint contracture
	Viscoelastic property ↑	Relief of joint stiffness
Nervous system	Ia afferent discharges ↑	Relief of muscle spasm
	II afferent discharges ↓	
	Ib afferent discharges ↑	
	Analgesic effect ↑	Relief of pain
	Sedative effect ↑	General relaxation
Vascular system	Local blood flow ↑	Relief of active inflammation

pressure (Petrofsky and Phillips, 1986). Dynamic exercise usually causes increase of cardiac output but little change in blood pressure. Isokinetic (constant velocity) exercise is a newly developed technique for muscle training and muscle testing. Some of the postulated advantages of isokinetic exercise include safety, accommodating resistance, and the facility for muscle force analysis (Osternig, 1986).

Exercise Training for the Elderly. Shephard (1986a) has pointed out the advantages of physical fitness in the elderly. These include: (1) prolonged independence in activities of daily living due to increase of muscular and cardiopulmonary fitness; (2) improved general lifestyle; (3) opportunities for social interaction, with an elevation of mood; and, most importantly, (4) a lessened risk of certain medical disorders including obesity (Buskird, 1986; Lampman *et al.*, 1986; Pacy *et al.*, 1986), adult-onset diabetes (Richter and Galbo, 1986), hypertension (Tipton, 1984), bone demineralization (Stillman *et al.*, 1986; Smith, 1981; Aloia, 1981), coronary heart disease (Shephard, 1986b; Sidney, 1981; Long, 1980; Clausen, 1977), and chronic obstructive lung disease (Shayevitz and Shayevitz, 1986).

The absolute training response over the short term is smaller in an older person than in a young one. However, the percentage increment of an index such as oxygen transport, relative to baseline scores, remains at least 10 to 15 percent, which is comparable to that seen in younger subjects (Shephard, 1986a).

Physiologic Basis of Thermal Therapy. (Table 26–4): Lehman and De Lateur (1982) described the physiologic effects of therapeutic heat as follows:

a. increased extensibility of collagen tissues (for treatment of joint contracture);
b. decreased viscoelastic properties of tissues (for treatment of joint stiffness);
c. increased Ia primary afferent discharges but decreased most of II secondary afferent discharges from muscle spindles, and increased Ib afferent discharges from Golgi tendon organs (for treatment of muscle spasms);
d. increased local blood flow probably owing to autonomic nervous system reflex or a local mechanism, such as a direct effect on vascular smooth musculature, stimulation from histamine-like substances and bradykinin, increase of metabolic rate, or axonal reflex;
e. analgesic and sedative effects probably due to local influences on free nerve endings or other indirect effects;
f. facilitated resolution of inflammatory reactions (subacute or chronic);
g. increased enzyme activity and chemical reaction rate.

TYPE OF THERMAL THERAPY

a. Conductive heat transfer devices—Hot packs, electric heating pad, hot-water bottles, Aqua-K pads and hot paraffin wax belong to this category. They are easy to apply, but the effects are limited to superficial or to reflex phenomena.
b. Convective heat—Hot water hydrotherapy with either whirlpool or Hubbard tank is helpful in many musculoskeletal disorders particularly when it is applied in conjunction with therapeutic exercise.
c. Radiation heat modalities—Infrared or

radiant heat provides only superficial heating effects.

Deep Heat. Short wave diathermy and microwave diathermy are the only two modalities of electromagnetic energy used in physical medicine. Ultrasound heat therapy is the application of mechanical energy to generate heating effects to the deep tissue. Both forms of deep heat therapy are used to treat arthritis or soft tissue lesions such as bursitis, capsulitis, tendinitis, sprain, and strain. However, the application of electromagnetic energy on an area with metallic implantation is contraindicated as tissue burns may occur easily.

HEAT THERAPY FOR THE ELDERLY PATIENT

Heat therapy is frequently prescribed for the geriatric individual frequently owing to the increased incidence of degenerative arthritis and soft tissue lesions, but should be applied carefully for the following reasons:

a. some aged subjects may have reduced thermal sensation and may develop burns easily;
b. subjects with heart failure or other cardiac disease may not be able to tolerate increased metabolism from generalized heat therapy such as hot water hydrotherapy;
c. subjects with generalized edema may have an exacerbation from vigorous heat therapy;
d. subjects with a bleeding disorder may have the risk of a massive bleed if the heat therapy is applied over the active hemorrhage site;
e. subjects with malignancy may have the risk of rapid growth or spread of the malignant cells if heat is applied directly over the area with malignant growth;
f. subjects with local infections may risk bacteremia or septicemia if the heat is applied directly over the site of infection;
g. heat applied to an ischemic area such as in peripheral vascular disease may precipitate gangrene due to a rise in local metabolism without concomitant increase in local blood flow and oxygenation of the local tissue.

THERAPEUTIC ELECTROGMAGNETIC ENERGY

Electricity—Electrical Stimulation. The application of electricity in clinical medicine for therapeutic purposes includes muscle, nerve, or bone stimulation. Modern electrical stimulators can generate direct or alternating currents of various intensities, durations, and frequencies. The minimal duration of an effective stimulus for muscle is about 1 msec, and that for nerve is only about 0.03 msec (Jacobs *et al.,* 1983; Liberson, 1984). Therefore, in most cases of electric stimulation, the nerve or the nerve endings are stimulated before the muscle itself is excited if the innervation of the muscle is intact. The duration of the current should be long enough to stimulate the denervated muscles.

Stimulation of the denervated muscle is applied to prepare for reinnervation, to prevent complications such as muscle fibrosis, muscle contracture, or deep vein thrombosis, and for neuromuscular re-education (Jacobs *et al.,* 1983). Stimulation of the sensory nerve is widely used for pain relief, such as transcutaneous electrical nerve stimulation (TENS) or acupuncture (Liberson, 1984; Thorsteinsson, 1983).

Motor nerve stimulation is applied for treatment of spasticity in spinal cord injury by using strong tetanizing current (Mooney *et al.,* 1969), of scoliosis with implanted electrodes in the paraspinal muscles (Bobechko *et al.,* 1979), phrenic nerve stimulation (diaphragm pacing), and functional electrical stimulation (FES). Liberson was the first to apply functional electrical stimulation on the peroneal nerve of the hemiplegic patient to prevent footdrop during ambulation (electrophysiologic orthosis), and later, he and others developed various techniques including an upper-extremity functional splint and multichannel stimulation to produce the desired motor pattern (Gracanin, 1982; Liberson, 1984).

The applications of electrotherapy for the neurogenic bladder include bladder stimulation with an implanted electrode (Merrill, 1979), and intraanal pelvic floor stimulation to treat urinary incontinence (Godec *et al.,* 1976).

Bone may be electrically stimulated to facilitate healing of nonunion fractures

Table 26–5. PHYSIOLOGIC BASIS OF THERAPEUTIC ELECTRICITY

SITE OF STIMULATION	PHYSIOLOGIC EFFECTS	CLINICAL APPLICATION
Skeletal muscle stimulation	Maintain normal function	Retard atrophy in denervated muscles
	Full range of muscle fiber contraction	Prevent muscle contracture in denervated muscle
	Maintain muscle pumping	Prevent deep-vein thrombosis in flaccid paralytic limb
Sensory nerve stimulation	Large fiber impulses ↑ Small fiber impulses ↓ (Gate control)	Relief of pain
Motor nerve stimulation	Contraction of partially paralyzed muscles, or upper-motor-neuron-induced paralyzed muscles	Diaphragm pacing, correction of scoliosis, electrophysiologic splint, treatment of neurogenic bladder

(Brighton *et al.*, 1981; de Haas *et al.*, 1980). Most studies use DC current or a time-varying magnetic field induced current.

The physiologic bases of electrotherapy (see Table 26–5) are:

a. Electrical stimulation of the denervated muscle: Electrical stimulation may retard denervation atrophy, improve local circulation, and offer a full range of muscle fiber contraction.

b. Sensory nerve stimulation: The analgesic effect of the TENS or acupuncture can be explained by the gate-control theory of pain (Melzack and Wall, 1965). The low-frequency TENS (or acupunturelike stimulation) may be modulated by the supraspinal endorphine-dependent mechanism (Thorsteinsson, 1983).

c. Motor nerve stimulation: Computerized electric stimulation allows the performance of more delicate activities, such as enabling the paraplegic to walk or the amputee to use the prosthesis selectively. The intensity, duration, and speed of muscle contraction can be adjusted as desired.

Ultraviolet Therapy. Effects of ultraviolet therapy include erythema, pigmentation, exfoliation, sterilization, antirachitic effect, and counterirritation (Stillwell, 1982; Scott, 1983). Traditionally, ultraviolet therapy was used in a variety of conditions including many dermatological lesions. However, it is now not used as often as it used to be. This is partly because it can be substituted by other more convenient or more effective methods of therapy. It is now still used clinically for treatment of chronic skin ulcer, psoriasis, and sterilization.

Magnetotherapy. In the late 19th and early 20th century, magnetotherapy with static magnetic field was very popular in Europe for the treatment of chronic pain. It is no longer used in this country, as heat therapy is simple and effective in pain management. The mechanism of magnetotherapy is still unknown, although nerve excitability is increased by exposure to high density static magnetic field (Hong *et al.*, 1986).

Diathermy. See Therapeutic Heat.

MASSAGE

The physiologic effects of massage may be classified as reflex and mechanical (Knapp, 1982). The reflex effects are induced by skin stimulation and are transmitted through the spinal cord or higher centers of the central nervous system. The final effects are sedation, relaxation of muscles, and vasomotor changes (either vasoconstriction or vasodilation). The direct mechanical effects consists of: (1) an increase of flow of blood and lymph in the deep tissues; and (2) intramuscular motion to stretch adhesions between muscle fibers and to mobilize accumulations of fluid (Knapp, 1982; Wakim, 1980).

MANIPULATION

Manipulation is the mechanical restoration of the joint or soft tissue by a second party, either gently and slowly (so-called mobilization) or forcefully and quickly with dynamic thrust (Tobis and Hoehler, 1986; Maigne, 1980; Mennel, 1975). The physiologic basis of manipulation is considered to be the stretching of spasmodic muscles (Tobis and Hoehler, 1986; Maigne, 1980). Geriatric patients have a high incidence of degenerative and demineralized changes in the spine. Therefore, spinal manipulation to these subjects should be performed cautiously.

DEVICES, EQUIPMENT, ORTHOSIS AND PROSTHESIS

In order to help the disabled patient become more independent in activities of daily living (ADL), various devices may be prescribed. The following items are those prescribed more frequently in rehabilitation medicine: wheelchair, crutches, cane, walker, ADL equipment (such as reacher, feeding devices, etc.), splints, hemisling, braces, spinal support, shoe arch support, and prosthesis. The purposes of using these devices are either for energy conservation or for substitution of lost function. The energy cost (KCal/min) of ambulation (Fisher and Gullikson, 1978) using various devices or equipment is listed in Table 26–6. One can see how important is the wheelchair to save the energy of transportation for patients with impaired cardiopulmonary function.

PHARMACOLOGICAL TOOLS

Some medications commonly used in rehabilitation medicine to enhance the effectiveness of physical medicine modalities are listed in Table 26–7.

DIAGNOSTIC TOOLS IN PHYSICAL MEDICINE

Evaluation of the physiologic state and correct diagnosis of intercurrent diseases are indispensable tools to formulate effective preventive and/or therapeutic regimens. This is true at all ages, but particularly in the elderly with their considerable variation in function and increased occurrence of pathologies. In physical medicine a number of tools have been especially useful, including electromyography, for the study of muscle and nerve including orthotic and prosthetic devices, and pharmacological agents. While the latter are discussed in Chapter 24, some properties and usefulness of the former tools are summarized in the following paragraphs and in the corresponding tables and figures.

Electromyography. The electromyographic (EMG) technique is used to study the electrical activity of muscle fibers in order to detect the disorder involved at any site of the motor unit (the lower motor neuron, its axon and neuromuscular junction, and its innervated muscle fibers). This is accomplished by inserting a needle electrode into the muscle. The muscle action potential is recorded extracellularly from the needle tip and transmitted through a preamplifier. The recorded electrical signal is magnified by the EMG amplifier and displayed on the oscilloscope. The sound

Table 26–6. ENERGY COST OF AMBULATION

TYPE OF DISABILITY	SPEED (M/MIN)	ENERGY EXPENDITURE PER UNIT TIME (KCAL/MIN/KG B.W.)	ENERGY EXPENDITURE PER UNIT DISTANCE (CAL/M/KG B.W.)
Normal (no disability)	80	0.04–0.06	0.6–0.8
BK* amputee with prosthesis	50–60	0.04–0.07	1.0–1.2
AK* amputee with prosthesis	40–60	0.05–0.08	1.0–1.7
Hemiplegics—no brace	40	0.04–0.06	1.0–1.5
Hemiplegics with brace	50	0.07	1.4
Paraplegics with brace and crutches	20–30	0.05–0.09	2.3–2.4
Wheelchair (disabled)	67	0.04	0.5

*BK, below knee; AK, above knee.

Table 26–7. DRUGS TO ENHANCE THE EFFECTIVENESS OF PHYSICAL MEDICINE

ACTION	DRUG CATEGORIES
I. Drugs to improve physical performance through:	
A. Relief of inflammation	Antiinflammatory—steroid, nonsteroid
B. Relief of pain	Analgesic—nonnarcotic, narcotic
C. Removal of causal factors of 2nd weakness	
1. for infection	Antibiotics
2. for anemia	Iron supplement, vitamin supplement
3. for neuromuscular diseases	Anticholinesterase (for myasthenia)
D. Relief of abnormal muscle tone:	
1. for spasticity	
a. systemic	Diazepam, baclofen, dantrium
b. motor point block or nerve block	Phenol
2. for rigidity	Anticholinergics, L-Dopa
II. Drugs to improve mental performance through:	
A. Relief of depression	Antidepressants
B. Relief of anxiety	Tranquilizers
C. Decrease of agitation	Haloperidol
III. Drugs to improve social performance through:	
A. Improvement of bladder function	
1. for hypotonic bladder	Cholinergics—urecholine
2. for hypertonic bladder	Anticholinergics
3. for tight sphincter	Sympatholytics—alpha blockers
B. Improvement of bowel function	
1. for constipation	Stool softeners
2. for diarrhea	Anticholinergics

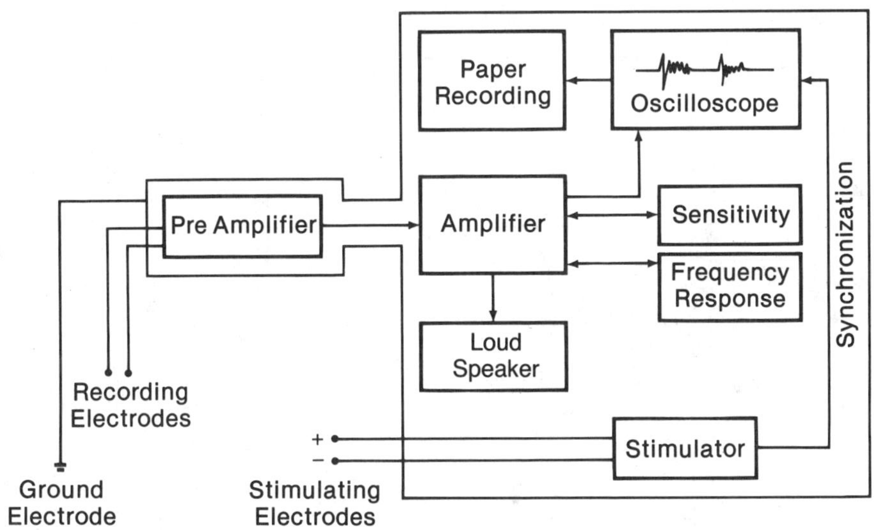

Figure 26–6. *Basic components of an electromyographic machine.*

of the waves of the electrical activity can also be recorded and magnified through the loudspeaker (Figure 26–6). For each sampling, several parameters are observed during an EMG test, as summarized in Table 26–8 (Kimura, 1984).

NERVE CONDUCTION STUDY

To study the motor nerve conduction using an EMG machine, the nerve is stimulated at two or more points along its course and a compound muscle action potential is recorded from the muscles innervated by this nerve (Figure 26–7). The latency from the time of stimulation to the onset of the compound action potential can be measured for each point of stimulation. The nerve conduction velocity (NCV) can be calculated easily by dividing the distance

Table 26–8. ELECTROMYOGRAPHIC (EMG) TEST

			NEUROGENIC LESION		MYOGENIC LESION		
PROCEDURES	ITEMS EXAMINED	NORMAL EMG	ACUTE	CHRONIC	DYSTROPHY	MYOTONIA	POLYMYOSITIS*
Needle insertion	Insertional activity	Few hundred msec	Increased	Decreased	Increased	Increased	Increased
Rest	Resting potential	Silent	Fibrillation, positive sharp waves	Fibrillation, positive sharp waves, (less) fasciculation	Silent	Myotonic discharges	Fibrillation, positive sharp waves
Minimum contraction	Motor unit potentials (MUPs):						
	Size	0.1–3.0 mV	Normal	Large	Small	Small	Small
	Form	2–4 phases	Normal	Polyphasic	Polyphasic or normal	Polyphasic or normal	Polyphasic or normal
	Motor unit recruitment	Early-slow MUPs, later-fast MUPs, gradual increase of number of MUPs	Early-fast MUPs	Early-fast MUPs	Early full	Early full	Early full
			Early decrease of number of MUPs	Early decrease of number of MUPs	Early increase of number of MUPs	Early increase of number of MUPs	Early increase of number of MUPs
Maximum contraction	Interference pattern	100% (full)	Reduced	Reduced	Full	Full	Full

*Inflammation of several muscles.

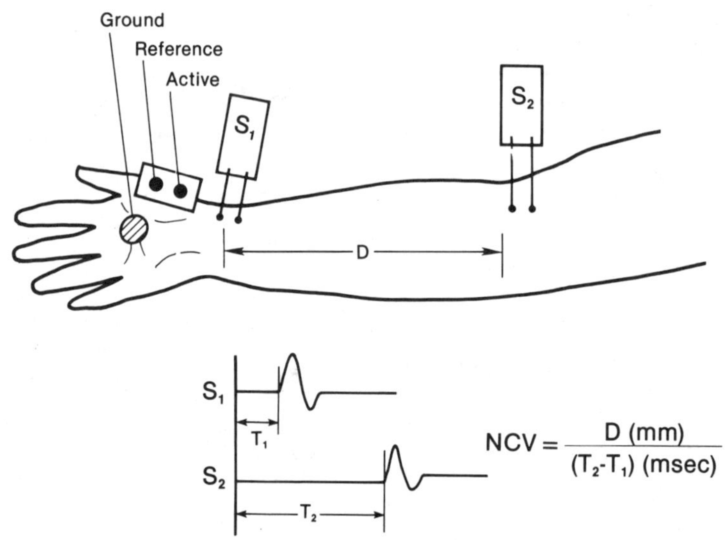

Figure 26–7. *Motor nerve conduction study on the median nerve.*

between any two points of stimulation by the difference in latencies between these two points. The sensory nerve conduction study follows the same principle, but the nerve action potential is recorded rather than the muscle action potential as in the motor nerve conduction study (Figure 26–8).

Many neurological lesions can be identified or confirmed by performing EMG and

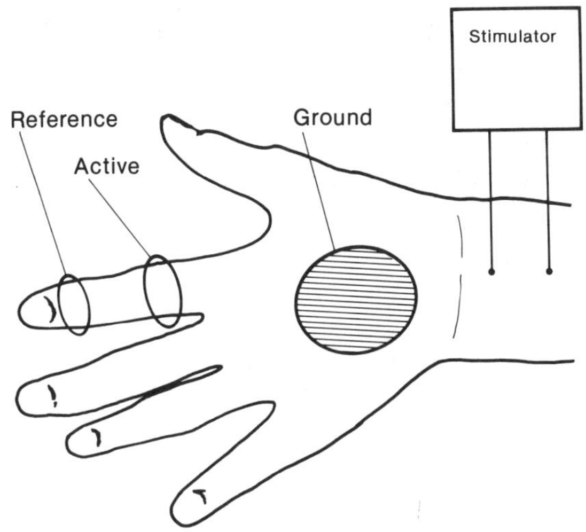

Figure 26–8. *Sensory nerve conduction study on the median nerve.*

nerve conduction studies (Kimura, 1984) (Table 26–9, Figure 26–9).

REHABILITATION IN NEUROLOGICAL DISORDERS

The rehabilitation program for someone with various neurological disorders is summarized in Table 26–10. Although there are some common basic principles applicable in general for each condition, it is very important to assess and treat each person as an individual.

REHABILITATION FOR PATIENT WITH BRAIN LESION

The rehabilitation program for a disabling brain injury or disease varies with the phase of recovery. In the acute stage, the functional disability is either due to extensive inflammatory process, such as brain edema, or due to neuronal and/or axonal damage. The rehabilitation program is directed toward facilitation of functional recovery and prevention of complications of bedrest such as contracture or pressure sores or circulatory complications, due to immobilization (Tobis and Lowenthal, 1960). It is also important to deal with psychosocial distress to the patient and family.

In the later stage, the anatomical lesion causing functional impairment becomes more clear-cut. The regeneration of the dead neurons is very limited, or unlikely. However, correction of reversible damage (such as edema) may result in significant functional recovery. Further neurologic recovery may depend on the unmasking of previously unused pathways (Yu, 1982a,b). But regeneration of axons (axon sprouting) may also occur in the central nervous system (Lynch *et al.*, 1976) although it may be less effective as in the peripheral nervous system, especially in the elderly. The prognosis for axonal lesions is usually better than for neuronal lesions. This is well demonstrated in a hemiplegic patient due to middle cerebral artery infarction. The paralysis of the upper extremity in this lesion is due to pyramidal cell damage in the motor cortex, but the paralysis of the lower extremity is due to a pyramidal tract lesion in the internal capsule. This is alleged to be the explanation why the motor recovery of the lower extremity is usually better and faster than that of the upper extremity, since the fibers are affected in the former and the neurons in the latter. In this stage, both neurologic facilitation and compensatory mechanism are important for the rehabilitation therapies. Finally, some adaptive equipment may be required in order to achieve independent living.

The rehabilitation goal depends on the anatomical lesion (assessed by CT scan or MRI), the residual neurological function, the cognitive deficit, the general medical status and other related factors.

Table 26–9. ELECTROMYOGRAPHIC (EMG) AND NERVE CONDUCTION TESTS FOR DIFFERENTIAL DIAGNOSIS

		NERVE CONDUCTION STUDY			
DIAGNOSIS	EMG FINDINGS: PATTERN AND DISTRIBUTION	NERVE CONDUCTION VELOCITY	AMPLITUDE OF EVOKED POTENTIAL	WAVEFORM OF EVOKED POTENTIAL	DISTRIBUTION OF ABNORMALITY
Upper-motor-neuron lesion	Normal except for reduced recruitment and interference	Normal	Normal	Normal	—
Motor neuron disease	Neurogenic pattern, diffuse	Normal	Reduced	Normal	Diffuse
Radiculopathy	Neurogenic pattern in muscles innervated by specific root	Normal	Reduced	Normal	In nerves derived from involved root
Polyneuropathy—axonopathy	Neurogenic pattern in distal muscles of all limbs	Normal	Reduced	Normal	In distal nerve segment of all limbs
Polyneuropathy—demyelinative	Normal	Slow	Reduced	Temporal dispersion	In all nerves
Polyneuropathy—combined	Neurogenic pattern in distal muscles of all limbs	Slow	Reduced	Temporal dispersion	In all involved nerves
Mononeuropathy—entrapment	Neurogenic pattern in muscles innervated by certain nerve	Slow	Reduced	Temporal dispersion	In the nerve segment with lesion
Myopathy	Myopathic pattern	Normal	Normal or reduced	Normal	—

Rehabilitation for Patient with Spinal Cord Lesion

It is unlikely for a patient with an established complete spinal cord lesion to have significant neurologic recovery. Therefore, the rehabilitation program emphasizes training for compensatory mechanisms rather than neurologic facilitation. A complete paraplegic patient can be trained to become totally independent in daily living at the wheelchair level. Ambulation with crutches is not a priority in terms of mechanical efficiency and cost effectiveness. Some complications from neurologic deprivation, such as pressure sores, problems from neurogenic bowel and bladder, orthostatic hypotension, autonomic hyperreflexia, heterotropic ossification, spasticity, and loss of normal thermoregulatory mechanism, should be prevented carefully.

Rehabilitation for Patient with Peripheral Nerve Lesion

Peripheral nerve has a higher potential regeneration than does the axon of the central nervous system. In a recent animal study, the recovery of conduction of injured nerve could be facilitated by ultrasound deep heat therapy. However, its application on human nerve lesion is still unclear (Hong *et al.*, 1986). The rehabilitation program for peripheral nerve lesion focuses on prevention of complications such as muscle contracture.

Rehabilitation for Patient with Degenerative Neurologic Disorders

Since the neurologic lesion progressively deteriorates, rehabilitation programs are not expected to provide neurologic recovery. Rehabilitation is undertaken to prevent rapid functional loss in order to improve the quality of life.

REHABILITATION IN MUSCULOSKELETAL DISORDERS

Rehabilitation in Arthritis and Allied Conditions

The majority of geriatric patients experience episodic arthralgia (i.e., joint pain) in

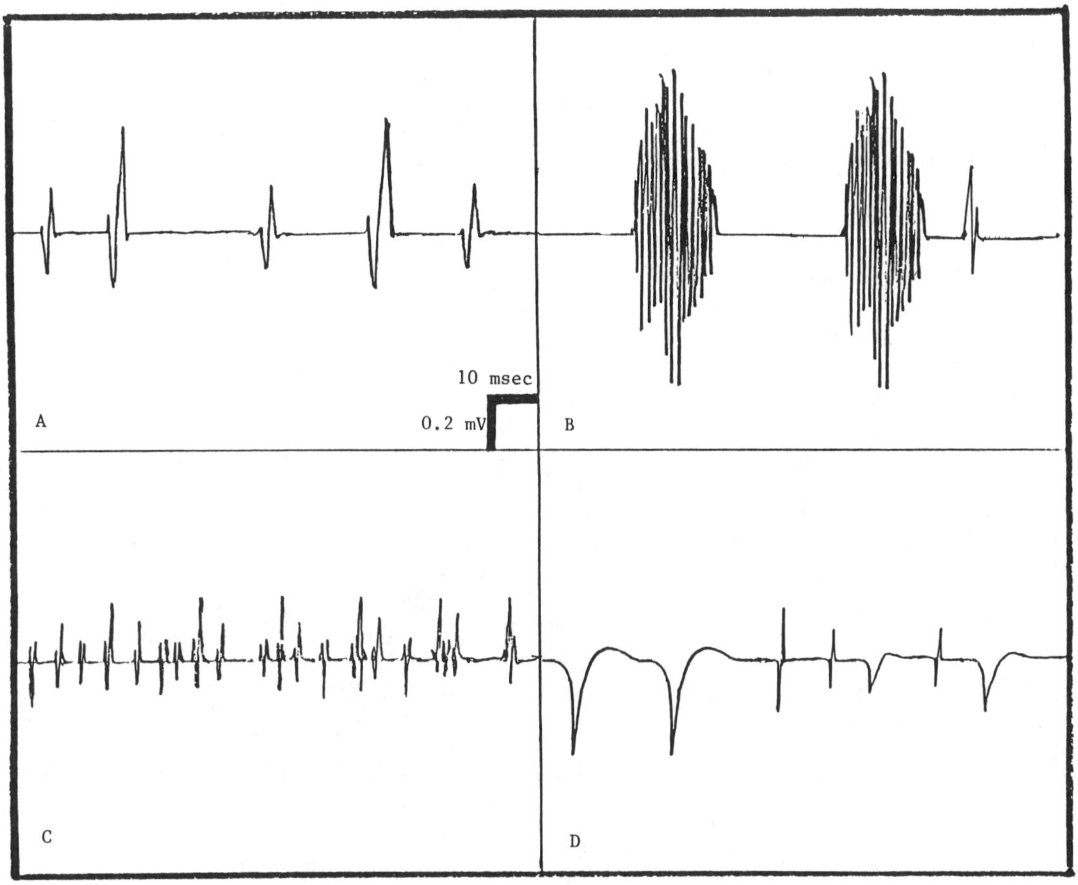

Figure 26–9.

EMG tracings: *A*. Normal motor unit potentials. *B*. Large polyphasic motor unit potentials in chronic neuropathy. *C*. Small short-duration motor unit potential in myopathy. *D*. Positive sharp waves and fibrillation potentials in acute denervation.

Table 26–10. REHABILITATION FOR NEUROLOGIC DISORDERS[a]

POSSIBLE DISABILITIES	REHABILITATION PROGRAMS
1. Impairment of motor function	
• weakness, paralysis	Therapeutic exercise, orthosis
• ataxia, poor balance	Exercise
• spasticity	Medicine, cold, heat, exercise, intramuscular neurolysis (motor point block)
2. Impairment of perceptual function	Perceptual training (OT)
3. Impairment of cognitive function	Cognitive training (OT, psychology, speech therapy, rehab nurse)
4. Impairment of speech and language function	Speech therapy
5. Impairment of sphincter function	Bladder and bowel training (rehab nurse)
6. Impairment of activities of daily living (ADL)	ADL training (OT, rehab nurse)
7. Poor adjustment to disability	Psychologic assessment and management
8. Others	

[a]Diseases: cerebrovascular accident, head injury, parkinsonism, spinal cord injury, multiple sclerosis, amyotrophic lateral sclerosis, peripheral neuropathy, polymyositis, muscular dystrophy, etc. OT: occupational therapist.

the spine or limbs (Chapter 22). The main cause is degenerative arthritis. The etiology is unknown. It is not curable. The rehabilitation goal is to maintain motor function (to avoid deterioration), to relieve discomfort (to relieve pain and stiffness), and to use residual function for compensation (body mechanics, energy saving techniques, and functional orthosis). It is cost effective to educate the patient to participate in a home program.

For acute arthritis such as exacerbation of inflammatory arthritis (rheumatoid arthritis, gouty arthritis, etc.), systemic medication may be more important than physical medicine modalities. However, a rehabilitation regimen is still very helpful for pain relief, maintenance of range of motion of the joint, and prevention of disuse atrophy.

Rehabilitation in Soft Tissue Lesions

Acute Sprain/Strain. Elderly people are vulnerable to minor traumatic soft tissue lesions due to the high incidence of falling (Tobis *et al.,* 1985). Early treatment for an acute traumatic lesion may reduce the subsequent complications. Cold therapy with an ice pack or ice massage is usually very helpful for both hemostasis (i.e., arrest of hemorrhage) and analgesia (i.e., blockage of pain) in the acute stage. The timing for gradual therapeutic exercise depends on the severity and site of trauma. For a first degree injury (mild tearing of muscle fibers or ligament, with only microhemorrhage), therapeutic exercise combined with heat therapy may be given if there is no evidence of a progressively expanding inflammatory reaction. If the injury is more than second-degree (i.e., significant swelling with ecchymosis or hemotoma due to extensive tearing of muscle fibers, tendons, or ligaments), immobilization for more than 48 hours is necessary. Therapeutic exercise and heat may be given at least 48 hours after if no further evidence of swelling or bleeding is noticed. *Myofascial pain syndrome*. Myofascial pain syndrome is a common problem in geriatric patients (Travell and Simons, 1983). It refers to the pain resulting from inflammation of a muscle and its fascia (i.e., connective envelope of the muscle) particularly at the facial insertion of muscle to bone. It is characterized by pain and/or autonomic phenomena referred from active myofascial trigger points (TPs) with associated dysfunction. The TP is a focus of hyperirritability in a tissue that, when compressed, is locally tender and, if sufficiently hypertensive, gives rise to referred pain and tenderness, and sometimes to referred autonomic phenomena and distortion of proprioception. The myofascial TP is always located on taut muscle fibers (taut band or nodule). When a snap palpation is applied to the TP, the taut muscle fibers contract and this phenomenon is called a "local twitch response" (LTR). LTR is a very useful objective sign for confirmation of a TP. The electromyographic recording of LTR has been well described (Dexter and Simons, 1981) and reveals both a local and reflex pathway that may be involved in the propagation of LTRs from the TP to the contractile apparatus of muscle (Hong *et al.,* 1986).

The perpetuating factors of myofascial pain syndrome include mechanical stress, nutritional inadequacies (especially vitamins B and C), metabolic and endocrine inadequacies, chronic infection, radiculopathy, and psychologic factors. It is important to correct the perpetuating factors to avoid the recurrence of the pain syndrome.

Therapeutic heat, therapeutic exercise, massage, spray and stretch to the tight muscle fibers, and trigger point injection with a local anesthetic with or without steroids are effective in most cases.

Rehabilitation in Orthopedic Lesions

Fracture or dislocation may be associated with falling in the geriatric patient. Care may require either open reduction or external fixation. Physical medicine modalities are helpful to facilitate recovery, to relieve pain, to maintain range of motion and strength, and to prevent other complications such as thrombophlebitis. The rehabilitation programs that may be helpful to patients with musculoskeletal disorders are listed on Table 26–11.

Table 26–11. REHABILITATION FOR MUSCULOSKELETAL DISORDERS[a]

POSSIBLE DISABILITIES	REHABILITATION PROGRAMS
1. Pain	Cold, heat, massage, traction, manipulation, TENS, acupuncture, exercise, local steroid injection, nerve block, medicine
2. Impairment of motor function	
• limited range of motion	Exercise, traction, manipulation, orthosis
• weakness (disuse)	Exercise, orthosis
• focal muscle spasm	Cold, heat, traction, manipulation, massage, exercise, medicine
• deformities	Exercise, orthosis
• gait impairment	Gait training, orthosis
• amputation	Prosthesis, exercise
3. Others	

[a]Diseases: arthritis, "low back pain," sprain, strain, myofascial pain syndrome, fracture, dislocation, subluxation, etc.

Table 26–12. REHABILITATION FOR CARDIOPULMONARY DISORDERS[a]

POSSIBLE DISABILITIES	REHABILITATION PROGRAMS
1. Impairment of cardiopulmonary fitness	Assessment of fitness level and general conditioning exercise with the following principles: 1. Submaximal rather than maximal 2. Aerobic rather than anaerobic 3. Dynamic (isotonic) rather than static (isometric) 4. Intermittent rather than continuous 5. Large group muscle activities
2. Impairment of ADL	ADL training, energy-saving techniques
3. Others	

[a]Diseases: coronary artery diseases, chronic obstructive lung diseases, congestive heart failure, etc.

REHABILITATION IN CARDIOPULMONARY DISORDERS

CARDIAC REHABILITATION

Disability from heart disease in the geriatric patient is usually related to reduced cardiac fitness due to the hemodynamic impairment of the heart or general deconditioning from prolonged bedrest (Chapters 17 and 22). Well programmed therapeutic exercise is one of the most important aspects in cardiac rehabilitation. Physiologic effects of exercise on the myocardium have been mentioned in the previous section. The quality and quantity of the exercise should be prescribed carefully to obtain optimal results and avoid risks. The general principles of the exercise prescription for the cardiac patient are (1) a readily accessible program with practical and simple protocols, with little or no exercise equipment required, (2) avoidance of excessive stress to the myocardium, and (3) measurable data to document improvement and to adjust the exercise programs. The types of exercise in cardiac rehabilitation programs are (1) dynamic rather than static, (2) aerobic rather than anaerobic, (3) intermittent rather than continuous, and (4) submaximal rather than maximal (Zohman and Tobis, 1970).

PULMONARY REHABILITATION

In general, the principles of cardiac rehabilitation can also be applied in pulmonary rehabilitation, as the heart is always involved in the advanced stage of pulmonary disease in the geriatric patient. In addition, breathing training exercises improve the efficiency of respiratory excursion by utilizing improved diaphragmatic abdominal control. Research has shown that the pulmonary patient can improve work ca-

Table 26–13. PHYSICAL MEDICINE IN PAIN MANAGEMENT

MODALITIES	PHYSIOLOGIC EFFECTS	CLINICAL APPLICATION
Heat therapy	Analgesic effect, sedative effect, relief of muscle spasm, relief of inflammation	Relief of chronic pain or pain due to chronic muscle spasm or inflammation
Cold therapy	Analgesic effect, relief of inflammation	Relief of acute or chronic pain or pain from acute inflammatory reaction
Transcutaneous electrical nerve stimulation	Increase of large-fiber impulses and decrease of small-fiber impulses	Relief of acute or chronic pain
Acupuncture	Unknown	Relief of acute or chronic pain
Massage	Sedative effect, muscle relaxation	Relief of acute or chronic pain of soft tissue lesions
Traction	Stretching of spasmodic muscles, increase of disc space (?)	Relief of acute or chronic pain from muscle spasm or discogenic diseases
Manipulation	Stretching of spasmodic muscles, mobilization of joints	Relief of acute or chronic pain from muscle spasm or soft tissue lesions

pacity in an exercise training program (Shayevitz and Shayevitz, 1986). Training also alleviates the emotional problems and social isolation frequently present in the geriatric patient with cardiopulmonary disease. The outline of cardiopulmonary rehabilitation programs is shown in Table 26–12.

PAIN MANAGEMENT

The most important aspect of pain management is the treatment of the etiological factors. However, in many cases, in the geriatric patient, this is unlikely either because the etiological factor is unclear, such as some chronic pain syndromes or because the etiological factor is not curable, such as pain from cancer. Physical medicine becomes an important tool in treating such kinds of pain. The common modalities used for the treatment of pain are listed in Table 26–13.

References

Aloia, J. F.: Exercise and skeletal health. *J. Am. Geriatr. Soc.*, **29:**104–107, **1981.**

Astrand, P- O., and Rodahl, K.: Physical training. In Astrand, P- O., and Rodahl, K. (eds.): *Textbook of Work Physiology,* 2d ed., McGraw-Hill, New York, **1977.**

Baldwin, K. M.: Effects of chronic exercise on biochemical and functional properties of the heart. *Med. Sci. Sports Exerc.*, **17:**522–528, **1985.**

Basmajian, J. V.: Biofeedback in therapeutic exercise. In Basmajian, J. V. (ed.): *Muscles Alive, Their Functions Revealed by Electromyography,* Williams & Wilkins, Baltimore, **1984.**

Bobechko, W. P.; Herbert, M. A.; and Friedman, H. G.: Electrospinal instrumentation for scoliosis: Current status. *Orthop. Clin. North Am.*, **10:**927–941, **1979.**

Booth, F. W.: Effect of limb immobilization on skeletal muscle. *J. Appl. Physiol.: Respir. Environ. Exercise Physiol.*, **52:**1113–1118, **1982.**

Brighton, C. T.; Black, J.; Friedenberg, Z. B.; Esterhai, J.; Day, L. J.; and Connolly, J. F.: A multicenter study of the treatment of non-union with constant direct current. *J. Bone Joint Surg.*, **63(A):**2–13, **1981.**

Buskirk, E. R.: Introduction to the symposium: Exercise in the treatment of obesity. *Med. Sci. Sports Exerc.*, **18:**1–2, **1986.**

Clausen, J. P.: Circulatory adjustments to dynamic exercise and effect of physical training in normal subjects and in patients with coronary artery disease. In Sonnenblick, E. H., and Lesch, M. (eds.): *Exercise and Heart Disease,* Grune & Stratton, New York, **1977.**

DeHaas, W. G.; Watson, J.; and Morrison, D. M.: Noninvasive treatment of ununited fractures of the tibia using electrical stimulation. *J. Bone Joint Surg.*, **62:**465–470, **1980.**

Dexter, J., and Simons, D.: Local twitch response in human muscle evoked by palpation and needle penetration of a trigger point. *Arch. Phys. Med. Rehabil.*, **62:**521–522, **1981.**

Fisher, S., and Gullickson, G.: Energy cost of ambulation in health and disability: Literature review. *Arch. Phys. Med. Rehabil.*, **59:**124–133, **1978.**

Godec, C.; Cass, A. S.; and Ayala, G. F.: Electrical stimulation for incontinence. *Urology,* **7:**388-397, **1976.**

Gracanin, F.: Functional electric stimulation. In Kottke, F. J.; Stillwell, G. K.; and Lehmann, J. F.: *Krusen's Handbook of Physical Medicine and Rehabilitation,* 3rd ed., W. B. Saunders, Philadelphia, **1982.**

Granger, C. V.: A conceptual model for functional assessment. In Granger, C. V., and Gresham, G. E. (eds.): *Functional Assessment in Rehabilitation Medicine,* Williams & Wilkins, Baltimore, **1984.**

Gullickson, G., and Licht, S.: Definition and philosophy of rehabilitation medicine. in Licht, S. (ed.): *Rehabilitation and Medicine,* Waverly Press, Baltimore, **1968.**

Hammond, H. K., and Froelicher, V. F.: The physiologic sequelae of chronic dynamic exercise. *Med. Clin. North Am.*, **69**(1):21–39, **1985.**

Harris, F. A.: Facilitation techniques and technological adjuncts in therapeutic exercise. In Basmajian, J. V. (ed.): *Therapeutic Exercise,* 4th ed., Williams & Wilkins, Baltimore, **1984.**

Haskell, W. L.: The influence of exercise on the concentration of triglyceride and cholesterol in human plasma. *Exercise Sport Sci. Rev.*, **12**:205–244, **1984.**

Herbison, G. J., and Gordon, E. E.: Exercise of normal muscles—Biochemical effects. *Arch. Phys. Med. Rehabil.*, **54**:409–415, **1973.**

Holloszy, J. O.; Rennie, M. J.; Hickson, R. C.; Conlee, R. K.; and Hagberg, J. M.: Physiological consequences of the biochemical adaptations to endurance exercise. *Ann. NY Acad. Sci.*, **301**:440–450, **1977.**

Hong, C- Z.; Harmon, D.; and Yu, J.: Static magnetic field influence on rat tail nerve function. *Arch. Phys. Med. Rehabil.*, **67**:746–749, **1986.**

Hong, C- Z., and Lien, I- N.: Metabolic effects of exhaustive training of athletes. *Arch. Phys. Med. Rehabil.*, **65**:362–365, **1984.**

Hong, C- Z.; Liu, H.; and Yu, J.: Ultrasound thermotherapy: Its effect on the recovery of nerve conduction in experimental compression neuropathy. *Arch. Phys. Med. Rehabil.*, **67**:618, **1986.**

Hong, C- Z.; Simons, D.; and Statham, L.: Electromyographic analysis of local twitch responses of human extensor digitorum communis muscle during ischemic compression over the arm. *Arch. Phys. Med. Rehabil.*, **67**:680, **1986.**

Jacobs, S. R.; Jaweed, M. M.; Herbison, G. J.; and Stillwell, G. K.: Electrical stimulation of muscle. In Stillwell, G. K. (ed.): *Therapeutic Electricity and Ultraviolet Radiation,* 3rd ed., Williams & Wilkins, Baltimore, **1983.**

Kimura, J.: Nerve conduction studies and electromyography. In Dyck, P.; Thomas, P. K.; Lambert, E. H.; and Bunge, R. (eds.): *Peripheral Neuropathy,* 2nd ed. W. B. Saunders, Philadelphia, **1984.**

Knapp, M. E.: Massage. In Kottke, F. J.; Stillwell, G. K.; and Lehmann, J. F. (eds.): *Krusen's Handbook of Physical Medicine and Rehabilitation,* 3rd ed., W. B. Saunders, Philadelphia, **1982.**

Lampman, R. M.; Schteingart, D. E.; and Foss, M. L.: Exercise as a partial therapy for the extremely obese. *Med. Sci. Sports Exerc.*, **18**:19–24, **1986.**

Lehmann, J. F., and De Lateur, B. J.: Therapeutic heat. In Lehmann, J. F. (ed.): *Therapeutic Heat and Cold,* 3rd ed., Williams & Wilkins, Baltimore, **1982.**

Leon, A. S.: Physical activity levels and coronary heart disease—Analysis of epidemiologic and supporting studies. *Med. Clin. North Am.*, **69**(1):3–20, **1985.**

Liberson, W. T.: Electrotherapy. In Ruskin, A. P. (ed.): *Current Therapy in Physiatry,* W. B. Saunders, Philadelphia, **1984.**

Licht, S.: History. In Basmajian, J. V. (ed.): *Therapeutic Exercise,* 4th ed., Williams & Wilkins, Baltimore, **1984.**

Long, C.: Exercise in the prevention and rehabilitation of ischemic heart disease. In Long, C. (ed.): *Prevention and Rehabilitation in Ischemic Heart Disease,* Williams & Wilkins, Baltimore, **1980.**

Lynch, G. S.; Smith, R. L.; and Cotman, C. W.: Recovery of function following brain damage: A consideration of some neural mechanisms. In Buerger, A. A., and Tobis, J. S. (eds.): *Neurophysiologic Aspects of Rehabilitation Medicine,* Charles C Thomas, Springfield, IL, **1976.**

Maigne, R.: Manipulation of the spine. In Rogoff, J. B. (ed.): *Manipulation, Traction and Massage,* 2d ed., Williams & Wilkins, Baltimore, **1980.**

Martin, R. P.; Haskell, W. L.; and Wood, P. D.: Blood chemistry and lipid profiles of elite distance runners. *Annu. Rev. Physiol.*, **39**:345–360, **1977.**

Melzack, R., and Wall, P. D.: Pain mechanisms: A new theory. *Science,* **150**:971–979, **1965.**

Mennell, J. M.: History of the development of medical manipulative concepts; medical terminology. In Goldstein, M. (ed.): NINDS Monograph no. 15: The research status of spinal manipulative therapy, US Department of Health, Education and Welfare, NIH, Bethesda, **1975.**

Merrill, D. C.: Electrical vesical stimulation. In Stillwell, G. K. (ed.): *Therapeutic Electricity and Ultraviolet Radiation,* 3rd ed., Williams & Wilkins, Baltimore, **1983.**

Mooney, V.; Wileman, W.; and McNeal, D. R.: Stimulation reduces spastic activity. *JAMA*, **207**:2199–2200, **1969.**

Morganroth, J., and Marion, B. J.: The athlete's heart syndrome: A new perspective. *Ann. NY Acad. Sci.*, **301**:931–941, **1977.**

Osternig, L. R.: Isokinetic dynamometry: Implications for muscle testing and rehabilitation. *Exercise Sport Sci. Rev.*, **14**:45–80, **1986.**

Pacy, P. J.; Webster, J.; and Garrow, J. S.: Exercise and obesity. *Sports Med.*, **3**:89–113, **1986.**

Petrofsky, J. S., and Phillips, C. A.: The physiology of static exercise. *Exercise Sport Sci. Rev.*, **14**:1–44, **1986.**

Richter, E. A., and Galbo, H.: Diabetes, insulin and exercise. *Sports Med.*, **3**:275–288, **1986.**

Saltin, B.; Henriksson, J.; Nygaard, E.; and Andersen, P.: Fiber types and metabolic potentials of skeletal muscles in sedentary man and endurance runners. *Ann. NY Acad. Sci.*, **301**:3–29, **1977.**

Scheuer, J., and Tipton, C. M.: Cardiovascular adaptations to physical training. *Annu. Rev. Physiol.*, **39**:221–251, **1977.**

Scott, B. O.: Clinical uses of ultraviolet radiation. In Stillwell, G. K. (ed.): *Therapeutic Electricity and Ultraviolet Radiation,* 3rd ed., Williams & Wilkins, Baltimore, **1983.**

Shayevitz, M. B., and Shayevitz, B. R.: Athletic training in chronic obstructive pulmonary disease. *Clin. Sports Med.*, **5**:471–491, **1986.**

Shephard, R. J.: Physical training for the elderly. *Clin. Sports Med.*, **5**:515–533, **1986a.**

Shephard, R. J.: Exercise in coronary heart disease. *Sports Med.*, **3**:26–49, **1986b.**

Sidney, K. H.: Cardiovascular benefits of physical activity in the exercising aged. In Smith, E. L., and Serfass, R. C. (eds.): *Exercise and Aging: The Scientific Basis,* Enslow Publishers, Hillside, NJ, **1981.**

Smith, E. L.: Bone changes in the exercising older adult. In Smith, E. L., and Serfass, R. C. (eds.): *Exercise and Aging: The Scientific Basis,* Enslow Publishers, Hillside, NJ, **1981.**

Stillman, R. J.; Lohman, T. G.; Slaughter, M. H.; and Massey, B. H.: Physiological activity and bone mineral content in women aged 30 to 85 years. *Med. Sci. Sports Exerc.*, **18**:576–580, **1986.**

Stillwell, G. K.: Ultraviolet therapy. In Kottke, F. J.; Stillwell, G. K.; and Lehman, J. F. (eds.): *Krusen's Handbook of Physical Medicine and Rehabilitation,* 3rd ed., W. B. Saunders, Philadelphia, **1982.**

Sutton, J. R.: Introduction to the symposium: Endorphins in exercise. *Med. Sci. Sports Exerc.*, **17**:73, **1985.**

Taylor, N. A. S., and Wilkinson, J. G.: Exercise-induced skeletal muscle growth: Hypertrophy or hyperplasia? *Sports Med.*, **3**:190–200, **1986.**

Thomas, D. P.: Effects of acute and chronic exercise on myocardial ultrastructure. *Med. Sci. Sports Exerc.*, **17**:546–553, **1985.**

Thorsteinsson, G.: Electrical stimulation for analgesia. In Stillwell, G. K. (ed.): *Therapeutic Electricity and Ultraviolet Radiation,* 3rd ed., Williams & Wilkins, Baltimore, **1983.**

Tipton, C. M.: Exercise, training and hypertension. *Exercise Sports Sci. Rev.*, **12**:245–306, **1984.**

Tobis, J. S.: Rehabilitation of the geriatric patient. In

Rossman, I. (ed.): *Clinical Geriatrics,* 2d ed., J. B. Lippincott, Philadelphia, **1979.**

Tobis, J. S., and Hoehler, F.: *Musculoskeletal Manipulation, Evaluation of the Scientific Evidence,* Charles C Thomas, Springfield, IL, **1986.**

Tobis, J. S., and Lowenthal, M.: *Evaluation and Management of the Brain-Damaged Patient,* Charles C Thomas, Springfield, IL, **1960.**

Tobis, J. S.; Reinsch, S.; Swanson, J. M.; Byrd, M.; and Scharf, T.: Visual perception dominance of fallers among community-dwelling older adults. *J. Am. Geriatr. Soc.,* **33:**330–333, **1985.**

Travell, J., and Simons, D.: *Myofascial Pain and Dysfunction: The Trigger Point Manual,* Williams & Wilkins, Baltimore, **1983.**

Wakim, K. G.: Physiologic effects of massage. In Rogoff, J. B. (ed.): *Manipulation, Traction and Massage,* 2d ed., Williams & Wilkins, Baltimore, **1980.**

Yu, J.: Neuromuscular recovery with training after central nervous lesions: An experimental approach. In Ince, I. P. (ed.): *Behavioral Psychology in Rehabilitation Medicine: Clinical Applications,* Williams & Wilkins, Baltimore, **1980.**

Yu, J.: Instrumental conditioning and plasticity of motor function. In Morrison, A. R., and Strick, P. L. (eds.): *Changing Concepts of the Nervous System,* Academic Press, New York, **1982a.**

Yu, J.: Animal models of recovery with training after central nervous system lesions. *Int. Rehab. Med.,* **4:**190–194, **1982b.**

Zohman, L. R., and Tobis, J. S.: *Cardiac Rehabilitation,* Grune & Stratton, New York, **1970.**

CHAPTER

27 AN AGENDA FOR HEALTHFUL AGING

Life Extension Sciences

The major purpose of this book has been to present an overall, systematic view of physiologic aging, not only in humans but also, for comparison and elucidation, in experimental animals and cultured cell models. References to medical illness are intended primarily as a recognition of the increased incidence of disease with aging, and a few diseases have been selected for brief discussion as examples of how pathology influences physiologic adjustments with advancing age. Limitations of time, space, and lack of expertise by this writer have prevented incursions into areas not specifically biomedically oriented but nevertheless extremely important for the promotion and maintenance of the quality of life in the elderly. Thus, in drawing the physiologic profile of an aged individual, the contribution of nonbiologic factors to good health status has been deliberately omitted, with little attention to the contribution to physiologic decline of social losses, preexistent personality, and sociocultural variables. Effective socioeconomic support networks and public health community programs do appear to play as important a role in determining the quality of life at all ages as medical care does. Biomedical progress in the United States and in all Western countries has allowed us to live many years longer than our parents and ancestors. We are now at the cutting edge of rapid biotechnologic advances and we should exploit, in full, our knowledge of these new techniques to treat the diseases of old age and to prolong and improve the lifespan. Some of the new directions of research, grouped under so-called life extension sciences, are briefly presented below.

Maintenance of the quality of life with old age is not merely a matter of improving physical fitness, but social, cultural, economic, and emotional factors must also be considered. We know that individuals, including old individuals, do not always see health as the most important issue in their lives. So far the increase in life expectancy witnessed in this country has been primarily attributed as much to improvements in hygiene, better nutrition, and the rising standard of living as to the successful eradication of a number of infectious diseases. Further breakthroughs in gerontology/geriatrics should be based on the effective articulation of biologic measures with socioeconomic policy.

WELLNESS AND HEALTH PROMOTION

At all ages, the condition of well-being or wellness (a term considerably abused by faddists and alternative health worshippers but retained here for its original and simplest meaning) depends on good physical and mental health in a favorable environment. Senescence, in contrast, is characterized by declining physiologic competence and increasing incidence and severity of disease, under the everyday stresses of life. Therefore, maintenance or restoration of wellness, with advancing age, depends both on strengthening physiologic responses and on eliminating disease (Dychtwald, 1986). With considerable effort some success has been achieved in the prevention and elimination of some diseases, particularly acute infections. However, the increasing incidence of chronic degenerative diseases in the aged population underlines the need for continuing research toward elimination of disease. Much less, indeed very little, has been done to strengthen physiologic competence and prevent, delay, or repair its decline with aging. This is an area that requires concerted effort as physiologic integrity is the nexus not only for well-being, but also for disease prevention. For an effective strengthening of physiologic competence, however, the molecular and cellular mechanisms of the aging process, and their role in the regulation of systemic function, must be understood. Therefore, maintenance of good health in the elderly requires a multifaceted approach.

Toward a New Image of Aging. As already discussed in Chapter 2, a number of erroneous myths and age-related stereotypes pervade our culture. These myths obscure the facts about the later years of life and undermine the truth of a possible vigorous and healthy senescence: "At eighty I believe I am a far more cheerful person than I was at twenty or thirty. I most definitely would not want to be a teenager again. Youth may be glorious, but it is also painful to endure. Moreover, what is called youth is not youth; it is rather something like premature old age" (Miller, 1977). It is essential that these myths be disavowed for the real picture of physiologic aging to emerge (Dychtwald, 1986). A brief list will identify the most common and insidious of these myths: old age starts at 65 years (although Picasso said, "One starts to get young at the age of sixty, and then it's too late"); old age is a disease; old age always brings mental impairment; the elderly represent a homogeneous group characterized by equal physiologic decline; old people are poor; old people are powerless; nothing can be done to modify aging, future elderly will have the same problems as current elderly; the United States have always been a youth-focused culture. These statements are incorrect and must be dispelled by intensive educational programs initiated at an early age with emphasis on the following: (1) good health is important during early ages as a forerunner of good health in old age; (2) considerable advances have been achieved in prolongation of life expectancy and in prevention and treatment of many diseases and similar advances may be expected in the future; (3) quality of life in old age depends on several complex factors and its improvement must be reached by a concerted effort of biomedical as well as socioeconomic and educational measures.

Concepts of wellness are illustrated in Table 27–1 presenting selected common conditions that affect the elderly and that depend on physical, emotional, and social circumstances that can be approached by a multipronged attack. Nutrition and exercise have been selected as they are physiologic parameters easily modified (Chapter 25); and smoking and alcohol, as they are two commonly met abuses. It emerges clearly that there is no single approach to the promotion of wellness, but rather a combination of medical, social, economic, and psychologic interventions is necessary.

Among the factors that can be modified to positively improve the quality of life are medical care, income, nutrition, housing, social integration, and education. The latter is worthy of greater emphasis than it has heretofore received. Inasmuch as aging must be viewed as a continuation of previous experiences, knowledge of physical makeup and environment is essential for programming lifestyles capable of generating an ongoing satisfactory quality of life.

Several programs are currently offered and more are planned to educate the elderly and increase their awareness of aging-related diseases and means of prevention and treatment. Useful as these educational programs may be, they belie the need for a broader view, that is, beginning education about aging during the school years; it is at an early age that initiation of regimens for good health will yield the greatest benefit for better quality of future life.

Another important role for education is to provide the skills to enable the individual to choose more effectively his/her position in society and to take advantage of opportunities and options. Indeed, "control of one's own destiny" rather than economic status may determine the quality of health and length of lifespan. It is possible that "formal" education is a key to improving control of one's destiny. While this is not a startling or original concept, formal education is rarely a top priority of any programs organized for the benefit of the elderly. A number of observations in support of this role of education in disease prevention and life improvement have been reviewed by Syme (1987). Only one example will be presented here to underline that socioeconomic status as a risk factor must be interpreted in a broader context than the mere restrictive difference of poverty versus nonpoverty. In this study, British civil servants were studied for the incidence of coronary heart disease and factors that might influence disease incidence. In all groups, after adjusting for the usual risk factors (serum cholesterol, smoking, obesity, and so forth), the rate of coronary heart disease was three times higher in employees at the bottom than in those at the top of the civil service hierarchy (Rose and Marmot, 1981). Most interesting was the presence of

Table 27–1. FACTORS AFFECTING THE ELDERLY AND AMENABLE TO MULTIFACTORIAL INTERVENTIONS[a]

CONDITION	UNDERLYING CAUSE	CONTROL
	Nutrition	
Reduced calcium absorption; loss of lean body mass and bone mass; low levels of vitamins K and D; muscle weakness and tetany	Inadequate caloric intake; little variety; excess processed food; lack of nutrition knowledge; alcohol, drugs; low income, social status; illness; physical difficulty in daily activities	Improved economics and education leading to adequate diet; improved physical condition leading to increased daily activities and greater social interactions
Hypertension; obesity; increased insulin resistance; high cholesterol; low HDL	Excess salt; excessive food intake; high caloric food intake; inactivity	Hormonal therapy; antihypertensive drugs; anticholesterol drugs
	Exercise	
Reduced muscle strength and endurance; loss of lean body mass; increased fat	Inactivity due to lack of stimulation in the environment; retirement	Education for need to exercise; improved social contacts; improved safety
Poor neurologic control; reduced coordination, balance; mental impairment	Confinement due to fear of crime; lack of knowledge for need to exercise	Treatment of underlying medical conditions
Reduced joint mobility, bone mass	Joint and bone discomfort; cardiovascular disease; respiratory disease	
	Drugs, Smoking, and Alcohol	
Polypharmacy; improper therapeutic drug dosage; drug addiction	Lack of knowledge of geriatric pharmacology; inaccurate diagnosis; noncompliance; unawareness of side effects; cost of drugs; lack of health insurance	Adequate diagnosis and treatment; surveillance of appropriate intake and side effects of drugs; economic support; rehabilitation from addiction
Respiratory insufficiency; loss of task capacity	Mass media; sex image; peer pressure	Stop smoking; support group
Impaired hepatic function; neurologic symptoms	Addiction: sex image social condition; heredity	Stop drinking; peer and family support

[a]Adapted, with permission, from Minkler and Pasick (1986).

a "gradient" among the different groups, with the high-level administrators having the lowest rate, followed by the professionals and executives with an intermediate rate, and the clerical workers having the highest rate. Clearly all subjects enjoyed a standard of living above poverty level, and therefore the differential incidence of the disease was to be ascribed to some still unidentified aspect, other than income, of the social and work status. The concept that the lower the position of an individual in the social structure and the fewer the resources and training for options of type of work and style of life, the greater the incidence of disease must be supported by future research. If it proves to be of value, then we would have available, through strengthening education, an avenue for intervention that is more precise and understandable than simply suggesting that we intervene in "socioeconomic status."

Health Programs for the Elderly. For the elderly, many programs have been and are being designed in the United States and most countries of the world, including the developing nations where the lifespan expectancy is rapidly rising and the percentage of elderly is increasing. Among the major programs capable of improving health, some strive to eliminate premature disease and to manage late degenerative disease—primarily the task of geriatricians. Others focus on the improvement of funding, social policy, social security programs, establishment of federal and state health care insurance, and tax exemptions—primarily the task of policy makers. Still others emphasize the physical and mental fitness by promoting programs in nutrition, exercise, personal safety, establishing senior citizen centers, centers for long-term care, and programs for stress management—primarily the task of the individual and the community.

A number of programs for the elderly concerned with health care, social policy, funding, senior center, community-based health care, and education are continually being proposed, established, and tested. How effective they are and which health strategies are most likely to benefit the elderly remain to be clarified by vigorous and sound research. Compassion and desire to help the elderly are not sufficient qualifications to ensure success. Improvements in the rational care of the elderly, and, incidentally, better cost-effectiveness, will depend ultimately on improvement in governmental health policy and the concerted effort of educators, health care providers, community and family support, and the elderly themselves.

FUTURE PERSPECTIVES IN BIOMEDICAL GERONTOLOGY: THE LIFE EXTENSION SCIENCES*

The life extension sciences include both classic and innovative biomedical areas such as interventive gerontology, cryonics, cloning, transplantation, resuscitation, artificial organs, and regeneration. Through the studied development and employment of these technologies, the course of aging and senescence, its ultimate culmination in morbidity and mortality, will be dramatically altered.

Experiments in nutritional gerontology indicate that the rate of aging can be modified in laboratory rodents. Maximum lifespans of rats and mice, usually 3.5 years, have been extended up to 5 years. Rats, usually infertile after 15 months, placed on a restricted dietary regimen early in life and maintained thereon for years, have borne litters at ages approaching 3 years. In addition, the age-related increase in tumor incidence, decline in homeostatic capability, and even the senescent deterioration of the coat have been delayed (Segall *et al.*, 1983; Timiras *et al.*, 1984). (See also Chapter 25.) These findings show that mammalian aging, once believed to be somehow inexorable, can be manipulated in the laboratory.

Substantial efforts are currently underway to determine the mechanisms underlying delayed aging in underfed rodents. We can eventually expect a comprehensive understanding of why food restriction produces its effects. With such knowledge will come the ability to even more profoundly influence the rate of aging, delay and even reverse senescent changes, and prolong lifespan. Such efforts may extend beyond the laboratory and into the area of clinical medicine. Treatments and strategies will become available that profoundly affect aging and lifespan in humans.

Parallel to these developments, advances in deep hypothermia and cryonics can be expected to facilitate prophylactic intervention in nonterminal situations. Surgical procedures are becoming available that permit hours of ice-cold bloodless perfusion and thereby may make possible surgical removal and specific organ-directed chemotherapeutic destruction of conventionally inoperable tumors, more effective transplantation of vital organs and tissues, and the implantation of a wide variety of prosthetic devices. These strategies will allow us to more successfully counteract the effects of senescence.

Cryopreservation. Several species of frogs overwinter in the partially frozen state. These animals have been known to survive up to 1 month in the laboratory at $-2°C$ with 35 to 50 percent of their body water frozen as ice. In order to restrict freezing to the extracellular compartment, and to avoid intracellular ice formations, these animals produce and circulate to their tissues large quantities of glucose or glycerol, which act as cryoprotectants (Storey and Storey, 1987). Hamsters have been revived following partial freezing at temperatures between -1 and $-3°C$ for 1 to 3 hours. In these animals, as in the frogs, up to 50 percent of their body water (presumably, the extracellular component) was frozen into ice. As these hamsters lacked cryoprotectant, they could not endure longer periods of freezing or lower temperatures (Smith, 1956).

Recent studies have shown that hamsters, and even dogs, can survive periods of near-total replacement of their blood with a synthetic blood substitute at temperatures very near the ice-point. A few hamsters have been revived following circulation of a blood substitute containing an amount of glycerol approaching the concentration of this cold-protecting chemical present in the blood of overwintering frogs. Attempts are currently in progress to revive such cryoprotected hamsters from partial freezing (Segall *et al.*, 1987).

When such revival from partial freezing becomes available in brain-dead humans, multiorgan transplant donors could be stored for periods long enough to allow maximum utilization of all

* This section (pages 452–454) was contributed by P. E. Segall, Department of Physiology-Anatomy, University of California, Berkeley, California.

their organs. This technology will provide for an increased availability of organs for transplantation. Advances in immunosuppression, already impressive since the discovery of cyclosporin A, coupled with increased organ availability, will qualify older patients as transplant recipients.

New forms of cryopreservation are now emerging. The most notable of these is vitrification, a technique in which tissues are saturated with high concentrations of chemical agents, subjected to pressures approaching and exceeding 1000 atmospheres, and frozen to cryogenic temperatures for indefinite storage. Mouse embryos have survived vitrification and liquid nitrogen storage and have been brought back to term following implantation in surrogate mothers (Rall and Fahy, 1985). Workers in the field are currently attempting to extend this technique to the cryogenic storage of vital organs for transplantation. The eventual goal is the reversible cryonics suspension of terminal patients or individuals with incurable degenerative disease, such as Alzheimer's disease, until a time when a cure is available.

Differentiated amphibian somatic cell nuclei, such as those from adult eye lens and adult red blood cells, have been transplanted into enucleated amphibian eggs and the transplanted embryos have been raised to tadpole stage. When tadpole intestinal cells were used as the nuclear donor, a small number of transplant embryos reached adulthood and were capable of reproduction. Application of such cloning techniques as nuclear transplant in mammals has not progressed as far, but successful transplantation of nuclei from one-, two-, and eight-cell-stage embryos of mice, sheep, and cows has been reported (McKinnell, 1985; Willadsden, 1986).

Cloning. When mammalian nuclear transplant technology produces the development of mature adults using nuclei transplanted from adult somatic cells, it may be possible to develop genetically identical bodies using single cells from an older patient. These "cloned" bodies could then be used as a source of young organs, which could be back-transplanted to replace those failing in the older individual. During the development of such a "parts clone," the prosencephalon could be removed and stored in liquid nitrogen. This would prevent the parts clone from developing into a sentient human being. After removal of the cells responsible for higher brain formation, the embryo would develop into the ethical equivalent of a brain-dead individual. Once matured by rapid hormone-stimulated growth, it could serve as a tissue and organ donor to supply healthy youthful parts.

The embryonic nerve cells from the forebrain removed during early development can eventually be used to replace analogous cells damaged by aging. With such cloning technology, it may be possible to nearly completely "renovate" an aging individual using genetically identical and, therefore, immunologically compatible parts. Such a technique, using cells, tissues, and organs from a parts clone, could ultimately be used to rescue older individuals placed in cryonics suspension due to Alzheimer's disease, terminal cancer or extreme debilitation secondary to advanced aging.

Another means to increase lifespan in the aging population involves rapid progress in emergency and critical-care medicine. Cardiovascular and pulmonary disorders leading to terminal conditions are more prevalent in the older patient, responsible for a disproportionate number of emergency calls. Improvements in resuscitation technology will add years to their life expectancy, as well as improve their quality of life by reducing morbidity from cerebral ischemia. Some recent innovations in this area include: the use of calcium channel blockers to prevent arterial constriction in the microcirculation; removal of leukocytes in blood used for reperfusion, employing manitol to augment blood flow and decrease postischemic tissue swelling; and the exploration of hypothermia in revival following cardiac arrest (Safar, 1986).

Coincidental with these advances is progress in the development of artificial internal organs such as the artificial kidney (renal dialysis), the artificial heart, and the extracorporeal membrane oxygenator (Cauwels, 1986). Advances of techniques for direct sustenance of tissues through the use of total parenteral nutrition allow those whose digestive functions have been impaired to survive until these functions return (Irving, 1986).

A revolution in medical visualization technology, including computer-assisted tomography (CAT scanning), positron emission tomography (PET scanning), magnetic resonance imaging (MRI), and ultrasonics, coupled with the use of semimicro multianalyses of physiologic chemistry allows early and accurate diagnosis of life-threatening situations and permits planning appropriate surgical, pharmacologic, and other forms of intervention.

Newly found growth factors, along with drugs or even electric and electromagnetic fields, which some have indicated may spur regeneration, could lead to techniques for revitalizing aged, damaged, or diseased tissues and organs. A preliminary example of these is the use of pulsed electromagnetism to heal cracks in bones (common in older individuals often compromised by osteoporosis) (Basset *et al.,* 1974; Barker *et al.,* 1984). Let us not minimize the importance of improving the self-image as through continuing progress in plastic surgery, cosmetic dermatology, and pharmacology (such as the use of minoxidil to stimulate hair growth).

* * *

Emphasis in achieving longevity and wellness in old age has, so far, focused primarily on prevention and treatment of disease and less often on enhancement of physiologic competence. Reducing risks and avoiding hazards represent yet another means, perhaps as effective as biomedical research, of achieving these goals. Risk assessment is an interesting and constructive first step in attempting to minimize mistakes (e.g., car accidents, cigarette smoking, radiation exposure) that may endanger the length and quality of life (Wilson and Crouch, 1987). However, ranking of such risks seems to remain quite difficult (Ames *et al.,* 1987), as are the perception of risk (Slovic, 1987) and the measures taken for correction (Russell and Gruber, 1987; Lave, 1987). Thus, "a zero risk society is not yet in the scientific cards" (Koshland, 1987).

While some of the predictions for life extension may sound like science fiction, this century has produced such monumental changes that these predictions should not be considered outrageous. Seeking "immortality in the arduous old-fashioned way, doing good deeds and tak[ing] care of [one's] children" (Koshland, 1987) remains a goal worthy of pursuit. It should not detract from efforts of continuing to improve and lengthen life. Aging and death remain, indeed, the last sacred enemies, particularly frustrating to 20th-century man who has circled the moon, harnessed nuclear energy, artificially reproduced DNA, and significantly extended life expectancy. Such a man can be expected to continue to strive to improve the quality of life at all stages, including old age, as well as extend the duration of life, as Tolstoy (1906) suggested when he wrote in a letter to a friend, "Don't complain about old age. How much good it has brought me that was unexpected and beautiful" and concluded "that the end of old age and of life will be just as unexpectedly beautiful. . . ." Here, again, we are emphasizing the biomedical; however, all of this is of little avail unless we also consider ethical, moral, economic, and cultural implications for the elderly population. To be successful, aging depends on the cooperation of the individual, who is responsible for the well-being of his/her own body; on the community, including the family, who are responsible for a supportive network; and on the government, which must provide a legal and monetary support for this segment of the population (Rowe and Kahn, 1987).

References

Ames, B. N.; Magaw, R.; and Gold, L. S.: Ranking possible carcinogenic hazards. *Science,* **236**:271–280, **1987.**

Barker, A. T.; Dixon, R. A.; Sharrard, W. J. W.; and Sutchliffe, M. L.: Pulsed magnetic field therapy for tibial non-union. *Lancet,* **1**:994–996, **1984.**

Basset, C. A. L.; Rawluck, R. J.; and Pilla, A. A.: Augmentation of bone repair by inductively coupled electromagnetic fields. *Science,* **184**:575–577, **1974.**

Cauwels, J. M.: *The Body Shop Bionic Revolution in Medicine,* C. V. Mosby, St. Louis, **1986.**

Dychtwald, K.: *Wellness and Health Promotion for the Elderly,* Aspen Systems Corp., Rockville, MD, **1986.**

Irving, M.: ABC of nutrition. Enteral and parenteral nutrition. *Br. Med. J.,* **291**:1404–1408, **1986.**

Koshland, D. E.: Immortality and risk assessment. *Science,* 236:241, **1987.**

Lave, L. B.: Health and safety risk analyses: Information for better decisions. *Science,* **236**:291–295, **1987.**

McKinnell, R. G.: *Cloning of Frogs, Mice and Other Animals,* rev. ed., University of Minnesota Press, Minneapolis, **1985.**

Miller, H.: In Sampson, A., and Sampson, S. (eds.): *The Oxford Book of Ages,* Oxford University Press, **1985,** p. 151, from: *Sextet.* Copyright **1977** by Henry Miller. Reprinted by permission of Capra Press, Santa Barbara, CA.

Minkler, M., and Pasick, R. J.: Health promotion and the elderly: A critical perspective on the past and future. In Dychtwald, K. (ed.): *Wellness and Health Promotion for the Elderly,* Aspen Systems Corp., Rockville, MD, **1986.**

Rall, W. F., and Fahy, G. M.: Ice-free cryopreservation of mouse embryos at −196 degrees by vitrification. *Nature,* **313**:573–575, **1985.**

Rose, G., and Marmot, M. G.: Social class and coronary heart disease. *Br. Heart J.*, **45**:13–19, **1981.**

Rowe, J. W., and Kahn, R. L.: Human aging: usual and successful. *Science*, **237**:143–149, 1987.

Russell, M., and Gruber, M.: Risk assessment in environmental policy-making. *Science*, **236**:286–290, **1987.**

Safar, P.: Cerebral resuscitation after cardiac arrest: A review. *Circulation*, **74**:138–141, **1986.**

Segall, P. E.; Timiras, P. S.; and Walton, J.: Low tryptophan diets delay reproductive ageing. *Mech. Ageing Dev.*, **23**:245–252, **1983.**

Segall, P. E.; Waitz, M. D.; Sternberg, H.; Steinberg, R.; Young, G. W.; Bellport, V.; Strack, D.; Cain, G.; Schertel, E. R.; Breznock, A. L.; and Breznock, E. M.: Ice-cold bloodless dogs revived using protocol developed in hamsters. *Fed. Proc.*, **46:**1338, **1987.**

Slovic, P.: Perception of risk. *Science*, **236**:280–285, **1987.**

Smith, A. U.: Studies on golden hamsters during cooling to and rewarming from body temperature below 0°C. *Proc. R. Soc.*, **145**:391–442, **1956.**

Storey, K. B., and Storey, J. M.: Freeze tolerance and intolerance as strategies of winter survival in terrestrially-hibernating amphibians. *Comp. Biochem. Physiol.*, **83**:613–617, **1986.**

Syme, L.: Social determinants of disease. *Ann. Clin. Res.*, **19**:44–52, 1987.

Timiras, P. S.; Hudson, D. B.; and Segall, P. E.: Lifetime brain serotonin: Regional effects of age and precursor availability. *Neurobiol. Aging*, **5**:235–242, **1984.**

Tolstoy, L.: In Sampson, A., and Sampson, S. *The Oxford Book of Ages*, Oxford University Press, **1985**, p. 148.

Willadsen, S. M.: Nuclear transplantion in sheep embryos. *Nature*, **320:**63–65, **1986.**

Wilson, R., and Crouch, E. A. C.: Risk assessment and comparisons: An introduction. *Science*, **236**:267–270, **1987.**

Index